Handbook of Dialysis

Third Edition

Handbook of Dialysis

Third Edition

Editors

John T. Daugirdas, M.D.
Professor of Medicine, University of Illinois at Chicago; Associate Chief of Staff for Research, VA Chicago Hospital Westside, Chicago, Illinois

Peter G. Blake, M.B., F.R.C.P.C., F.R.C.P.I.
Associate Professor, Department of Medicine, University of Western Ontario; Staff Nephrologist, Director of Peritoneal Dialysis and Co-Director, Optimal Dialysis Research Unit, London Health Sciences Centre, London, Ontario, Canada

Todd S. Ing, M.D.
Professor of Medicine, Loyola University Chicago, Stritch School of Medicine; Program Director, Renal and Hypertension Section, Veterans Affairs Hospital, Hines, Illinois

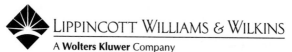

LIPPINCOTT WILLIAMS & WILKINS
A **Wolters Kluwer** Company
Philadelphia · Baltimore · New York · London
Buenos Aires · Hong Kong · Sydney · Tokyo

Acquisitions Editor: Timothy Y. Hiscock
Developmental Editor: Ellen DiFrancesco
Production Editor: Emily Lerman
Manufacturing Manager: Colin J. Warnock
Cover Designer: Patricia Gast
Compositor: Circle Graphics
Printer: RR Donnelley, Crawfordsville

© 2001 by John T. Daugirdas, Peter G. Blake, Todd S. Ing
Published by Lippincott Williams & Wilkins
530 Walnut Street
Philadelphia, PA 19106 USA
LWW.com

Library of Congress Cataloging-in-Publication Data

Handbook of dialysis/editors, John T. Daugirdas, Todd S. Ing, Peter G. Blake.—
    3rd ed. p. ; cm.
    Includes bibliographical references and index.
    ISBN 0-316-17381-9 (alk. paper)
    1. Hemodialysis—Handbooks, manuals, etc. I. Daugirdas, John T. II. Ing, Todd S. III. Blake, Peter G.
    [DNLM: 1. Hemodialysis—Handbooks. WJ 39 H2355 2000]
RC901.7.H45 H36 2000
617.4′61059—dc21
                                                                              00-030163

Care has been taken to confirm the accuracy of the information presented and to describe generally accepted practices. However, the authors, editors, and publisher are not responsible for errors or omissions or for any consequences from application of the information in this book and make no warranty, expressed or implied, with respect to the currency, completeness, or accuracy of the contents of the publication. Application of this information in a particular situation remains the professional responsibility of the practitioner.

The authors, editors, and publisher have exerted every effort to ensure that drug selection and dosage set forth in this text are in accordance with current recommendations and practice at the time of publication. However, in view of ongoing research, changes in government regulations, and the constant flow of information relating to drug therapy and drug reactions, the reader is urged to check the package insert for each drug for any change in indications and dosage and for added warnings and precautions. This is particularly important when the recommended agent is a new or infrequently employed drug.

Some drugs and medical devices presented in this publication have Food and Drug Administration (FDA) clearance for limited use in restricted research settings. It is the responsibility of the health care provider to ascertain the FDA status of each drug or device planned for use in their clinical practice.

10 9 8 7 6 5

Contents

III. Peritoneal Dialysis

IV. Special Problems in the Dialysis Patient

V. Special Problems Pertaining to Various Organ Systems

This book is dedicated to Oliver M. Wrong, M.D., F.R.C.P.,
whose pioneering work on renal tubular acidosis
has inspired generations of students.

Contributing Authors

Stephen R. Ash, M.D., *Department of Comparative Medicine, Purdue University, West Lafayette, Indiana 47906; St. Elizabeth Medical Center and Home Hospital, Lafayette, Indiana 47901*

Joanne M. Bargman, M.D., *Associate Professor, Faculty of Medicine, University of Toronto; Staff Nephrologist, Department of Medicine, The Toronto General Hospital, 200 Elizabeth Street, Toronto, Ontario M5G 2C4, Canada*

Cyril H. Barton, M.D., *Associate Professor, Department of Medicine, University of California, Irvine, Irvine, Calfornia 92697; Director UCI Renal Dialysis Center, Department of Medicine, UCI Medical Center, 101 The City Drive, Orange, California 92868*

Robert L. Benz, M.D., *Clinical Professor of Medicine, Thomas Jefferson University; Chief, Division of Nephrology, Main Line Health, 100 Lancaster Avenue, Wynnewood, Pennsylvania 19096*

Anatole Besarab, M.D., *Chief of Nephrology, Department of Medicine, Ruby Memorial Hospital; Professor, Department of Medicine, West Virginia University, 1 Medical Drive, Morgantown, West Virginia 25606*

Peter G. Blake, M.B., F.R.C.P.C., F.R.C.P.I., *Associate Professor, Department of Medicine, University of Western Ontario; Staff Nephrologist, Director of Peritoneal Dialysis, and Co-Director, Optimal Dialysis Research Unit, London Health Sciences Centre, London, Ontario N6A 4G5, Canada*

Michael J. Blumenkrantz, M.D., *Director, Division of Dialysis, Los Angeles Dialysis Training Center, 10780 Santa Monica Boulevard; Staff Nephrologist and Internist, Division of Nephrology, Cedars-Sinai Medical Center, 8700 Beverly Boulevard, Los Angeles, California 90048*

James T. Boag, B.S.M.E., *Biomedical Engineering Consultant Specializing in Dialysis (deceased)*

Juan P. Bosch, M.D., *Professor, Department of Medicine, George Washington University Medical Center, 2150 Pennsylvania Avenue, NW; Director, Division of Renal Diseases and Hypertension, George Washington University Hospital, 901 23rd Street, NW, Washington, DC 20007*

Harold Bregman, M.D., *Director, Division of Nephrology, Lutheran General Hospital, 1775 Dempster Street, Park Ridge, Illinois 60068*

Ralph J. Caruana, M.D., *Professor and Interim Chair, Department of Medicine, Medical College of Georgia; Interim Chief, Department of Medicine, Medical College of Georgia Hospital and Clinics, 1120 15th Street, Augusta, Georgia 30912*

John T. Daugirdas, M.D., *Professor of Medicine, University of Illinois at Chicago; Associate Chief of Staff for Research, VA Chicago Hospital Westside, Chicago, Illinois 60612*

Marc E. DeBroe, M.D., Ph.D., *Professor of Medicine, Department of Nephrology, University of Antwerp, Universiteitsplein 1, B-2610 Wilrijk; Chief, Department of Nephrology, University Hospital Antwerp, Wilrijkstraat 10, B-2650 Edegem, Antwerp, Belgium*

James A. Delmez, M.D., *Professor of Medicine, Department of Internal Medicine, Washington University School of Medicine, St. Louis, Missouri 63130*

Patrick C. D'Haese, Ph.D., *Associate Professor, Department of Nephrology, University of Antwerp, Universiteitsplein 1, B-2610 Wilrijk; Associate Professor, Department of Nephrology, University Hospital Antwerp, Wilrijkstraat 10, B-2650 Edegem, Antwerp, Belgium*

Jose A. Diaz-Buxo, M.D., *President, Peritoneal Dialysis Services, Fresenius Medical Care North America, 95 Hayden Avenue, Lexington, Massachusetts 02420-9192*

George Dunea, M.D., *Professor of Medicine, University of Illinois College of Medicine; Chairman, Division of Nephrology, Cook County Hospital, Chicago, Illinois 60612*

Richard N. Fine, M.D., *Professor and Chairman, Department of Pediatrics, University Medical Center, State University of New York at Stony Brook, Health Sciences Center T11, Stony Brook, New York 11794-8111*

Steven Fishbane, M.D., *Associate Professor of Medicine, State University of New York at Stony Brook, School of Medicine, Stony Brook, New York; Director of Dialysis Services, Winthrop University Hospital, 222 Station Plaza North, Mineola, New York 11501*

Eli A. Friedman, M.D., *Distinguished Teaching Professor, State University of New York Health Science Center at Brooklyn College of Medicine; Chief, Renal Disease Division, University Hospital of Brooklyn, Brooklyn, New York 11203*

Vasant C. Gandhi, M.D., *Professor of Medicine, Loyola University of Chicago Stritch School of Medicine; Director, Dialysis Unit, Renal and Hypertension Section, Veterans Affairs Hospital, Hines, Illinois 60141*

Susan Grossman, M.D., *Associate Professor of Clinical Medicine, New York Medical College; Director, Internal Medicine Residency Program, St. Vincent's Medical Center of Richmond, Staten Island, New York 10301*

Raymond M. Hakim, M.D., Ph.D., *Adjunct Professor of Medicine, Division of Nephrology, Vanderbilt University, S-3307 Medical Center North; Division of Nephrology, Vanderbilt University Medical Center, 1211 22nd Avenue South, Nashville, Tennessee 37232*

Jessie E. Hano, M.D., *Emeritus Professor of Medicine, Loyola University Chicago, Stritch School of Medicine, Maywood, Illinois 60153*

Joachim Hertel, M.D., *Former Associate Professor, Department of Medicine, Medical College of Georgia, 1120 15th Street, Augusta, Georgia 30912; Attending Physician, Department of Medicine, Southeast Georgia Regional Medical Center, 3100 Kemble Avenue, Brunswick, Georgia 31520*

Susan Hou, M.D., *Professor of Medicine, Loyola University Chicago, Stritch School of Medicine, 2160 South First Avenue, Maywood, Illinois 60153*

Todd S. Ing, M.D., *Professor of Medicine, Loyola University Chicago, Stritch School of Medicine; Program Director, Renal and Hypertension Section, Veterans Affairs Hospital, Hines, Illinois 60141*

Nuhad Ismail, M.D., *Associate Professor of Medicine, Department of Internal Medicine, Vanderbilt University School of Medicine, S-3223 Medical Center North, Nashville, Tennessee 37232*

Allen M. Kaufman, M.D., *Associate Professor of Clinical Medicine, Albert Einstein College of Medicine; Chief, Division of Nephrology and Hypertension, Beth Israel Medical Center, 170 East End Avenue at 87th Street, New York, New York 10128*

Jonathan Kay, M.D., *Assistant Clinical Professor of Medicine, Harvard Medical School, Boston, Massachusetts; Director, Rheumatology Research and Senior Staff Rheumatologist, Department of Rheumatology, Lahey Clinic, 41 Mall Road, Burlington, Massachusetts 01805*

Michael Kaye, M.Div., M.B., *Professor of Medicine, McGill University Faculty of Medicine; Nephrologist, Montreal General Hospital, Montreal, Quebec H3G 1A4, Canada*

Dawn M. Keep, M.S.N., R.N., C.N.N., *Nurse Manager, Hemodialysis Unit, Medical College of Georgia, 1120 15th Street, Augusta, Georgia 30912*

Paul L. Kimmel, M.D., *Professor of Medicine, George Washington University Medical Center, 2150 Pennsylvania Avenue, NW; Attending Physician, Department of Medicine, George Washington University Hospital, 901 23rd Street, NW, Washington, DC 20037*

Petras V. Kisielius, M.D., *Instructor in Urology, Northwestern University Medical School; Consultant in Urology, Mercy Hospital, Chicago, Illinois; Elmhurst Memorial Hospital, Elmhurst, Illinois 60126*

Chagriya Kitiyakara, M.B., *Instructor, Department of Medicine, Ramathibodi Hospital, Mahidol University, Rama Vi Road, Bangkok 10400, Thailand*

Carl M. Kjellstrand, M.D., Ph.D., *Clinical Professor, Department of Medicine, Loyola University Chicago, Stritch School of Medicine, 2160 South First Avenue, Maywood, Illinois 60153; Vice President of Medical Affairs, Aksys Ltd., Two Marriott Drive, Lincolnshire, Illinois 60069*

Stephen M. Korbet, M.D., *Professor, Department of Medicine, Rush Medical College, 600 South Paulina; Associate Director of Nephrology, Rush Presbyterian-St. Luke's Medical Center, 1653 West Congress Parkway, Chicago, Illinois 60612*

Nouhad O. Kronfol, M.D., *Clinical Assistant Professor of Medicine, University of Mississippi School of Medicine Jackson, Mississippi; Nephrologist, Department of Medicine, Delta Regional Medical Center, Greenville, Mississippi 38703*

David J. Leehey, M.D., *Associate Professor, Department of Medicine, Loyola University Chicago, Stritch School of Medicine, 2160 South First Avenue, Maywood, Illinois 60153; Section Chief, Renal and Hypertension, Veterans Affairs Hospital, Hines, Illinois 60141*

Joseph R. Lentino, M.D., Ph.D., *Professor, Department of Medicine, Loyola University Chicago, Stritch School of Medicine, 2160 South First Avenue, Maywood, Illinois 60153; Chief, Infectious Diseases, Veterans Affairs Hospital, Hines, Illinois 60141*

Nathan W. Levin, M.D., *Professor of Clinical Medicine, Albert Einstein College of Medicine, 1300 Morris Park Avenue, Bronx, New York 10461; Attending Physician, Beth Israel Medical Center, First Avenue at 16th Street, New York, New York 10003*

Norman B. Levy, M.D., *Professor of Psychiatry, Medicine, and Surgery, and Director, Liaison Psychiatry Division, New York Medical College, Valhalla, New York 10595*

Susie Q. Lew, M.D.,   *Professor, Department of Medicine, George Washington University Medical Center, 2150 Pennsylvania Avenue, NW; Associate Director, Division of Renal Diseases and Hypertension, George Washington University Hospital, 901 23rd Street, NW, Washington, DC 20037*

Victoria S. Lim, M.D.,   *Professor of Medicine, Department of Internal Medicine, University of Iowa College of Medicine, Iowa City, Iowa 52242*

Susan R. Mendley, M.D.,   *Assistant Professor, Department of Pediatrics and Medicine, University of Maryland, 655 West Baltimore Street; Chief, Department of Pediatric Nephrology, University of Maryland Medical System, 22 South Greene Street, Baltimore, Maryland 21201*

Roxana Neyra, M.D.,   *Instructor of Medicine, Midwestern University, Arizona College of Osteopathic Medicine; Nephrologist, Advanced Cardiac Specialists, 1205 South 7th Avenue #101, Phoenix, Arizona 85007*

Anthony J. Nicholls, M.D.,   *Honorary Clinical Tutor, Postgraduate Medical School, University of Exeter; Director, Kidney Unit, Royal Devon and Exeter Hospital, Exeter, Devon EX4 4QJ, United Kingdom*

Allen R. Nissenson, M.D.,   *Professor of Medicine and Director, Dialysis Program, University of California, Los Angeles, 200 Medical Plaza, Los Angeles, California 90095*

Dimitrios G. Oreopoulos, M.D., Ph.D.,   *Professor of Medicine, University of Toronto; Director, Peritoneal Dialysis Program, The Toronto Hospital, Western Division, 399 Bathurst Street, Suite 6EW-539, Toronto, Ontario M5T 2S8, Canada*

Emil P. Paganini, M.D.,   *Professor of Clinical Medicine, Medical College of Pennsylvania State University; Head, Section of Dialysis and Extracorporeal Therapy, Division of Nephrology and Hypertension, The Cleveland Clinic Foundation, 9500 Euclid Avenue, Cleveland, Ohio 44195*

Mark R. Pressman, Ph.D.,   *Director, Sleep Medicine Services, Lankenau Hospital; Director, Sleep Medicine Services, Paoli Hospital; Clinical Professor, Department of Medicine, Thomas Jefferson Medical College, Philadelphia, Pennsylvania 19107*

Sarah S. Prichard, M.D.,   *Professor, Department of Medicine, McGill University Health Centre; Nephrologist, Division of Nephrology—Medicine, Royal Victoria Hospital, 687 Pine Avenue West, Montreal, Quebec H3A 1A1, Canada*

Rasib M. Raja, M.D.,   *Professor, Department of Medicine, Temple University School of Medicine; Chief, Kraftsow*

Division of Nephrology, Albert Einstein Medical Center, 5501 Old York Road, Philadelphia, Pennsylvania 19141

Panduranga S. Rao, M.D., *Assistant Professor, Department of Medicine, Medical College of Ohio, 3120 Glendale Avenue; Staff Nephrologist, Department of Medicine, Medical College of Ohio Hospital, 3000 Arlington, Toledo, Ohio 43614*

Michael V. Rocco, M.D., *Associate Professor, Department of Internal Medicine and Nephrology, Wake Forest University School of Medicine, Medical Center Boulevard, Winston-Salem, North Carolina 27157-1053*

Edward A. Ross, M.D., *Associate Professor of Medicine, University of Florida College of Medicine and Shands Teaching Hospital; Director, End-Stage Renal Disease Program, Division of Nephrology, Hypertension, and Transplantation, Shands Teaching Hospital, Gainesville, Florida 32611*

Raouf Sayegh, M.D., *Nephrologist, 67 School Street, Hopkinton, Massachusetts 01748*

Anthony J. Schaeffer, M.D., *Herman L. Kretschner Professor of Urology, Northwestern University Medical School; Chairman, Department of Urology, Northwestern Memorial Hospital, Chicago, Illinois 60611*

Miles H. Sigler, M.D., *Clinical Professor of Medicine, Thomas Jefferson University Medical College, 1025 Walnut Street; Program Director, Division of Nephrology, Lankenau Hospital and Lankenau Institute for Medical Research, City Line and Lancaster Avenue, Philadelphia, Pennsylvanina 19096*

Michael I. Sorkin, M.D., *Professor, Department of Medicine, West Virginia University, Morgantown, West Virginia 26506-9165*

Brendan P. Teehan, M.D., *Clinical Professor, Department of Medicine, Jefferson Medical College, Sansom Street, Philadelphia, Pennsylvania; Division of Nephrology, Department of Medicine, Lankenau Hospital, 100 East Lancaster Avenue, Wynnewood, Pennsylvania 19096*

Amir Tejani, M.D., *Professor, Department of Pediatrics, New York Medical College, Valhalla, New York 10595*

Antonios H. Tzamaloukas, M.D., *Professor of Medicine, University of New Mexico, 2201 Lomas NE; Chief, Renal Section, New Mexico VA Health Care System; 1501 San Pedro SE, Albuquerque, New Mexico 87108*

John C. Van Stone, M.D., *Professor, Department of Medicine, University of Missouri Medical School, 1 Hospital Drive, Columbia, Missouri 65201*

N.D. Vaziri, M.D.,   *Professor, Department of Medicine,
University of California, Irvine, Irvine, California 92697;
Chief, Division of Nephrology and Hypertension, Department
of Medicine, UCI Medical Center, 101 The City Drive, Orange,
California 92868*

Beat von Albertini, M.D.,   *Nephrologist, Centre de Dialyse
Cecil, Av. de Savoie 10, 1003 Lausanne, Switzerland*

James F. Winchester, M.D.,   *Professor of Medicine,
Director of Dialysis Programs, and Associate Chief, Division of
Nephrology and Hypertension, Georgetown University Medical
Center, 3800 Reservoir Road, NW, Washington, DC 20007*

Edward T. Zawada, Jr., M.D.,   *Freeman Professor and
Chairman, Department of Internal Medicine, University of
South Dakota School of Medicine, 1400 West 22nd Street;
Co-Director, Dialysis Unit, Sioux Valley Hospital and
University Medical Center, 1100 South Euclid Avenue,
Sioux Falls, South Dakota 57105*

Carmine Zoccali, M.D.,   *Professor, Centro di Fisiologia Clinica
del Consiglio Nazionale delle Ricerche; Director, Renal and
Hypertension Research Unit, Ospedal Riuniti, via Sbarre
Inferiori, 39-89131, Reggio Calabria, Italy*

Preface

Six years have passed since the publication of *Handbook of Dialysis, Second Edition*. These years have been marked by great progress in the field of dialysis. Great strides have been made in examining national databases such as that compiled by the United States Renal Data systems, as well as that compiled by the Renal Networks working with Health Care Financing Administration (HCFA). The NIH HEMO study has provided much needed information about dialysis quantification, and will shortly weigh in on outcomes as a function of membrane flux and urea-based Kt/V. The anemia-iron area has seen much activity, including the availability of new intravenous iron products. In the study of bone disease, the increased recognition of adynamic bone disease, the near-complete abandonment of aluminum use as a phosphorus binder, and the availability of new phosphorus binding compounds are among the advances that have occurred. In the acute dialysis field, controversy continues about the potential beneficial effects of continuous versus intermittent therapy, use of biocompatible membranes, and use of more frequent dialysis. Daily hemodialysis is now the *avant garde* of dialysis, along with its variant, nocturnal hemodialysis. The approach to vascular access has been an active area with measurement of access blood flow by various direct and indirect methods having become commonplace. In peritoneal dialysis, we have seen a much greater emphasis on the achievement of higher clearances and a consequent major change in prescription practices, with increased use of larger dwell volumes and, in particular, of automated peritoneal dialysis. New solutions based on osmotic agents other than glucose have become available in many countries with the potential to improve ultrafiltration and nutrition. In the United States, we now have practice guidelines compiled by panels of experts pertaining to adequacy, anemia management, vascular access, and nutrition with more on the way regarding bone disease. The role of inflammatory mediators, in raising dialysis mortality, as heralded by C-reactive protein, is becoming increasingly appreciated.

Several new authorities have contributed to the *Handbook of Dialysis, Third Edition*, although many of the original authors also participated in the revision of their chapters. With the burgeoning increase in knowledge in the peritoneal dialysis field, we have added the expertise of Dr. Peter Blake. Dr. Blake has completely revised the peritoneal dialysis section of the book. In the hemodialysis area, many changes, including the addition of the DOQI guidelines, have been made in the adequacy section and vascular access section to reflect progress that has been made. The emphasis on urea kinetics has been increased slightly, although care was taken not to overload the reader with formulas and equations. The acute dialysis chapter has been rewritten to highlight potential benefits of more frequent intermittent dialysis, including slow intermittent therapies. Several of the chapters were discontinued or combined with others for greater clarity and compactness. We continued the format of a pocket-sized handbook and have resisted the notion of putting in a large drug table.

Drugs, with their relevant dosing recommendations, continue to be listed by organ- or system-specific chapters as in the previous editions.

We thank each of the contributors for the present group of chapters for their truly wonderful efforts, along with authors of chapters from previous editions; it is on the foundation of their work that the present, Third edition has been developed.

John T. Daugirdas, M.D.

Peter G. Blake, M.D.

Todd S. Ing, M.D.

Indications for Dialysis

Initiation of Dialysis

Edward T. Zawada, Jr.

I. **Uremic syndrome.** The uremic syndrome consists of symptoms and signs that result from toxic effects of elevated levels of nitrogenous and other wastes in the blood.

A. **Symptoms.** Uremic patients commonly become nauseated and often vomit soon after awakening. They may lose their appetite such that the mere thought of eating makes them feel ill. They often feel fatigued, weak, and/or cold. Their mental status is altered; at first, only subtle changes in personality may appear, but eventually, the patients become confused and, ultimately, comatose.

B. **Signs.** The classic uremic physical findings of a sallow coloration of the skin due to accumulation of urochrome pigment (the pigment that gives urine its yellow color) and of an ammonia-like or urine-like odor to the breath are rarely seen unless the degree of uremia is severe. A pericardial friction rub or evidence of pericardial effusion with or without tamponade reflects uremic pericarditis, a condition that urgently requires dialysis treatment. Foot- or wrist-drop may be evidence of uremic motor neuropathy, a condition that also responds to dialysis. Tremor, asterixis, multifocal myoclonus, or seizures are signs of uremic encephalopathy. Prolongation of the bleeding time occurs and can be a problem in the patient requiring surgery.

C. **Signs and symptoms: uremia versus anemia.** Several of the symptoms and signs previously ascribed exclusively to uremia may be partially due to the associated anemia. For example, when the anemia of dialysis patients is corrected with erythropoietin, they experience a marked decrease in fatigue and a concomitant increase in sense of well-being and exercise tolerance. The bleeding time may also improve, and there may be improvement in angina pectoris and a reduction in left ventricular hypertrophy. There are improvements in cognitive function as well.

D. **Relationship between uremic syndrome and creatinine clearance.** The uremic syndrome predictably develops when the creatinine clearance falls below 10 mL per minute per 1.73 m^2. Diabetic individuals appear to be especially susceptible and frequently require earlier initiation of chronic dialysis (e.g., when creatinine clearance falls to 15 mL per minute per 1.73 m^2). However, in chronic renal failure, decreased spontaneous protein intake, anemia, and derangements in Ca/PO$_4$/PTH homeostasis are already demonstrable when clearance is still 30–40 mL per minute per 1.73 m^2.

II. **Acute renal failure**

A. **Common indications.** The indications for dialysis for acute renal failure are listed in Table 1-1. The most common indication for acute dialysis is the presence of uremic signs or symptoms in the setting of laboratory evidence of renal impairment. In particular, pericarditis is an urgent indication for

Table 1-1. Indications for acute dialysis

A. In patients with laboratory evidence of impaired renal function
   (e.g., creatinine clearance <20–25 mL/min/1.73 m^2):
   1. Symptoms known to be associated with uremia:
      a. Nausea, vomiting, impaired nutrition because of poor
         appetite; other gastrointestinal symptoms, including gas-
         tritis with hemorrhage, ileus, and colitis with or without
         hemorrhage
      b. Altered mental status (e.g., lethargy, somnolence, malaise,
         stupor, coma, or delirium) or signs of uremic encephalopa-
         thy (asterixis, tremor, multifocal myoclonus, seizures)
      c. Pericarditis (high risk of hemorrhage and/or tamponade)
         (*urgent indication*)
      d. Bleeding diathesis associated with uremic platelet dys-
         function (*urgent indication*, although this may respond to
         increasing hematocrit to >30%)
   2. Refractory or progressive fluid overload
   3. Uncontrollable hyperkalemia
   4. Severe metabolic acidosis, especially in an oliguric patient
B. Steady worsening of renal function, with blood urea nitrogen
   exceeding 70–100 mg/dL (25–36 mmol/L) or measured (urine collection) creatinine clearance <15–20 mL/min (ideally factored by
   1.73 m^2 body surface area)

dialysis, as it may lead to effusion and life-threatening tamponade. Hyperkalemia, severe acidosis, and fluid overload that
cannot be managed with drugs are other common indications.
Dialysis is customarily initiated prophylactically in patients
with acute renal failure when the serum urea nitrogen level
reaches 70–100 mg/dL (25–36 mmol/L) or when the creatinine
clearance decreases to less than 15–20 mL per minute (ideally,
factored per 1.73 m^2 body surface area). In acute renal failure
patients, there is less emphasis on the serum urea nitrogen
level, as this may vary enormously depending on the protein
nitrogen appearance rate, the presence of gastrointestinal bleeding, the use of antianabolic drugs, and so forth. The creatinine
clearance should be the primary measure followed, and it should
be determined from urine collection rather than from the serum
creatinine level because formulas estimating clearance from the
serum creatinine level assume steady-state conditions, which as
a rule do not hold in this setting.

In the absence of any of the clinical manifestations of uremia
and with acceptable serum levels of potassium and bicarbonate,
acute dialysis does not necessarily have to be performed when
the serum urea nitrogen level or creatinine clearance crosses
these boundaries. For example, patients with a prerenal component and high serum urea nitrogen levels but adequate creatinine clearances often can be managed expectantly. On the
other hand, in patients with decreased urea generation due to
poor nutrition or to liver disease, manifestations of the uremic
syndrome may appear when the serum urea nitrogen level is
well below 50 mg per dL (18 mmol per L) or lower.

B. Less common indications. Less common indications for dialysis therapy include the following: drug intoxication (hemoperfusion for certain drugs), hypothermia, hypercalcemia, hyperuricemia, and metabolic alkalosis (special dialysis solution required).

III. Choice of a therapeutic modality. For acute dialysis, the choice is among hemodialysis, peritoneal dialysis, and one of the "slow continuous" procedures described in Chapter 10.

A. Hemodialysis. Hemodialysis is by far the most common method employed for acute renal failure management in the United States. Hemodialysis offers a more rapid change in plasma solute composition and the possibility of more rapid removal of excess body water than peritoneal dialysis or the slow continuous procedures. However, because hemodialysis is applied episodically, the daily requirement for fluid removal and solute alteration must be fulfilled over a short time interval; rapid removal of fluid often is poorly tolerated by very ill patients in an intensive care setting.

B. Peritoneal dialysis. Peritoneal dialysis is rarely used to treat acute renal failure in the United States unless a cuffed peritoneal catheter has been implanted previously. A cuffed catheter can be implanted acutely, and peritoneal dialysis has some theoretical advantages. Although peritoneal dialysis is approximately one-eighth as efficient as hemodialysis in altering blood solute composition and about one-fourth as efficient in terms of fluid removal, it can be applied continuously, 24 hours a day, whereas hemodialysis is usually given for a maximum of 4 hours per day. Thus, on a daily basis, the efficacy of peritoneal dialysis in effecting changes in solute and fluid status is not markedly different from that of hemodialysis. The continuous nature of peritoneal dialysis allows changes in blood solute and total body water to be made gradually, making peritoneal dialysis an attractive option for patients who are hemodynamically unstable.

In some patients, peritoneal dialysis cannot be performed due to the state of the abdomen. The presence of extensive adhesions from previous abdominal surgery can render catheter insertion or drainage of dialysate next to impossible. Recent abdominal surgery that involved a bowel anastomosis or that has left open drains in the abdominal wall is another relative contraindication to peritoneal dialysis. The presence of a fresh intra-abdominal vascular graft is a relative contraindication because of the possible spread of dialysis-associated peritonitis (should it occur) to the graft material, but peritoneal dialysis has been done in patients with remote intra-abdominal graft placement without complication.

C. Slow continuous procedures. These are described in Chapter 10. They offer a gradual change in plasma solute composition and gradual removal of excess fluid similar to that obtained with peritoneal dialysis. The principal advantage is increased hemodynamic stability. The main disadvantages are the need for specialized training of the nurses in the intensive care unit, the need for continuous monitoring of the extracorporeal circuit for safety reasons, problems with device malfunction/clotting (especially during the night shift), and increased expense.

D. Mortality. Mortality statistics are difficult to evaluate because of patient selection. There appears to be no clear-cut advantage for intermittent hemodialysis versus acute peritoneal dialysis. The only large multicenter randomized trial comparing intermittent hemodialysis with the slow continuous therapies for acute renal failure failed to show any benefit of the latter approach (Mehta et al, 1996), although severely hypotensive patients were excluded from this trial by design.

IV. Chronic dialysis

A. Predialysis care. Survival of end-stage renal disease (ESRD) patients on dialysis depends to a large extent on their condition at the time dialysis was first initiated. Accordingly, it is important to pay attention to control of blood pressure, anemia, calcium/phosphorus intake, and nutrition during the predialysis period, as well as timely insertion of an arteriovenous fistula. When this is done using a multidisciplinary predialysis program that includes patient and family education, early choice of appropriate modality, and elective creation of dialysis access, the advantages have been fewer urgent dialyses, fewer hospital days in the first month after beginning dialysis, and a \$4,000 estimated cost savings per patient at the time of commencing dialysis (Levin et al, 1997). Little can be accomplished unless there is timely referral to the nephrologist during the pre-ESRD period.

B. Indications

1. Medicare reimbursement constraints. In the United States, the decision to start chronic dialysis is now monitored by the US Health Care Finance Administration (HCFA) and regional peer review organizations (networks). Medicare reimbursement is contingent on meeting a federally approved creatinine clearance criterion (submitted via HCFA Form 2728) of less than 10 mL per minute for non-diabetics or less than 15 mL per minute for diabetics (not adjusted for body size). This clearance can either be measured via urine collection or estimated from the serum creatinine level using the Cockcroft and Gault formula (Table 1-2). If the patient's clearance does not meet these benchmarks, then the treating physician must justify the decision to start dialysis to the regional network. If the justification is rejected, then payment for dialysis is not approved.

2. Problems with Medicare reimbursement constraints. Problems with such criteria that are limited to clearance measures occur in patients with renal impairment who have problems with fluid overload, hyperkalemia, or "failure to thrive" that are out of proportion to their creatinine clearance. For example, patients with advanced age and cognitive impairment may be poorly compliant with taking high-dose diuretics or potassium-lowering agents. Patients with advanced cardiac disease and borderline creatinine clearances may have trouble with refractory fluid retention. Patients without financial resources or insurance may have trouble paying for high-dose diuretics and antihypertensives to achieve good fluid and potassium control. Such patients may present frequently to emergency facilities with pulmonary edema, hyperkalemia, and worsening azotemia, which

Table 1-2. Estimating creatinine clearance or glomerular filtration rate from serum creatinine level

A. Cockcroft and Gault formula (creatinine clearance, not corrected to 1.73 m²):

Basis: Regression equations that estimate 24-h urine creatinine excretion based on sex, age, and weight. DO NOT USE in acute renal failure, as the formula assumes a steady-state serum creatinine level!

$$\text{Creatinine clearance} = \frac{(140 - \text{age}) \times \text{weight (kg)}}{72 \times \text{serum creatinine (mg/dL)}}$$

$$\text{Creatinine clearance} = \frac{(140 - \text{age}) \times \text{weight (kg)}}{0.81 \times \text{serum creatinine (}\mu\text{mol/L)}}$$

Adjustments: The calculated clearance is reduced by 15% for women. In spinal cord patients, reduce by 20% for paraplegics and 40% for quadriplegics. In African American males, increase by 12% (Goldwasser et al. *Am J Kidney Dis* 1997;30:16–22). There are no data in African American females. HCFA criteria do not incorporate the correction for African American males as of the year 2000.

Examples:

1. Consider two patients with same weight and serum creatinine level, one 80 years old, the other 20 years old. Creatinine clearance for the 80-year-old patient (140 – age = 60) is half that for the 20-year-old patient (140 – age = 120).
2. Consider two patients with serum creatinine values of 5 mg/dL. Patient 1, a 68-year-old diabetic woman weighing 50 kg, would have an estimated clearance of (140 – 68) × 50 × 0.85 divided by 72 × 5 = 8.5 mL/min. This patient qualifies for long-term dialysis. Patient 2 is a 30-year-old 70-kg white man with a serum creatinine value of 5 mg/dL. The estimated clearance is (140 – 30) × 70 divided by 72 × 5 = 21 mL/min. This patient does not yet qualify for long-term dialysis.

B. MDRD formula (GFR, corrected to 1.73 m²)

This equation is more complex and requires knowledge of race. Several variants have been published. One equation is described in Levey AS, et al. *J Am Soc Nephrol* 2000;11: in press

$$\text{GFR (mL/min/1.73m}^2) = 186 \times \text{Pcr}^{-1.154} \times \text{age}^{-0.203}$$
$$\times 1.212 \text{ if black} \times 0.742 \text{ if female}$$

The MDRD equation is marginally better than the Cockcroft and Gault formula. If the latter were adjusted for black race (see above), it is not clear that the MDRD formula would be any better. As it estimates GFR instead of creatinine clearance, the MDRD formula gives slightly lower values than Cockcroft and Gault. Also, the MDRD equation is normalized to 1.73 m² body surface area.

HCFA, Health Care Finance Administration; MDRD, Modification of Diet in Renal Disease study; GFR, glomerular filtration rate; Pcr, plasma creatinine.

improve after short hospitalization or even after several hours in the emergency room and treatment with appropriate medications. Once these patients are initiated on dialysis, frequent dialysis therapy prevents fluid and potassium problems, and the emergency room visits and hospital admissions often decrease markedly or cease altogether. Delay in initiation of dialysis for such patients until their creatinine clearances fall into the mandated range may have an adverse effect on their long-term survival.

3. Concept of early or "timely" initiation of dialysis. Current guidelines from the Dialysis Outcomes Quality Initiative (DOQI) suggest that dialysis should be started at a creatinine clearance of 9–14 mL per minute per 1.73 m^2 in all patients, irrespective of their diabetic status, or earlier if their protein intake is less than 0.8 g per kg per day, or if they have uremic (see DOQI internet references).

The rationale for this approach is that ultimate survival on dialysis depends greatly on nutritional status and serum albumin status at the time dialysis is initiated. Patients started early on dialysis (at higher creatinine clearance levels) have higher serum albumin levels. Furthermore, spontaneous protein intake begins to fall early in chronic renal insufficiency (when creatinine clearance is still above 25 mL per minute). Observational uncontrolled studies by Bonomini et al (1985) and from the CANUSA (Canada-United States) study (McCusker et al, 1999; CANUSA Study Group, 1996), although unadjusted for lead time bias, suggest that mortality is lower in patients who begin dialysis at a higher initial level of residual creatinine clearance.

The DOQI dialysis initiation guidelines are set in terms of weekly Kt/V_{urea} (they suggest starting dialysis when weekly Kt/V_{urea} falls below 2.0). This level of urea clearance is supposed to correspond to a creatinine clearance of 9–14 mL per minute per 1.73 m^2, but weekly Kt/V_{urea} and creatinine clearance correlate somewhat poorly (Mujais, et al. 1999). Use of a urea target ties together the concepts of minimum amount of peritoneal dialysis clearance (weekly Kt/V_{urea} of 2.0) in patients already on dialysis, and laboratory criteria for when to start dialysis (also when Kt/V_{urea} is less than 2.0). Currently, these new concepts are directly in conflict with HCFA reimbursement policy, as many such patients will have creatinine clearances greater than 10 mL per minute. At present, it is unclear how this situation will be resolved.

a. Computing weekly Kt/V_{urea} in pre-ESRD patients. The DOQI guidelines for initiation of dialysis are in terms of weekly Kt/V urea. How is this calculated? A 24-hour urine sample is collected in the usual fashion and analyzed for urea as well as creatinine. The urea clearance is determined in the usual fashion [like creatinine clearance, using the UV/P equation, where U = urine urea concentration, V = urine flow rate, and P = plasma (serum) urea concentration]. For example, one may come up with a urea clearance of 10 mL per minute and a creatinine clearance of

17 mL per minute. One now multiplies the urea clearance in milliliters per minute by the number of minutes in a week (10,080) and divided by 1,000 to convert to liters per week. This yields a value of 100.8 L per week of urea clearance. This is the $K \times t$ term of the Kt/V. To convert to Kt/V, one then needs to estimate V from an anthropometric equation (see Table A-2.) Assume $V = 35$ L. Then weekly Kt/V urea is $101/35 = 2.9$. This is greater than 2.0, suggesting that this patient may not yet require dialysis.

C. Modality selection. Choices for therapy for chronic renal failure include:

  1. In-center hemodialysis, staff-dependent.
  2. In-center hemodialysis, self-care.
  3. Home hemodialysis.
  4. Home continuous ambulatory peritoneal dialysis (CAPD).
  5. Home continuous cycling peritoneal dialysis (CCPD).

D. Patients for whom peritoneal dialysis is favored over hemodialysis for chronic renal failure include:

  1. Infants or very young children.
  2. Patients with severe cardiovascular disease.
  3. Patients with difficult vascular access (e.g., diabetics).
  4. Patients who desire greater freedom to travel.
  5. Patients who wish to perform home dialysis but do not have a suitable partner to assist them.

E. The principal contraindication to chronic peritoneal dialysis is an unsuitable peritoneum due to presence of adhesions, fibrosis, or malignancy. The principal cause of abandonment of peritoneal dialysis is the occurrence of frequent episodes of peritonitis, although patient burnout is also a factor. Some patients simply prefer a hemodialysis schedule of three or more well-defined periods a week during which they can get their dialysis "over with," leaving them free of any other dialysis responsibility.

Creation of an arteriovenous fistula during the pre-ESRD period for patients in whom hemodialysis is planned is very important, as this obviates risks of venous catheter placement at time of dialysis initiation.

F. Excluding patients from dialysis. Are there any patients who should be routinely excluded from dialysis for chronic renal failure?

  1. Elderly. In the United States and elsewhere, the fastest growing age group presenting for dialysis is the "oldest old" (patients older than 80 years). Access placement in this group is not particularly difficult, and cuffed venous catheters have been used with success in difficult cases. Time constraints are not a problem, and these individuals often arrive eager for their treatments. Transportation is often available from assisted-living providers, retirement community staff, or municipal programs. A high rate of compliance with all aspects of treatment often offsets a higher prevalence of comorbid (cardiac, vascular, malignancies) conditions in achieving a good outcome. As a result, many elderly patients placed on dialysis continue to enjoy a good quality of life and benefit from documented improvement in a variety of health outcome measures.

2. Patients with multiorgan disease or malignancy. Patients with advanced disease in an organ system other than the kidneys, or those with malignancy, have sometimes been excluded from chronic dialysis. For example, those with advanced liver disease might have ascites, encephalopathy, bleeding diathesis, and hypotension. These concomitant problems may make access difficult, and the dialysis treatments may create too much hypotension or fail to correct the accompanying fluid overload. In some such patients, dialysis may be futile. Futility is an ethical principle on which one can make a reasonable decision not to initiate dialysis. On the other hand, some such patients may achieve good quality of life and "remission" of failure of the other organ system with the fluid removal, electrolyte balance, and improved nutrition provided by the multidisciplinary support available through ESRD management.

SUGGESTED READINGS

Adequacy of dialysis and nutrition in continuous peritoneal dialysis: association with clinical outcomes. Canada-USA (CANUSA) Peritoneal Dialysis Study Group. 1996.

Arora P, et al. Prevalence, predictors, and consequences of late nephrology referral at a tertiary care center. *J Am Soc Nephrol* 1999;10: 1281–1286.

Bonomini V, et al. Benefits of early initiation of dialysis. *Kidney Int* 1985;17(Suppl):S57–S59.

Cockcroft DW, Gault MH. Prediction of creatinine clearance from serum creatinine. *Nephron* 1976;16:31–35.

Harris LE, et al. Effects of multidisciplinary case management in patients with chronic renal insufficiency. *Am J Med* 1998;105: 464–471.

Ifudu O, et al. Excess morbidity in patients starting uremia therapy without prior care by a nephrologist. *Am J Kidney Dis* 1996;28: 841–845.

Ikizler TA, et al. Spontaneous dietary protein intake during progression of chronic renal failure. *J Am Soc Nephrol* 1995;6:1386–1391.

Levin A, et al. Multidisciplinary predialysis programs: quantification and limitations of their impact on patient outcomes in two Canadian settings. *Am J Kidney Dis* 29:1997;533–540.

McCusker FX, et al. How much peritoneal dialysis is required for the maintenance of a good nutritional state? Canada-USA (CANUSA) Peritoneal Study Group. *Kidney Int Suppl* 1996;56:S56–S61.

Mehta R, et al, for the Collaborative ARF Group. Continuous versus intermittent dialysis for acute renal failure in the ICU: results from a randomized multicenter trial. *J Am Soc Nephrol* 1996;7:1457 (abstr).

Mujais SK, et al. Discordance between Kt/V and creatinine clearance thresholds for dialysis initiation in DOQI-NFK guidelines. *J Am Soc Nephrol* 1999;10:335A (abstr).

National Kidney Foundation. NKF–DOQI clinical practice guidelines for peritoneal dialysis adequacy. *Am J Kidney Dis* 1997;30(3 Suppl 2): S67–S136.

Obrador GT, et al. Prevalence of and factors associated with suboptimal care before initiation of dialysis in the United States. *J Am Soc Nephrol* 1999;10:1793–1800.

Oreopoulos DG. Dialyzing the elderly: benefit or burden? *Periton Dial Int* 1997;17(Suppl 2):S7–S11.

Soucie JM, McClellan WM. Early death in dialysis patients: risk factors and impact on incidence and mortality rates. *J Am Soc Nephrol* 1996;7:2169–2175.

Tattersall J, Greenwood R, Farrington K. Urea kinetics and when to commence dialysis. *Am J Nephrol* 1995;15:283–289.

Internet References

NKF-DOQI guidelines (http://www.kidney.org)

HCFA Form 2728 (http://www.hdcn.com/hd/hcfa.htm)

Timely initiation of dialysis links (http://www.hdcn.com/hd/timely.htm)

GFR, urea, creatinine clearance calculators (http://www.hdcn.com/hd/gfrcalc.htm)

Hemodialysis

2

Physiologic Principles and Urea Kinetic Modeling

John T. Daugirdas and John C. Van Stone

Dialysis is a process whereby the solute composition of a solution, A, is altered by exposing solution A to a second solution, B, through a semipermeable membrane. Conceptually, one can view the semipermeable membrane as a sheet perforated by holes or pores. Water molecules and low molecular weight solutes in the two solutions can pass through the membrane pores and intermingle, but larger solutes (such as proteins) cannot pass through the semipermeable barrier, and the quantities of high molecular weight solutes on either side of the membrane will remain unchanged.

I. Mechanisms of solute transport. Solutes that can pass through the membrane pores are transported by two different mechanisms: diffusion and ultrafiltration (convection).

   A. Diffusion. The movement of solutes by diffusion is the result of random molecular motion. In Fig. 2-1, as a solute molecule in solution A moves about, it will from time to time collide with the membrane. If the solute molecule happens to encounter a membrane pore of sufficient size, the molecule will pass through the membrane into solution B. Likewise, a low molecular weight solute in solution B can pass through the membrane in the reverse direction into solution A.

     1. Importance of concentration gradient. The relative rates of passage of a given solute (call it solute [x]) from solution A to solution B and back again will depend on the frequency of collisions between solute [x] molecules and each side of the membrane. The collision frequency will, in turn, be related to the relative concentrations of solute [x] on each side of the membrane. For example, if the concentration of solute [x] in solution A is 100 mM and in solution B is 1.0 mM, the probability of a solute [x] molecule colliding with the A side of the membrane (and of hitting a pore and moving through the membrane into solution B) will be much higher than the probability of a solute [x] molecule colliding with the B side of the membrane (and moving into solution A). Thus, the net rate of transfer of a given solute from solution A to solution B will be greatest when the concentration gradient between the two solutions for that particular solute is highest.

     2. Importance of molecular weight. The larger the molecular weight of a solute, the slower will be its rate of transport across a semipermeable membrane. The reasons for this pertain to speed and size.

      a. Speed. The velocity of a molecule in solution is inversely related to the weight of the molecule. For example, the velocity of a molecule weighing 200 d will be less than the velocity of a molecule weighing 100 d. Small molecules, moving about at high velocity, will collide with the

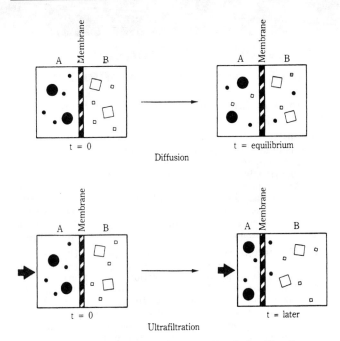

Figure 2-1.   The processes of diffusion (*top*) and ultrafiltration (*bottom*). As shown, in both processes, low molecular weight solutes can cross the semipermeable membrane, whereas larger solutes are held back.

membrane often, and their rate of diffusive transport through the membrane will be high. Large molecules, even those that can fit easily through the membrane pores, will diffuse through the membrane slowly because they will be moving about at low velocity and colliding with the membrane infrequently.

   b.   Size. The molecular weight of a solute correlates highly with its size. The membrane will partially or completely inhibit passage of a solute as its molecular size approaches and exceeds the size of the membrane pores.

3.   Importance of membrane resistance

   a.   Membrane resistance due to the membrane itself. The resistance of the membrane to solute transport will be high if the membrane is thick, if the number of pores is small, or if the pores are narrow.

   b.   Membrane resistance due to "unstirred" fluid layers next to the membrane. Unstirred layers of fluid on either side of the membrane inhibit diffusion because they act to decrease the "effective" concentration gradient at the membrane surface. The thickness of these unstirred layers is affected by dialysis solution and blood flow rates and by dialyzer design.

B.   Ultrafiltration. The second mechanism of solute transport across semipermeable membranes is ultrafiltration (convective transport). Water molecules are extremely small and can pass through all semi-permeable membranes. Ultrafiltration occurs when water driven by either a hydrostatic or an osmotic force is pushed through the membrane (Fig. 2-1). (Analogous processes are wind in the atmosphere and current in the ocean.) Those solutes that can pass easily through the membrane pores are swept along with the water (a process called "solvent drag"). The water being pushed through the membrane is accompanied by such solutes at close to their original concentrations. Larger solutes, especially those that are larger than the membrane pores, are held back. For such large solutes, the membrane acts as a sieve.

    1.   Hydrostatic ultrafiltration

      a.   Transmembrane pressure. During hemodialysis, water (along with small solutes) moves from the blood to dialysate in the dialyzer as a result of a hydrostatic pressure gradient between the blood and dialysate compartments. The rate of ultrafiltration will depend on the total pressure difference across the membrane (calculated as the pressure in the blood compartment minus the pressure in the dialysate compartment).

      b.   Ultrafiltration coefficient (K_{Uf}). The permeability of dialyzer membranes to water, though high, can vary considerably and is a function of membrane thickness and pore size. The permeability of a membrane to water is indicated by its ultrafiltration coefficient, K_{Uf}. K_{Uf} is defined as the number of milliliters of fluid per hour that will be transferred across the membrane per mm Hg pressure gradient across the membrane.

    2.   Osmotic ultrafiltration. Osmotic ultrafiltration is described in **Chapter 13.**

    3.   Implications of ultrafiltration on solute clearance

      a.   Hemofiltration and hemodiafiltration. Whereas diffusive removal of a solute depends on its size, all ultrafiltered solutes below the membrane pore size are removed at approximately the same rate. This principle has led to the development of hemodialysis techniques whereby a large amount of ultrafiltration (more than is required to restore euvolemia) is coupled with infusion of a replacement fluid.

      Extracorporeal therapy whereby ultrafiltration is used as an important adjunct to solute removal is called *hemofiltration* or *hemodiafiltration* (hemofiltration combined with hemodialysis). Although hemodialysis and hemofiltration often have comparable removal of small solutes such as urea (MW = 60), hemofiltration can effect much higher removal of larger, poorly diffusible solutes, such as inulin (MW = 5,200).

C.   Removal of protein-bound compounds. The normal kidney detoxifies protein-bound organic acids and bases. Being protein-bound, they are filtered to only a small extent and so bypass the glomerulus. However, in the peritubular capillary network, these substances are somehow removed from albumin and taken up by proximal tubular cells. Then they are secreted into the tubular lumen, to be excreted in the urine. Other protein-bound compounds (bound to albumin and small proteins) are filtered into the glomerulus along with their carrier proteins. In the proximal tubule, the filtered proteins are catabolized along with their bound compounds.

Some of the derangements associated with uremia may be due to accumulation of protein-bound compounds. Removal of protein-bound compounds by hemodialysis depends on the percentage of the "free" fraction of the compound in plasma (the fraction that is exposed to dialysis). Also, removal depends on how quickly the free fraction is replenished by the protein-bound pool. Substances that are tightly bound to proteins with a low free fraction in the plasma will be removed to only a negligible extent by hemodialysis. Use of charcoal hemoperfusion is quite effective in lowering the blood concentration of protein-bound compounds but is not being done on a routine long-term basis to treat uremia.

II. Clinical applications of diffusion and ultrafiltration: solute removal from the dialyzer perspective

A. Diffusion

1. **Hemodialysis circuit.** In clinical use, the box containing two solutions in Fig. 2-1 becomes the dialyzer, containing blood and dialysis solution. The latter consists of highly purified water into which sodium, potassium, calcium, magnesium, chloride, bicarbonate, and dextrose have been introduced. The low molecular weight waste products that accumulate in uremic blood are absent from the dialysis solution. For this reason, when uremic blood is exposed to dialysis solution, the flux rate of these solutes from blood to dialysate is initially much greater than the back flux from dialysate to blood. Eventually, if the blood, and dialysate were left in static contact with each other via the membrane, the concentration of permeable waste products in the dialysate would become equal to that in the blood, and no further net removal of waste products would occur. Transport back and forth across the membrane would continue, but the rates of transport and back transport would be equal. In practice, during dialysis, concentration equilibrium is prevented, and the concentration gradient between blood, and dialysate is maximized, by continuously refilling the dialysate compartment with fresh dialysis solution and by replacing dialyzed blood with undialyzed blood. Normally, the direction of dialysis solution flow is opposite to the direction of blood flow (Fig. 2-2). The purpose of "countercurrent" flow is to maximize the concentration difference of waste products between blood and dialysate in all parts of the dialyzer.

2. **Dialyzer whole-blood clearance.** The blood leaving the dialyzer has a lower concentration of waste products than the blood entering the dialyzer. For example, if the plasma urea nitrogen level at the dialyzer inlet is 100 mg per dL, at the dialyzer outlet the level may be 25 mg per dL. However, the "work" that the dialyzer is doing is not well represented by the extent to which it reduces the blood concentration of a given waste product. If the blood flow is slow, then

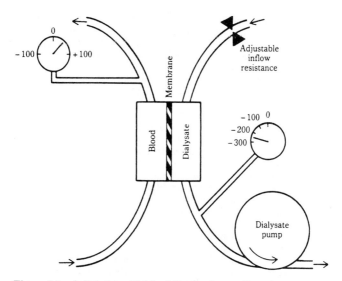

Figure 2-2. A dialyzer with blood flowing in one direction and dialysis solution flowing in the opposite direction. Hydrostatic pressure across the membrane (and ultrafiltration) is adjusted by varying the resistance to inflow of dialysis solution. The position of the gauges monitoring pressure at the blood and dialysate outflow ports is also shown, along with typical operating pressures. In this case, the transmembrane pressure is about 300 mm Hg (+50 mm Hg at the blood outlet, −[−250 mm Hg] at the dialysate outlet).

very little urea is being removed. To better characterize dialyzer work, the percentage reduction in the blood concentration of a given waste product is multiplied by the blood flow rate through the dialyzer to obtain a hypothetical volume of blood that is being totally "cleared" of that waste product each minute. In the above example, the reduction in plasma urea nitrogen concentration from 100 to 25 mg per dL translates to a 75% reduction. If the blood flow is 200 mL per minute, then 150 mL per minute of blood (0.75 × 200) is being totally cleared of urea.

One strength of the clearance concept is its independence from the concentration of the waste product in the inflowing blood. For example, if the inflowing urea concentration is decreased to 50 mg per dL, the urea concentration in the outflowing blood will decrease proportionately, from 25 to 12.5 mg per dL. The percentage removal, however, will still be 75 {100 × (50−12.5)/50}, and the urea clearance will remain 150 mL per minute.

    a. Effect of erythrocytes. In the concept of clearance described above, the blood was treated as a simple fluid. However, this is not the case. A blood flow of 200 mL per minute is really a plasma flow rate of 140 mL per minute and an erythrocyte flow rate of 60 mL per minute (at a hematocrit of 30%). What is measured at the dialyzer inlet and outlet are the plasma levels of a given waste product.

For urea, the presence of erythrocytes is not a major problem because urea diffuses into and out of erythrocytes quickly. For example, if the outlet plasma urea nitrogen level is 25 mg per dL, the urea concentration in erythrocytes will have been reduced to about that level also.

For creatinine and many other solutes, the problem is more complex because these substances do not equilibrate quickly between plasma and erythrocytes. Many other substances, such as phosphate, are present in different concentrations in plasma and erythrocytes. For such substances, the whole-blood clearance method using plasma levels is not a good approximation of removal rate during dialysis.

(1) Computing the blood water urea clearance. Urea is dissolved in erythrocytes and plasma water. Approximately 93% of plasma is water (depending on its protein concentration), and about 72% of an erythrocyte is water. However, because some urea associates with the nonwater portion of erythrocytes, one normally considers urea to be dissolved in a volume equal to 80% of the erythrocyte volume. If the blood flow rate is 200 mL per minute at a hematocrit of 30%, the effective blood water flow rate for urea can be estimated as follows:

Whole-blood flow rate = 200 mL per minute; hematocrit = 30%;
Plasma flow rate = $200 \times (1 - 0.30) = 140$ mL per minute;
Plasma water flow rate = 0.93×140 mL per minute = 130 mL per minute;
Erythrocyte flow rate = $200 \times 0.30 = 60$ mL per minute;
Erythrocyte water flow rate = 0.80×60 mL per minute = 48 mL per minute;
Blood water flow rate = plasma water flow rate + erythrocyte water flow rate = $130 + 48 = 178$ mL per minute.

The correction for blood water becomes important when using the dialyzer clearance to compute how much urea is being removed during a dialysis session. Generally, not making the blood water correction will cause overestimation of the amount of urea removal by about 10%. The correction commonly used to account for blood water content of both plasma and erythrocytes together is to multiply the whole-blood clearance by 0.894 (see Table A-1).

(2) Effect of hematocrit on blood water urea clearance. Increasing the hematocrit (e.g., from 20% to 40%) causes only a trivial reduction of the blood water urea clearance because the effective urea distribution volume in erythrocytes (80%) is closely similar to that in plasma (93%).

(3) Effect of hematocrit on clearance of creatinine and phosphorus. Increasing the hematocrit will cause a reduction in the dialyzer clearances of creatinine and phosphorus. Creatinine may not be removed from erythrocytes to the same extent as from the plasma during passage through the dialyzer. As the hematocrit is increased from 20% to 40%, creatinine removal decreases by about 8%. For phosphorus, the reduction will be about 13% because the amount of phosphorus available for transport out of red cells is smaller than the amount in plasma, and also because the rate of transport of phosphorus out of red cells during their passage through the dialyzer is slow (Lim et al, 1990).

3. **Factors affecting the blood water urea clearance (K_w).** The principal determinants of the blood water clearance during dialysis are the blood flow rate, the dialysis solution flow rate, and the efficiency of the dialyzer used.

a. **Effect of the blood flow rate.** One might think that the blood clearance increases in direct proportion to the blood flow rate, given that clearance is computed as the blood flow rate times percentage reduction across the dialyzer in the plasma urea nitrogen level. This is only partially true. As the blood flow rate increases, the dialyzer is unable to remove urea with the same degree of efficiency. As a result, the plasma urea nitrogen level at the dialyzer outlet rises.

Consider an example where the blood flow rate is 200 mL per minute, the inlet plasma urea nitrogen level is 100 mg per dL, and the outlet level is 25 mg per dL. The clearance is 200 mL × (100 − 25)/100 = 150 mL per minute. If the blood flow rate is now increased to 400 mL per minute, the outlet plasma urea nitrogen level will increase (how much depends on the efficiency of the dialyzer), typically from 25 to about 50 mg per dL. Now the clearance is 400 × (100 − 50)/100 = 200 mL per minute. Thus, a 100% increase in the blood flow rate (from 200 to 400 mL per minute) will have raised the blood urea clearance by only 33%, from 150 to 200 mL per minute.

For dialysis of normal-size adults, the blood flow rate is usually set between 200 and 600 mL per minute, with flow rates of 350 to 500 mL per minute being used for most patients in the United States (many European countries prefer to use a lower average blood flow rate).

b. **Effect of dialysis solution flow rate.** Clearance of urea depends on the dialysis solution flow rate as well. A faster dialysis solution flow rate increases the efficiency of diffusion of urea from blood to dialysate; however, the effect is usually not large. The usual dialysis solution flow rate is 500 mL per minute. A flow rate of 800 mL per minute will increase urea clearance by about 12% when a high-efficiency dialyzer is used and when the blood flow rate is greater than 350 mL per minute.

c. **Effect of dialyzer efficiency.** A high-efficiency dialyzer with a thin, large-surface-area membrane, wide pores, and a design that maximizes contact between blood and dialysate will remove a higher percentage of waste products than a low-efficiency dialyzer. For example, at a blood flow rate of 200 mL per minute, the blood leaving a high-efficiency dialyzer may have a urea nitro-gen level of only 5 mg per dL (if the inlet serum urea nitrogen, or SUN, is 100 mg per dL). The extraction percentage will be 95% instead of 75%, and the dialyzer urea clearance will be 0.95 [×] 200 = 190 mL per minute (not corrected for blood water).

(1)   The dialyzer mass transfer area coefficient, KoA. The efficiency of a given dialyzer in removing any solute can be described by a constant referred to as *KoA*. This constant determines the height of the curve relating blood and dialysate flow rates to clearance (Fig. 2-3).

One can think of the *KoA*, which is measured in milliliters per minute, as the maximum possible clearance of a given dialyzer at infinitely large blood and dialysate flow rates. Dialyzers of usual efficiency have in vitro *KoA* values for urea of 500–700 mL per minute; high-efficiency dialyzers have *KoA* values greater than 700 mL per minute. In practice, these maximum clearance levels are never achieved because it is not possible to approach the large blood and dialysate flow rates that would be necessary.

Once the *KoA* of a dialyzer is known, a nomogram (see Fig. 2-3) or an equation (Table A-1) can be used to predict the blood water urea clearance (K) at any combination of blood (Q_B) and dialysate (Q_D) flow rates.

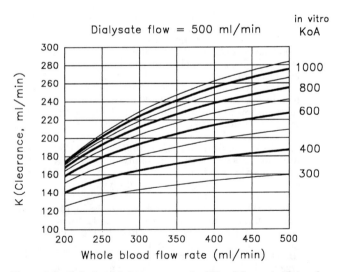

Figure 2-3.   Relationship between nominal blood flow rate (Q_B) and blood water urea clearance (K) as a function of dialyzer efficiency (KoA). K was computed as per the equations in Table A-1. Clearance values from this nomogram will still overestimate true in vivo clearances slightly, but will correspond to urea volumes estimated by anthropometric equations.

EXAMPLE:

K

KoA	Qb200	Qb400	% change in K
400	137	173	+26%
800	166	235	+42%

If a low-*KoA* dialyzer is used (*KoA* = 400 mL per minute, row 1), doubling the blood flow rate from 200 to 400 will only increase the blood water urea clearance (*K*) by 173/137, or 26%. However, with a high-*KoA* dialyzer (*KoA* = 800), *K* will increase by 235/166, or 42%. The clinical point is that one needs to use a high-efficiency dialyzer to obtain a substantial increase in clearance with a higher blood flow rate. A formal set of equations to compute *K* from Q_B, Q_D, *KoA,* and the ultrafiltration rate is given in Table A-1.

(2)   **Effect of dialysate flow rate on *KoA*.** In theory, the *KoA* (maximum dialyzer clearance) depends only on the permeability constant of the membrane material for a given solute (*Ko*) multiplied by the effective surface area (*A*). The *KoA* should be constant for all levels of blood and dialysate flow rate. In practice, whereas the *KoA* of a dialyzer does not change at various blood flow rates, the *KoA* does increase substantially when dialysate flow rate is increased from 500 to 800 mL per minute (Cheung et al, 1997). This apparent increase in the surface area of the dialyzer at high dialysate flow rate is probably due to better penetration of the dialysate into the hollow-fiber bundle, resulting in an expansion of the dialyzer effective surface area.

(3)   **Computing the dialyzer *KoA*.** The *KoA* urea is the maximum height of the urea clearance curve. The curve has a known mathematical shape, which is similar for all dialyzers. Thus, if one knows the actual clearance at any given blood and dialysate flow rates, one can mathematically compute the peak height of the clearance curve, or the *KoA*. A method of doing this is described in the next chapter, and a calculator to compute *KoA* exactly is available on the Internet (see "Internet References").

d.   Effect of molecular weight on diffusive clearance. Because high molecular weight solutes move slowly through solutions, they diffuse poorly through the membrane. As a result, whereas urea (MW 60) may be removed from blood with an efficiency of 75% (e.g., concentration of outflow blood 25 mg per dL, with inflow blood of 100 mg per dL), creatinine (MW 113) may be removed with an extraction efficiency of only 60%; that is, if the inflow blood level of creatinine is 10 mg per dL, the outflow level may be as high as 4 mg per dL. Thus, the clearance for creatinine at 200 mL per minute blood flow may be only 0.6 [×] 200 = 120 mL per minute.

For even larger solutes, such as vitamin B_{12} (MW 1355), the solute level at the blood outlet might be 75% of the level at the blood inlet. Thus, the percentage removed is 25%, and the clearance at 200 mL per minute blood flow would be 0.25 [×] 200 = 50 mL per minute. With vitamin

B_{12}, the dialyzer limits are reached early, and raising the blood flow rate above 200 mL per minute has only a modest effect on increasing clearance of such larger molecules.

    e. Very large molecules. Very large molecules, such as β_2-microglobulin (MW 11,800), cannot get through the pores of standard (low-flux) dialysis membranes at all. Thus, dialyzer clearance of β_2-microglobulin will be zero! However, "high-flux" membranes have pores of sufficient size to pass this molecule. Also, some dialysis membranes remove β_2-microglobulin by adsorption. Whether or not such high-flux membranes result in improved clinical outcome is a matter of ongoing research.

B. Ultrafiltration

    1. Need for fluid removal. Ultrafiltration during dialysis is performed for the purpose of removing water accumulated either by ingestion of fluid or by metabolism of food during the interdialytic period. Typically, a patient being dialyzed thrice weekly will gain 1–4 kg of weight between treatments (most of it water), which will need to be removed during a 3- to 4-hour period of dialysis. Patients with acute fluid overload may need more rapid fluid removal. Thus the clinical need for ultrafiltration usually ranges from 0.5 to 1.5 L per hour.

III. Clinical application of diffusion and ultrafiltration: solute removal from the patient perspective

    A. Importance of urea. Solute removal during hemodialysis focuses on urea. Urea is manufactured by the liver from amino acid nitrogen via ammonia and is the principal way in which nitrogenous waste products are excreted from the body. Urea is a small molecule, with a molecular weight of 60. It is only slightly toxic. Urea generation occurs in proportion to protein breakdown, or the protein nitrogen appearance rate (PNA). In stable patients, the PNA is proportional to dietary protein intake. Using a mathematical model known as urea kinetics, one can compute both the rate of removal and production of urea. The extent of urea removal gives us a measure of the adequacy of dialysis, whereas the amount of urea nitrogen generation gives an estimate of dietary protein intake.

    B. The weekly SUN profile. As a result of dialysis, the predialysis SUN level is typically reduced by about 70%, so that postdialysis SUN is 30% of the predialysis value. During the subsequent interdialytic period (assuming a thrice-weekly dialysis schedule), the SUN will rise to almost the same level as that seen prior to the first treatment. The result is a sawtooth pattern. The time-averaged SUN (TAC) level can be computed mathematically as the area under the sawtooth curve divided by time. Both the predialysis SUN and TAC SUN levels reflect the balance between urea production and removal. For a given level of dialysis therapy, predialysis SUN and TAC SUN will rise if urea nitrogen generation (g) is increased or will fall if g is decreased. Also, for any given rate of urea nitrogen generation, predialysis SUN and TAC SUN levels will rise if the amount of dialysis is decreased or will fall if the amount of dialysis is increased.

    C. Pitfalls in analyzing the predialysis or TAC SUN. Early attempts to model dialysis adequacy focused on predialysis or TAC SUN. Therapy was thought to be adequate as long as predialysis or TAC SUN was appropriately low. However, low predialysis or TAC SUN levels were found to be associated with a high mortality rate and were found to most often reflect inadequate protein intake rather than adequate dialysis.

D.   Indices of urea removal

1.   Urea reduction ratio (URR). The current primary measure of dialysis adequacy is the treatment-related urea reduction ratio, or URR. This is computed as follows: Assume that predialysis SUN is 60 mg per dL and postdialysis SUN is 18 mg per dL. The relative reduction in SUN (or urea) level is $(60–18)/60 = 42/60 = 0.70$. By convention, URR often is expressed as a percentage, so the value of the URR can be said to be 70%.

2.   Definition of spKt/V (single-pool Kt/V). Most published studies of dialysis adequacy have used the spKt/V ratio as a measure of urea removal. The spKt/V was popularized by Gotch and Sargent in their reanalysis of the National Cooperative Dialysis Study (1985). In that study, an spKt/V value less than 0.8 was found to be associated with a high likelihood of morbidity and/or treatment failure. Since that time, a number of additional studies have been published or presented suggesting that the delivered spKt/V is related to mortality in dialysis patients.

The spKt/V is a dimensionless ratio representing fractional urea clearance. K is the dialyzer blood water urea clearance (L per hour), t is dialysis session length (hours, hr), and V is the distribution volume of urea (liters, L).

$$K \times t = \text{L/hr} \times \text{hr} = \text{L}$$
$$V = \text{L}$$
$$(K \times t)/V = \text{L/L} = \text{dimensionless ratio}$$

If we deliver an spKt/V of 1.0, this implies that $K \times t$, or the total volume of blood cleared during the dialysis session, is equal to V, the urea distribution volume.

3.   How URR is related to spKt/V

a.   Holding tank model. To understand how the URR is related to Kt/V, one first needs to consider the hypothetical example of fluid flowing through a dialyzer that completely clears the fluid of waste solute in a single pass (Fig. 2-4A). In such a case, the clearance "K" of this perfect dialyzer will be equal to the fluid flow through the device because the dialyzer outlet solute concentration is zero, and the extraction ratio will be 100%. Cleared fluid leaving the dialyzer is temporarily collected in a holding tank outside of the "body" until dialysis stops. At the end of dialysis, the dialyzed fluid in the holding tank is mixed back with any remaining fluid in the body that has not yet passed through the dialyzer.

Because the dialyzed fluid is not routed back to the body until the end of dialysis, the inlet SUN concentration (80 mg per dL in this example) will remain constant throughout dialysis (Fig. 2-4B). The dialyzer outlet SUN concentration will always be zero. The volume of fluid cleared by the dialyzer and collected in the holding tank will be $K \times t$. If we assume that V is 40 L and that K is 10 L per hour, then $K \times t$ will be 40 L when 4 hours has elapsed. At that time, a volume $(K \times t)$ equal to the body water (V) will have

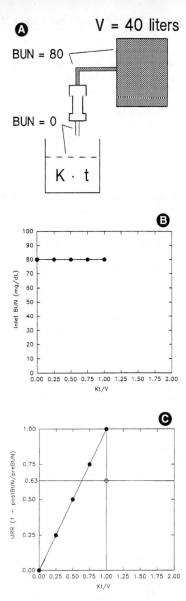

Figure 2-4. (A) A fixed-volume model of urea removal (no urea generation) in which fluid from the dialyzer is routed to a holding tank and is mixed with the source "body" tank only at the end of dialysis. In this cartoon, blood flow rate = dialyzer clearance as we are assuming a perfect dialyzer. B: The dialyzer inlet SUN (i.e., BUN) remains constant (80 mg per dL in this example) throughout dialysis. C: In this model, Kt/V = URR and Kt/V = 1.0 represents a perfect dialysis (all toxins removed). (Reproduced with permission from Daugirdas JT. Urea kinetic modeling tutorial. *Hypertens Dial Clin Nephrol* [HDCN] http://www.hdcn.com)

passed through the dialyzer. $K \times t$ will be equal to V, and hence $K \times t$ divided by V, or Kt/V, will be equal to 1.0. When $Kt/V = 1.0$, the total-body water will have been completely cleared of waste solutes, and the urea reduction ratio, this time expressed as a fraction, and not as a percentage (URR = 1 – post-SUN/pre-SUN) will be URR = 1 – 0/80 = 1.0. In this idealized situation, a Kt/V of 1.0, thus, represents a "perfect" dialysis, impossible to improve upon.

At Kt/V values less than 1.0, the URR will be linearly related to Kt/V. For example, after only 2 hours at a K of 10 L per hour, $K \times t$ will be 20 L, and the Kt/V ratio will be 20 : 40 = 0.5. At that time, one-half of the total V will have been cleared of waste solute by passing through this ideal dialyzer. Because 20 L will have been cleared (SUN = 0 mg per dL) and 20 L will remain (SUN = 80 mg per dL), on mixing these volumes at the end of dialysis, the postdialysis SUN will be 40 mg per dL, and the URR (1 – 40/80) will be 0.50. Similarly, Kt/V values of 0.25 and 0.75 will result in URR values of 0.25 and 0.75, respectively. Thus, when the dialyzer outlet is routed to a holding tank during dialysis, $Kt/V = $ URR. This relationship is shown graphically by the solid circles in Fig. 2-4C.

b. Dialyzer outlet fluid returned continually during dialysis. In practice, there is no holding tank, and fluid leaving the dialyzer outlet is continually returned to the body or source tank throughout the dialysis session (Fig. 2-5A). As a result, the inlet SUN does not stay constant as in Fig. 2-4B but falls continually during dialysis, as shown in Fig. 2-5B. Dialyzer clearance (K) remains the same (i.e., equal to flow through the dialyzer). However, less urea is removed because the amount of urea in the blood that is being presented to the dialyzer now decreases as dialysis progresses. For this reason, the system with continuous fluid return is far less efficient than when fluid is kept in a holding tank until the end of dialysis. With this new arrangement, even after running all 40 L through our ideal dialyzer ($Kt/V = 1.0$), even though the outlet SUN has been zero, there still will be urea left in the tank. As shown by the hollow circles in Fig. 2-5C, the URR will be 0.63 instead of 1.0 at a Kt/V value of 1.0. Even if we run all 40 L through a second ($Kt/V = 2.0$) and a third ($Kt/V = 3.0$) time, the postdialysis SUN still will not be zero (Fig. 2-5C). The SUN in the body will decline in an exponential fashion as a function of Kt/V (which can be thought of as the number of "passes" through an ideal dialyzer). The mathematical equation expressing the relationship between Kt/V and URR (i.e., 1 – post-SUN/pre-SUN) is:

$$Kt/V = -\ln(1 - \text{URR})$$

where ln represents a function called the "natural logarithm."

If the URR is 0.63, then

$$Kt/V = -\ln(1 - 0.63)$$
$$= -\ln(0.37)$$
$$= 1.0$$

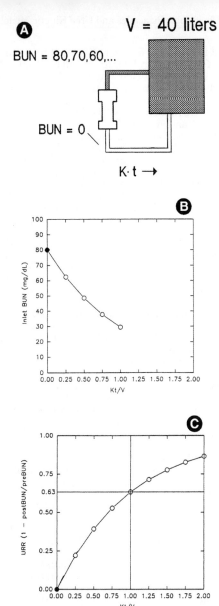

Figure 2-5. A: Another fixed-volume model, except this time the dialyzer outlet fluid is continually returned to the source tank throughout dialysis. As shown in B, the inlet serum urea nitrogen (SUN) now falls exponentially during dialysis, reducing dialysis efficiency. C: With continuous outlet return a urea reduction ratio (URR) of only 0.63 is reached when the total tank volume (V) is passed through the dialyzer, making Kt/V = 1.0. (Reproduced with permission from Daugirdas JT. Urea kinetic modeling. *Hypertens Dial Clin Nephrol* [HDCN] http://www.hdcn.com)

as shown in Fig. 2-5C. This means that if the URR is 0.63, the entire volume of the "tank" will have been passed through an ideal dialyzer, and $Kt/V = 1.0$. From this point on, we will be using $\mathrm{sp}Kt/V$ where "sp" signifies "single-pool".

c. spKt/V versus URR: Correction for urea generation (g). In fact, there is a small amount of urea generated during dialysis, such that if you dialyze to a spKt/V of 1.0, the postdialysis SUN will drop from 100 mg per dL to only about 40 instead of from 100 to 37, and the URR at sp$Kt/V = 1.0$ will be 0.60 rather than 0.63 (see top two nomogram lines in Fig. 2-6). The 0.03 shortfall in the expected URR is due to urea generated during the treatment.

d. spKt/V versus URR: Correction for ultrafiltrate volume removed. At any given URR, ultrafiltration during dialysis increases the amount of urea removed because by convention spKt/V is based on a postdialysis value for V. Assume two patients. Both have a pre- and post-SUN levels of 100 and 40 mg per dL, and both have postdialysis values for V of 40 L. However, patient A had 10% of body weight removed during dialysis. Predialysis V was therefore 44 L, ultrafiltration (UF) volume was 4 L, and UF/V was 4/40 = 0.10. In patient B, UF was zero. It is obvious that although URR was 0.60 for both patients, more urea nitrogen was removed from patient A: predialysis UN content was 44 L $\times$ 1 g per L = 44 g; postdialysis content was 40 L $\times$ 0.4 g per L = 16 g, for a removal of 28 g. In patient B, predialysis UN content was 40 L $\times$ 1 g per L = 40 g and removal was 40 − 16 = 24 g.

4. Deriving spKt/V from the URR. The effects of g and UF on the basic relation between spKt/V and URR can be corrected for. The basic equation linking spKt/V and URR, as described above, was

$$\mathrm{sp}Kt/V = -\ln(1 - \mathrm{URR})$$

Now, if we define R as post-SUN/pre-SUN, then $R = 1 - \mathrm{URR}$, and the equation becomes:

$$\mathrm{sp}Kt/V = -\ln(R)$$

The adjusted equation (Daugirdas, 1995) is as follows:

$$\mathrm{sp}(Kt/V) = \underbrace{-\ln(R - 0.008 \times t)}_{\text{adjust for } g} + \underbrace{(4 - 3.5 \times R) \times 0.55\ \mathrm{UF}/V}_{\substack{\text{Adjust for} \\ \text{volume reduction}}}$$

where t is the session length (in hours), UF is the volume of fluid removed during dialysis (in liters), and V is the postdialysis urea distribution volume (in liters). The $0.008 \times t$ term adjusts the post-/pre-SUN ratio, R, for urea generation and is a function of session length. For a session length of 3–4 hours, the generation term is about 0.024–0.032. The second adjustment term accounts for the added spKt/V due to reduction in postdialysis V and usually adds about 10% to the unadjusted spKt/V term. If V is not known, an anthropometric estimate can be used (see Table A-2) or, alternatively, V can be assumed

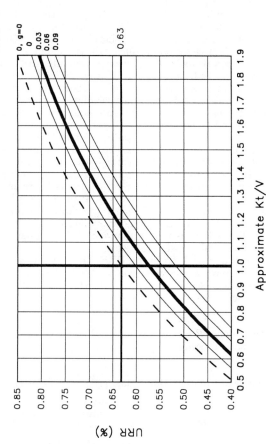

Figure 2-6. Actual relationship between *Kt/V* and URR, taking into account urea generation and the effects of volume contraction. We now see that a *Kt/V* of 1.0 corresponds to a URR of 0.60 instead of 0.63, due to urea generation. In fact, depending on how much fluid is removed as a percent of the body weight, a *Kt/V* of 1.0 can be attained with URR values as low as 0.52, with an average URR of 0.57 (heavy line represents the usual UF/W of 3%). (Reproduced with permission from Daugirdas JT. Urea kinetic modeling. *Hypertens Dial Clin Nephrol* [HDCN] http://www.hdcn.com)

to be 55% of the postdialysis weight (W). The expression then simplifies to

$$sp(KtV) = -\ln (R - 0.008 \times t) + (4 - 3.5 \times R) \times UF/W$$

as $0.55 \times UF/V$ is approximately equal to UF/W. A nomogram based on this equation is shown in Fig. 2-6. From this nomogram, it is apparent that to reach an $spKt/V$ of 1.0, the URR must be about 60% when no fluid is removed, but the URR need be only 52% when 9% of the postdialysis weight ($UF/W = 0.09$) is removed during dialysis. The lower URR reflects the added urea removal associated with volume contraction. Similarly, a URR of 0.60, which corresponds to an $spKt/V$ of 1.0 when no fluid is removed, corresponds to an $spKt/V$ of greater than 1.2 when a large amount of fluid is removed during dialysis.

Thus, both the URR and $spKt/V$ are mathematically linked, and both are determined primarily from the pre- and postdialysis SUN levels. The $spKt/V$ also takes into account ultrafiltration and urea generation. Neither is superior to the other as a measure of outcome (Held et al. 1996).

5. Multipool models, urea inbound, and rebound. The model shown in Fig. 2-5 assumes that urea is contained in a single body compartment. This assumption leads to a monoexponential decline in the SUN during dialysis, as per hollow circles in Fig. 2-5B, and to a minimal rebound after dialysis has been discontinued. In fact, the SUN profile during dialysis deviates from the exponential decrease shown in Fig. 2-5B, usually being lower than expected (Fig. 2-7). Also, following dialysis, SUN rebounds to levels that cannot be explained on the basis of urea generation (Fig. 2-7). These observations suggest that urea is being sequestered somewhere during dialysis, as shown in Fig. 2-7. Because urea is being removed from a smaller apparent volume during the early part of dialysis, the SUN during the initial part of dialysis falls more quickly than expected. We have designated this unexpected fall in intradialytic SUN as urea **inbound**. Toward the end of dialysis, as a concentration gradient develops between the sequestered compartment and the accessible compartment, the fall in SUN slows. After dialysis is complete, continued movement of urea from the sequestered to the accessible compartment causes the postdialysis urea **rebound** (Fig. 2-7).

a. Regional blood flow model. An idea in vogue until recently was that urea sequestration occurred primarily intracellularly. It has now been shown that urea is sequestered during dialysis in tissues, primarily muscle, that contain a high percentage of total-body water, and hence urea, but receive a low percentage of the cardiac output. Because of the low ratio of blood flow through these tissues to their urea content, the transfer rate of urea from these tissues to the blood during dialysis is slow, causing urea sequestration.

b. Implications of urea inbound and rebound on measures of adequacy

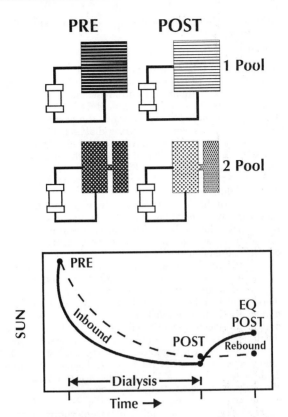

Figure 2-7. The effects of urea sequestration on the intradialytic fall
in SUN (urea inbound) and the postdialysis increase in SUN
(rebound). When there is sequestration, the intradialytic SUN level
falls more quickly than expected (inbound) due to initial removal
from a smaller apparent space. However, after dialysis is complete,
continued entry of urea from the sequestered space to the proximal
space causes urea rebound to occur. (Reproduced with permission
from Daugirdas JT. Urea kinetic modeling. *Hypertens Dial Clin
Nephrol* [HDCN] http://www.hdcn.com)

**(1) Single-pool urea kinetics overestimates
amount of urea removal.** Why is this so? Urea kinetics
can be used to compute the amount of urea removed during dialysis, as the time-averaged SUN during a dialysis
session multiplied by the liters of plasma cleared.

Example: Assuming that the predialysis SUN is 100
and postdialysis SUN 30, the time-averaged value during dialysis (t.a.d.) is about 55 mg per dL. [For reasons
beyond the scope of this handbook, the time-averaged
SUN during dialysis (t.a.d.) is less than the arithmetic

mean (65 mg per dL) of the pre- and post-dialysis SUN.]
Urea nitrogen removed is then equal to liters of plasma
cleared × t.a.d. – SUN concentration.

Problem: Assume that 57 liters of plasma are cleared
during this dialysis treatment (e. g., 238 mL per min ×
240 min): How much urea nitrogen should be removed
using the single-pool model?

Solution: We first convert all quantities to grams and
liters, so t.a.d. – SUN = 0.55 g per L, and urea nitrogen
removed = 57 L × 0.55 g per L = 32 g.

However, if one collects the dialysate, and if one then
multiplies the dialysate urea nitrogen concentration ×
volume of dialysate to compute the amount of urea
nitrogen in the spent dialysate, one may find only 28 g
of urea nitrogen in the tank, despite the fact that the
blood-sided analysis predicted that 32 g should have
been recovered. Why the discrepancy?

One reason for the error in computations is urea inbound. Due to urea sequestration during dialysis, the
actual time-averaged level of urea nitrogen "seen" by the
dialyzer was substantially lower than 55 mg per dL.
Actual measurement of the intradialytic SUN profile to
get the true time-averaged SUN value multiplied by the
liters of plasma cleared would give the correct urea nitrogen removal amount of 28 g per treatment.

(2)   The concept of equilibrated Kt/V (eKt/V).
Most of the postdialysis urea rebound resulting from
compartment effects is over with by 30–60 minutes.
One can measure the postdialysis SUN at this time and
compute a "true" or equilibrated URR, which will be
less than the URR based on an immediate postdialysis
sample. The equilibrated URR can be translated into an
equilibrated Kt/V. One uses the 30- to 60 minute post-
SUN to compute R_{eq} or the equilibrated post-/pre-SUN
ratio. R_{eq} is used instead of R in the Kt/V equation:

Example: Pre-SUN 100, post-SUN 35, equilibrated
post-SUN 44, $t = 3$ hours, UF/V = 0.06 (e.g., 3 kg removed
from a patient with $V = 50$ L).

$eKt/V = -\ln (R_{eq} - 0.008 \times t) + (4 - 3.5 \times R_{eq}) \times 0.55 \times UF/V$
$= -\ln (0.44 - 0.008 \times 3) + (4 - 3.5 \times 0.44) \times 0.55 \times 0.06$
$= 0.877 + 0.081$
$= 0.96$

$spKt/V = -\ln (R - 0.008 \times t) + (4 - 3.5 \times R) \times 0.55 \times UF/V$
$= -\ln (0.35 - 0.008 \times 3) + (4 - 3.5 \times 0.35) \times 0.55 \times 0.06$
$= 1.12 + 0.091$
$= \mathbf{1.21}$

The eKt/V is typically about 0.2 Kt/V unit lower than
the $spKt/V$, but this depends on the efficiency, or rate of
dialysis, as discussed below.

We can compare eKt/V with $spKt/V$ as follows:

$eKt/V = spKt/V - \text{rebound}$

Note that, in the above case, rebound is about 1.21 –
0.96 = 0.25 Kt/V units.

(3) Predicting postdialysis urea rebound. The amount of urea rebound depends on the intensity or rate of dialysis that was given. The rate of dialysis can be expressed as the number of Kt/V units per hour, or (Kt/V) divided by t in hours. A formula has been designed and validated that can predict the amount of rebound based on the rate of dialysis. This "rate equation" avoids the requirement of having to draw a postdialysis SUN level 30–60 minutes after the completion of dialysis. The rate equation (Daugirdas and Schneditz, 1997) predicts that:

Rebound = $0.6 \times$ rate of dialysis $- 0.03$ (arterial access)
Rebound = $0.47 \times$ rate of dialysis $- 0.02$ (venous access)

Substituting $(\text{sp}Kt/V)/t$ for (rate of dialysis), we have:

$eKt/V = \text{sp}Kt/V - 0.6 \times (\text{sp}Kt/V)/t + 0.03$ (arterial access)
$eKt/V = \text{sp}Kt/V - 0.47 \times (\text{sp}Kt/V)/t + 0.02$ (venous access)

In these equations, t is in hours, and $\text{sp}Kt/V$ divided by t simplifies to K/V (expressed as hr^{-1}). For example, if a $\text{sp}Kt/V$ of 1.2 is being delivered using an arterial access over 6, 3, or 2 hours:

spKt/V	t(hr)	spKt/V per hr	Rebound	eKt/V
1.2	6	0.2	0.09	1.11
1.2	3	0.4	0.21	0.99
1.2	2	0.6	0.33	0.87

then eKt/V will be about 1.1, 1.0, or 0.9, depending on whether these 1.2 $\text{sp}Kt/V$ units were delivered over 6, 3, or 2 hours.

(a) Why two formulas for eKt/V for arterial versus venous access? During dialysis an arteriovenous (AV) gradient for urea develops in the following fashion: Once dialysis is begun, the dialyzer returns dialyzed blood to the heart, which mixes in the heart with blood returning from tissues, diluting it and lowering the arterial urea level. Subsequently, as the arterial blood passes through the tissues, its urea level again increases, setting up the AV gradient. Usually, the magnitude of this AV gradient is on the order of 5% to 10%. Once dialysis is stopped, the AV urea gradient rapidly begins to close because the dialyzer is no longer feeding dialyzed blood to the heart.

Postdialysis urea rebound computed using the ($0.6 \times$ rate of dialysis $- 0.03$) equation above is based on total rebound from a postdialysis **arterial** blood sample. About 30% of the total post-dialysis urea rebound is due to rapid closure of the AV gradient. If venous blood is sampled post dialysis, then 30% of the total rebound will have been accounted for, and the AV urea gradient must be subtracted from the total urea rebound. For this reason, there are two formulas to estimate eKt/V: one for arterial postdialysis blood and one for venous postdialysis blood.

(b) Sampling method for postdialysis blood.
With an arterial access, blood is usually sampled soon after stopping dialysis (e.g., within 15 seconds), at a time when the AV urea gradient due to dialysis has not had a chance to dissipate. With an arterial access, if blood is sampled 2 minutes after slowing of dialysis, the AV gradient for urea will have largely closed, and the "venous access" formula for eKt/V should be used. Arterial blood samples taken 20 seconds to 2 minutes after dialysis will reflect partial closure of the dialysis-associated AV urea gradient, and then the rebound will be somewhere between the points computed using arterial and venous rebound equations. With a venous access, sampling time within the 15-second to 2-minute postdialysis period is not critical because closure of the AV gradient is not a factor. For venous access, the venous formula for eKt/V can be used for samples taken 15 seconds to 2 minutes after dialysis.

4. Access recirculation (AR)

a. Definition. Normally blood flow through an AV access averages about 1 L per minute. The blood pump, which normally routes a portion of this flow through the dialyzer, usually is set to take a flow of 350–500 mL per minute. Because upstream (relative to the arterial needle entry point) access supply normally exceeds the demand of the blood pump, usually there is no AR. Exceptions occur when the access needles are placed too close to one another, or when the needle positions have been inadvertently reversed, so that the venous needle returns blood upstream to the arterial needle.

In some fistulas, and also in failing AV grafts, flow through the access can decrease to the range of 200–450 mL per minute, particularly toward the end of dialysis. Under such conditions, upstream (relative to the arterial needle entry point) flow may be less than the blood pump flow rate.

In such instances, the blood pump begins to draw blood from both the upstream and downstream access segment (relative to the arterial needle). The shortage of upstream supply causes flow to be reversed between the two access needles.

Some portion of the blood flow leaving the dialyzer outlet then goes back retrograde to the dialyzer inlet without picking up additional urea from the tissue bed. This phenomenon is called AR.

b. Impact of AR on dialysis adequacy. The impact of AR on dialysis adequacy has to do with the resultant lowering of the urea concentration of the blood flowing into the dialyzer. When AR occurs, the urea concentration in the blood entering the dialyzer may be reduced by 5%–40% or more relative to that in the upstream arterial blood because of admixture with urea-poor blood from the dialyzer outlet. The amount of urea removed in the dialyzer is equal to the volume of blood cleared × dialyzer inflow urea concentration. Although dialyzer clearance remains unchanged, the amount of urea removed is reduced because of the reduced urea concentration at the dialyzer inlet throughout dialysis.

c. **Impact of AR on apparent URR or spKt/V.** In patients with AR, if blood at the end of dialysis is drawn from the inlet blood line, the urea level in this blood will be lower than that in the patient's upstream blood, the latter representing the true postdialysis SUN concentration. Hence, if postdialysis SUN is artifactually low, the URR and, consequently, the spKt/V will be overestimated.

Stopping the blood pump prior to drawing the sample does not prevent this problem, as the admixed blood in the inlet blood line is simply "frozen" in place. A sample taken from the inlet blood line after stopping the pump still reflects admixed blood.

To ensure that blood being sampled reflects patient blood, one needs to slow the blood pump to a flow rate (e.g., less than 100 mL per minute) that is assuredly below the access flow rate for a short period of time (10–20 seconds). The length of the slow-flow period depends on the dead space between the tip of the arterial needle and the sampling port (usually about 9 mL in most adult blood lines) and should be sufficient to allow the column of nonadmixed blood to reach the sampling port (100 mL per minute = 100/60 = 1.7 mL per second; in a 10- to 20-second slow-flow period, 17–34 mL of blood will have advanced into the arterial blood line). Postdialysis blood should always be drawn after a short slow-flow period for this reason.

5. **Cardiopulmonary recirculation**

a. **Definition.** A recirculation can be defined broadly to occur whenever blood leaving the dialyzer outlet returns to the inlet without first having traversed the peripheral urea-rich tissues. In AR, the recirculation occurs via the short access segment between the venous and arterial needles. Cardiopulmonary recirculation occurs through the heart and lungs (which contain negligible amounts of urea) when the dialyzer is fed from the arterial circulation (e.g., via an AV access). During dialysis, cleared blood from the dialyzer outlet returns to the heart. In the aorta, the cleared blood is partitioned; some of it get routed to the non-access arteries that lead it to the tissues to pick up more urea, but a fraction goes directly back through the access to the dialyzer without having traversed a peripheral capillary bed. When a dialyzer is fed from a venous access, cardiopulmonary recirculation cannot occur. Although an AV urea gradient is still present, all of the blood leaving the dialyzer must go through the peripheral capillary bed before it sees the dialyzer again.

b. **Impact of cardiopulmonary recirculation on dialysis adequacy.** During dialysis using either an AV or venous access, there is an AV gradient for urea that is established. With an AV access, the dialyzer "rides" the arterial intradialytic urea nitrogen concentration curve, which is 5% to 10% lower than the venous intradialytic urea nitrogen concentration curve. Hence, dialysis with an AV access is inherently less efficient (by about 5%–10%) than that using a venous access. This effect usually is outweighed by the lower blood flow rates achievable with venous accesses and the higher associated access (catheter) recirculation rate.

6.   Urea modeling of urea distribution volume
   a.   Definitions. Urea modeling can be used to determine the patient's apparent urea space, V. The principle
is straightforward. Using blood-sided modeling, a value of
spKt/V is determined from the URR and the degree of volume contraction, UF/V or UF/W (Fig. 2-6). Then an estimate is made for dialyzer blood water clearance, K (from
the dialyzer KoA, blood flow rate, and dialysate flow rate,
as per Fig. 2-3) or Table A-1. spKt/V is known, and now t
and K are known, so V can be computed algebraically.
   Problem: URR is 60% with UF/W = 0. t is 4 hours.
Dialyzer KoA is 800 mL per minute. Dialysate flow rate is
500 mL per minute. Blood flow rate is 450 mL per minute.
What is V?
   Solution: From Fig. 2-6, spKt/V is 1.0. From the equations in Table A-1 or the nomogram in Fig. 2-3, K_w is 250 mL
per minute (15 L per hour). So by algebra, we know that K
(15 L per hour) $\times t$ (4 hours) divided by V (L) is 1.0. V then is
equal to $K \times t$ or to $15 \times 4 = 60,000$ mL, or 60 L.
   b.   Use of modeled volume (V). Initially, the modeled
V can be compared to expected values (usually 55% of body
weight in men and 50% of body weight in women). An anthropometric estimate (Watson or Hume Weyers) of V can
also be used (Table A-2). The modeled volume should be
within about 25% of the anthropometric value for V. A more
powerful use of V is to follow the modeled value over time.
Although values for V have a substantial variation from
treatment to treatment, a large change in V may reflect an
error in blood sampling technique, an unrecorded change in
the amount of dialysis ($K \times t$) given, or the presence of AR.
   (1) V much smaller than usual. In this case, the
URR is higher than expected, as is the spKt/V. Because
the modeling program is told that K and t have not
changed, the high spKt/V causes the program to conclude
that the patient must have shrunk, as a smaller than
usual value for V is calculated. Most often, if the V is
reduced by about 100%, the problem is that postdialysis
blood sample was drawn from the outlet line instead of the
inlet. Other potential causes are discussed in Chapter 6.
   (2) V much larger than normal. The URR and
spKt/V are lower than expected, and so the program con-
cludes that if K and t are unchanged, then the patient
must have somehow expanded to account for such a low
URR. In fact, the real problem is that either K or t is lower
than recorded. Most common problems include treatment
interruption (full duration not given), or lowering of blood
flow rate due to technical problems (K lower than expected), or some sort of dialyzer performance problem
resulting in reduced dialyzer clearance. AR can also cause
this because the inflow blood urea level is lower than
upstream blood, reducing effective access clearance. One
caveat: The effects of AR on V will *only* be seen if blood is
drawn properly (e.g., after a slow-flow period). If admixed
blood is drawn post dialysis, then the URR will be artifactually increased. The expected lowering of URR due to AR
then may not be seen, and modeled V may be unchanged!

(3) **Effect of URR on V.** The V computed using single-pool modeling does not take into account all phases of rebound, especially compartment effects. By a mathematical coincidence, the single pool V approximates the true V at a URR of about 65%–70%. At lower levels of URR, single-pool V is lower than the true V, and at higher levels of URR, single-pool V is more than true V. Unless one is using very low levels of URR (e.g., for daily hemodialysis), this error in V is usually trivial, on the order of less than 5%, and not usually detectable in individual patients (Daugirdas and Smye, 1997).

7. Urea nitrogen generation rate and the nPNA

a. Utility of nPNA. One of the benefits of urea modeling is that the generation rate of urea nitrogen (g) can be estimated from the urea nitrogen removal rate and the time-averaged plasma level. Because urea production comes from protein breakdown, a regression estimate can be used to derive the protein nitrogen appearance rate normalized to modeled V (nPNA) based on g. The actual clinical utility of g or nPNA is debatable. nPNA is not a very robust predictor of mortality (once serum albumin and creatinine are controlled for). Generally, outcome is poor when nPNA is low, as this usually reflects poor dietary intake. Before one can make the assumption that a low nPNA reflects a low dietary protein intake, one needs to exclude marked anabolism. Similarly, a high nPNA may be due to hypercatabolism rather than to a good dietary protein intake.

b. Methods of computing g (and thereby nPNA). In standard urea kinetic modeling, there are two approaches to calculating g or nPNA: the three-point method and the two-point method.

(1) **Three-point method.** The three-point method is more useful in an acute situation, as it does not depend on any steady-state assumptions. One simply measures the SUN before dialysis, after dialysis, and at some third point during the interdialytic interval (usually 44–68 hours later). Once V is known (estimated from Kt/V, K, and t during dialysis), one knows (a) the size of the box and (b) the increase in concentration of urea nitrogen during some or all of the inter-dialytic interval. It is simple algebra to compute how much material must be added to a box of size V to result in an increase in concentration from value 1 to value 2. The actual computation is a bit more complex because the value for g affects the URR, and this has a small effect on spKt/V and therefore on the initial estimate of V. Therefore, in practice, an iterative (going back and forth) mathematical approach is used to first estimate V assuming a g of about 6 mg per minute; then, based on the first estimate of V and two interdialytic SUN values, one computes a second, better estimate for g. Then one goes back using this more accurate estimate for g to compute a better estimate for V, and so on, until going back and forth no longer changes the answer. Fluid gain during the interdialytic interval dampens the increase in SUN, and this factor is also taken into consideration in urea kinetic modeling programs.

Problem: Postdialysis V is 60 L and postdialysis SUN is 30 mg per dL. A SUN value measured 48 hours later is 78 mg per dL. What is g?

Solution (simplified calculation neglecting volume changes): $78 - 30 = 48$ mg per dL increase in SUN over 48 hours = 1 mg per dL per hour. This is 10 mg per L per hour $\times$ 60 L = 600 mg of urea nitrogen generated per hour = 10 mg urea nitrogen per minute. $g = 10$ mg per minute.

(2)   Two-point method. In the two-point modeling method, a predialysis and postdialysis SUN only are obtained. There is no third SUN sample taken during the interdialytic interval prior to the next dialysis. However, a value for g (and therefore nPNA) is computed. How can this be done?

(a)   Analogy to creatinine clearance.

With urea kinetics, we can ask the computer to generate a weekly sawtooth SUN plasma profile, from which we can compute a time-averaged SUN. This is analogous to the serum creatinine level. With creatinine clearance, we know the creatinine generation rate (from a 24-hour urine collection), and we use this plus the serum creatinine level to compute clearance. In UKM, we go the other way. We know the urea clearance (from the dialysis session spKt/V and residual renal urea clearance), and we know the time-averaged urea level. From these two quantities, the urea nitrogen generation rate can be computed. The relationships between urea removal (spKt/V), the predialysis SUN, and the urea generation rate (expressed as PNA rate normalized to V, or nPNA), are shown in Fig. 2-8. For any level of urea removal (spKt/V and K_{ru}), there will be a direct linear relationship between urea generation (expressed as nPNA) and the predialysis SUN.

(b)   How a two-point urea modeling program computes the nPNA. The computer generates a series of sawtooth SUN patterns based on the measured spKt/V and various hypothetical values of g. As the values for g are increased, the height of the sawteeth will rise. For each value of g, the computer assumes that every dialysis has the same spKt/V (except for ultrafiltration) and runs the simulation until the predialysis SUN (computed for either Monday, Wednesday, or Friday) stabilizes. The computer then compares the stabilized predialysis SUN with the actual measured value. If the value is too high, the computer inputs a lower value of g and redoes the computation. The computer keeps adjusting the value for g until the predicted predialysis SUN value matches the actual value. For example, in the Fig. 2.8, identify the line where sp$Kt/V = 1.2$. If the nPNA is only 0.6 g per kg per day, then the height of the sawtooth (pre-SUN) at the first dialysis day of the week (after the 2-day interval) will only be 41 mg per dL. If the nPNA increases to 1.2 g per kg per day, then the height of the first-of-week pre-SUN sawtooth will stabilize at about 90 mg per dL (Fig. 2-8).

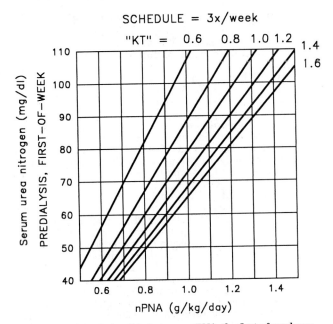

Figure 2-8. The relationship between nPNA, the first-of-week predialysis SUN, and *Kt/V* for patients undergoing dialysis three times
per week. Similar nomograms have been devised for midweek (see
Fig. A-3) and end-of-week predialysis SUN, and for twice-weekly
schedules. "KT" = Kt/v adjusted for residual renal function (see Fig.
A-3). (Reproduced with permission from Daugirdas JT. Urea kinetic
modeling. *Hypertens Dial Clin Nephrol* [HDCN] http://www.hdcn.com)

    (c)   Formulas to obtain nPNA from sp*Kt/V* **and
predialysis SUN.** These are given in Depner and
Daugirdas (1996). A formal computation can be made
by a urea kinetic modeling program. One such program is available through the internet (see "Internet
References").

  8.   Residual renal function. Residual renal function in
end-stage renal disease patients can be approximated as the
average of the creatinine and urea clearances. Urea clearance
(K_{ru}) underestimates GFR due to proximal tubular urea reabsorption, whereas creatinine clearance (K_{rc}) overestimates
GFR because of tubular secretion. It is well established that
end-stage renal disease (ESRD) patients with substantial
residual renal function (K_r) live longer, and so it is important
to attempt to preserve residual function and to minimize
potential injury to the ESRD kidney (e.g., by avoiding nephrotoxic drugs and by minimizing intradialytic hypotension).

    a.   Measuring the K_{ru}. For this, one needs to collect all
urine during a 24-hour period of the interdialytic interval.

Usually, the patient starts the collection 24 hours before coming to the dialysis unit and then reports to the unit with the urine container and gives a sample of blood to measure the SUN. If the patient is receiving a usual amount of dialysis, and if the collection interval is 24 hours prior to dialysis, one can assume that the average serum urea level during the collection is 90% of the predialysis SUN (Daugirdas, unpublished observations). The K_{ru} calculation is then:

$$K_{ru} = \frac{\text{UUN}}{\text{SUN}} \times \text{urine flow rate} \ (\text{mL/min})$$

Where UUN is the urine urea nitrogen concentration.

The units for the UUN and SUN do not matter, but they must be the same, as they cancel each other out. Typically, K_{ru} values of 0–8 mL per minute will be obtained.

Problem: If urine flow rate is 0.33 mL per minute, or 20 mL per hour, over 24 hours one would collect 480 mL of urine. Assume that the urine urea concentration is about 800 mg per dL and that the collection was during the 24-hour interval immediately preceding a dialysis. Predialysis SUN for that dialysis is 56 mg per dL. What is the K_{ru}?

Solution: First, compute the estimated mean SUN during the 24-hour collection interval. As discussed above, the estimated mean SUN during the collection period is 90% of the predialysis SUN, or $0.9 \times 56 = 50$ mg per dL. So K_{ru}= (800 mg per dL × 0.33 mL per minute)/50 mg per dL = 5.3 mL per minute.

b. Adding the residual renal urea clearance to *Kt/V*-urea in peritoneal dialysis and in hemodialysis

(1) In peritoneal dialysis, *Kru* and Kt from *Kt/V* are additive. In peritoneal dialysis patients, as both residual renal urea clearance (K_{ru}) and peritoneal urea clearance (K_{pu}) are operative during a steady-state situation, K_{ru} and K_{pu} can be simply added. One milliliter per minute of K_{ru} mathematically approximates 10.08 L of urea clearance per week, as there as 10,080 minutes in a week. This is discussed further in the peritoneal dialysis physiology chapter.

(2) In hemodialysis, *Kru* cannot be simply added to *Kt/V*. For hemodialysis, one cannot add dialyzer urea clearance (K_{totw} in Table A-1) and residual urea clearance (K_{ru}), as the dialyzer urea clearance is operative during a period of changing SUN and hence is less efficient in terms of urea removal than K_{ru}.

c. The concept of equivalent urea clearance (e*Kru*). One can compute the equivalent clearance for any given dialysis regimen using the same principle as computing a creatinine clearance: If one knows the generation rate (24-hour collection in the case of creatinine) and the mean plasma level, one can compute clearance as ratio of the two. Using any of a number of computer programs or a simplified equation (Depner and Daugirdas, 1997), one can compute both the urea nitrogen generation rate (g) and the time-averaged urea nitrogen level (TAC urea), and compute the ratio of the two to get an equivalent renal clearance.

$$\mathrm{Cr_{cl}} - \frac{UV}{P}$$

$$eK_{ru} = \frac{g}{\mathrm{TAC}}$$

Where $\mathrm{Cr_{cl}}$ is creatinine clearance (see Chapter 1), and eK_{ru} is the equivalent urea clearance, g is the urea nitrogen generation rate, and TAC is the time averaged urea nitrogen level. This basic approach was first popularized by Casino and Lopez (1996).

Problem: The recommended minimum spKt/V for thrice-weekly dialysis is 1.2 per session. What is the equivalent renal urea clearance?

Solution: Assume this is given over 3 hours. Rebound using the rate equation (see above) will be about 0.2 Kt/V units. So eKt/V will be 1.0 per session. Using the Casino and Lopez nomogram (see their paper), this translates to an eK_{ru} of about 11 mL per minute.

d.   Going from eK_{ru} (in mL per minute) to weekly Kt/V. Theoretically, one can take any hemodialysis prescription, compute g and TAC using a modeling program, and then convert it to eK_{ru}. This value can be added to the measured residual renal urea clearance. The resulting eK_{ru} can be expressed either in milliliters per minute, or in liters per week. When expressed as liters per week, eK_{ru}, which is not equivalent to $(K \times t)$, or volume of plasma cleared during the week, can be further divided by V to arrive at a weekly Kt/V-urea.

Problem: In a patient with $V = 35$ L, eK_{ru} is 11 mL per minute. What is the weekly Kt/V-urea?

Solution: 11 mL per minute $\times$ 10,080 mL per week divided by 1,000 to convert milliliters to liters gives a weekly volume of plasma cleared of 110 L per week. This is the $K \times t$ term of Kt/V. Dividing by $V = 35$, we get weekly Kt/V urea = 3.14.

e.   Problems with the Casino/Lopez eK_{ru} and its resultant weekly Kt/V-urea. One problem with this approach is that, as shown above in sections c and d, a thrice-weekly spKt/V of 1.2, or an eKt/V of 1.0, translates into an eK_{ru} of about 11 mL per minute, or a weekly $K \times t$ of about 110 L, or a weekly Kt/V of about 110/35, assuming $V = 35$ L, or 3.1. This suggests that a weekly Kt/V-urea of 3.1 is required as a minimum standard in patients being treated with intermittent hemodialysis. But we know from the peritoneal dialysis outcomes literature that a weekly Kt/V-urea (derived as the sum of residual renal and peritoneal urea clearance) of about 2.0–2.2 is a reasonable minimum target level of adequacy.

So the Casino–Lopez–derived eK_{ru} does not appear to be equivalent to either peritoneal dialysis Kt/V-urea or to residual renal urea clearance in terms of outcome.

The reasons for this difference in weekly Kt/V-urea outcomes target between hemodialysis and peritoneal dialysis are speculative. One explanation is that urea may be less compartmentalized than other low molecular weight solutes. In such a case, equivalent amounts of urea removal where one therapy is highly intermittent may not represent equivalent therapy.

f.   The Gotch adjusted eK_{ru}. Gotch has proposed a new equation for eK_{ru} for hemodialysis regimens to correct this problem (National Kidney Foundation, 1997). Whereas the Casino–Lopez idea is to divide g by the time-averaged urea level (TAC urea), Gotch computes an adjusted eK_{ru} as being equal to g divided by the mean weekly predialysis plasma urea level.

Example: Thrice-weekly hemodialysis schedule. $g = 6$ mg per minute per 35 L; TAC urea = 40 mg per dL; peak urea values for Mon, Wed, Fri 65, 60, 55 mg per dL; mean predialysis urea = (65 + 60 + 55)/3 = 60 mg per dL. In this case, we can see that the Gotch adjusted eK_{ru} will be about one-third lower than the Casino–Lopez eK_{ru}:

eK_{ru} (Casino–Lopez) $= g$/TAC-SUN =
(6 mg/min) / (40 mg/dL)
= 0.15 dL/min
= 15 mL/min

eK_{ru}(Gotch) g/(mean pre-SUN) = 6/60
= 0.10 dL/min
= 10 mL/min

Using the Gotch approach, a standard thrice-weekly hemodialysis regimen (spKt/V = 1.2) will yield an eK_{ru} of about 7 mL per minute, or 70 L per week, which in a person with $V = 35$ L translates into a weekly Kt/V urea of about 2.0. Thus, the Gotch modification of the eK_{ru} allows consistency and perhaps additivity among hemodialysis, peritoneal dialysis, and residual renal urea continuous-clearance equivalents.

It should be emphasized that the Gotch eK_{ru} is an intentionally down-regulated number and that it cannot be used directly in the computation of nPNA. For that purpose, the Casino–Lopez $eK_{ru}(g$/TAC) must be used).

g.   Graded (partial)–dose hemodialysis or peritoneal dialysis. According to DOQI guidelines, one should normally begin ESRD replacement therapy when the weekly Kt/V-urea is about 2.0. One could theoretically use the concepts of the Gotch adjusted eK_{ru} to start patients out on either hemodialysis or peritoneal dialysis at other than a full dose.

An approximation of the required thrice-weekly Kt/V can be found using a nomogram proposed by Gotch (Fig. A-4), found in the Peritoneal Dialysis DOQI guidelines. Details are beyond the scope of this handbook (see Appendix A).

IV.   Acid–base aspects

A.   Acid–base balance. Acid production is a function of PNA (protein intake in noncatabolic patients). In nonuremic patients, acid production rate can be estimated at 0.77 [x] PNA and is about 60 mmol per day (420 mmol per week) for a 70-kg patient.

Recent evidence, however, suggests that acid production in hemodialysis patients is reduced to the range of 28 mmol per day for reasons that are not completely clear (Uribarri, 1998).

B. Predialysis HCO₃ level. Metabolic acidosis has been linked to adverse effects on protein metabolism. However, outcome studies do not show an adverse effect of acidosis until the predialysis serum HCO_3 level decreases to less than 16 mEq per L. Attempts to maintain hemodialysis patients at predialysis HCO_3 levels in the mid-20s instead of 20 or less have yielded no benefit in terms of increases in serum albumin or in anthropometric measures of muscle mass.

C. Proper dialysate bicarbonate level. During hemodialysis, alkali is delivered to the patient from the dialysis solution in the form of bicarbonate. The usual dialysis solution bicarbonate level is 35–38 mEq per L. Once predialysis acidosis has been largely corrected, further use of dialysis solution with a bicarbonate concentration of 38 mEq per L may cause postdialysis alkalemia; postdialysis plasma bicarbonate levels of greater than 30 mEq per L with pH values greater than 7.55 have been reported. For this reason, the postdialysis plasma bicarbonate level should be monitored, and the dialysis solution bicarbonate concentration should be reduced if necessary; a reasonable target value for the postdialysis plasma bicarbonate level would be in the vicinity of 27 mEq per L. Not all machines are capable of easily delivering a lower than standard (35–38 mEq per L) bicarbonate dialysate.

1. Effect of ultrafiltration and interdialytic weight gain. The amount of bicarbonate transfer to the patient is greatly reduced at high ultrafiltration rates. For this reason, higher than usual dialysis solution bicarbonate levels often must be used in patients with large interdialytic weight gains. Another reason for this is that such patients often are found to a have high PNA. Whether this is due to high dietary protein intake or to negative nitrogen balance has not been ascertained. However, the high PNA per se engenders increased generation of acid equivalents.

2. Effect of dialysis adequacy. Dialyzer bicarbonate uptake generally is proportional to (but less than) urea clearance (Kt/V). For this reason, underdialysis, as reflected by a poor Kt/V urea, usually results in predialysis acidosis as well.

Acknowledgment: The urea kinetic modeling update of this chapter has been adapted from the urea kinetic modeling tutorial on *Hypertens Dial Clin Nephrol,* with permission.

SELECTED READINGS

Casino FG, Lopez T. The equivalent renal urea clearance. A new parameter to assess dialysis dose. *Nephrol Dial Transplant* 1996;11: 1574–1581.

Daugirdas JT. Simplified equations for monitoring Kt/V, PCRn, eKt/V, and ePCRn. *Adv Ren Replace Ther* 1995;2:295–304.

Daugirdas JT, Schneditz D. Overestimation of hemodialysis dose depends on dialysis efficiency by regional blood flow but not by conventional two pool urea kinetic analysis. *ASAIO J* 1995;41: M719–M724.

Depner TA, Daugirdas JT. Equations for normalized protein catabolic rate based on two-point modeling of hemodialysis urea kinetics. *J Am Soc Nephrol* 1996;7:780–785.

Depner TA, Daugirdas JT. Simplified equations for mean BUN (TAC) and the continuous equivalent of urea clearance (EKR) from Kt/V and PCRn. *J Am Soc Nephrol* 1997;8:281a (Abstr).

Gotch FA, Sargent JA. A mechanistic analysis of the National Cooperative Dialysis Study (NCDS). *Kidney Int* 1985;28:526–534.

Held et al. *Kidney Int* 1996;50:550–556.

HEMO Study Group (prepared by Daugirdas JT, et al). Methods of estimating the equilibrated Kt/V: data from the HEMO study. *Kidney Int* 1997;52:1395–1405.

Leypoldt JK, et al. Hemodialyzer mass transfer-area coefficients for urea increase at high dialysate flow rates. The Hemodialysis (HEMO) study. *Kidney Int* 1997;51:2013–2017.

Lim VA, Flanigan MJ, Fangman J. Effect of hematocrit on solute removal during high efficiency hemodialysis. *Kidney Int* 1990;37:1557.

National Kidney Foundation. NKF–DOQI clinical practice guidelines for peritoneal dialysis adequacy. *Am J Kidney Dis* 1997 Sept;30 (3 Suppl 2):S67–S136.

Schneditz D, et al. Cardiopulmonary recirculation during dialysis. *Kidney Int* 1992;42:1450.

Schneditz D, Daugirdas JT. Formal analytical solution to a regional blood flow and diffusion-based urea kinetic model. *ASAIO J* 1994;40:M667–M673.

Uribarri J, et al. Acid production in chronic hemodialysis patients. *J Am Soc Nephrol* 1998;9:114–120.

Internet References

Urea kinetic modeling tutorial/questions (http://www.hdcn.com/hd/ukmtutor.htm)

Urea kinetic modeling calculators (http://www.hdcn.com/hd/ukmcalc.htm)

Urea kinetic modeling links (http://www.hdcn.com/hd/ukmlinks.htm)

Hemodialysis Apparatus

John T. Daugirdas, John C. Van Stone,
and James T. Boag

I.   The dialyzer. The dialyzer shell is a box or tube with four ports. Two ports communicate with a blood compartment and two with a dialysate compartment. The semipermeable membrane separates the two compartments. The boundary area between the two compartments is maximized by using a membrane divided into multiple hollow fibers or parallel plates.

A.   Hollow-fiber versus parallel-plate construction

1.   Structure. In the hollow-fiber (also called capillary) dialyzer, the blood flows into a chamber at one end of the cylindrical shell. From there, blood enters thousands of small capillaries tightly bound in a bundle (Fig. 3-1). The dialyzer is designed so that blood flows through the fibers, and dialysis solution flows around the outside. Once through the capillaries, the blood collects in a chamber at the other end of the cylindrical shell and is then routed back to the patient.

In parallel-plate dialyzers, the blood is routed between sheets of membranes laid on top of one another (Fig. 3-1). The dialyzer is configured so that blood and dialysis solution pass through alternate spaces between the membrane sheets. Parallel-plate dialyzers are no longer commonly used in the United States.

B.   Membranes

1.   Membrane material. There are four types of membranes currently used in dialyzers: cellulose, "substituted" cellulose, cellulosynthetic, and synthetic.

a.   Cellulose. The cellulose is obtained from processed cotton. Cellulose membranes go by various names, such as regenerated cellulose, cuprammonium cellulose (Cuprophane), cuprammonium rayon, and saponified cellulose ester.

b.   Substituted cellulose. The cellulose polymer has a large number of free hydroxyl groups at its surface. In the cellulose acetate, cellulose diacetate, and cellulose triacetate membranes, a substantial number of these groups are chemically bonded to acetate.

c.   Cellulosynthetic. To make this, a synthetic material (a tertiary amino compound) is added to liquefied cellulose during formation of the membrane. As a result, the surface of the membrane is altered, and biocompatibility is greatly increased. This membrane goes under the trade names of Cellosyn or Hemophan.

d.   Synthetics. These membranes are not cellulose-based, and materials used include polyacrylonitrile (PAN), polysulfone, polycarbonate, polyamide, and polymethylmethacrylate (PMMA).

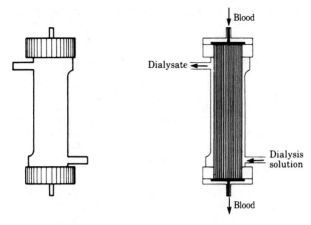

Hollow-fiber dialyzer

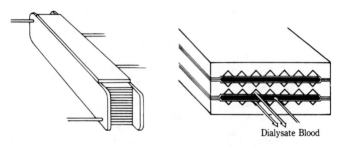

Parallel-plate dialyzer

Figure 3-1.   Blood and dialysis solution flow pathways through a hollow-fiber and parallel-plate dialyzer. (Modified from Man NK, Jungers P. Hemodialysis equipment. In: Hamburger J, Crosnier J, Grunfeld JP, eds. *Nephrology.* New York: Wiley, 1979:1206, 1207.)

    2.   Complement activation with different membrane materials. During dialysis using membranes made from unsubstituted cellulose, the free hydroxyl groups on the membrane surface activate the complement system in blood flowing through the dialyzer. The consequences of complement activation during dialysis are discussed in Chapter 7. Complement activation is reduced with unsubstituted cellulose membranes when they are reused (provided they have not been exposed to bleach) because of protein coating of the membrane surface during initial use. Complement activation occurs to a much lesser extent with substituted cellulose membranes and with cellulosynthetic and synthetic membranes.

3. Membrane permeability to solutes and to water.
The permeability to solutes and water of each of the four
membrane types can be altered markedly by adjusting the
thickness of the membrane and the pore size.

   a. Membrane efficiency versus flux. The ability of a
dialyzer to remove small molecular weight solutes, such as
urea, is primarily a function of its membrane surface area
(plus a minor component due to dialyzer and membrane
design). A high-efficiency dialyzer is basically a big dialyzer
that by virtue of its high surface area has a high ability
to remove urea. High-efficiency dialyzers can have small
or large pores, and thus can have either high or absent
clearance for larger molecular weight solutes, such as
β_2-microglobulin (MW 11,800).

   High-flux membranes have large pores that are capable of
passing larger molecules, such as β_2-microglobulin. Usually,
β_2-microglobulin clearances are not reported in standard dialyzer specification charts. High-flux membranes also have
high water permeability, with coefficient of ultrafiltration
(K_{Uf}) values greater than 10 mL per hour per mm Hg, and
usually greater than 20 mL per hour per mm Hg. In a reuse
situation, the permeability of some high-flux membranes to
β_2-microglobulin can decrease or increase markedly, depending on the reuse procedure employed (see Chapter 8).

   b. Interpreting a dialyzer specification sheet (Table
3-1). Information usually provided about dialyzers includes
K_{Uf}; clearance of substances such as urea, creatinine, vitamin B_{12}, and phosphate (and occasionally β_2-microglobulin);
membrane surface area; priming volume; fiber length; and
fiber thickness.

   (1) K_{Uf}. The ultrafiltration coefficient, as defined in
Chapter 2, is the milliliters per hour of ultrafiltration
effected by each mm Hg of transmembrane pressure
(TMP). If the K_{Uf} is 2.0, the permeability to water is low.
To remove 1,000 mL per hour, 500 mm Hg TMP will be
needed. If the K_{Uf} is 4.0, the permeability to water is
moderate, and the required TMP will be only 250 mm
Hg. If the K_{Uf} is 8.0, the TMP will have to be only 125 mm
Hg. Certain synthetic membranes are noted for their
extremely high permeability to water, with K_{Uf} values in
the range of 10–60 mL per hour per mm Hg. When the
K_{Uf} is large (when water permeability is high), small
errors in setting the TMP will result in large errors in
the amount of ultrafiltrate removed. For this reason, dialyzers with a K_{Uf} greater than 6.0 (certainly those with a
K_{Uf} greater than 8.0) should be used only with dialysis
machines that contain special pumps and circuits that
directly control the ultrafiltration rate.

   The K_{Uf} values reported by dialyzer companies are
usually in vitro values. In practice, the in vivo K_{Uf} is
often somewhat lower (5%–30%). Some companies pub-
lish both an in vitro K_{Uf} and an "expected in vivo"
K_{Uf} value. The numbers listed in Table 3-1 are mostly
in vitro values.

Table 3-1. Specifications of some commonly used dialyzers

Company	Model	Membrane	Type	Steril	K_{Uf}	In Vitro KoA Urea	Cl. Urea Q_B=300	Cl. B$_{12}$ Q_B=200	Priming Vol.	Surface Area
Althin	Altra Nova 140	Cellulose acetate	HF	ETO	5.9	407[a]	193[a]	55	78	1.4
Althin	Altra Nova 170	Cellulose acetate	HF	ETO	6.7	518[a]	214[a]	58	102	1.8
Althin	Altra Nova 200	Cellulose acetate	HF	ETO	9.0	637[a]	231[a]	82	123	2.2
Althin	Altrex flux 140	Cellulose acetate	HF	GAM	13.0	483[a]	208[a]	83	83	1.4
Althin	Altrex flux 170	Cellulose acetate	HF	GAM	18.0	472[a]	206[a]	95	95	1.7
Althin	Altrex flux 200	Cellulose acetate	HF	GAM	19.0	645[a]	232[a]	116	116	2.2
Althin	MCA-130	Cellulose acetate	HF	ETO	3.3	512[a]	212[a]	74	74	1.3
Althin	MCA-180	Cellulose acetate	HF	ETO	5.0	637[a]	231[a]	107	107	1.8
Althin	MCA-200	Cellulose acetate	HF	ETO	6.3	778[a]	246[a]	118	118	2.1
Asahi	50H	Cellulose	HF	GAM	4.8	575	223	54	59	1.0
Asahi	50M	Cellulose	HF	GAM	3.9	550	219	51	59	1.0
Asahi	50U	Cellulose	HF	GAM	6.2	635	231	61	59	1.0

continued

Table 3-1. *Continued*

Company	Model	Membrane	Type	Steril	K_{Uf}	In Vitro KoA Urea	Cl. Urea $Q_B=300$	Cl. B_{12} $Q_B=200$	Priming Vol.	Surface Area
Asahi	65H	Cellulose	HF	GAM	6.2	730	242	66	75	1.3
Asahi	65U	Cellulose	HF	GAM	7.7	840	251	73	75	1.3
Asahi	75U	Cellulose	HF	GAM	9.3	1000	263	85	90	1.5
Asahi	90U	Cellulose	HF	GAM	11.0	1065	266	90	102	1.8
Asahi	AM-B10-50	Modified cellulose	HF	GAM	5.7	538	219	54	63	1.0
Asahi	AM-B10-65	Modified cellulose	HF	GAM	7.8	670	237	66	78	1.3
Asahi	AM-B10-75	Modified cellulose	HF	GAM	8.8	755	246	74	94	1.5
Asahi	AM-B10-100	Modified cellulose	HF	GAM	12.0	1065	266	89	123	2.0
Asahi	AM-NR-50U	Modified cellulose	HF	GAM	6.8	616	231	61	63	1.0
Asahi	AM-NR-65H	Modified cellulose	HF	GAM	6.4	715	242	66	78	1.3
Asahi	AM-NR-65U	Modified cellulose	HF	GAM	8.8	806	251	73	78	1.3
Asahi	AM-NR-75U	Modified cellulose	HF	GAM	10.3	973	263	85	94	1.5
Asahi	AM-NR-100U	Modified cellulose	HF	GAM	13.6	1090	270	100	123	2.0

Baxter	CA-050	Cellulose acetate	HF	ETO	2.5	245	148	26	35	.5
Baxter	CA-070	Cellulose acetate	HF	ETO	3.6	330	174	34	45	.7
Baxter	CA-090	Cellulose acetate	HF	ETO	4.0	426	197	41	60	.9
Baxter	CA-110	Cellulose acetate	HF	ETO	4.8	515	212	50	70	1.1
Baxter	CA-150	Cellulose acetate	HF	ETO	6.8	675	236	63	95	1.5
Baxter	CA-170	Cellulose acetate	HF	ETO	7.9	780	246	69	105	1.7
Baxter	CA-210	Cellulose acetate	HF	ETO	9.3	990	262	82	125	2.1
Baxter	CT-110G	Cellulose triacetate	HF	GAM	24.0	950	261	113	70	1.1
Baxter	CT-190G	Cellulose triacetate	HF	GAM	36.0	1220	273	143	115	1.9
Baxter	DICEA 090G	Cellulose diacetate	HF	GAM	6.8	530	214	60	60	.9
Baxter	DICEA 110G	Cellulose diacetate	HF	GAM	8.4	630	229	69	70	1.1
Baxter	DICEA 150G	Cellulose diacetate	HF	GAM	11.4	760	248	90	95	1.5
Baxter	DICEA 210G	Cellulose diacetate	HF	GAM	15.5	1110	268	105	125	2.1
Baxter	PSN-120	Polysynthane	HF	ETO	6.7	620	228	61	75	1.2

continued

Table 3-1. *Continued*

Company	Model	Membrane	Type	Steril	K_{Uf}	In Vitro KoA Urea	Cl. Urea Q_B=300	Cl. B_{12} Q_B=200	Priming Vol.	Surface Area
Baxter	PSN-150	Polysynthane	HF	ETO	7.8	760	246	72	85	1.5
Baxter	PSN-170	Polysynthane	HF	ETO	9.0	865	256	80	106	1.7
Baxter	PSN-210	Polysynthane	HF	ETO	10.7	1003	265	91	123	2.1
Baxter	Tricea 110G	Cellulose triacetate	HF	GAM	25.0	840	259	119	65	1.1
Baxter	Tricea 150G	Cellulose triacetate	HF	GAM	29.0	1130	278	142	90	1.5
Baxter	Tricea 190G	Cellulose triacetate	HF	GAM	37.0	1330	284	151	115	1.9
Baxter	Tricea 210G	Cellulose triacetate	HF	GAM	39.0	1520	287	164	125	2.1
Cobe	400-HG	Cell-syn (Hemophan)	HF	GaM	4.5	490	209	54	47	.9
Cobe	500-HG	Cell-syn (Hemophan)	HF	GAM	6.4	650	233	66	58	1.1
Cobe	600-HE	Cell-syn (Hemophan)	HF	ETO	8.7	815	251	85	88	1.5
Cobe	700-HE	Cell-syn (Hemophan)	HF	ETO	9.9	930	258	93	113	1.9
Cobe	Filtral 20	PAN	HF	ETO	78.0	785	245	105	142	1.9
Fresenius	F-50	Polysulfone	HF	ETO	30.0	577	223	110	63	.9
Fresenius	F-60A	Polysulfone	HF	ETO	40.0	760	244	118	82	1.3

Fresenius	F-60B	Polysulfone	HF	ETO	38.0	760	244	110	82	1.3
Fresenius	F-60-M	Polysulfone	HF	ETO	19.0	760	244	100	82	1.3
Fresenius	F-80A	Polysulfone	HF	ETO	65.0	945	259	135	110	1.8
Fresenius	F-80B	Polysulfone	HF	ETO	52.0	945	259	133	110	1.8
Fresenius	F-80-M	Polysulfone	HF	ETO	27.0	890	255	110	110	1.8
Fresenius	F5	Polysulfone	HF	ETO	4.2	556	220	45	63	.9
Fresenius	F6	Polysulfone	HF	ETO	5.5	660	234	56	83	1.2
Fresenius	F8	Polysulfone	HF	ETO	8.1	800	248	76	120	1.8
Gambro	Alwall GFE-09	Cellulose	HF	ETO	4.0	340	180	39	45	0.9
Gambro	Alwall GFE-11	Cellulose	HF	ETO	5.3	450	205	48	60	1.1
Gambro	Alwall GFE-12	Cellulose	HF	ETO	6.0	545	221	51	65	1.3
Gambro	Alwall GFE-15	Cellulose	HF	ETO	6.4	640	234	56	75	1.5
Gambro	Alwall GFE-18	Cellulose	HF	ETO	8.3	665	240	70	95	1.8
Gambro	Alwall GFS Plus 1	Cellosyn (Hemophan)	HF	STM	5.5	450	205	48	60	1.1
Gambro	Alwall GFS Plus 1	Cellosyn (Hemophan)	HF	STM	6.8	550	222	60	70	1.3
Gambro	Alwall GFS Plus 1	Cellosyn (Hemophan)	HF	STM	9.4	655	240	72	95	1.7
Gambro	Alwall GFS Plus 2	Cellosyn (Hemophan)	HF	STM	11.4	660	242	84	100	1.8

continued

Table 3-1. *Continued*

Company	Model	Membrane	Type	Steril	K_{Uf}	In Vitro KoA Urea	Cl. Urea $Q_B=300$	Cl. B_{12} $Q_B=200$	Priming Vol.	Surface Area
Gambro	Alwall GFS-12	Cellulose	HF	STM	6.5	545	221	51	65	1.3
Gambro	Alwall GFS-16	Cellulose	HF	STM	8.8	780	248	72	95	1.8
Gambro	Lundia Alpha 400	Cellulose	PP	ETO	4.8	400	194	41	62	0.7
Gambro	Lundia Alpha 500	Cellulose	PP	ETO	6.1	575	223	52	72	1.0
Gambro	Lundia Alpha 600	Cellulose	PP	ETO	8.3	605	232	60	96	1.3
Gambro	Lundia Alpha 700	Cellulose	PP	ETO	11.2	725	246	74	13	1.3
Gambro	Lundia Aria 550	Cellosyn (Hemophan)	PP	ETO	6.5	605	232	55	90	1.0
Gambro	Lundia Aria 700	Cellosyn (Hemophan)	PP	ETO	8.5	730	244	71	120	1.3
Gambro	Lundia Pro 500	Gambrane	PP	ETO	7.0	410	200	72	80	1.0
Gambro	Lundia Pro 600	Gambrane	PP	ETO	9.0	475	211	82	105	1.3
Gambro	Lundia Pro 800	Gambrane	PP	ETO	11.0	740	240	98	130	1.6
Gambro	Polyflux 11S	Polyamide	HF	STM	53.0	600	224	110	81	1.1

Manufacturer	Model	Material	Type	Sterilization	K_{UF}	KoA	Cl-Urea	Cl-B12	Priming vol	Surface area
Gambro	Polyflux 14S	Polyamide	HF	STM	62.0	750	242	125	102	1.4
Gambro	Polyflux 17S	Polyamide	HF	STM	71.0	890	254	136	121	1.7
Gambro	Polyflux 21S	Polyamide	HF	STM	83.0	1110	267	149	152	2.1
Terumo	10-NL	Cellulose	HF	STM	4.5	472	206	46	64	1.0
Terumo	12-NL	Cellulose	HF	STM	6.1	563	221	52	79	1.2
Terumo	15-NL	Cellulose	HF	STM	6.9	654	233	60	90	1.5
Terumo	NT-120-L	Cellulose	HF	ETO	6.0	707	239	63	88	1.2
Terumo	NT-150-L	Cellulose	HF	ETO	7.5	757	244	77	107	1.5
Terumo	NT-175-L	Cellulose	HF	ETO	8.8	824	250	82	62	1.8
Terumo	T-150	Cellulose	HF	ETO	5.4	730	242	71	101	1.5
Terumo	T-175	Cellulose	HF	ETO	6.0	930	257	79	120	1.7
Terumo	T-220	Cellulose	HF	ETO	8.0	1130	268	87	148	2.2
Toray	B3-0.8-A	PMMA	HF	GAM	35.9	410	190	61	49	0.8
Toray	B3-1.0-A	PMMA	HF	GAM	7.0	505	212	70	61	1.0
Toray	B3-1.0-A	PMMA	HF	GAM	8.8	635	231	70	76	1.3
Toray	B3-1.6-A	PMMA	HF	GAM	58.7	705	236	88	95	1.6
Toray	B3-2.0-A	PMMA	HF	GAM	11.0	900	254	101	118	2.0
Toray	BK-1.6-U	PMMA	HF	GAM	14.0	745	245	108	94	1.6
Toray	BK-2.1-U	PMMA	HF	GAM	19.0	980	263	125	135	2.1

PMMA, polymethylmethacrylate; HF, hollow-fiber; PP, parallel-plate; ETO, ethylene oxide; STM, steam-sterilized; GAM, gamma ray sterilized; K_{UF}, ultrafiltration coefficient; KoA, mass transfer area coefficient for urea; Q_B, blood flow rate.

Units: K_{UF}, mL/hr per mm Hg; KoA, mL per min; Cl-Urea, mL per min; Cl-B12, mL per min; priming vol, mL; surface area, m².

[a] In vivo values. Althin does not provide in vitro clearance information for their dialyzers.

With reuse, K_{Uf} will tend to increase when bleach is employed in the reuse procedure, whereas K_{Uf} may remain unchanged or even decrease in reuse methods that do not use bleach. The effects of reuse on K_{Uf} have not been well studied; they depend on the exact combination of chemicals used in the reuse procedure and the type of membrane material.

(2) Clearance

(a) Urea. The clearance values provided by the manufacturer for urea (MW 60) are in vitro values. Clearances are usually reported at "blood" flow rates of 200, 300, and 400 mL per minute. The values in the specification sheet for urea clearance overestimate values obtained during actual dialysis but are useful for comparing dialyzers.

The dialyzer mass transfer area coefficient for urea, *KoA*, is a measure of dialyzer efficiency in clearing urea and solutes of similar molecular weight. The *KoA* is the maximum theoretical clearance of the dialyzer in milliliters per minute for a given solute at infinite blood and dialysate flow rates. For any given membrane, *KoA* will be proportional to the surface area of the membrane in the dialyzer, although there is a drop-off in the gain in *KoA* as membrane surface area becomes very large.

Dialyzers with *KoA* values less than 500 should be used only for "low-efficiency" dialysis or for small patients. Dialyzers with *KoA* values of 500–700 represent moderate-efficiency dialyzers, useful for routine therapy. Dialyzers with *KoA* values greater than 700 are used for "high-efficiency" dialysis, although such dialyzers may be necessary for an adequate amount of dialysis to be given to a large patient even when a 4-hour dialysis session is used.

i) Obtaining the dialyzer *KoA*. The KoA, or maximum theoretical clearance of any dialyzer, can be computed from the urea clearances on a dialyzer specification sheet, according to Fig. A-5. A more exact computation is given in Table A-3.

Once the dialyzer *KoA* is known, Fig. A-1 can be used to estimate the in vivo urea clearance at any given blood flow rate when the dialysate flow rate is 500 mL per minute. For more precise values, and when Q_d (dialysate flow rate) is other than 500 mL per minute, use the equations in Table A-1. The urea clearances predicted by either of these methods will be substantially lower than the in vitro clearances on dialyzer specification sheets. For this reason, in vitro dialyzer urea clearances should never be used to predict actual urea clearance for the purposes of urea kinetic modeling.

(b) Creatinine. Some manufacturers provide creatinine (MW 113) clearance values. The dialyzer creatinine clearance is usually about 80% of the urea clearance and provides no clinically useful additional information, as the clearances for the two molecules are almost always in the same proportion, regardless of membrane or dialyzer type.

(c) **Vitamin B_{12} and β_2-microglobulin.** In vitro clearance of vitamin B_{12} (MW 1,355) is an indication of how well the membrane allows the passage of larger molecular weight solutes. Recently, it has become customary to consider the clearance of β_2-microglobulin (MW 11,800) rather than vitamin B_{12} to characterize the flux of a dialyzer. In vitro measures of β_2-microglobulin are problematic and are not usually reported. Most unsubstituted cellulose membranes, cellulose acetate, and Hemophan membranes have β_2-microglobulin clearances of zero, although there are some exceptions, and membranes in each of these three categories have been manufactured that are true high-flux membranes with substantial clearance of β_2-microglobulin. Typically, many cellulose diacetate and most cellulose triacetate membranes have substantial β_2-microglobulin clearance and are therefore high-flux dialyzers. Polysulfone can be manufactured as either a low-flux membrane (e.g., Fresenius F6, F8) or a high-flux membrane (e.g., Fresenius F60, F80). PMMA can also be made in a low-flux or high-flux configuration. PAN and AN69, a PAN-related membrane; are high-flux membranes that adsorb β_2-microglobulin, thus augmenting its removal by dialysis.

The clinical importance of removal of high molecular weight solutes by dialysis, and hence, the benefit of using high-flux dialyzers, is controversial.

(3) The membrane surface area is usually 0.8–2.1 m^2. Large surface area dialyzers normally have high urea clearances, although dialyzer design and thinness of the membrane are also important. When an unsubstituted cellulose membrane is used, a large membrane surface area is an undesirable feature because the degree of complement activation is proportional to the membrane surface area. Surface area is not as important an issue with regard to complement activation with membranes in which the degree of complement activation is small (e.g., substituted cellulose or synthetic membranes).

(4) The priming volume is usually 60– 120 mL and is related to the membrane surface area. The slight increase in volume in parallel-plate dialyzers during ultrafiltration is due to bulging of the membrane sheets. It should be remembered that the priming volume of the blood lines is about 100–150 mL. Hence, total extracorporeal circuit volume will be 160–270 mL. In the typical adult patient, the presence of 10 or 20 mL more or less in the dialyzer is of little clinical importance.

(5) **Fiber length and thickness.** This information is of no clinical usefulness.

C. **Mode of sterilization.** The most common mode of dialyzer sterilization is exposure to ethylene oxide gas. The use of this sterilant is being reevaluated because of the rare but serious occurrence of anaphylactic reactions during dialysis in occasional patients who are allergic to ethylene oxide. Two alternative sterilization methods, using either γ-irradiation or steam autoclaving, are becoming more popular.

II. Water for dialysis treatment. Patients are exposed to about 120 L of water during each dialysis treatment. All small molecular weight substances present in the water have direct access to the patient's bloodstream as if they had been administered by intravenous injection. For this reason, it is very important that the purity of the water used for dialysis be known and controlled. The Association for the Advancement of Medical Instrumentation has developed minimum standards for the purity of water used in hemodialysis.

A. Important contaminants in water. Several contaminants sometimes present in water used to make dialysis solution are detrimental to patients. Aluminum contamination can cause bone disease, progressive neurologic deterioration, and anemia. Excessive amounts of copper in dialysis solution (the result of leaching of the metal from copper plumbing) can cause hemolytic anemia. Hemolytic anemia also can occur as a result of exposure to chloramine in dialysis solution. Chloramine is a chemical frequently added to municipal water supplies to control bacterial contamination. Fatal fluoride intoxication can occur from fluoride that accumulates in deionizers that are not changed at appropriate intervals and that then leaches into the product water stream, ultimately reaching the patient.

B. Methods of purifying water for dialysis. Several methods are used to purify water for hemodialysis. Often softening of the water to remove most of the calcium and magnesium is the first step. Then, passage through a carbon filter is done to remove organics and other impurities such as chloramine and chlorine. Next, the concentration of dissolved solutes is markedly reduced by pushing the water through a semipermeable membrane with pores small enough to restrict passage of even small molecular weight solutes, such as urea, sodium, and chloride. Reverse osmosis removes more than 90% of the impurities and, depending on the initial degree of water contamination, frequently produces water sufficiently pure for dialysis. Deionizers, which exchange charged solutes for hydrogen and hydroxyl ions, thereby removing charged solutes from water, can be used either as an alternative to reverse osmosis or to "polish" water initially treated with a reverse osmosis system.

C. Sterility. Water for dialysis need not be completely sterile because the dialyzer membrane is normally an effective barrier to both bacteria and endotoxins. However, the bacterial counts should be kept below 100 colonies per milliliter in the water (below 500 colonies per milliliter in the final dialysis solution) by periodically disinfecting the water treatment system with appropriate disinfectants and by using bacteriologic filters in some instances. Limits for endotoxin for water and final dialysate are 2 and 5 IU per milliliter, respectively (see "Internet References").

Several outbreaks of pyrogen reactions with severe clinical manifestations have been reported in association with the use of bicarbonate-containing dialysis solution concentrate and the use of high-flux membranes. The problem appears to be multifactorial: Some bicarbonate powders and concentrates may be heavily contaminated with bacteria or endotoxins initially. With dialysis machines incorporating complex hydraulic ultra-filtration control pathways, it becomes especially important to clean the dialysis circuit properly between dialysis treatments; otherwise, high bacterial counts can develop in the dialysis solution pathway. Finally, use of certain high-flux membranes may permit easier access of endotoxins and other bacterial products to the circulation.

Recent work suggests that insufficient attention has been paid to removal of bacteria and bacterial products from dialysis solutions: Some bacterial products in the dialysis solution apparently can stimulate blood monocytes to produce interleukin-1. High circulating levels of interleukin-1 can then result in pyrexia and possibly other as yet undefined symptoms and side effects.

Some dialysis machines incorporate an optional hollow-fiber ultrafilter in the dialysis solution line that serves to remove bacteria and most endotoxins. The clinical necessity and benefits of such dialysis solution sterilization have not yet been proved by well-controlled clinical studies. In hemodiafiltration, a substantial amount of the fluid removed by ultrafiltration is replaced by dialysate that is back-filtered across the dialyzer membrane. In machines that perform hemodiafiltration, at least two, and sometimes three, in-line serial ultrafilters are used to sterilize the dialysis solution being administered to the patient in this fashion.

III. Dialysis solution

A. Liquid concentrates. A typical composition of bicarbonate-containing dialysis solution is shown in Table 3-2. The composition can be varied substantially in special clinical circumstances. High concentrations of calcium, magnesium, and bicarbonate cause the precipitation of calcium and magnesium carbonate. To circumvent the problem of calcium

Table 3-2. Components of standard bicarbonate-containing dialysis solution

Component	Bicarbonate Containing (mEq/liter)
Sodium	135–145
Potassium	0–4.0
Calcium	2.5–3.5
Magnesium	0.5–0.75
Chloride	98–124
Acetate[a]	2–4[a]
Bicarbonate	30–40
Dextrose	11
P_{CO_2}(mm Hg)	40–110
pH	7.1–7.3

[a] The acetate is in the form of acetic acid in the "acid" component. On mixing with the bicarbonate component, the hydrogen in acetic acid reacts with an equimolar amount of bicarbonate to form CO_2.

and magnesium precipitation, a bicarbonate-based dialysate generating system utilizes two concentrate components, a "bicarbonate" component and an "acid" component, the latter containing a small amount of lactic, acetic, or citric acid plus sodium, chloride, potassium (if needed), dextrose (optional), and all of the calcium and magnesium. Specially designed dialysis machines mix the two components simultaneously with purified water to make the product dialysis solution. During mixing, the small amount (usually 4 mM) of organic acid in the "acid" component reacts with an equimolar amount of bicarbonate in the "bicarbonate" component to generate carbon dioxide. The carbon dioxide that is generated forms carbonic acid, which lowers the pH of the final bicarbonate-containing solution to approximately 7.0–7.4. In such a pH range and in the lower concentrations present in the final mixture, calcium and magnesium remain in solution.

B. Dry (powder) concentrates. To avoid the problems of bacterial growth in bicarbonate concentrate and to reduce shipping and storage costs, several companies now offer the bicarbonate concentrate, or both the bicarbonate and acid concentrate as canisters containing the chemicals in powdered form, which are reconstituted with treated water at the time dialysis is taking place.

IV. Dialysis machines. The modern dialysis machine consists of a blood pump, dialysis solution delivery system, and appropriate safety monitors.

A. Blood pump. The blood pump moves blood from the access site through the dialyzer and back to the patient. The usual flow rate for adult patients is 350–500 mL per minute.

B. Dialysis solution delivery system

1. Central versus individual proportioning. These are the two major types of dialysis solution delivery systems. With the central delivery system, all of the solution used for the dialysis unit is produced by a single machine (by mixing concentrates with purified water), and the final dialysis solution is pumped through pipes to each dialysis machine. With the individual system, each dialysis machine proportions its own dialysis solution concentrate with purified water. The central delivery system has the advantages of a lower initial equipment cost and reduced labor costs. Individual dialysis systems have the advantage of permitting modification of the dialysis solution composition for a given patient (either by choosing a different concentrate or by altering the mixing ratio of concentrate to water).

2. Heating and degassing. In both systems, the dialysis solution must be heated by the machine to the proper temperature (usually 35–37°C) prior to being pumped to the dialyzer. Water obtained from city water supplies is invariably pressurized and contains a large amount of dissolved air. The dialysis machine must remove this air from the water before use. Degassing is usually done by exposing the heated water to a negative pressure.

3. Negative pressure. In dialysis machines without an ultrafiltration controller, the dialysis solution pump is located on the line leading from the dialyzer to the drain (see Fig. 2-2).

This location allows the machine to create a negative pressure in the dialysate compartment of the dialyzer to perform ultrafiltration. The negative pressure is generated by partially occluding the line routing dialysis solution to the dialyzer (adjustable inflow resistance).

4. Disinfection. Dialysis machines routinely are rinsed after each use and commonly are disinfected at the end of the day. Disinfection may be using heat or bleach, and often is preceded by a vinegar rinse to remove carbonate encrustations and buildup in the tubing passages. Maximum allowed residual levels of various disinfectants in water used for dialysis can be found in the internet references.

C. Monitoring devices. An important aspect of the dialysis machine is its monitoring function.

1. Blood circuit (Fig. 3-2).

a. Pressure monitors. T tubes attached to the blood line permit monitoring of pressure at various points in the blood circuit. Frequent locations for these pressure monitors are proximal to the blood pump and just distal to the dialyzer. The pressure monitor proximal to the blood pump is placed here to guard against excessive suction on the vascular access site by the blood pump. The pressure monitor distal

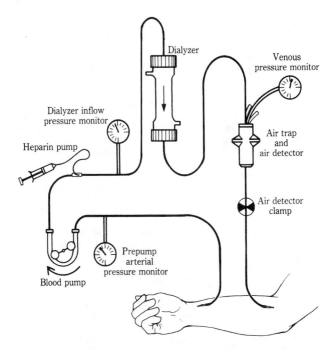

Figure 3-2. The blood circuit showing the usual location of the pressure monitors. The alternative location of the "arterial" pressure monitor between the blood pump and the dialyzer is also shown.

to the dialyzer ("venous" monitor) guards against excessive resistance to return of blood in the venous limb of the vascular access site. The pressure reading at the venous monitor is also used to estimate the dialyzer blood compartment pressure. Either of these monitors can be adjusted to alarm or to shut off the blood pump when the desired pressure limits are exceeded (see Chapter 5 for more information on monitor use).

In some machines, the "arterial" monitor is located distal to the blood pump and just proximal to the dialyzer. This monitor is used to detect clotting in the dialyzer and to help the machine more precisely estimate the pressure in the blood compartment of the dialyzer (used in automatic calculation or control of the ultrafiltration rate). Pressure monitors also help protect the patient in the event of an accidental blood line separation; when a line separation occurs, the pressures in the blood lines usually rapidly approach zero, exceeding the allowable limits of a properly set pressure monitor, causing it to activate an alarm and shut off the blood pump.

b.   Venous air trap and air detector. These are located just distal to the venous pressure monitor. A filter is sometimes placed here as well. The purpose of the air trap and detector is to prevent air that may have inadvertently entered the blood circuit from being returned to the patient. The air detector is attached to a relay switch, which automatically clamps the venous blood line and shuts off the blood pump if air is detected.

2.   Dialysis solution circuit

a.   Dialysis solution conductivity. If the proportioning system that dilutes the concentrate with water malfunctions, an excessively dilute or concentrated dialysis solution can be produced. Exposure of blood to a severely hyperosmolar dialysis solution can lead to hypernatremia and other electrolyte disturbances. Exposure to a severely hypoosmolar dialysis solution can result in rapid hemolysis or hyponatremia. Because the primary solutes in dialysis solution are electrolytes, the degree of concentration of dialysis solution will be reflected by its electrical conductivity, and proper proportioning of concentrate to water can be monitored by a meter that continuously measures the conductivity of the product dialysis solution as it is being fed to the dialyzer.

b.   Dialysis solution temperature. Malfunction of the heating element in the dialysis machine can result in the production of excessively cool or hot dialysis solution. Use of cool dialysis solution is not dangerous unless the patient is unconscious, in which case hypothermia can occur. A conscious patient will complain of the cold and shiver. On the other hand, use of a dialysis solution heated to greater than 42°C can lead to hemolysis. A temperature sensor in the machine continuously monitors dialysis solution temperature.

c.   Bypass valve. If either the dialysis solution conductivity or temperature is found to be out of limits, a bypass valve is activated to divert the dialysis solution around the dialyzer directly to the drain.

d. Blood leak detector. The blood leak detector is placed in the dialysate outflow line. If this detector senses blood, as occurs when a leak develops through the dialyzer membrane, the appropriate alarm is activated.

e. Dialysate outflow pressure monitor. In machines that do not have special pumps and circuitry to control the ultrafiltration rate directly, the pressure at this location can be used in conjunction with the pressure at the blood outflow line to calculate TMP and thereby estimate the ultrafiltration rate.

D. Options

1. Heparin pump. A heparin pump allows the continuous infusion of heparin into the patient for anticoagulation.

2. Adjustable bicarbonate. One often encounters patients who are relatively alkalemic, especially in an acute-dialysis setting. With machines that do not have an adjustable bicarbonate option, the final dialysate bicarbonate concentration can be changed only by altering the composition of the bicarbonate concentrate. Practically, this means that, with commercially available concentrates, a final dialysate bicarbonate concentration lower than 32–35 mM cannot be achieved. Machines with a variable bicarbonate option work by altering the proportioning of bicarbonate concentrate to water. They allow delivery of final bicarbonate concentrations as low as 20 mM. Such machines are very useful to treat nonacidotic patients or patients either with frank alkalemia or who are at high risk of developing respiratory alkalosis.

3. Variable sodium. This option permits rapid alteration of the dialysis solution sodium concentration by simply turning a dial. The sodium concentration is usually altered by changing the proportions of "acid concentrate" and water. Changing the dialysis solution sodium level in this manner will also change the concentration of all other solutes present in the concentrate. The variable sodium option allows for the individualization of the dialysis solution sodium concentration on a patient-by-patient basis and also allows for the sodium concentration to be changed during the dialysis procedure.

4. Controlled ultrafiltration. There are several different methods by which the ultrafiltration rate can be precisely controlled. The hydraulics involved are often complex and beyond the scope of this manual. Suffice it to say that precise ultrafiltration control is a desirable feature for a dialysis machine to have and that manual efforts to determine the ultrafiltration rate by estimating the TMP are fraught with potential errors.

The most advanced method of ultrafiltration control is the so-called volumetric method. Such volumetric circuitry is incorporated into many advanced dialysis machines. With these machines, even dialyzers that are very water permeable (K_{Uf} greater than 10 mL per hour per mm Hg) can be used safely.

5. Programmable ultrafiltration. Normally, ultrafiltration is performed at the same rate throughout the dialysis session. Some believe that a constant rate of fluid removal is not necessarily the best approach, especially when the sodium concentration is being varied during the dialysis session. Some dialysis machines allow for the bulk of the ultrafiltration to be performed during the initial portion of a dialysis session and also allow the operator to devise any form of ultrafiltration profile desired. The clinical benefits of programmable ultrafiltration have not been demonstrated by controlled studies.

6. Dialysate urea sensor (on-line Kt/V monitor). At least two manufacturers have developed urea sensors that measure urea concentration in the spent dialysate at multiple time points during dialysis. The sensors use this information to calculate the amount of urea removed per treatment and also can generate a dialysate side equivalent to the equilibrated Kt/V discussed in Chapter 2.

There is no systematic difference between dialysate side and blood side equilibrated Kt/V values. However, if such sensors were part of the dialysis machine proper, they would be quite useful to monitor in real time the amount of dialysis that has been delivered, avoiding the need for monthly pre- and post-dialysis blood sampling.

7. Blood temperature control module. This module monitors the temperature of incoming and exiting blood, as well as dialysate. It allows for control of thermal balance during dialysis. One can set the machine to add or remove heat from the patient during dialysis or to keep the body temperature constant. This module is particularly useful in providing low-temperature dialysates for increased hemodynamic stability. The module may also be used to measure access recirculation or blood flow as described below.

8. Modules to measure access recirculation or access blood flow. These all work on the dilution principle (Fig. 3-3). The composition of the blood leaving the dialyzer is quickly altered by (a) injecting 5 mL of isotonic or hypertonic saline,

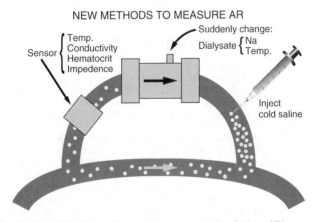

NEW METHODS TO MEASURE AR

Figure 3-3. **Principles of measuring access recirculation (AR) (Reproduced from Daugirdas JT.** *Hypertens Dial Clin Nephrol 1997;* http://www.hdcn.com)

(b) acutely changing the dialyzer ultrafiltration rate to promote hemoconcentration, or (c) acutely changing the dialysate temperature to cool the returning blood. A sensor attached to the blood inflow line seeks to detect the resulting change in hematocrit, conductivity, or temperature. If there is access recirculation, the perturbation caused in the outflow line will almost immediately be detected in the inflow line sensor, and the magnitude of the perturbation will reflect the degree of recirculation. To measure access flow, the lines are deliberately reversed, such that the inflow (arterial) needle is drawing blood from the access "downstream" to the outflow (venous) needle. In this manner, access recirculation is induced. The degree of recirculation is then measured as above. The degree of recirculation is proportional to the ratio of flows in the extracorporeal circuit and access. Once the degree of recirculation has been measured, the extracorporeal blood flow is known, and the amount of access recirculation can be calculated (Krivitski, 1995).

9. Blood volume monitors. These use an ultrasonic or optical sensor operating on the inflow blood line to detect changes in hematocrit during dialysis. Normally, in the course of fluid removal, the hematocrit increases, and the amount of increase reflects the degree of plasma volume reduction. One touted feature of such monitors is to be able to anticipate and prevent a hypotensive episode by reducing ultrafiltration whenever a limiting increase in hematocrit during dialysis has occurred or when a "crash crit," identified during previous sessions, is being approached. Another potential use is to identify patients with covert fluid overload by recognizing that such patients tend to have no increase in hematocrit during dialysis despite fluid removal. Careful controlled study is needed to establish the usefulness of blood volume monitors during dialysis.

10. On-line clearance monitors. Because sodium clearance is similar to urea clearance, it can be used to estimate the urea clearance of a dialyzer just prior to use. Typically, the machine initiates a momentary change in dialysate inflow sodium concentration and measures the resultant change in conductivity of dialysate outflow level. This is a useful method of ensuring at the point of dialysis that the urea clearance of a reused dialyzer is still in the clinically acceptable range.

E. Single blood pathway ("single-needle") devices. Most hemodialysis treatments are performed using two separate blood pathways: one to obtain blood from the patient and another to return blood to the patient. Several systems allow dialysis to be performed using a Y-shaped single blood pathway. Description and discussion of single-needle devices is beyond the scope of this book as they are used only rarely in the United States.

SELECTED READINGS

Canaud BJM, Mion CM. Water treatment for contemporary hemodialysis. In: Jacobs C, et al, eds. *Replacement of renal function by dialysis,* 4th ed. Dordrecht; Kluwer Academic Publishers, 1996:231–255.

Krivitski NM. Theory and validation of access flow measurement by dilution technique during hemodialysis. *Kidney Int* 1995;48:244–250.

Pass T, et al. Culture of dialysis fluids on nutrient-rich media for short periods at elevated temperatures underestimate microbial contamination. *Blood Purif* 1996;14:136.

Core Curriculum for the Dialysis Technician. Medical Media Publishing, 1999.

Vorbeck-Meister I, et al. Quality of water used for haemodialysis: bacteriological and chemical parameters. *Nephrol Dial Transplant* 1999; 14:666–675.

Internet References

Dialyzer *KoA* calculator (www.hdcn.com/calc.htm)
Expanded dialyzer clearance table (www.hdcn.com/calc.htm)
Residual disinfectant standards (www.hdcn.com/hd/disinfect.htm)
Water quality standards for dialysis (www.hdcn.com/hd/wquality.htm)
Dialysis machine add-ons (www.hdcn.com/hd/hdmacadd.htm)

4

Vascular Access for Hemodialysis

Anatole Besarab and Rasib M. Raja

The necessity for vascular access in patients with renal failure can be temporary or permanent. The necessity for temporary access may vary from several hours (single dialysis) to months [if used to dialyze while waiting for an arteriovenous (AV) fistula to mature]. Temporary access is established by the percutaneous insertion of a catheter into a large vein (internal jugular, femoral, or, less desirably, subclavian). Construction of a permanent vascular access permits repeated angioaccess for months to years.

An ideal permanent access delivers a flow adequate for the dialysis prescription, lasts a long time, and has a low complication rate. The autologous AV fistula comes closest to satisfying these criteria because it has the best 5-year patency rate and during this period requires many fewer interventions than other access methods. Prosthetic accesses (AV grafts) are constructed by the insertion of a subcutaneous tube in a straight, curved, or loop configuration between an extremity artery and vein. Placement of a cuffed double-lumen silicone elastomer catheter (e.g., Perm-Cath device) or a pair of cuffed single-lumen catheters (e.g., Tesio catheter) into an internal jugular vein for permanent access is also done in selected circumstances.

Although the autologous AV fistula is clearly the desired access for patients initiating hemodialysis, there is disproportionate use of AV grafts in the United States and an increasing dependence on cuffed indwelling central venous catheters. Guidelines developed by the National Kidney Foundation Dialysis Outcomes Quality Improvement initiative promote the increased construction of AV fistulas and earlier referral of patients to nephrologists, permitting early-access evaluation and early construction of an AV fistula or graft, thereby minimizing the use of venous catheter access (see "Internet References"). A second goal of the guidelines is to promote detection of access dysfunction prior to access thrombosis.

I. Venous access
A. Indications
   1. **Temporary access.** Venous catheters are commonly used for acute angioaccess in the following patients: (a) those with acute renal failure; (b) those requiring hemodialysis or hemoperfusion for overdose or intoxication; (c) those with end-stage renal failure needing urgent hemodialysis but without available mature access; (d) those on maintenance hemodialysis who have lost effective use of their permanent access and require temporary access until permanent access function can be reestablished; (e) patients requiring plasmapheresis or hemoperfusion; (f) peritoneal dialysis patients whose abdomens are being rested prior to new peritoneal catheter placement (usually for severe peritonitis that required

peritoneal dialysis catheter removal); and (g) transplant recipients needing temporary hemodialysis during severe rejection episodes.

2. Permanent access. Cuffed venous catheters are evolving into an alternative form of long-term vascular access for patients in whom an AV access cannot be readily created.

Such patients include small children, some diabetic patients with severe vascular disease, patients who are morbidly obese, and, patients who have undergone multiple AV access insertions and in whom additional sites for AV access insertion are not available. Additional indications include patients with cardiomyopathy unable to sustain adequate blood pressures or access flows, and patients who require more frequent blood access (daily nocturnal home hemodialysis). However, survival rates for cuffed double-lumen catheters are about 60% at 6 months and 40% at 1 year if revisions are included (Shaffer et al, 1992). Inadequate blood flow through cuffed venous catheters is a significant problem with catheters. Nominal flow greater than 400 mL per minute (actual flow 350 mL per minute) can rarely be obtained, and usually flow is limited to a range closer to 300 mL per minute. This limits use of permanent cuffed venous catheters in larger patients and results in a lower average urea reduction ratio (URR) or fractional urea clearance (Kt/V).

B. Catheter types and design

1. Dual-lumen versus coaxial dual-lumen design. Dual-lumen venous catheters are available in two basic cross-sectional configurations: a "double-D" configuration (Fig. 4-1A) and one in which the two blood pathways are configured as coaxial cylinders. The former design has been shown to deliver a higher blood flow rate (Sands et al, 1997).

2. Cuffed versus uncuffed. Use of an uncuffed catheter for periods of time beyond several weeks results in a relatively high rate of infection. Bonded felt or Dacron cuffs were

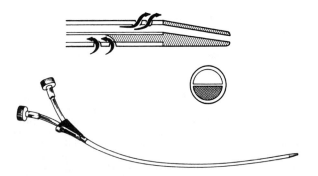

Figure 4-1A. Diagram of a double-lumen cannula designed for percutaneous insertion into the subclavian, femoral, or internal jugular vein. (Reproduced from Krupski WC, et al. Access for dialysis. In: Cogan MG, Garovoy MR, eds. *Introduction to dialysis.* New York: Churchill Livingstone, 1985:52.)

designed to extend the use of venous catheters from weeks to several months by reducing the incidence of line-related infection and of catheter migration, but such cuffs require surgical tunneling for placement. Unequivocal demonstration that cuffs prevent infection has not been shown (Marr et al, 1997). Use of cuffed catheters is especially useful when one is planning or has just placed an AV fistula, which requires several months to mature properly. Some centers use cuffed catheters routinely for most cases of acute renal failure when the duration is expected to extend beyond 1 week.

3. Antiseptic impregnation. Catheters impregnated with chlorhexidine and silver sulfadiazine are available and may be associated with a lower rate of blood-borne catheter-related infection (Maki et al, 1997), but studies in dialysis patients are still preliminary.

4. Twin cuffed silicone catheters (Tesio and Ash Split-Cath). Recent interest has focused on use of twin silicone rubber catheters (Tesio et al, 1994; Fig. 4-1B), each with its own cuff for either long-term temporary or permanent access. In some studies, a higher flow rate with these catheters is claimed, although mean flow rates still are in the range of 400 mL per minute nominal (blood pump setting) flow, 360 mL per minute actual ultrasonographically measured flow (Prabhu et al, 1997). In one study, flow with Tesio catheters was no higher than with the double-D dual-lumen design. Other touted advantages of Tesio catheters are increased patient comfort (the catheters are soft and less bulky than a dual-lumen catheter), less positional dysfunction (as the outlet ports are wound spirally around the distal parts of each catheter), and perhaps increased longevity, with a lower incidence of perforations, mural thromboses, etc. However, none of these

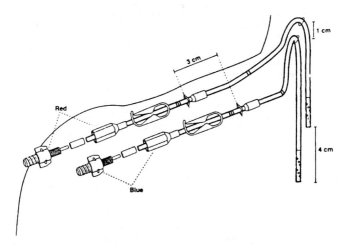

Figure 4-1B. Schematic drawing of Tesio twin-catheter positioning. (Reproduced from American Roentgen Ray Society. *AJR Am J Roentgenol* 1995;164:1519–1520.)

claims has been proven in randomized trials. The Split-Cath is a single dual-lumen double-D catheter in which the internal portion has been split to increase compliance and decrease recirculation.

5. Tunneling. The optimal tunnel design has not been clearly established. An important aspect is the location of the venotomy relative to the exit skin site. Curved tunnels permit smooth passage of the catheter to the anterior chest wall (superior vena cava location) or to the lateral abdominal wall (inferior vena cava location). They therefore provide comfort to the patient and minimize kinking. Cuffs on catheters are commonly used but are not required as long as the catheter is secured to prevent migration.

C. Insertion location. The merits of the various insertion locations are listed in Table 4-1. The usual insertion site is the internal jugular vein, with the femoral vein as an occasional alternative site. The subclavian site should generally be avoided because it is associated with a higher incidence of insertion-related complications (pneumothorax, hemothorax, subclavian artery perforation, brachial plexus injury) and, more importantly, a higher incidence (up to 40%) of delayed central venous stenosis. The principal disadvantage of the jugular vein approach is that the catheter is difficult to fix to the skin in this position and neck mobility is impaired. These disadvantages can be overcome by tunneling over the clavicle to a skin exit site to the anterior chest wall. Catheterization of the femoral vein is a good choice when the need for hemodialysis (or hemoperfusion or plasmapheresis) is expected to be short (less than 1 week). The femoral approach is useful for performing the initial hemodialysis treatment in patients who present with acute pulmonary edema because the patient's head and chest can be elevated during insertion.

D. Insertion technique

1. Use of ultrasonographic guidance. Use of a portable ultrasound monitor to guide catheter insertion is very useful. The central veins of the neck exhibit anatomic variability, and occasionally one of them may be absent. Atypical or ectatic carotid arteries are also a problem. With the use of one such bedside ultrasound device (Site-Rite II), the rate of successful

Table 4-1. Insertion sites for temporary catheters: advantages and disadvantages

Site	Advantages	Disadvantages
Femoral vein	Insertion ease; low insertion risk	Patient immobility; higher infection risk; high recirculation unless 18-cm-length catheter used
Subclavian vein	Patient comfort; extended use	Highest vein stenosis and insertion complication rate
Internal jugular vein	Extended use; lower risk	More difficult to insert

internal jugular puncture on first attempt increased from 36 to 83%, and the rate of carotid artery punctures was reduced from 8% to 0% (Farrell and Gellens, 1997).

2. General. The catheter should be inserted using an aseptic technique, with the operator wearing a sterile surgical gown and gloves. At the time of catheter placement, skin disinfection with 2% aqueous chlorhexidine is superior to that of povidone–iodine. For double-lumen catheters, a probing 16-gauge needle attached to a 10 cm^3 syringe filled with heparinized saline is used to enter the vein. A single-lumen catheter is probed with an 18-gauge needle. Gentle aspiration during advancement of the needle is required. Entry of dark red blood into the needle indicates entry into the vein. Once the vein is entered with the probing needle, a guide wire is promptly inserted, which should pass easily into the vein and advance freely for 10–15 cm. If the wire does not advance easily, it must be withdrawn and venous puncture with the probing needle attempted again. After the guide wire has been introduced, it is held in place while the probing needle is removed. The point of entry of the guide wire into the skin is enlarged using a no. 11 scalpel blade. A dilator to enlarge the tract is used for double-lumen catheters (10–11F). Single-lumen (8F) catheters can be introduced without a dilator. Stiff catheters (polyurethane, polyethylene, polytetrafluoroethylene) are always inserted over the guide wire in the appropriate vein. Care should be taken to control the guide wire externally while placing the catheter over the guide wire. Silicone rubber catheters are inserted while using a peel-away sheath.

The ports to the catheter should be occluded with a finger as soon as the guide wire is removed to prevent inadvertent air embolism. After insertion, the catheter is filled with heparinized saline if it is to be used within an hour, or otherwise, the catheter is filled with 1,000 units per mL heparin, with the amount determined by the volume of each catheter lumen. The hub of the catheter is fixed to the skin near the skin exit site by one or more sutures. A sterile dressing is then applied. The catheter can be used immediately if a chest radiograph has confirmed proper positioning and the absence of pneumothorax or hemothorax (Table 4-2). It is important to verify the position of the catheter tip at the second to third intercostal space by fluoroscopy. It is also important to align the arterial port at the catheter tip toward the center of the vena cava to reduce suction against the caval wall during dialysis.

3. Jugular vein approach. Respiratory status permitting, the patient is placed in a supine head-down (Trendelenburg) position of about 15 degrees to distend the neck veins. The head is extended and turned away from the side of venipuncture. The right side is preferred for a variety of reasons, including the fact that the dome of the lung and pleura is lower on the right side than on the left. The right internal jugular vein travels in a relatively straight path to the atrium. The thoracic duct, which is on the left, is not endangered. One of three approaches to the internal jugular vein can be used: central, posterior, or anterior. The choice depends on the experience and preference of the operator. The central approach may be the easiest of the three. (See Figs. 4-2A to 4-2C for a guide to

Table 4-2. Complications of central venous catheterization

Immediate complications	Delayed complications
Arterial puncture	Thrombosis
Pneumothorax	Infection
Hemothorax	Vascular stricture
Arrhythmias	Arteriovenous fistula
Air embolism	
Perforation of vein or cardiac chamber	
Pericardial tamponade	**Injury to adjacent structures:**
	Brachial plexus
	Trachea
	Recurrent laryngeal nerve

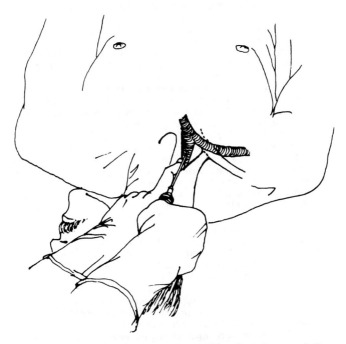

Figure 4-2A.   Central approach to internal jugular vein cannulation.
The triangle formed by the two heads (sternal and clavicular) of the
sternomastoid and the clavicle is located by palpation. With large or
obese patients, asking the patient to lift the head slightly may accen-
tuate the muscles and define the triangle more clearly. The needle is
inserted at the apex of the triangle (formed by the two heads of the
sternomastoid muscle) and directed caudally and laterally toward
the ipsilateral nipple at an angle of 45–60 degrees with the frontal
plane. The vein is entered within a few centimeters of the puncture
site. To minimize the risk of puncturing the carotid artery, the needle should not be directed medially. (Reproduced from *Textbook of
Advanced Cardiac Life Support*, 2nd ed. 1990. Copyright © American
Heart Association.)

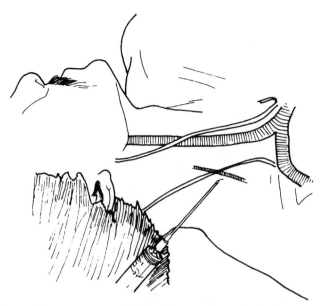

Figure 4-2B. Posterior approach. The needle is introduced under the sternomastoid muscle at its lateral (posterior) border, at the junction of the middle and lower thirds of the posterolateral border, about 5 cm above the clavicle. The needle is aimed at the suprasternal notch at a 45-degree angle to the horizontal plane and a 15-degree forward angulation in the frontal plane. The vein should be entered within 5–7 cm of the insertion site. (Reproduced from *Textbook of Advanced Cardiac Life Support*, 2nd ed. 1990. Copyright © American Heart Association.)

insertion technique.) Some authorities advocate subcutaneous tunneling of the catheter to a new exit site away from the jaw (for patient comfort), but this is generally not needed for catheters intended for short term (less than 3 weeks) use.

4. Subclavian vein approach. The procedure can be safely performed in the dialysis unit by skilled staff. Unless jugular venous distention is present, the Trendelenburg position is recommended. The patient's head is turned 45 degrees away from the side of insertion. The shoulders are kept back by insertion of a longitudinally rolled towel between the scapulae. The skin just below the clavicle at the junction of the middle and inner thirds is anesthetized. A more lateral needle entry site is associated with a higher risk of arterial injury and pneumothorax.

Aiming for the jugular notch, the probing needle is advanced under the clavicle and mild suction applied to the syringe as it is inserted. Both aiming the needle toward the floor or a more lateral needle entry site are associated with a higher risk of arterial injury and pneumothorax. [Some initially probe with

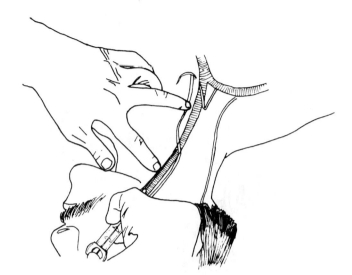

Figure 4-2C.   Anterior approach. The carotid artery is palpated and retracted medially away from the anterior border of the sternomastoid, 5 cm above the clavicle. The needle is introduced at this point, aimed toward the ipsilateral nipple, forming an angle of 30–45 degrees with the frontal plane. (Reproduced from *Textbook of Advanced Cardiac Life Support*, 2nd ed. 1990. Copyright © American Heart Association.)

a smaller (22-gauge) needle and upon entry into the vein note its position, withdraw it, and replace it with an 18- or 16-gauge needle. Use of the smaller needle may minimize complications since the resultant hole in the artery wall from inadvertent puncture of the subclavian artery is small and hemostasis more readily achieved than with a larger needle.]

As for intrajugular punctures, some authorities advocate subcutaneous tunneling of the catheter to a new exit site lower down on the chest wall, but this again is generally not needed for catheters intended for short term (less than 3 weeks) use.

5.   Femoral vein approach. The patient is placed flat on the back with the knee slightly flexed and leg abducted and rotated outward. The groin is shaved, cleansed, painted with antiseptic, and draped. The femoral vein should be initially located 2–4 cm below the inguinal ligament using a 22-gauge needle filled with heparinized saline or with local anesthetic. The latter can be infiltrated around the vein to prevent subsequent venous spasm. Once the vein is located, the small-gauge needle is withdrawn and replaced with an 18-gauge (for single-lumen catheters) or 16-gauge (for double-lumen catheters) probing needle. A guide wire is inserted through the needle into the vein. It is important for the guide wire to be freely movable back and forth after it is fully inserted. If it is not, the guide wire should be withdrawn completely, the angle of the needle in the vein changed (sometimes the needle hub has to be lowered to the skin level to almost parallel the vein), and the guide wire reinserted. Only after free to-and-fro movement of the inserted guide wire is achieved is the probing needle removed and the catheter inserted. Catheters with a minimal length of 18 cm are preferred since they reach the inferior vena cava providing better blood flow with less recirculation. Even so, recirculation is higher with femoral dual-lumen catheters than with their internal jugular or subclavian counterparts, probably because flow in the lower inferior vena cava is still lower than in the superior vena cava.

An uncuffed femoral catheter may be used several times within a 2- to 4-day period. The patient must remain at bed rest as long as the catheter is in place. After 72 hours, the catheter should generally be removed, although extended use of cuffed femoral catheters has been reported (Weitzel et al, 1993).

6. Insertion of cuffed catheters, especially Tesio catheters. The insertion technique for cuffed dual-lumen catheters is beyond the scope of this book but is similar to the techniques described for insertion of uncuffed catheters (see Bour et al, 1990). Insertion methods for cuffed Tesio catheters are detailed in Prabhu et al (1997), from which the following is paraphrased with permission: Briefly, under ultrasound guidance, the internal jugular vein is punctured with a 21-gauge needle. A guide wire followed by a 6F dilator is then inserted. A second puncture is made 1 cm inferior to the first and the process is repeated. Using a guide wire and fluoroscopic guidance, the correct lengths of the two catheters are determined and the catheters trimmed to fit. The lengths are adjusted, so the aspiration catheter (red hub) is located 4 cm cephalad to the return catheter (blue hub). The latter is located at the superior portion of the right atrium. After further dilatation of the venotomies, the catheters are inserted through peel-away sheaths. After placing and threading through the tunnels, kinks are reduced by pulling gently on the catheter with the patient's head turned to one side. A 0.089-cm hydrophilic-coated guide wire is inserted into each catheter to reduce kinks.

7. Insertion-related complications. These include arterial puncture, pneumothorax, hemothorax, air embolism, mediastinal hemorrhage, pericardial tamponade, and brachial plexus injury (Table 4-2). Arrhythmias can also occur as a result of endocardial irritation, especially when the catheter or guide wire has been advanced too deeply. Rarely, erosion of the superior vena cava can occur. The sum of all early major complications should not exceed 5% of all central venous catheter placements.

E. Care and use of venous catheters

1. Dressings. During catheter connect and disconnect procedures, both dialysis staff and patient should wear a surgical mask or face shield. The lumen and catheter tips should never remain open to air. A cap or syringe should always be placed on or in the catheter lumen while maintaining a clean field under the catheter connectors. Catheter lumens must be kept sterile: Interdialytic infusions through the catheter are forbidden.

After each dialysis, catheter hubs or blood line connectors should be soaked in povidone–iodine for 3–5 minutes, then dried prior to separation. Povidone–iodine ointment, chlorhexidine patch, or other polymicrobial gel is applied to the catheter exit site and the catheter covered with a sterile dry dressing. Nonbreathable or nonporous transparent film dressings should be avoided as they pose a greater threat of exit site colonization than dry dressings.

   2.   Heparin. After each dialysis, the dead space of each lumen is filled with heparin (1,000–5,000 units per mL) through the catheter injection ports. The dead space of each catheter lumen varies among manufacturers and length of catheter. It is important to record this information on the patient's chart, so it is readily available to the dialysis staff. Injection of a volume of heparin solution larger than necessary should be avoided as it results in some degree of systemic anticoagulation that may be hazardous to patients at risk for bleeding. Prior to each dialysis, the heparin in each lumen is aspirated, the catheter flushed with heparinized saline (100 units per mL) and hemodialysis initiated.

   3.   Bathing and showering. The exit site should never be immersed in bath water. Showering is best done prior to coming to the dialysis unit, where a new dressing and antibacterial ointment will be promptly applied.

F.   Infection. Infection is the leading cause of catheter loss and increases morbidity and mortality. Infection usually arises from the migration of the patient's own skin flora through the puncture site and onto the outer catheter surface, although it can also result from contamination of the catheter connectors, lumen contamination during dialysis, or from infused solutions. Catheters can also become colonized from more remote sites during bacteremia. Gram-positive bacteria (usually *Staphylococcus* species) are the most common culprits.

   1.   Prevention
      a.   Aseptic insertion and handling of the catheters. As discussed above under "Care and Use of Venous Catheters."
      b.   Minimize duration of cannulation. The incidence of infection of central uncuffed catheters is generally under 8% by 2 weeks. By 1 month, 25% of uncuffed central catheters become infected, and this figure doubles by the end of the second month. Catheter-related septicemia may occur in 2%–20% of catheters. The most important factor in minimizing the incidence of infection is limitation on the duration of a catheter use.

      To reduce infection risk, uncuffed femoral catheters should be removed after 2–4 days of use in mobile patients, whereas uncuffed internal jugular or subclavian catheters may remain in place for several weeks. Cuffed catheters can be left in place for an indefinite period, and some centers routinely insert a cuffed catheter initially in a majority of patients requiring acute dialysis (Prabhu et al, 1997).

      c.   Prophylactic antibiotics. These should be given for procedures likely to produce bacteremia (dental procedures, sigmoidoscopy, colonoscopy, endoscopic retrograde cholangiopancreatography). They are not given routinely prior to cuffed catheter insertion.

2. **Diagnosis and treatment**
   a. **Infections in uncuffed catheters**
      (1) **Localized exit site infection.** If there is erythema and/or crust but no purulent discharge, one can usually treat with appropriate antibiotics for up to 2 weeks. The catheter must be removed if systemic signs of infection develop (leukocytosis or temperature greater than 38°C), if pus can be expressed from the tract of the catheter, or if the infection persists or recurs after an initial course of antibiotics. If blood cultures are positive and a false-positive result due to contamination is believed unlikely, then the catheter should be removed.

      (2) **Tunnel infection.** Purulent exudate can often be expressed, and pain/warmth is present along the tunnel. Initial catheter removal is indicated with administration of antibiotics for 2 weeks. Infrequently, the tunnel infection is severe enough to require unroofing.

      (3) **Systemic infection.** Initial presentation is typically with fever and leukocytosis. Leukocyte counts obtained during dialysis using a cellulose membrane during the first hour are unreliable due to complement-induced leukopenia. The degree of fever may increase during dialysis, and this is not necessarily a sign of pyrogenic reaction. Signs of exit site or tunnel infection are common but on occasion may be absent.

      In some patients, another source for infection will be present (e.g., pneumonia, urinary tract infection, wound infection). In such cases, the distant infection can be treated, and the catheter may be left in place cautiously with close continued surveillance. On the other hand, if initial history, physical examination, or radiologic studies show no other apparent source, catheter infection should be presumed and the catheter should generally be promptly removed. Blood cultures should be obtained from a peripheral vein and through the catheter prior to removal. On removal, the catheter tip should be cultured using special technique (Table 4-3). The duration of antibiotic treatment depends on clinical response. In general, antibiotic therapy should be continued for a minimum of 2–3 weeks.

      (4) **Placement of a new catheter.** A new catheter can be inserted at another site 48 hours after catheter removal if repeat blood cultures are negative. A new catheter should not be inserted as long as blood cultures are positive.

   b. **Infections in cuffed catheters.** Treatment is similar to that used for temporary catheters, with the following additional considerations. Whereas bacteremia with a temporary catheter is usually an indication for catheter removal, in patients with a permanent catheter in place, the catheter and the venous site may represent the last readily available form of access. Thus, an initial attempt at salvage is justified. Tunnel infections can be given a quick trial of parenteral

Table 4-3.   Central venous catheter culture methods

There are at least four methods currently in use. All have similar sensitivity. The first (Maki) tip-roll method has the lowest specificity.

1. Maki tip-roll technique:
   After wiping off antibiotic ointment at the skin exit site, cut distal 5-cm tip and roll over a plate containing 6% sheep blood agar, then culture tip in trypticase soy broth. When there is ≥15 cfu on the plate, it is read as positive.[a]
2. Endoluminal brush method (>100 cfu per mL).[b]
3. Modified tip-flush method (>100 cfu per mL).[b]
4. Gram-stain and acridine-orange leukocyte cytospin (AOLC) method (presence of any microorganisms within the cellular monolayer).[c]

[a] Maki DG, Weise CE, Sarafin HW. A semiquantitative culture method for identifying intravenous-catheter-related infection. *N Engl J Med* 1977;296:1305–1309.
[b] Kite P, et al. Evaluation of a novel endoluminal brush for the in situ diagnosis of catheter related sepsis. *J Clin Pathol* 1997;50:278–282.
[c] Kite P, et al. Rapid diagnosis of central-venous-catheter-related bloodstream infection without catheter removal. *Lancet* 1999;354:1504–1507.

antibiotics, but failure to respond requires prompt catheter removal and replacement through a new tunnel and exit site. In catheter-related bacteremia, an initial course of parenteral antibiotics can be given if there is no evidence of tunnel infection and no clinical signs of sepsis. The catheter should be removed in all patients who are still symptomatic after 36–72 hours of parenteral therapy. In patients who become asymptomatic and who continue to have no tunnel or exit site infection, the catheter may be left in place with continued monitoring. An alternative is to change a cuffed catheter over a guide wire (Carlisle, 1991). Blood cultures should be repeated periodically. The salvage rate of cuffed catheters is relatively low at 32% (Marr et al, 1997), and attempts at salvage did not increase the complication rates (osteomyelitis, septic arthritis, endocarditis). The newly inserted catheter should be removed if signs and symptoms of bacteremia recur.

   c.   **Complications of catheter infection.** Delay in therapy or prolonged attempts to salvage an infected cuffed catheter can lead to serious complications, including endocarditis, osteomyelitis, suppurative thrombophlebitis, and spinal epidural abscess. The last is a rare but serious neurologic complication in hemodialysis patients. In one series, 50% of cases were associated with attempted salvage of an infected cuffed venous catheter (Kovalik et al, 1996). Presenting complaints are fever, backache, local spinal tenderness, leg pain and weakness, sphincter dysfunction, paresis and/or paralysis. For diagnosis, magnetic resonance imaging appears to be less sensitive (80%) than computed tomography-myelography. Plain computed tomographic scanning without myelography has low sensitivity and can give misleading results (e.g., disk protrusion). Early (immediate) decompressive surgery usually is advised, although rare patients can be treated with antibiotics only.

G. Catheter dysfunction

1. Early. Initial dysfunction of internal jugular and sub-clavian catheters is due usually either to malposition or to intracatheter thrombosis. Many dysfunctional catheters exhibit positional occlusion during dialysis.

a. Intracatheter thrombosis. Most simple thromboses will respond to intraluminal thrombolytic injection of urokinase as described in Table 4-4 or tissue plasminogen activator (tPA) as described in Table 4-5.

b. Malposition, catheter tip thrombus. Persistent low flow despite urokinase treatment requires examination under fluoroscopy, with or without contrast injection, to diagnose malposition or catheter tip thrombus. Large catheter tip thrombi may require systemic thrombolysis (urokinase 20,000 units per hour for 6 hours or streptokinase

Table 4-4. Open-catheter protocol using urokinase[a]

1. Attach a syringe filled with urokinase (5,000 IU/mL) to the clamped catheter. Unclamp the catheter and slowly instill 1.0 mL volume of urokinase solution followed by an amount of heparinized saline that equals the dead space of the catheter lumen less the 1.0 mL of urokinase injected (a 1.9-mL catheter requires 0.9 mL of heparinized saline). Most catheters have a dead space greater than 1.0 mL. The urokinase must reach the distal tip of the catheter to be effective. Half-life of urokinase (2–3 min) precludes any significant systemic effect from the small doses of urokinase to be injected systemically.
2. Reclamp the catheter and leave attached to it a syringe containing an additional 1.0 mL of heparinized saline (to prevent contamination).
3. Leave urokinase in the catheter for 5–10 min.
4. Unclamp the catheter, inject 0.3 mL of the heparinized saline, and reclamp.
5. Repeat step 4 two more times. The total amount of urokinase injected systemically is less than 5,000 U per lumen.
6. Aspirate 4–5 mL of blood. If blood can be aspirated easily, flush the catheter with heparinized saline and use the catheter for hemodialysis.
7. If blood cannot be aspirated, repeat steps 1–6.
8. Other causes of catheter malfunction should be considered if the second urokinase instillation fails to restore patency. If the catheter has been in place for less than a week and the exit site is not inflamed, the clotted catheter can be replaced by a new one inserted through the same skin exit site with minimal risk of infection. A flexible guide wire is inserted through the clotted catheter, the clotted catheter is removed, and a fresh catheter is threaded over the guide wire.

[a] The procedure is similar for femoral, subclavian, or internal jugular vein catheters, including the PermCath device. See also the high-dose intradialytic urokinase protocol by Twardowski (*Am J Kidney Dis* 1998;31:841–847). Urokinase is temporarily not available in the United States due to FDA concerns about the safety of the production process. Recombinant urokinase is anticipated to be available soon.

Table 4-5. Dosing of tissue plasminogen activator (tPA) and urokinase for occluded catheters (drug injected into catheter)

Indications	Dose of Alteplase/tPA	Dose of Urokinase
Thrombosis in tunneled catheters or central vein	High dose: 5 mg × 3 doses at 3- to 10-min intervals, followed by 3.5 mg/hr × 4 hr, then 1 mg/hr × 12 hr. Concomitant heparin.	High dose: 4,400 U/kg bolus, followed by 4,400 U/kg/hr for 12 hr
	Medium dose: 10 mg over 10 min, followed by 0.05 mg/kg/hr (or 3.5 mg/hr) × 6–12 hr. Consider concomitant heparin.	Medium dose: 120,000–250,000 U as bolus, followed by 2,000 U/min × 6–12 hr
	Low dose: 2 mg/port, repeat once	Low dose: 5,000 U per port
Intra-arterial thrombosis in patient undergoing thrombo-embolectomy	5 mg over 15 min × 3 doses (maximum 15 mg)	

3,000 units per hour for up to 24 hours). If a thrombus is absent, the catheter can be changed over a guide wire, but the problem is likely to recur.

2. Late dysfunction (more than 5 days)

a. Fibrin sleeves and mural thrombi. In addition to malposition and simple intracatheter or catheter tip thrombus, formation of a fibrin sleeve or a mural thrombus may be the cause of "late" catheter dysfunction. Almost all catheters inserted into a central vein develop a fibrin sleeve within one to several weeks after insertion. Such fibrin sleeves are initially clinically silent until they obstruct the ports at the distal end of the catheter. Generally, saline infuses into a port but aspiration is difficult. Fibrin sleeves can serve as a nidus for infection as well. A catheter venogram should be performed to confirm the diagnosis. The following methods can be used to deal with fibrin sheaths.

b. Systemic thrombolytics. One can give urokinase 20,000 units per hour for 6 hours or streptokinase 3,000 units per hour for up to 24 hours. An alternative, high-dose, intra-dialytic urokinase protocol has recently been proposed by

Twardowski et al (1998). Several medium- and high-dose tPA and urokinase protocols are described in Table 4-5.

   c. Snare catheter stripping. This procedure requires cannulation of the femoral vein and advancement of the snare up the inferior vena cava to the occluded catheter. The operator then pulls away the adherent fibrin sleeve/thrombus from the catheter, after which the removed material usually embolizes into the lung. Clinically evident pulmonary embolism has been reported to result from this procedure but is unusual. The potential delayed effects of multiple iatrogenic pulmonary embolizations on long-term pulmonary function are of theoretical concern.

   d. Exchange of the catheter over a guide wire. This will solve many problems and has been shown to be as effective as snare catheter stripping in the case of fibrin sleeve formation.

   3. Prevention. The incidence of early dysfunction due to malposition may be strongly dependent on the experience of the person performing the insertion. Tesio-type silicone catheters may have a lower incidence of positional dysfunction due to the spiral winding of their exit holes around the distal 3.5 cm of each catheter. Also, fibrin formation may be less around silicone catheters.

   The use of warfarin or other anticoagulants on a chronic basis may limit fibrin sleeve formation and catheter thrombus formation. However, use of anticoagulants for this purpose has not been studied in a systematic fashion. When used, systemic anticoagulation is required with an international normalized ratio of 2–2.5 (personal experience).

H. Embolic complications. Large clots adherent to the end of the catheter or to the vessel wall can be clinically silent or can give rise to embolic events. Large mural thrombi also can proceed to stenosis and central vein thrombosis as described below. Treatment options for a ball thrombus or a catheter-associated right atrial thrombus include simple catheter removal, systemic or catheter fibrinolytic therapy (Tables 4-5 and 4-6) and, rarely, thoracotomy with thrombectomy.

I. Central vein stenosis, thrombosis, stricture

   1. Incidence. Central venous stenosis arises from endothelial injury at the site of catheter–endothelial contact through the release of a variety of growth factors. The incidence increases with the use of stiff, nonsilicone catheters; use of the subclavian approach (presumably because of higher angular stresses on the catheter in the subclavian position); and in patients with previous catheter-related infections.

   2. Presentation/diagnosis. A stenosis may be asymptomatic and clinically silent until unmasked by the creation of an AV fistula. Symptoms then are invariably those of gross edema (often explosive) of the entire arm and in extreme cases the development of venous skin ulcers. When the stenosis develops after an access has been placed, development of the edema is slower.

   3. Treatment. Ligation of the vascular access produces the most rapid improvement but sacrifices the access. Initial anticoagulation (with heparin followed by warfarin) and elevation may ameliorate the symptoms and signs if thrombosis is present, but more definitive therapy can be avoided in only a minority of such cases. Balloon angioplasty has been used for stenosis, but the lesion tends to recur. Stent placement combined with angioplasty is indicated in elastic central vein lesions or if the stenosis recurs within a 3-month period. Some patients may be candidates for surgical axillary–internal jugular bypass of the affected subclavian vein. .

II.   Arteriovenous access. Characteristics of the patient's arterial, venous, and cardiopulmonary system determine the access most suitable for that patient. Life expectancy may also influence type and access location.

A.   Preoperative evaluation

1.   History. Crucial features in the history are the previous placement of a central venous catheter or transvenous pacemaker because of the possibility of vein stenosis. Any AV access may alter the hemodynamics and cardiac function in a patient with congestive heart failure. History of peripheral vascular disease (arterial or venous) or the presence of diabetes mellitus may limit the options for access construction. Previous surgery or trauma to the arm, chest, or neck may limit access site construction. Comorbid conditions, such as severe coronary artery disease or malignancy limiting life expectancy, may preclude use of anything but a cuffed catheter as permanent access. Patients in whom live donor transplantation is planned for the near future may not require a permanent vascular access.

2.   Physical examination. Usually, examination of the arterial and venous systems is sufficient supplemented by hand-held Doppler when necessary. Blood pressure should be measured in both arms, the Allen test performed, and arm sizes compared. The patient should be examined for evidence of previous central or venous catheterization and for trauma or surgery of the arm, chest, or neck. Some surgeons perform tourniquet venous mapping to select the best veins for access. The presence of a 6-cm segment of cephalic vein at the wrist is needed to create a wrist AV fistula.

3.   Radiologic studies

a.   Doppler venous ultrasonography or venography. Doppler ultrasonography or venography may be required to exclude central vein stenosis. Indications include previous central vein catheterization, especially for dialysis access or a transvenous pacemaker, edema in the extremity, presence of collateral veins around the shoulder or on the chest wall, and unequal extremity size. Previous AV access construction in the extremity also may warrant such studies. Doppler venous studies may also identify suitable veins for AV construction not readily visible on the surface.

b.   Arteriography. Indicated when pulses in the desired access location are markedly diminished or absent.

c.   Doppler evaluation. Brachial artery flow can easily be measured. A flow greater than 80 mL per minute is predictive of successful maturation of an AV fistula.

4.   Anticipating the need for AV fistula. In patients with progressive renal failure, one should minimize venipuncture or placement of intravenous catheters into the forearm veins, especially the cephalic vein of the nondominant arm. The dorsum of the hand should be used when venipuncture of the nondominant arm cannot be avoided.

The AV fistula should be created 4–6 months prior to the initiation of hemodialysis; the latter time point can be anticipated from the rate of rise of the plasma creatinine level. In general, patients should be referred to the surgeon when the serum creatinine is higher than 4 mg per dL. Surgical consensus promotes the use of the nondominant arm.

With the increased ability to tide peritoneal dialysis patients through a period of temporary loss of peritoneal access (from catheter obstruction, infection, leakage, or hernia) by use of percutaneous venous catheters, the previous common practice of creating an AV fistula in patients planning to start peritoneal dialysis has been abandoned by many centers. However, the high incidence of peritoneal catheter malfunction, peritonitis, and technique failure places these patients at risk every time a venous catheter has to be placed; such risks are avoided by the creation of an AV fistula (Hakim and Lazarus, 1995).

B. AV fistula

    1. Characteristics. An AV fistula consists of a subcutaneous anastomosis of an artery to an adjacent vein. It is the safest and the longest lasting permanent vascular access. Its advantages over other access types include excellent patency, lower morbidity associated with its creation, and lower complication rates (infection, stenosis, and steal). For equivalent degrees of assisted patency, the AV fistula requires three- to fourfold fewer procedures.

    Disadvantages include the long maturation time as well as failure in some cases to develop a blood flow sufficient to support the dialysis prescription. Creation of an adequate AV fistula may not be possible in some patients with arterial disease (e.g., due to diabetes or severe atherosclerosis), in the markedly obese, in patients with small or deep veins, in older patients, and in patients whose veins have been damaged by multiple venipunctures. Doppler ultrasonography mapping studies may identify veins not readily apparent to the nephrologist or surgeon.

    2. Location. Wrist radiocephalic (Brescia-Cimino; Fig. 4-3) and elbow brachiocephalic AV fistula are the two types most often created. Other options include a snuff-box fistula, wrist ulnar-basilic, and a transposed elbow brachiobasilic fistula.

    The fistula is usually created in the nondominant arm both to facilitate self-dialysis and to limit the consequences of any functional disability that may occur. One should begin as distally as possible, moving up the arm proximally as accesses fail and have to be replaced. When all sites in the nondominant arm have been exhausted, the dominant arm can be used.

    3. Construction. The anastomosis can be made either side-of-artery to side-of-vein or side-of-artery to end-of-vein. In both instances, distal blood flow through the artery is preserved. With the side-to-side method (Fig. 4-3), higher pressure may sometimes be transmitted to the veins in the hand, resulting in venous hypertension and swelling. The side-of-artery to

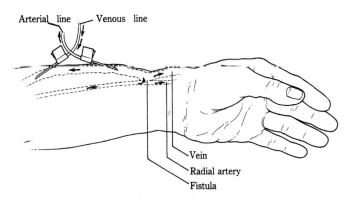

Figure 4-3.   The radiocephalic arteriovenous (AV) fistula, showing blood flow and the usual position of the access needles.

end-of-vein anastomosis prevents venous hypertension of the hand because the distal vein is tied. The surgery is usually performed in the operating room under regional anesthesia. The details of the operative technique are beyond the scope of this book.

   4.   Postoperative care and maturation. The arm should initially be kept elevated. Tight circumferential dressings should be avoided. The fistula blood flow should be checked daily (more frequently initially) by feeling for a thrill at the fistula site and by listening for an associated bruit. The fistula should never be used for venipuncture. Regular hand exercises with or without a lightly applied tourniquet may aid in access maturation. Maturation, a process of dilatation and thickening of the wall of the venous limb of the fistula permitting repeated insertion of dialysis needles, may require 1–6 months.

   An AV fistula should not be used before it is mature. Failure to mature the superficial veins of the fistula may result from poor brachial artery inflow or an inadequate anastomosis but also results from the presence of side branches in the venous segment. Ligation of these may result in successful maturation. Premature access cannulation is associated with infiltration and compression of the vessel and with permanent loss of the fistula. Infiltrated fistulas should be rested.

C.   AV graft
   1.   Characteristics. When an adequate AV fistula cannot be created, an AV connection can be made using a tube graft made from synthetic material. Synthetic polytetrafluoroethylene tubes provide superior performance in comparison with biologic bovine heterografts and are the preferred material. AV grafts have the following advantages over AV fistula: (a) large surface area, (b) easy cannulation, (c) short maturation time, and (d) easy surgical handling characteristics. However, the long-term patency of an AV graft is inferior to that of an AV fistula despite a fourfold increase in the number of salvage procedures.

2. Configuration and location. Grafts may be placed in straight, looped, or curved configurations (Fig. 4-4). Patient-specific features as well as the projected time on dialysis determine location. As with AV fistulas, the nondominant arm is used initially. Placement more distally preserves potential future graft placement sites, but such grafts can experience more frequent bouts of thrombosis. A distal graft (e.g., straight forearm graft from radial artery to an antecubital fossa vein) can sometimes be used to mature an upstream vein for future AV fistula construction. The most common initial sites for AV graft placement use the nondominant forearm: a straight graft from the radial artery at the wrist to the basilic vein (Fig. 4-4 A); a loop graft in the forearm from the brachial artery to the basilic vein (see Fig. 4-4, B) or an upper arm graft from brachial artery to axillary vein. The anastomoses in all instances are made between the end of the graft and the side of the vein or artery to minimize interference with blood flow through the native vessels. The axillary artery can be used as the source of a loop graft in the upper extremity; the

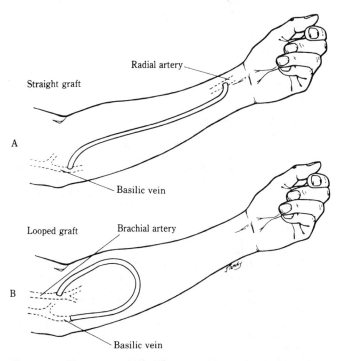

Figure 4-4. **The two most common types of AV grafts. A: The straight graft between the radial artery and basilic vein. B: The loop graft between the brachial artery and basilic vein. (Modifed from Larson E, et al. *Development of the clinical nephrology practitioner.* St. Louis: Mosby, 1982.)**

graft can extend from the arm to the internal jugular vein to bypass a subclavian stenosis on the same side. Grafts can also be placed in the thigh, but with a higher associated complication rate. Long-term dialysis patients frequently have had both upper extremities used for access. In extreme cases, chest wall (necklace) grafts have been constructed.

3.   Surgical placement. AV grafts are placed in the operating room under regional anesthesia (with general anesthesia backup) by a surgeon who should be skilled in performing vascular anastomoses. Prophylactic antibiotics (e.g., second-generation cephalosporins) are commonly administered immediately prior to the operation. Short grafts have no advantage over long grafts in terms of patency and longevity and should not be constructed. Postoperative care of grafts is the same as that for fistulas. The extremity is kept elevated for several days, and graft function is checked regularly by assessing for venous pulsation, thrill, and bruit. Most graft placements are now performed on an outpatient basis.

4.   Maturation. Although some advocate immediate use of a AV graft for dialysis, adhesion of the subcutaneous tunnel and graft requires about 2–3 weeks. Potential hematoma (from early cannulation in the tunnel) may compress and ruin the access. Thus, use of an AV graft should be delayed for 2–3 weeks if at all possible to allow for healing of the subcutaneous tunnel. Temporary catheters can be used if urgent dialysis is needed. A graft is considered mature when edema and erythema have resolved and the graft course is easily palpable. Cannulation of a graft that cannot be easily palpated or is edematous invites inaccurate needle insertions, leading to hematoma formation or frank laceration.

   a.   Early-use grafts. Grafts with additional layers of fiber windings have been marketed with the idea that one might be able to cannulate almost immediately (within 5 days) after insertion, as the extra windings limit the extravasation of blood on needle withdrawal and hence the risk of perigraft hematoma formation. This may obviate the need for a venous catheter access as a bridge. Despite initial enthusiasm, however, at least the first such early-use grafts have not been widely adopted; they are more difficult to insert because of their increased thickness, and they have a lower patency rate and possibly a higher rate of infection.

D.   Cannulation

1.   Anesthesia. In pain-sensitive patients, a topical anesthetic cream can be applied to the skin prior to puncture; however, local anesthetics are infrequently used.

2.   Needle size. During the initial use of a permanent vascular access, some nephrologists recommend the use of small (16-gauge) needles and low blood flow rates, particularly in AV fistula. In mature accesses, larger (15-gauge) needles are needed to support the required blood flow rates (more than 350 mL per minute) for high-efficiency dialysis.

3.   Needle orientation. Two needles are placed in the dilated vein(s) of the fistula or into the graft. The arterial needle leading to the dialyzer blood inlet is always placed in the more distal segment but at least 3 cm away from the AV (or arterial graft) anastomotic site. The arterial needle may point toward either the heart or the hand. Pointing the arterial needle toward the heart is popular in some countries, the rationale being, that the "flap" left behind when the needle is withdrawn tends to close more naturally with the flow of blood. However, there is no controlled evidence to suggest that this is the case. The venous needle should be inserted pointing toward the heart approximately 5 cm proximal to the arterial needle (to minimize recirculation). Some caregivers rotate each needle 180° along the needle axis after insertion, with the idea that injury to the deep wall of the vessel by the needle is then less likely. Again, this issue has not been systematically studied.

Special care must be taken when cannulating forearm loop grafts. In more than 80% of such grafts, the arterial limb will be medial (ulnar), but in the remainder the arterial limb may lie on the radial side of the forearm (as in Fig. 4-4). For reference, a "road map" of the access from the surgeon is very useful. Reversal of needle placement may occur unless the dialysis unit staff knows that blood in this particular graft flows in the opposite-to-usual direction. Reverse needle placement substantially increases the amount of recirculation (to more than 20%) and can result in inadequate delivery of dialysis. This happens more commonly than one would expect, as patients may be operated on at another center and a diagram of the inserted access might not be readily available. When in doubt, a careful physical examination with transient occlusion of the access and palpation on either side of the occluding finger will reveal the direction of blood flow in most cases.

4. Needle placement strategies. The manner in which needles are inserted affects the long-term patency and survival of accesses, particularly AV fistula. The "ladder" or rotational approach uses the entire length of the access without localizing needle sticks to any two areas. Grouping needle sticks in one or two specific areas weakens the wall, producing an aneurysm. In AV fistula, a less commonly used alternative is the "buttonhole" method. With this method, the AV fistula is always punctured through a limited number of sites, the use of which is rotated. The needle must be placed precisely through the same needle tract used previously. Ideally, special "dulled" needles should be used to minimize laceration of the buttonhole tract. There is no published experience with the buttonhole method in AV grafts, and it should probably not be tried in AV graft without further study.

5. Hemostasis. This is achieved by direct pressure following needle removal. One must prevent hematoma formation at the access site as well as control bleeding at the skin exit site. Pressure must be held for at least 10 minutes before checking the needle site for bleeding. Prolonged bleeding (more than 20 minutes) may indicate increased intra-access pressure (PIA) and is common in patients on therapeutic doses of warfarin. Adhesive bandages should not be applied until complete hemostasis is achieved.

E. Complications of AV access. Complications related to vascular access are a common reason for hospitalization in chronic dialysis patients. In the United States, access failure is the most common cause for hospitalization and in some centers accounts for the largest number of hospital days in end-stage renal disease patients.

1. Stenosis. More than 85% of AV graft thromboses are associated with a hemodynamically significant stenosis. The most common cause of stenosis in AV grafts is myointimal hyperplasia, which usually occurs at or just distal to the graft–vein anastomosis. At present, there is no way of preventing this process, although pharmacologic and irradiative approaches are being investigated. In AV fistula, the cause of stenosis tends to be more varied and may be due to turbulence, pseudoaneurysm formation, and needle-stick injury. Early detection permits correction of stenosis (by angioplasty or surgical revision) prior to thrombosis and extends the useful life of the access. Monitoring of vascular access for stenosis also helps maintain adequate blood flow to prevent underdialysis.

a. Clinical indicators. Recurrent clotting (twice a month or more), difficult needle placement (strictures), difficulty with hemostasis on needle withdrawal (intra-access hypertension), and a persistently swollen arm are all suggestive that stenosis may be present. However, these indicators, as well as indicators of underdialysis (reduced URR and Kt/V), are generally very late manifestations of access dysfunction.

Physical examination of the access should be performed at regular intervals, and the patient should be educated to do this as well, although the predictive value of physical findings to detect access stenosis has not been critically assessed. A palpable thrill at the arterial, body, and venous segments of an AV graft predict a flow greater than 450 mL per minute. A present pulse with an absent thrill suggests a lower flow. A discontinuous, systolic, harsh, high-pitched bruit over the access site may be suggestive of stenosis. This contrasts with the continuous, soft, low-pitched bruit heard over a well-functioning access site. Another sign of stenosis is a discontinuous, water-hammer type of pulse over the graft.

During dialysis, if gentle occlusion of the graft segment between the dialysis needles results in a marked rise in venous chamber pressure or an increase in the negativity of the prepump arterial pressure, this finding suggests that recirculation (and thereby stenosis) is present.

b. Access flow measurements

(1) Relation to risk of thrombosis. To what extent low access flow reflects stenosis and the risk of thrombosis depends on the type of access. The usual flow through a native AV fistula commonly averages 500–800 mL per minute, and in grafts, flow is somewhat higher, about 1,000 mL per minute (but may range up to 3 L per minute!). Native AV fistula may maintain patency at flows as low as 200 mL per minute, whereas AV grafts begin to thrombose at access flows between 600 and 800 mL per minute—flows that often provide adequate dialysis but offer few clinical premonitory signs that the access is at risk for thrombosis.

(2) How intra-access pressure (PIA) and venous drip chamber pressure reflect access flow

(a) PIA in AV grafts. Flow, pressure, and resistance are mathematically related. In an AV graft, the intragraft pressure (PIA) is normally less than 50% of the mean arterial pressure (MAP). Most of this pressure drop occurs at the anastomosis, unless there is an intragraft stenosis. When outflow stenosis develops (e.g., due to neointimal hyperplasia at or downstream from the graft-vein anastomosis), PIA rises and flow decreases (Fig. 4-5). When PIA rises above 50% of the MAP (PIA/MAP greater than 0.50), graft flow commonly has decreased into the thrombosis-prone range of 600–800 mL per minute, and the presence of stenosis is likely.

(b) AV grafts and fistulas compared. Venous outlet stenotic lesions in AV grafts are more likely to

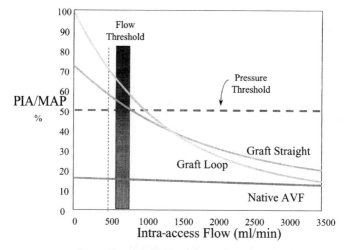

Figure 4-5. The relationship of intra-access pressure to flow in permanent vascular access. Pressure in the access (PIA) is normalized by the mean arterial pressure (MAP). The profiles differ between the AV fistula (AVF) and AV grafts. Normalized PIA is independent of access flow in AVF *(solid black line)* even if stenosis develops because blood can flow out through collateral channels. In contrast, PIA increases proximal to the recording needle in both loop and straight AV grafts *(gray lines)*. Threshold values for venous limb pressures in grafts are shown by the horizontal dashed line. Access flows associated with thrombosis in grafts are depicted by the vertical shaded area, which is to the right of usual dialyzer blood flows *(dashed vertical line)*. Not illustrated is the fact that low PIA/MAP ratios (e.g., less than 0.35) also may be associated with low flows, presumably due to poor inflow resulting from inadequate anastomosis or proximal stenosis).

manifest increased PIAs than those in native vein fistulas. The pressure flow characteristics differ in AV fistulas and AV grafts. In AV fistulas, blood entering the venous system returns via multiple collateral veins. This lowers basal PIA in an AV fistula, and prevents a major increase in PIA with outlet stenosis (Fig. 4-5). In contrast, AV graft outlet stenosis usually occurs at or just downstream to the graft–vein anastomosis. There are no accessory veins between the outflow stenosis and the graft, so outflow stenosis reliably causes an increase in intragraft pressure.

   (c) **Importance of a low PIA/MAP ratio.** If a stenosis develops in the body of the graft between the areas used for arterial and venous limb cannulation, PIA at the venous needle remains normal or even decreases, despite the decrease in flow. Inflow stenosis does not increase intragraft pressures and possibly decreases them. In fact, a PIA/MAP ratio lower than 0.35 may also be associated with low graft flow, presumably for this reason (Kapoian et al, 1997).

   (d) **Measuring equivalent PIA (EQPIA).** It is impractical to measure PIAs directly. However, one can estimate intragraft pressure using regular dialysis equipment as follows (Besarab et al, 1996): After placing the needles and priming all of the lines, the blood pump is stopped. A clamp is placed upstream to the venous drip chamber. After 30–40 seconds, the pressure in the venous drip chamber is read. This "static" pressure reflects intragraft pressure, assuming the transducer has been properly calibrated, but there will be an offset: namely, the vertical distance between the venous drip chamber height and that of the patient's fistula. One can measure this vertical distance and correct for it, thereby estimating the PIA (Table 4-6).

   The EQPIA is best normalized to the MAP. A value of EQPIA/MAP greater than 0.5 is highly specific for a 50% luminal outlet stenosis in an AV graft and is associated with decreased graft flow as well. In AV fistulas, the EQPIA/MAP ratio is low (about 0.20) and for reasons noted above does not usefully predict stenosis.

   (3) Venous drip chamber pressures measured with the blood pump running. Intragraft pressures can also be inferred from the pressure at the venous drip chamber with the blood pump running. The concept is that at any given blood flow rate, blood viscosity (hematocrit), and venous needle size there is a certain level of venous pressure at the drip chamber. Most of this pressure is due to resistance at the venous needle, and this value is primarily determined by the venous needle size used and the blood flow rate. However, access resistance downstream to the venous needle also contributes to this venous drip chamber pressure. A progressive increase in downstream access resistance causes the venous drip chamber pressures measured during dialysis to rise over time.

Table 4-6.   Measuring EQPIA/MAP ratio

Example:
1. Measure MAP: Assume that BP is 190/100. MAP is diastolic plus one-third of pulse pressure, or 130 mm Hg
2. Measure static intra-access pressure:
   a. With the blood pump off and the blood line upstream to the venous drip chamber clamped, the venous drip chamber pressure is 60 mm Hg.
   b. Compute offset using equation: offset (mm Hg) = $3.4 + 0.35 \times H$ (cm) where H is the height between the arm of the chair and middle of drip chamber. Assume H is 35 cm. Then offset = $3.4 + 12 = 15$ mm Hg.
   c. Add offset to compute EQPIA: EQPIA = $60 + 15 = 75$ mm Hg.
   d. Compute the EQPIA/MAP ratio. In this case, $75/130 = 0.58$, which is >0.5. This access is at risk for stenosis.

EQPIA, equivalent intra-access pressure; MAP, mean arterial pressure; BP, blood pressure.

One advantage of measuring venous drip chamber pressures with the blood pump running is that such pressures are routinely recorded during each dialysis anyway. One only needs to standardize the time at which they are recorded and the blood flow rate. Measurement is made at low dialyzer blood flow rates (200–225 mL per minute) because at higher blood flow rates, resistance in the venous needle accounts for the great majority of the total resistance in the circuit.

A baseline value should be established when the access is first used (new). The pressure should be measured within the first 2–5 minutes into dialysis, and the venous needles must be properly positioned within the lumen (e.g., not partially occluded by the vessel wall). The threshold pressure that triggers further access evaluation varies with needle gauge (Fig. 4-6); for 15-gauge needles, it is more than 115–120 mm Hg; for 16-gauge needles it is more than 150 mm Hg. The threshold must be exceeded on three consecutive dialysis treatments to be meaningful. Trend analysis is more important than any single value. Stenosis at the venous anastomotic site is suggested by progressive increase in this pressure over time.

Although the finding of a persistently elevated venous drip chamber pressure is an accepted means of screening for the presence of a functionally significant venous stenosis (Schwab et al, 1989), one study suggests that pressure measurements done at zero blood flow normalized to the MAP (EQPIA) are more sensitive and specific in detecting access stenosis (Dinwiddie et al, 1996).

(4)   Direct-flow measurements. It has now been repeatedly shown that in AV grafts, flows lower than 600–800 mL per minute are associated with a high risk of subsequent graft thrombosis. Apart from the pressure

Pressure Flow Relations

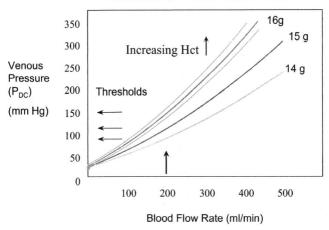

Figure 4-6. Drip-chamber venous pressure profiles as a function of blood pump flow. Needle gauge is a strong determinant of pressure, as shown by the horizontal arrows varying from 90 mm Hg for 14-gauge to 150 mm Hg for 16-gauge dialysis needles. The dotted lines show the effect of hematocrit (Hct) variation from 20 to 40 vol % with a 16-gauge needle. Note that at no-flow conditions, needle gauge does not affect the pressure.

methods mentioned above, several "direct" methods of measuring access blood flow have become available. It is anticipated that access flow and recirculation measurements will become routine in the near future as these devices are incorporated into dialysis machines.

(a) Ultrasonography (hematocrit) dilution/conductivity/temperature methods that require temporary reversal of blood flow lines during dialysis to measure access flow rate. The principle of the method (Krivitski, 1995) is as follows (Fig. 4-7):

1. During dialysis, the blood pump is stopped, and the blood lines are transiently reversed (at their connection to the tubings attached to the arterial and venous needles). The blood pump is then restarted. Reversal of the access lines forces an obligatory "recirculation" through the access, as the upstream blood line is now adding blood to the access. The percentage of this upstream blood from the dialyzer that is picked up into the downstream blood line depends on the ratio of the blood pump flow rate to the access blood flow rate. Once the percent "recirculation" under such reversed line conditions is calculated (because the blood pump flow rate is known) the access blood flow can be calculated algebraically.

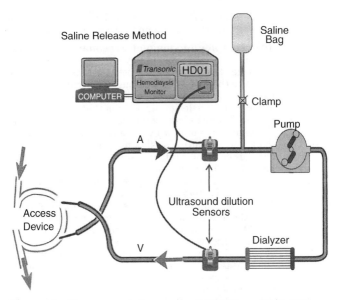

Figure 4-7. Measurement of access flow by dilution with blood line reversal (Krivitski's method). (Reproduced with permission from Promotional literature created by Transonics, Inc., Ithaca, New York.

2. To detect what percentage of blood from the upstream blood line enters the downstream blood line, a sensor is placed on the downstream blood line (which is the arterial blood line in this reversed configuration). The sensor detects hematocrit, conductivity, speed of an ultrasonographic pulse (ultrasonographic dilution), or temperature. Sometimes a similar sensor is placed on the upstream blood line for calibration purposes.

3. Using the dilution concept, a sudden perturbation in blood composition in the extracorporeal circuit is induced. With optical hematocrit or ultrasonographic sensors, the perturbation is a bolus of saline injected into the upstream blood line. This dilutes the blood going into the access, and the dilution effect is detected in the downstream blood line sensor. Another method suddenly increases the ultrafiltration rate in the dialyzer, which results in an increase in the hematocrit exiting the upstream blood line. Another method abruptly changes the dialysate temperature such that there is cooling of the blood entering the access from the upstream blood line. Yet another method requires infusion of concentrated saline into the upstream blood line. The principle remains the same: The extent of the perturbation in the upstream blood line that is

detected in the downstream blood line depends on the ratio of blood pump to access flow rates.

(b)   Doppler and magnetic resonance angiography. Doppler ultrasonography, though usually utilized to image stenotic lesions directly, can also be used to measure the rate of flow through a vascular access. A variety of machines can be used, and there are several different flow velocity algorithms that they use; as a result, there can be systematic underestimation and overestimation of flow by certain classes of machines (Sands et al, 1996). Also, flow measurement by Doppler depends on an accurate measure of velocity and vessel diameter. This may be difficult when flow is turbulent in an access. In such cases, flow is better measured at the brachial artery, where the vessel is a smooth cylinder of blood and where flow is non-turbulent. Almost all of the flow in the brachial artery (apart from about 60–80 mL per minute nutrient flow) is used to feed the vascular access, and brachial artery flow correlates very well with access flow rate (Besarab and Sherman, 1997). Magnetic resonance angiography can be used to measure access flow quite accurately but is too expensive for routine use.

c.   Recirculation

(1)   Dependence on access blood flow rate. Access recirculation does not develop until access flow decreases to a level equal to or less than that being drawn by the blood pump (Besarab and Sherman, 1997). Thus, barring inadvertent needle reversal or improper needle placement, access recirculation will not be present until access flow falls to the range of 350–500 mL per minute.

(2)   Implications for AV graft versus AV fistula. Recirculation tests are not a sensitive method of predicting stenosis or imminent thrombosis in AV grafts, as the risk of thrombosis in an AV graft begins to increase when flows fall to 600–800 mL per minute. At that graft flow rate, which is still well above the usual blood pump settings, recirculation measurements should still be zero. True recirculation in an AV graft that is not due to improper needle placement is an urgent indication to study the graft, as the risk of thrombosis at a graft flow rate of 350–500 mL per minute is quite high. Detection of unrecognized needle reversal by measuring recirculation is also clinically useful.

With a failing AV fistula, recirculation measurements are useful in detecting access dysfunction/stenosis, but continued patency of the AV fistula is likely even when recirculation is present (when flows are in the range of 350–500 mL per minute). The benefits of screening AV fistulas for access recirculation are relatively small in terms of preventing thrombosis, but screening for recirculation is useful to prevent underdialysis.

(3)   Methods of detecting access recirculation. Non–urea-based methods for measuring access recirculation have been developed and are identical to those described to measure access blood flow, except that the blood lines are not reversed. These non–urea dilution methods show that recirculation is zero (detection limit of 1%–2%) in the overwhelming majority of patients if the access is properly cannulated (Depner et al, 1995; Sherman et al, 1997). Urea-based methods for measuring access recirculation are described in Chapter 2. If one waits only 10 seconds to draw the sample at a "slow-blood flow rate" of 120 mL per minute), a calculated recirculation value greater than 5%–10% is highly predictive of actual access recirculation (Kapoian and Steward, 1997).

d.   Imaging the vascular access
(1)   Doppler ultrasonography. This noninvasive technique allows direct imaging of the flow pattern in AV grafts and fistulas. It has been useful in the detection of stenoses and the characterization of aneurysms. As lesions can develop within 2–3 months, Doppler ultrasonography flow measurements are prohibitively expensive for routine assessment. Their chief role is in the evaluation of flow and anatomy in accesses that have been screened by other techniques. Some centers refer patients with a high probability of stenosis as determined by low cost methods directly for angiography and balloon angioplasty, bypassing Doppler altogether.

e.   Intervention once access stenosis had been identified
(1)   Percutaneous transluminal catheter angioplasty (PTCA). A percutaneous technique via a 16-gauge dialysis needle inserted into the graft is used. A detailed description of the methods is beyond the scope of this handbook. Intervention with PTCA or surgical revision to correct stenosis before thrombosis occurs dramatically reduces thrombosis rates and the loss of AV grafts (Besarab et al, 1995; Safa et al, 1996). Successful angioplasty or surgical revision should be accompanied by a decrease in either dynamic (blood pump running) or static (blood pump off) access pressures into the normal range and an increase in the measured access flow rate. Restenosis is a frequent event. PTCA yields 90-day patency of 30%–40%, but the procedure can be repeated many times (Beathard, 1992). Surgical revision provides longer patency but utilizes veins. The restenosis rate for subclavian stenoses is considerably higher, with only 30% of treated subclavian veins functional at 6 months. Stents may have a role in a small subgroup with elastic stenoses or rapid recurrence.

2.   Thrombosis
a.   Predisposing factors and prevention. A number of dialysis patients may have subtle accentuation of hemostasis, including high fibrinogen levels, reduced levels of protein S or C, factor V Leiden mutation, or lupus anticoagulant. Whether or not these conditions are associated with increased access thrombosis is controversial. Apparently hematocrit levels greater than 40% are associated with

increased thrombotic risk (Besarab et al, 1998). Warfarin may be indicated for some of these patients, although in patients with protein S or C deficiency, use of warfarin may precipitate skin necrosis, and in patients with lupus anticoagulant, the prothrombin time is an unreliable measure of anticoagulation.

(1) **In AV fistulas.** Thrombosis of the fistula occurs either soon after construction or as a late event. Early thrombosis results from technical factors (and almost always requires surgical revision), although there may be inadvertent compression while sleeping. Poor flow precedes late thrombosis in most cases, but hypotension or hypercoagulability may also precipitate thrombosis.

Treatment of thrombosis is difficult. Neither surgical nor percutaneous methods using urokinase provide good results, but salvage should be attempted, especially when the fistulogram demonstrates a correctable obstruction in the venous limb after declotting (Oakes et al, 1997).

(2) **In AV grafts.** Thrombosis can be managed by surgical thrombectomy or by mechanical or pharmacomechanical thrombolysis (Vesely et al, 1999). The choice is left to the expertise of the medical center. However, it is essential that the following be considered: Treatment should be done within 48 hours to avoid the need for femoral vein catheterization for dialysis. The access should be evaluated after declotting with fistulography to detect residual stenosis (Beathard, 1994). Residual stenosis should be corrected with balloon angioplasty or surgical revision. The role of antiplatelet drugs or warfarin in patients with recurrent thrombosis is unknown (Diskin et al, 1993). Patients who clot with intra-access flows greater than 1,000 mL per minute should be educated about not applying pressure to their accesses, worked up for hypercoagulability, and/or examined for presence of delayed hypotension after dialysis.

(3) **Silent infection in thrombosed AV grafts.** A recent report has suggested that many chronically thrombosed grafts may become infected with few local signs (Ayus and Sheikh-Hamad, 1997), raising the question that perhaps such grafts should be electively removed if flow is not successfully reestablished. This area needs further study.

3. **Ischemia or edema of the graft extremity**
    a. **AV fistula**
       (1) **Ischemia of the hand.** Patients with diabetes, older persons with atherosclerosis, and those with vascular anomalies are at greatest risk. Ischemia distal to an AV access can occur at any time (hours to months) following access construction. Mild ischemia manifested by coldness or paresthesias but without sensory or motor loss can be managed expectantly. Pain of the hand on exercise, a "steal" effect (or in extreme instances even at rest), or the appearance of nonhealing ulcers usually requires surgical intervention. Severe ischemia with nerve injury is an emergency. With the usual radiocephalic side-to-side fistula, the radial artery anastomosis regularly steals

blood flow from the ulnar artery system. Converting the side-of-artery to an end-of-artery anastomosis can sometimes be used to treat ischemia due to steal.

   (2) Edema of the hand. This results from increased pressures in the veins draining the hand. Treatment consists of converting the anastomosis from a side-of-vein to an end-of-vein opening or by selectively tying off affected veins.

  b. AV graft

   (1) Ischemia of the hand. As with AV fistula, ischemia can develop with all of the same risk factors. However, because the access flow increases rapidly and is maximal within days of construction, the symptoms can develop rapidly and the danger of permanent nerve damage is greater.

   (2) Edema of the extremity. A small increase in circumference (2–3 cm) of the arm bearing the access is common. Larger increases indicate venous hypertension due to venous outlet stenosis often secondary to a partially occluded subclavian vein.

4. Pseudoaneurysm

  a. AV fistula. Pseudoaneurysm of the venous limb is much more common than a true aneurysm. It results from inadequate hemostasis and extravasation of blood following dialysis needle removal. Most pseudoaneurysms or true aneurysms are treated by observation only and puncturing the venous limb of the fistula away from the aneurysm site. When marked enlargement and compromise of the overlying skin develops, rupture may develop producing hemorrhage. Large lesions can prevent adequate needle placement and limit potential puncture sites.

  b. AV graft. These should be treated by resection and insertion of an interposition graft if they are (a) rapidly expanding, (b) more than 12 mm in diameter, and (c) threatening viability of the overlying skin.

5. Infections

  a. AV fistula. Infections are rare and usually staphylococcal in origin; they should be treated in the same manner as subacute endocarditis. Diagnosis is based on local signs of inflammation. Prompt therapy with antistaphylococcal antimicrobials after local and blood cultures have been obtained is often curative. Only septic embolus during therapy warrants removal of the fistula.

  b. AV graft. Graft infection occurs eventually in 5%–20% of grafts placed. Thigh grafts have a higher rate of infection. Prophylactic antimicrobials should be used when patients harboring vascular grafts undergo procedures capable of inducing bacteremia, such as dental extraction or genitourinary manipulation. Most graft infections are staphylococcal, but rarely gram-negative organisms such as *Escherichia coli* may be cultured. Initial antibiotic treatment should include drugs active against gram-negative and gram-positive organisms as well as against *Enterococcus.* Local infection of a graft can be treated with antibiotics (based on culture results) and by incision/resection of the infected portion. Extensive infection requires complete excision/removal.

Septicemia may occur without local signs. In such cases, a technetium-labeled leukocyte scan may help reveal a graft infection, but care must be taken to remove any blood-soaked dressings prior to scanning, as they may lead to a falsely positive result (Ghesani et al, 1996). Hemorrhage may occur due to rupture of an infected graft. A graft placed within 30 days that becomes infected should always be removed.

6.   Congestive heart failure. Blood flow rate through an AV fistula or graft can vary from barely adequate (400 mL per minute) to more than 2,000 mL per minute. Wrist and forearm accesses have lower flows than upper arm accesses. Accesses in the leg often have the highest flow rates. Congestive heart failure is unusual with a forearm access but may occur in patients with upper arm or femoral fistulas. Surgical narrowing or banding should be done only after cardiac studies have shown marked changes in cardiac output following transient occlusion of the fistula. Long-term cardiac function is generally unaffected by the presence of an AV access. In patients with unexplained high cardiac output states, the role of anemia and use of vasodilators, such as minoxidil or hydralazine, without concomitant β blockade should always be ruled out.

SELECTED READINGS

Ayus AC, Sheikh-Hamad D. Silent infections in clotted hemodialysis access grafts. *J Am Soc Nephrol* 1998;9:1314–1317.

Besarab A, et al. The effects of normal versus anemic hematocrit on hemodialysis patients with cardiac disease. *N Engl J Med* 1998; 339:584–590.

Beathard GA. Mechanical versus pharmacomechanical thrombolysis for the treatment of thrombosed dialysis access grafts: a controlled study. *Kidney Int* 1994;45:1401–1406.

Besarab A, et al. The utility of intra-access monitoring in detecting and correcting venous outlet stenoses prior to thrombosis. *Kidney Int* 1995;47:1364–1373.

Besarab A, et al. Simplified measurement of intra-access pressure. *ASAIO J* 1996;42:M682–M687.

Besarab A, Sherman R. The relationship of recirculation to access blood flow. *Am J Kidney Dis* 1997;29:223–229.

Bolz KD, et al. Catheter malfunction and thrombus formation on double-lumen hemodialysis catheters: an intravascular ultrasonographic study. *Am J Kidney Dis* 1995:25:597–602.

Bour ES, et al. Experience with the double lumen Silastic catheter for hemoaccess. *Surg Gynecol Obstet* 1990;171:33.

Carlisle EJF, et al. Septicemia in long-time jugular hemodialysis catheters: eradicating infection by changing the catheter over a guidewire. *Int J Artif Organs* 1991;14:150.

Crain MR, et al. Fibrin sleeve stripping for salvage of failing hemodialysis catheters: technique and initial results. *Radiology* 1996;198: 41–44.

Daiehagh P, et al. Efficacy of tissue plasminogen activator administration on patency of hemodialysis access catheters. *Am J Kidney Dis* 2000;36:75–79.

Depner TA, Krivitsky NM, MacGibbon D. Hemodialysis access recirculation measured by ultrasound dilution. *ASAIO J* 1995;41: M749–M753.

Dinwiddie LC, et al. Comparison of measures for prospective identification of venous stenosis. *ANNA J* 1996;23:593–600.

Dionisio P, et al. Monitoring of central venous dual-lumen catheter placement in haemodialysis: improvement in technique for the practicing nephrologist. *Nephrol Dial Transplant* 1995:10:874–876.

Diskin CJ, Stokes TJ, Pennell AT. Pharmacologic intervention to prevent hemodialysis vascular access thrombosis. Editorial review. *Nephron* 1993;64:1–26.

Farrell J, Gellens M. Ultrasound-guided cannulation versus the landmark-guided technique for haemodialysis access. *Nephrol Dial Transplant* 1997;12:1234–1237.

Ghesani M, et al. Importance of dressing removal before radiolabeled WBC imaging for musculoskeletal infection. *Clin Nuclear Med* 1996;21:537–540.

Hakim RM, Lazarus JM. Initiation of dialysis. *J Am Soc Nephrol* 1995:6:1319–1328.

Hung K-Y, et al. Infection associated with double lumen catheterization for temporary haemodialysis: experience of 168 cases. *Nephrol Dial Transplant* 1995;10:247–251.

Kanterman RY, et al. Dialysis access grafts: anatomic location of venous stenoses and results of angioplasty. *Radiology* 1995;195:135–139.

Kapoian T, Steward CA, Sherman RA. Validation of a revised slow flow/stop flow recirculation method. *Kidney Int* 1997;52:839–842.

Kite P, et al. Evaluation of a novel endoluminal brush for the in situ diagnosis of catheter related sepsis. *J Clin Pathol* 1997;50:278–282.

Kite P, et al. Rapid diagnosis of central-venous-catheter-related bloodstream infection without catheter removal. *Lancet* 1999;354: 1504–1507.

Kovalik EC, et al. A clustering of epidural abscesses in chronic hemodialysis patients: risks of salvaging access catheters in cases of infection. *J Am Soc Nephrol* 1996;10:2264–2267.

Krivitski NM. Theory and validation of access flow measurement by dilution technique during hemodialysis. *Kidney Int* 1995;48:244–250.

Lund GB, et al. Outcome of tunneled hemodialysis catheters placed by radiologists. *Radiology* 1996;198:467–472.

McLaughlin K, et al. Long-term vascular access for hemodialysis using silicone dual-lumen catheters with guidewire replacement of catheters for technique salvage. *Am J Kidney Dis* 1997;29:553–559.

Maki DG, et al. Prevention of central venous catheter-related bloodstream infection by use of an antiseptic-impregnated catheter. *Ann Intern Med* 1997;127:257–266.

Maki DG, Weise CE, Sarafin HW. A semiquantitative culture method for identifying intravenous-catheter-related infection. *N Engl J Med* 1977;296:1305–1309.

Marr KA, et al. Catheter-related bacteremia and outcome of attempted catheter salvage in patients undergoing hemodialysis. *Ann Intern Med* 1997;127:275–280.

Middlebrook MR, et al. Thrombosed hemodialysis grafts: percutaneous mechanical balloon declotting versus thrombolysis. *Radiology* 1995:196:73–77.

Moss AH, et al. Use of silicone dual-lumen catheter with a Dacron cuff as a long-term vascular access for hemodialysis patients. *Am J Kidney Dis* 1990;16:211–215.

Oakes DD, et al. Surgical salvage of failed radiocephalic arteriovenous fistulae: techniques and results in 29 patients. *Kidney Int* 1998;53: 480–487.

Prabhu PN, et al. Long-term performance and complications of Tesio twin catheter systems for hemodialysis access. *Am J Kidney Dis* 1997;30:213–219.

Safa AA, et al. Detection and treatment of dysfunctional hemodialysis access grafts: effect of a surveillance program on graft patency and the incidence of thrombosis. *Radiology* 1996;199:653–657.

Sands J, Jabayc P, Miranda C. Delivered blood flow in cuffed central venous dialysis catheters. *ASAIO J* 1997;43:69(abst).

Sands J, Glidden D, Miranda C. Access flow measured during hemodialysis. *ASAIO J* 1996;42:M530–M532.

Sands J, et al. Difference between delivered and prescribed blood flow in hemodialysis. *ASAIO J* 1996;42:M717–M719.

Schillinger F, et al. Post catheterization vein stenosis in haemodialysis. Comparative angiographic study of 50 subclavian and 50 internal jugular accesses. *Nephrol Dial Transplant* 1994;6:722–724.

Schwab SJ, et al. Prevention of hemodialysis fistula thrombosis. Early detection of venous stenosis. *Kidney Int* 1989;36:707–711.

Shaffer D, et al. Use of Dacron cuffed silicone catheters as long-term hemodialysis access. *ASAIO J* 1992;38:55–58.

Sherman R, et al. Recognition of the failing vascular access: a current perspective. *Semin Dial* 1997;10:1–5.

Skolnick ML. The role of sonography in the placement and management of jugular and subclavian central venous catheters. *AJR Am J Roentgenol* 1994:164:291–295.

Tanriover B, et al. Bacteremia associated with tunneled dialysis catheters: comparison of two treatment strategies. Kidney Int 2000; 57:2151–2155.

Tesio F, et al. Double catheterization of the internal jugular vein for hemodialysis: indications, techniques, and clinical results. *Artif Organs* 1994;18:301–304.

Trerotola SO, et al. Thrombosed dialysis access grafts: percutaneous mechanical declotting without urokinase. *Radiology* 1996;198:41–44.

Turmel-Rodrigues L, et al. Treatment of failed native arteriovenous fistulae for hemodialysis by interventional radiology. *Kidney Int* 2000;57:1124–1140.

Twardowski ZJ, et al. Blood recirculation in intravenous catheters for hemodialysis. *J Am Soc Nephrol* 1993;12:1978–1981.

Twardowski ZJ. High-dose intradialytic/urokinase to restore patency of permanent central vein hemodialysis catheters. *Am J Kidney Dis* 1998;31:841–847.

Uldall R. Permanent vascular access for hemodialysis. Percutaneous jugular vein cannulation for hemodialysis access in patients with end-stage renal failure: special points of technique. *Semin Dial* 1995;8:187–191.

Veseley TM, et al. Comparison of the Angiojet rheolytic catheter to surgical thrombectomy for the treatment of thrombosed hemodialysis grafts. Peripheral Angiojet Clinical Trial. *J Vasc Interven Radiol* 1999;10:1195–1205.

Weitzel WF, et al. Successful use of indwelling cuffed femoral vein catheters in ambulatory hemodialysis patients. *Am J Kidney Dis* 1993;22:426–429.

Ziegler TW, et al. Prolonging the life of difficult hemodialysis access using thrombolysis, angiography, and angioplasty. *J Assoc Ren Replace Ther* 1995;2:52–59.

Internet References

DOQI guidelines for vascular access (http://www.hdcn.com/hd/doqiva.htm)

Available venous catheters for hemodialysis (http://www.hdcn.com/hd/cathve.htm)

Abstract/article update: venous catheters for hemodialysis (http://www.hdcn.com/hd/venous.htm)

Abstract/article update: AV access (http://www.hdcn.com/hd/arterial.htm)

5

Acute Hemodialysis Prescription

John T. Daugirdas, Edward A. Ross, and Allen R. Nissenson

This chapter deals with intermittent hemodialysis only. Continuous therapies are available and should be part of the nephrologist's armamentarium. They are useful when daily obligatory fluid gain exceeds 3–4 L per day or when fluid overload is combined with a markedly hypotensive patient requiring vasopressors. The continuous therapies are discussed in Chapter 10.

I. The hemodialysis prescription. All patients are different, and the circumstances eventuating in the need for acute hemodialysis vary widely. The prescription for hemodialysis will change accordingly. As a teaching tool only, we present a "typical" prescription for an acute hemodialysis in a 70-kg adult.

R_x: Acute hemodialysis (not for initial treatment)
Session length: Perform hemodialysis for 4 hours
Blood flow rate: 350 mL per minute
Dialyzer:
Dialyzer membrane: your choice
Dialyzer K_{Uf}: your choice
Dialyzer efficiency: usually a dialyzer with a *KoA* of 500–800 is used
Dialysis solution composition (variable):
Base: bicarbonate 25 mEq per L
Sodium: 145 mEq per L
Potassium: 3.5 mEq per L
Calcium: 3.5 mEq per L
Magnesium: 0.75 mEq per L
Dextrose: 200 mg per dL
Phosphate: none
Dialysis solution flow rate: 500 mL per minute
Dialysis solution temperature: 35–36°C
Fluid removal orders:
Use ultrafiltration control device
Remove 2.2 L over 4 hours at a constant rate
Anticoagulation orders:
See Chapter 9

A. Determining dialysis session length and blood flow rate. The dialysis session length together with the blood flow rate are the most important determinants of the amount of dialysis to be given (dialyzer efficiency is also a factor).

1. Reduce the amount of dialysis for the initial one or two sessions. For the initial treatment, especially when the predialysis serum urea nitrogen (SUN) level is very high (e.g., greater than 130 mg per dL, the dialysis session length and blood flow rate should be reduced to result in a urea reduction ratio of about 40%. This usually means using a blood flow rate that is about three times the body weight in kilograms for adults (however, blood flow rate should be kept high when heparin-free dialysis is being used to prevent clotting), along with a 2-hour treatment time. A longer initial dialysis session or use of excessively high blood flow rates in the acute setting may result in the so-called disequilibrium syndrome, described more fully in Chapter 7. This neurologic syndrome, which includes the appearance of obtundation, or even seizures and coma, during or after dialysis, has been associated with excessively rapid removal of blood solutes. The risk of disequilibrium syndrome is increased when the predialysis serum urea nitrogen level is high. If a longer session is required for purposes of fluid removal, just before or after the dialysis session, dialysate flow can be routed to bypass the dialyzer for an additional period of isolated ultrafiltration (Chapter 10).

After the initial dialysis session, the patient can be reevaluated and should generally be dialyzed again the following day.

The length of the second dialysis session can usually be increased to 3 hours, provided that the predialysis serum urea nitrogen level is less than 100 mg per dL, and the third and subsequent dialysis sessions can often be up to 6 hours in length. The length of a single dialysis treatment rarely exceeds 6 hours unless the purpose of dialysis is treatment of drug overdose.

2. Dialysis frequency and dose for subsequent treatments and dialysis adequacy. It is difficult to deliver a large amount of dialysis in the acute setting. True delivered blood flow rate through a venous catheter rarely exceeds 350 mL per minute and often is substantially lower. Recirculation occurs in venous catheters and is greatest with catheters in the femoral position due to the low pericatheter venous flow rate. Often the treatment is interrupted due to hypotension. Furthermore, the degree of urea sequestration in muscle may be increased, as such patients often are on pressors, reducing blood flow to muscle and skin, which contain a substantial portion of urea and other dissolved waste products. Concomitant intravenous infusions, which often are given to patients in an acute setting, dilute the urea level in the blood, and reduce efficiency of dialysis. Recent data suggest that a typical 3- to 4-hour acute-dialysis session will deliver a single-pool Kt/V of only 0.9, with an equilibrated Kt/V of 0.7. Dialysate-side urea removal may be even lower (Evanson et al, 1999). This low level of Kt/V, if given three times per week, is associated with a high mortality in chronic, stable patients. Nevertheless, there are very few controlled studies relating amount of dialysis to survival in the acute setting, and in many centers, standard therapy is a 3- to 4-hour session given every other day.

One option is to dialyze sick patients with acute renal failure on a daily (six times per week) basis. Each treatment is then approximately 3–4 hours in length. Recent preliminary data by Schiffl et al (1997) suggest that mortality is reduced in patients with acute renal failure dialyzed daily as opposed to those receiving a similar amount of therapy every other day. If every-other-day dialysis is to be given, the treatment length should probably be set at 4–6 hours, to deliver at least a single-pool Kt/V of at least 1.2–1.3, as recommended for chronic therapy. Sustained low-efficiency dialysis (SLED), using 6–12 hour daily sessions with low dialysate and blood flow rates, is also becoming popular (see Chapter 10).

The amount of dialysis may need to be adjusted upwards in hypercatabolic patients, but a low predialysis SUN level should not be used as a justification to reduce the amount of dialysis given unless substantial residual renal urea clearance is documented.

B.   Choosing a dialyzer

  1.   Membrane. The differences among dialyzer membranes are discussed in Chapter 3.

  a.   Increased infections/mortality during use of unsubstituted cellulose membranes to treat acute renal failure. Two studies (Schiffl et al, 1994; Himmelfarb et al, 1998) initially suggested that use of unsubstituted cellulose membranes for acute dialysis might prolong the course of acute renal failure and increase the risk of oliguria, and also (in the Schiffl study) might increase mortality, especially due to infection. The hypothesis is that complement-activated neutrophils migrate to injured glomeruli and cause further damage by generating reactive oxygen compounds. However, two other randomized studies failed to find any deleterious effects of using unsubstituted cellulose membranes for acute dialysis (Kurtal et al, 1995; Jorres et al, 1999). Also, there is no evidence that the use of substituted cellulose membranes such as cellulose acetate, diacetate, or triacetate, or Hemophan, is harmful when treating acute renal failure in comparison with synthetic membranes (Gastaldello et al, 2000; Assouad et al, 1996).

  b.   High-flux membranes. The better results found by Hakim et al (1996) were obtained when using a low-flux biocompatible synthetic membrane. However, the better results found by Schiffl et al were based on use of a high-flux synthetic membrane, confounding issues of biocompatibility and flux. No recommendation favoring use of high-flux membranes for acute dialysis can be made at this time, as membrane flux has not been studied as a separate factor in any randomized study of acute dialysis.

  c.   Anaphylactoid reactions in patients taking angiotensin-converting enzyme (ACE) inhibitors. In patients taking ACE inhibitors (e.g., captopril, enalapril, lisinopril), acute anaphylactoid reactions have been reported during dialysis (Parnes and Shapiro, 1991). In most of the cases published to date, patients were being dialyzed with the AN69 membrane. AN69 is a copolymer of polyacrylonitrile and sodium methallyl sulfonate. The AN69 membrane is negatively charged. One hypothesis is that the surface negative charges may activate the bradykinin system. Activity of bradykinin and other kinins is enhanced in patients taking ACE inhibitors because ACE deactivates kinins.

  2.   Mode of sterilization. Most dialyzers available in the United States are sterilized with ethylene oxide. Rarely, patients manifest severe anaphylactic reactions during hemodialysis, usually on the basis of immunoglobulin E (IgE)-mediated hypersensitivity to ethylene oxide. Such reactions often occur the first time a new patient is dialyzed. The incidence of such reactions is quite low (3–5/100,00), but may be higher in atopic individuals and in those with blood eosinophilia. For such patients, use of a γ-irradiated or steam-sterilized dialyzer (see Table 3-1) might be appropriate. For all patients, special attention should be paid to rinse properly ethylene oxide-sterilized dialyzers prior to use.

3. Ultrafiltration coefficient (K_{Uf}). The desired water permeability of the dialyzer to be chosen depends on whether an ultrafiltration controller is available. The ultrafiltration controller accurately controls the ultrafiltration rate by means of special pumps and circuits. By and large, most of the machines with volumetric ultrafiltration controllers are designed to use dialyzers of high water permeability (e.g., K_{Uf} more than 6.0) and may lose accuracy if a high fluid removal rate is attempted using a dialyzer that is relatively impermeable to water.

If a dialysis machine with an ultrafiltration controller is not available, then a membrane with a relatively low water permeability (K_{Uf}) should be chosen, so that the transmembrane pressure (TMP) will have to be set at a relatively high level to remove the amount of fluid desired; then the inevitable errors in maintaining the desired TMP will have less impact on the rate of fluid removal.

Desired fluid removal rate	**Ideal in vivo dialyzer K_{Uf}**
<500 mL/hr	<3.0
500–1000 mL/hr	3.0–4.0
>1,000 mL/hr	4.0–5.0

When close monitoring of the fluid removal rate is required and a machine with advanced ultrafiltration control circuitry is not available, the fluid removal rate can be monitored by placing the patient on an electronic bed or chair scale and continuously following the weight during dialysis.

4. Dialyzer urea clearance. For the first couple of dialysis sessions, it is best to avoid using very high-efficiency dialyzers. A dialyzer with an in vitro KoA urea of about 500 mL per minute is recommended to minimize the risk of inadvertent overdialysis and of developing the disequilibrium syndrome. After that, particularly if a high blood flow rate is being used, the largest dialyzer that can economically be used should be chosen.

C. Choosing the dialysis solution. In our example, we have chosen a bicarbonate level of 25 mEq per L, with a sodium level of 145 mEq per L, a potassium level of 3.5 mEq per L, a calcium level of 3.5 mEq per L, a magnesium level of 0.75 mEq per L, a dextrose level of 200 mg per dL, and no phosphorus. Depending on the circumstances, this prescription may have to be altered in a given patient. It is important to recognize that for acute patients the dialysate composition should be tailored, and the "standard" composition designed for acidotic, hyperphosphatemic, hyperkalemic, chronic dialysis patients more often than not is inappropriate in an acute setting.

1. **Dialysis solution bicarbonate concentration.** In the sample prescription above, we have chosen to use a 25 mEq per L bicarbonate level. Standard, higher bicarbonate levels will, of course, be required in treating acidotic patients. However, acute patients often are relatively alkalotic for reasons described below. If the predialysis plasma bicarbonate level is 28 mEq per L or higher, or if the patient has respiratory alkalosis, standard dialysis solution containing 35 or 38 mEq per L bicarbonate should not be used. Rather, a custom dialysis solution should be mixed with an appropriately lower bicarbonate level (e.g., 20–28 mEq per L, depending on the degree of alkalosis).

   a.   Dangers of metabolic alkalosis. A dialysis patient with even a mild metabolic alkalosis (e.g., plasma bicarbonate level of 30 mEq per L) requires very little hyperventilation to increase blood pH to dangerous levels. In many respects, alkalemia (blood pH higher than 7.50) is more dangerous to the organism than acidemia. Dangers of alkalemia include soft-tissue calcification and cardiac arrhythmia (sometimes with sudden death). Alkalemia also has been associated with such adverse symptoms as nausea, lethargy, and headache.

   b.   Predialysis metabolic alkalosis. In dialysis patients, the most common causes of metabolic alkalosis are a reduced intake of protein, intensive dialysis for any reason (e.g., daily dialysis), and vomiting or nasogastric suction. Another common cause is administered lactate or acetate with total parenteral nutrition (TPN) solutions. Calcium carbonate and acetate are poorly absorbed and cause little alteration of acid–base balance. Coadministration of aluminum hydroxide with sodium polystyrene sulfonate resin can cause alkalosis because the resin binds aluminum, and the latter can no longer bind to and sequester bicarbonate secreted by the pancreas. The bicarbonate is reabsorbed, causing the alkalosis (Madias and Levey, 1983).

   c.   Predialysis respiratory alkalosis. Many patients who are candidates for acute dialysis have preexisting respiratory alkalosis. The causes of respiratory alkalosis are the same as in patients with normal renal function and include pulmonary disease (pneumonia, edema, embolus), hepatic failure, and central nervous system disorders. Normally, compensation for respiratory alkalosis is twofold. There is an acute decrease in the plasma bicarbonate level due to release of hydrogen ions from body buffer stores. In patients with normal renal function, there is a further delayed (2–3 days) compensatory fall in the plasma bicarbonate level due to excretion of bicarbonate in the urine. Renal bicarbonate excretion obviously cannot occur in dialysis patients. The therapeutic goal should always be to normalize the pH rather than the plasma bicarbonate level. In patients with respiratory alkalosis, the plasma bicarbonate level at which the blood pH will be normal may be as low as 17–20 mEq per L; the dialysis solution to use should contain less than the usual amount of bicarbonate to achieve a postdialysis plasma bicarbonate level in the desired subnormal range.

d. Achieving an appropriately low dialysate bicarbonate level. In certain machines, the proportioning ratio of concentrate to product water is fixed, and as a result the dialysate bicarbonate level can be reduced only by changing the concentrate bicarbonate level. With such machines the bicarbonate cannot be reduced below about 32 mEq per L. In machines where the concentrate/product water ratio can be changed, bicarbonate levels as low as 20 mEq per L usually can be delivered, but not lower. A low-base dialysis solution can be made using a batch system (i.e., mixing the solution from its component chemicals in a large tank). The problems of batch-mixing bicarbonate-containing dialysis solution (loss of Pco_2 and calcium and magnesium precipitation) are discussed in Chapters 2 and 3.

e. Patients with severe predialysis metabolic acidosis

(1) Dangers of excessive correction of metabolic acidosis. Excessive correction of severe metabolic acidosis (plasma bicarbonate level less than 10 mEq per L) can have adverse consequences, including paradoxical acidification of the cerebrospinal fluid and an increase in the tissue production rate of lactic acid. Initial therapy should aim for only partial correction of the plasma bicarbonate level; a target postdialysis plasma bicarbonate value of 15–20 mEq per L is generally appropriate.

(2) Respiratory acidosis. The normal compensation to respiratory acidosis is an acute buffer response, which can increase the plasma bicarbonate level by 2–4 mEq per L, followed by a delayed (3–4 days) increase in renal bicarbonate generation. Because the second response is obviated in dialysis patients, respiratory acidosis will have a more pronounced effect on blood pH than in patients with normal renal function.

2. Dialysis solution sodium level. The dialysis solution sodium level in the sample prescription is 145 mEq per L. This level is generally acceptable for patients who have normal or slightly reduced predialysis serum sodium concentrations. If marked predialysis hypernatremia or hyponatremia is present, the dialysis solution sodium level will have to be adjusted accordingly.

a. Hyponatremia. Hyponatremia is common in seriously ill patients requiring acute dialysis, primarily because such patients often have received large amounts of hyponatric intravenous solutions with their medications and parenteral nutrition. Hyponatremia is frequently seen accompanying severe hyperglycemia in diabetic dialysis patients. For every increase of 100 mg per dL in the serum glucose concentration, there is a corresponding initial decrease of 1.3 mEq per L in the serum sodium concentration due to osmotic shift of water from the intracellular to the extracellular compartment. Because osmotic diuresis secondary to the hyperglycemia does not occur, the excess plasma water is not excreted and hyponatremia is maintained. Correction of hyperglycemia by insulin administration reverses the initial water shift and thereby corrects the hyponatremia.

(1) Predialysis serum sodium level greater than 130 mEq per L. If the patient is to undergo an average-efficiency, 4-hour dialysis, then a postdialysis serum sodium level of 140 mEq per L can usually be achieved by setting the dialysis solution sodium concentration to 140 + (140 − predialysis serum sodium value). For example, if the predialysis serum sodium level is 130 mEq per L, to attain normonatremia the dialysis solution sodium concentration should be 150 mEq per L (140 + [140 − 130]). Overcorrection or undercorrection of the serum sodium level results if an unusually intense or mild dialysis treatment, respectively, is administered (e.g., by virtue of altered treatment length or blood flow).

(2) Predialysis serum sodium level less than 130 mEq per L. When the degree of predialysis hyponatremia is moderate to severe, and especially if the hyponatremia is of long duration, it may be dangerous to achieve normonatremia quickly. Rapid correction of hyponatremia has been linked to a potentially fatal neurologic syndrome known as osmotic demyelination syndrome (whether it is in fact linked is controversial). The maximum safe rate of correction of the serum sodium concentration in severely hyponatremic patients is controversial. At this stage of incomplete knowledge, it seems prudent when treating patients with severe, longstanding hyponatremia to set the dialysis solution sodium level no higher than 15–20 mEq per L above the plasma level, with the goal of correcting hyponatremia during multiple dialysis treatments performed over several days.

b. Hypernatremia. Hypernatremia is less common than hyponatremia in a hemodialysis setting but does occur, usually in a context of dehydration, osmotic diuresis, and failure to give sufficient electrolyte-free water. It is somewhat dangerous to attempt to correct hypernatremia by hemodialyzing against a low-sodium dialysis solution. Whenever the dialysis solution sodium level is more than 3–5 mEq per L lower than the plasma value, three complications of dialysis occur with increased incidence:

(1) Osmotic contraction of the plasma volume occurs as water shifts from the dialyzed blood (containing less sodium than before) to the relatively hyperosmotic interstitium, causing hypotension.

(2) The propensity to develop muscle cramps is increased.

(3) Water from the dialyzed, relatively hyponatremic blood enters cells, causing cerebral edema and exacerbating the disequilibrium syndrome.

The risk of disequilibrium syndrome is the most important one; use of low-sodium dialysis solution should certainly be avoided in situations in which the predialysis SUN level is high (e.g., greater than 100 mg per dL). The safest approach is to first dialyze a patient with a dialysis solution sodium level close (within 2 mEq per L) to that of plasma and then correct the hypernatremia by slow administration of slightly hyponatric fluids.

3. Dialysis solution potassium level. The usual dialysis solution potassium concentration for acute dialysis ranges from 2.0 to 4.5 mEq per L. An important number of patients requiring acute dialysis will have a plasma potassium value in the normal or even the subnormal range, especially in patients with nonoliguric acute renal failure and in oliguric patients if food intake is poor. Hypokalemia is also a complication of total parenteral nutrition. Correction of severe acidosis during dialysis causes a shift of potassium into cells, lowering the plasma potassium level further. Hypokalemia and arrhythmia can result.

Whenever the predialysis serum potassium level is less than 4.0 mEq per L, the dialysate potassium level should be 4.0 mEq per L or higher.

In patients with a predialysis plasma potassium level greater than 5.5 mEq per L, a dialysis solution potassium level of 2.0 is usually appropriate in stable patients, but the dialysis solution potassium concentration should be raised to 2.5 or 3.0 in patients at risk for arrhythmia or in those receiving digitalis. If the potassium level is higher than 7.0, some nephrologists will use a dialysis solution potassium level below 2.0 mEq per L. However, the plasma potassium level must be monitored hourly, and there is considerable danger of precipitating arrhythmia if the plasma potassium concentration is lowered too rapidly.

a. Potassium rebound. There is a marked rebound increase in the serum potassium level within 1–2 hours after dialysis. One should resist the temptation to treat a postdialysis hypokalemia with potassium supplements unless there are extenuating circumstances.

b. Acute hyperkalemia. Patients with very severe hyperkalemia present with alterations on the electrocardiogram (low P waves, peaked T waves, widening of the QRS, cardiac standstill), along with weakness and lethargy. Such patients should be treated immediately with intravenous infusion of calcium chloride or calcium gluconate or intravenous glucose plus insulin while arrangements for emergency hemodialysis are being made. The response to intravenous sodium bicarbonate in dialysis patients is suboptimal. Another therapy is intravenous or inhaled albuterol.

c. Subacute hyperkalemia. Treatment includes review of the diet and oral administration of a sodium–potassium exchange resin (e.g., as sodium polystyrene sulfonate, given orally or as an enema). The resin usually is given orally with sorbitol to prevent constipation or mixed with sorbitol as an enema. However, several reports of intestinal necrosis associated with sorbitol and oral sodium polystyrene sulfonate have been published (e.g., Gardiner, 1997). The risk of alkalosis with coadministration of sodium polystyrene sulfonate and aluminum hydroxide has been noted above.

d. Potassium removal and dialysis solution glucose. Potassium removal during dialysis using glucose-free dialysis solution may be 30% greater than potassium removal using a 200 mg per dL glucose solution because with glucose-free dialysis solution there may be decreased intradialytic translocation of potassium into cells (Ward et al, 1987). Use of a dialysis solution containing 100 mg per dL glucose may be the best option.

4. Dialysis solution calcium levels. The normal level for acute dialysis is 3.0–3.5 mEq per L, respectively. There is some evidence that dialysis solution calcium levels lower than 3.0 mEq per L predispose to hypotension during dialysis (van der Sande et al, 1998). In patients with predialysis hypocalcemia, unless a sufficiently high dialysate calcium level is used, correction of acidosis can result in further lowering of the ionized plasma calcium level (with possible precipitation of seizures). A recent study showed that QTc dispersion increased (potentially promoting arrhythmias) when a low calcium dialysis solution was used (Nappi et al, 2000). Routine use of 2.5 mEq per L calcium dialysate (now standard for treatment of chronic dialysis patients taking calcium-containing phosphorus binders) is conceptually inappropriate in the acute setting, where a decline in the ionized calcium concentration is usually undesirable.

   a. Dialytic treatment of acute hypercalcemia. Hemodialysis can be effective in lowering the serum calcium concentration in hypercalcemic patients. In most commercially prepared hemodialysis solutions, the calcium concentration ranges from 5 to 7 mg per dL (2.5–3.5 mEq per L). We prefer to add at least 2.5 mEq per L calcium to the hemodialysis solution to minimize the possibility of an overly rapid decrease in the serum ionized calcium (which can cause tetany or seizures). Frequent measurement of the serum ionized calcium concentration and physical examination of the patient should be performed during dialysis to avoid these complications.

5. Dialysis solution magnesium levels. The usual dialysate magnesium level ranges from 0.75 to 1.5 mEq per L. Even lower magnesium concentrations in dialysate have been used chronically in combination with magnesium carbonate as a phosphorus binder. Magnesium is a vasodilator, and in acute dialysis one preliminary report suggests that blood pressure is better maintained when a dialysate magnesium level of 0.75 mEq per L was used versus dialysate containing 1.5 mEq per L magnesium (Roy and Danziger, 1996).

   a. Hypomagnesemia. Hypomagnesemia occurs in malnourished dialysis patients and in dialysis patients receiving TPN (due to shifting of magnesium into cells during anabolism). Hypomagnesemia can cause cardiac arrhythmia and can impair the release and action of parathyroid hormone. Serum magnesium values should be carefully monitored in dialysis patients during TPN, and TPN fluids should be supplemented routinely with magnesium unless the serum magnesium level is high.

   b. Hypermagnesemia. Hypermagnesemia is usually caused by accidental or covert use of magnesium-containing laxatives, enemas, or antacids. Manifestations of hypermagnesemia include hypotension, weakness, and brady-arrhythmias. Treatment is cessation of ingestion of magnesium-containing compounds. Hemodialysis also is effective in lowering the serum magnesium level.

6. Dialysis solution dextrose level. Dialysis solution for acute dialysis should always contain dextrose (200 mL per dL). Septic patients, diabetics, and patients receiving β-blockers are at risk of developing severe hypoglycemia during dialysis. Addition of dextrose to the dialysis solution reduces the risk of hypoglycemia and may also result in a lower incidence of dialysis-related side effects. The interaction between dialysate solution glucose and potassium has been discussed above.

7. Dialysis solution phosphate levels. Phosphate is normally absent from the dialysis solution, and justifiably so, as patients in renal failure typically have elevated serum phosphate values. Use of a large surface area dialyzer and provision of a longer dialysis session increase the amount of phosphate removed during dialysis.

   a. Hypophosphatemia. Malnourished patients and patients receiving hyperalimentation may have low or low-normal predialysis serum phosphate levels. Predialysis hypophosphatemia may also be present in patients being intensively dialyzed for any purpose. In such patients, hypophosphatemia can be aggravated by dialysis against a zero-phosphate bath. Severe hypophosphatemia can cause respiratory muscle weakness and alterations in hemoglobin oxygen affinity. This can lead to respiratory arrest during dialysis. For patients at risk, phosphate can be added to the dialysis solution. Alternatively, phosphate can be given intravenously, although this must be done carefully to avoid overcorrection and hypocalcemia.

   b. Adding phosphorus to bicarbonate-containing dialysis solutions. For prevention of hypophosphatemia the phosphorus concentration in the final dialysis solution should be about 1.3 mmol per L (4 mg per dL).

   Phosphorus cannot be added to concentrate for acetate-containing dialysis solutions because of Ca-Mg-PO$_4$ solubility problems. Phosphorus can be added to the bicarbonate component of the concentrate (which does not contain calcium or magnesium).

   (1) Phosphosoda-buffered saline laxative (designed for oral consumption, manufactured by C. B. Fleet Co., Inc., Lynchburg, VA) is an inexpensive source of phosphorus. This product contains 0.48 g of sodium biphosphate (NaH$_2$PO$_4 \cdot$ H$_2$O) and 0.18 g of sodium phosphate (Na$_2$HPO$_4 \cdot$ 7H$_2$O) per mL, totaling 4.8 mmol per mL sodium and 4.2 mmol per mL phosphorus.

   (2) The amount added to the bicarbonate component of the concentrate depends on the dilution ratio. In most machines, the bicarbonate component is diluted 1:20. If such is the case, then addition of 60 mL of the above product to 9.5 L of bicarbonate component concentrate (the amount required to generate 190 L of final dialysis solution) results in a phosphorus level in the final dialysis solution of 1.3 mmol per L. (Additional information is given in Yu et al, 1992.) This use is not FDA-approved, and information about Fleet's phosphosoda content of aluminum and other trace elements is not available at this time.

D. Choosing the dialysis solution flow rates. For acute dialysis, the usual dialysis solution flow rate is 500 mL per minute.

E. Dialysis solution temperature. This is usually 35–37°C. The lower range should be used in hypotension prone patients (see Chapter 7).

F. Ultrafiltration orders. Fluid removal needs may range from 0 to 5 kg per dialysis session.

    1. Guidelines for ultrafiltration orders. Some guidelines to gauge the total amount of fluid that needs to be removed are as follows:

        a. Even patients who are quite edematous and in pulmonary edema, rarely need removal of more than 4 L of fluid during the initial session. Remaining excess fluid is best removed during a second session the following day.

        b. If the patient does not have pedal edema or anasarca, in the absence of pulmonary congestion, it is unusual to need to remove more than 2 liters over the dialysis session, In fact, the fluid removal requirement may be zero in patients with little or no jugular venous distention. If so, a dialyzer with a very low K_{Uf} (less than 2.5) should be chosen, or an ultrafiltration controller machine should be used to prevent inadvertent fluid removal (and resultant hypotension) during dialysis due to the unavoidable positive pressure in the blood compartment.

        c. The fluid removal plan during dialysis should take into account the 0.2 L that the patient will receive at the end of dialysis in the form of saline to rinse the dialyzer and any other fluid ingested or administered during the hemodialysis session.

        d. As noted above, if it is the initial dialysis, the length of the dialysis session should be limited to 2 hours. However, if a large amount of fluid (e.g., 4.0 L) must be removed, it is impractical and dangerous to remove such an amount over a 2-hour period. In such instances, the dialysis solution flow can initially be shut off and isolated ultrafiltration (see Chapter 10) can be performed for 1–2 hours, removing 2–3 kg of fluid. Immediately thereafter, dialysis can be performed for 2 hours, removing the remainder of the desired fluid volume. (If severe electrolyte abnormalities, such as hyperkalemia, are present, dialysis may have to be performed prior to isolated ultrafiltration.)

        An alternative approach is to dialyze such a patient for 4–5 hours at a reduced blood flow rate and remove the fluid at 1 L per hour. However, blood flow rates lower than 200 mL per minute through adult-size dialyzers may increase the risk of dialyzer clotting.

        e. In general, it is best to remove fluid at a constant rate throughout the dialysis treatment. This is best done by a dialysis machine that incorporates an ultrafiltration controller. If the dialysis solution sodium level has been set lower than the plasma value (e.g., in the treatment of hyper-natremia), the ultrafiltration rate should initially be reduced to compensate for the osmotic contraction of blood volume that will occur as the plasma sodium concentration is being rapidly lowered.

In patients with acute renal failure, it is extremely important to avoid hypotension at all times, including during dialysis. In a rat model of acute renal failure, Kelleher et al (1987) showed that the renal autoregulatory response to systemic hypotension is greatly impaired. They found that transient episodes of hypotension caused by blood withdrawal caused further renal damage and delay of functional renal recovery.

2. Impact of dialysis frequency on ultrafiltration needs. It is difficult in an acute setting to limit a patient's fluid gain to less than 2 L per day. Often 3 L per day is absorbed in patients receiving parenteral nutrition. Use of a daily (six times per week) dialysis schedule reduces the amount of fluid that must be removed with each dialysis, thereby lowering the risk of intradialytic hypotension and further ischemic damage to an already impaired set of kidneys.

II. Hemodialysis procedure

A. Rinsing and priming the dialyzer (single-use setting). Thorough rinsing of the dialyzer is important because it may reduce the incidence or severity of anaphylactic dialyzer reactions by virtue of removal of leachable allergens (e.g., ethylene oxide in ethylene oxide–sterilized dialyzers).

B. Obtaining vascular access

1. Percutaneous venous cannula. Clot or residual heparin is first aspirated from each catheter lumen. Patency of the catheter lumina is checked by irrigating with a saline-filled syringe. For acute dialysis, heparin-free dialysis is becoming more popular and is routinely used in some centers. If heparin is to be used, the heparin loading dose is administered in with saline. After 3 minutes (to allow heparin to mix with the blood), blood flow is initiated. (Some nephrologists administer the heparin into the arterial line leading to the dialyzer and start blood flow immediately thereafter.)

2. Arteriovenous (AV) fistula (see also Chapter 4). Both needles are placed in the vein central to the anastomosis. Flow through the venous limb is distal to proximal; hence, the arterial needle is placed distally. Some tips regarding needle placement are as follows:

a. In a patient with a poorly distended venous limb, brief application of a tourniquet may be helpful in defining its location. This tourniquet should be removed during dialysis, as its presence will encourage recirculation.

b. A 16-gauge (or 15-gauge) needle should be used.

c. Prepare the needle insertion sites with povidone–iodine for a full 10 minutes.

d. Arterial needle. Insert it first, at least 3 cm away from the site of the AV anastomosis. The needle should be inserted bevel up, at a 45-degree angle, pointing toward the anastomosis.

e.   Venous needle. Insert bevel up, at a 45-degree angle, pointing toward the heart. The insertion point should be at least 3–5 cm proximal to the arterial needle to minimize entry of dialyzed blood into the arterial needle (recirculation).

3.   AV graft. The anatomy of the graft should be known and preferably diagrammed in the chart. The guidelines for placing needles are the same as for the AV fistula. Use of a tourniquet is never necessary.

After the needles have been placed, if heparin is to be used, the heparin loading dose is given into the venous needle and flushed in with saline. After 3 minutes, flow through the blood circuit is initiated.

C.   Initiating dialysis. The blood flow rate is initially set at 50 mL per minute, then 100 mL per minute, until the entire blood circuit fills with blood. As the blood circuit fills, the priming fluid in the dialyzer and tubing can either be given to the patient or disposed of to drain. In the latter instance, the venous blood line is kept to drain until the blood column passes through the dialyzer and reaches the venous air trap. In unstable patients, the priming fluid is usually administered to the patient to help maintain the blood volume.

After the circuit is filled with blood and proper blood levels in the venous drip chamber are ensured, the blood flow rate should be increased promptly to the desired level (usually about 350 mL per minute for acute dialysis). The pressure level of the inflow (arterial) monitor between the access site and blood pump, and of the outflow (venous) monitor between the dialyzer and venous air trap are noted, and the pressure limits are set, slightly above and below the operating pressure to ensure that the blood pump will stop, and alarms will sound in the event of a line separation. If a line separation does occur, the pressure in the blood line will rapidly approach zero. As it does, it should trigger a properly set pressure limit switch. The lower pressure limit on the venous pressure gauge should be set within 10–20 mm Hg of the operating pressure; a larger gap can cause failure of the alarms to trigger with line separation (Dellanna et al., 1995).

The dialysis solution flow can now be initiated, and the transmembrane pressure (TMP), calculated as described in Chapter 3, is set by adjusting the pressure level at the dialysate outflow line. In machines with an ultrafiltration controller, the desired fluid removal rate is simply dialed in.

D.   Beeps, buzzers, and alarms. As introduced in Chapter 3, the monitors on the dialysis solution machine include the following:

Blood circuit	**Dialysis solution circuit**
Inflow pressure	Conductivity
Outflow pressure	Temperature
Air detector	Hemoglobin

1.   Blood circuit (see Fig. 3-2)

a.   Inflow (prepump) pressure monitor. Usually, the inflow pressure (proximal to the blood pump) is –80 to –200 mm Hg, with –250 mm Hg being considered the usual limit beyond which one does not go to avoid hemolysis.

If the access is not providing sufficient blood to the pump, the suction proximal to the blood pump will increase, and the alarm will sound, shutting off the blood pump. Once the blood pump is shut off, the suction will be relieved; the alarm will then deactivate, and the pump will resume operation until suction again builds up, repeating the cycle.

(1)   Causes of excessive inflow suction

(a)   Venous catheter access. Usually improper position or ball-valve thrombus or fibrin plug at the catheter tip.

(b)   AV access:

(i)   Improperly positioned arterial needle (needle not in vessel or up against vessel wall).

(ii)   Decrease in the patient's blood pressure (and hence flow through the access).

(iii)   Spasm of the access vessel (AV fistula only).

(iv)   Stenosis of the arterial anastomosis of an AV graft.

(v)   Clotting of the arterial needle or of the access.

(vi)   Kinking of the arterial line.

(vii)   Collapse of the access due to elevation of the arm (if this is suspected, sit the patient up, blood pressure permitting, until the access site is below heart level).

(viii)   Use of too small a needle for the blood flow rate being used. In general, 15-gauge needles should be used whenever a blood flow rate greater than 350 mL per minute is desired.

(2)   Management

(a)   Venous catheter. Check lines for kinking. Sometimes changing arm or neck position or moving the catheter slightly makes the catheter work. Reversing the catheter ports is another maneuver that sometimes works. If these initial steps do not work, subsequent steps include urokinase or tissue plasminogen activator infusion, checking catheter position in the radiology suite, or fibrin sleeve stripping as described Chapter 4.

(b)   AV access

(i)   Reduce blood flow rate to the point that inflow suction decreases and the alarm stays off.

(ii)   Verify that the patient's blood pressure is not unusually low. If the pressure is low, correct it by administering fluid or reducing the ultrafiltration rate.

(iii)   If a patient's pressure is not unusually low, untape the arterial needle, move it up or down slightly, or rotate it.

(iv)   Turn up blood flow rate to previous level. If inflow suction remains excessive, repeat (iii).

(v)   If improvement is not obtained, continue dialysis for a longer time at a lower blood flow rate or place a second arterial needle (leaving the original, flushed with heparinized saline, in place until the end of dialysis), and dialyze through the second needle.

(**vi**) If excessive inflow suction persists despite needle change, the inflow to the vascular access may be stenosed. Occlude the access between the arterial and venous needles by transient pressure with two fingers. If the negative pressure at the prepump monitor increases markedly when the intraneedle segment is occluded, this is a sign that some of the inflow was coming from the downstream access limb and that blood flow through the upstream limb of the access is inadequate.

b. Outflow (venous) pressure monitor. Usually, the pressure here is +50 to +250 mm Hg, depending on needle size, blood flow rate, and hematocrit.

(1) Causes of high venous pressure

(**a**) The pressure may be as high as 200 mm Hg when using an AV graft because the high arterial pressure in the graft is often transmitted to the venous line.

(**b**) High blood flow rate when using a relatively small (16-gauge) venous needle.

(**c**) Clotting in the venous blood line filter if one is being used. Clotting of the filter may be the first sign of inadequate heparinization and of incipient clotting of the entire dialyzer.

(**d**) Stenosis (or spasm) at the venous limb of the vascular access.

(**e**) Improperly positioned venous needle or kinked venous line.

(**f**) Clotting of the venous needle or venous limb of the vascular access.

(2) Management of high venous pressure

(**a**) If clotting of the venous blood line filter is at fault, the dialyzer should be rinsed with saline (by opening up the saline infusion line and briefly clamping the blood inlet line proximal to the saline infusion port). If the dialyzer is not clotted (fibers appear clear on saline rinse), then a new venous line can be rapidly primed with saline and substituted for the partially clotted line, and dialysis can be resumed after adjusting the heparin dose.

(**b**) The presence or absence of obstruction at the venous needle or in the venous limb of the access can be assessed by shutting off the blood pump, quickly clamping the venous blood line, disconnecting the venous blood line from the venous needle, and irrigating through the venous needle with saline and noting the amount of resistance.

(**c**) Occlude the access between the arterial and venous needles by pressing down gently with two fingers. If stenosis downstream is causing outflow obstruction through the vascular access, the positive-pressure measured at the venous monitor will increase further when the upstream access is occluded.

(3) Effects of high venous pressure on ultrafiltration rate. When an ultrafiltration controller is not used, high pressure in the blood compartment can result in excessive ultrafiltration. This is especially a problem when a dialyzer with a high permeability to water (high K_U) is used. To limit the amount of ultrafiltration, the pressure in the dialysate compartment should be increased to approach (but not exceed) the pressure in the blood compartment (in some older machines the pressure in the dialysate compartment cannot be increased above zero). The patient's weight and blood pressure should be carefully monitored, and intravenous fluids given as necessary.

    c. Air detector. The danger of inadvertent air entry is greatest between the vascular access site and the blood pump, where the pressure is negative. Common sites of air entry include the region around the arterial needle (especially if the inflow suction is very high), via leaky tubing connections, via broken blood tubing as it passes through the roller pump, or via the saline infusion set. Air can also enter the patient if air return is improperly performed at the end of dialysis. Many air emboli occur after the air detector has been turned off because of false alarms. This practice should be avoided. Air embolism can be fatal. Clinical manifestations of air embolism and its management are discussed in Chapter 7.

    d. Blood line kinking and hemolysis. Severe hemolysis may occur due to kinking of the blood line between the pump and dialyzer. High pressure in this segment will not be detected if the blood set being used has an inflow pressure monitoring configuration (blood lines usually are configured for only one pressure-monitoring segment in the arterial side). Blood line configures for prepump pressure will not alarm if high pressures are encountered in the segment between pump and dialyzer. Even if a postpump pressure monitor configuration blood line is being used, if the kink is proximal to the monitoring line, high pressure due to the kink will not be detected (Sweet, 1996).

  2. Dialysis solution circuit monitors. The dangers of dialyzing against an excessively concentrated, dilute, or hot dialysis solution have been discussed in Chapter 3.

    a. Conductivity. The most common cause of increased dialysis solution conductivity is either a kink in the tubing routing purified water to the dialysis machine, or low water pressure, resulting in insufficient water delivery to the machine. The most common cause of a reduced conductivity is an empty concentrate bottle. Otherwise, the cause is usually in the proportioning pump. The dialysis solution bypass valve is activated as soon as conductivity deviates from the specified limits, diverting the abnormal dialysis solution away from the dialyzer to the drain.

    b. Temperature. Abnormal temperature is usually caused by some malfunction in the heating circuit. Again, a properly functioning bypass valve protects the patient.

    c. Hemoglobin (blood leak). False alarms may be due to the presence of air bubbles in the dialysis solution, to dialysate bilirubin in jaundiced patients, or to a dirty sensor. The dialysate may not appear to be discolored to the naked eye. A blood leak alarm should be confirmed by testing the effluent dialysate with a test strip of the sort used for detecting hemoglobin in the urine.

If a leak is confirmed, the dialysate compartment pressure should be set to −50 mm Hg or lower to minimize entry of bacteria or their products from the dialysis solution into the blood side of the extracorporeal circuit. The blood should be returned and dialysis discontinued, although small leaks in hollow-fiber dialyzers may seal themselves off with continued dialysis.

E.   Patient monitoring and complications. The patient's blood pressure should be monitored as often as necessary, but at least every 15 minutes for an acute dialysis. The manifestations and treatment of hypotension and other complications during dialysis are discussed in Chapter 7.

F.   Termination of dialysis. The blood in the extracorporeal circuit can be returned using either saline or air. If saline is used, the patient usually receives 100–200 mL of this fluid during the rinse-back procedure, nullifying the corresponding amount of fluid removed by ultrafiltration. However, if the patient's blood pressure is low at the end of dialysis, the saline bolus will help to raise the blood pressure quickly. When air is used, the blood pump is first shut off, and the arterial blood line is clamped close to the patient. The arterial blood line is then disconnected just distal to the clamp, opening it to air. The blood pump is restarted at a reduced rate (20–50 mL per minute), and the air is allowed to displace the blood in the dialyzer. When the air reaches the venous air trap, or when air bubbles are first seen in the venous blood line, the venous line is clamped, the blood pump shut off, and the return procedure terminated. Use of air to return the blood increases the risk of air embolism, and the termination procedure should be extremely carefully supervised when air return is employed.

G.   Postdialysis evaluation

1.   Weight loss. The patient should be weighed after dialysis whenever possible, and the postdialysis weight compared with the predialysis weight. It is not uncommon for the weight loss to be greater or less than that anticipated based on the calculated ultrafiltration rate. Sources of error include the following:

a.   Use of a TMP that failed to account for the fact that the in vivo dialyzer water permeability (K_{Uf}) may be markedly less than the published in vitro value.

b.   Reduction in dialyzer water permeability because of coating of the membrane with protein or clot.

c.   Difficulty in maintaining the desired TMP during dialysis due to changes in venous resistance.

d.   Use of a dialyzer that is highly permeable to water, with small errors in the TMP translating into larger errors in fluid removal.

e.   Failure to take into account fluid administered to the patient during dialysis in the form of saline, medications, hyperalimentation, or oral fluid ingestion.

Errors a–d can be minimized by use of a dialysis machine with ultrafiltration controller circuitry.

2. Postdialysis blood values. Blood can be sampled immediately after dialysis to confirm the adequacy of urea nitrogen removal and correction of acidosis. For urea nitrogen, sodium, and calcium, the postdialysis specimen can be drawn 10 seconds to 2 minutes after dialysis, although a postdialysis increase in the plasma urea level of 10%–20% usually occurs within 30 minutes due to reequilibration of urea between various body compartments. In patients with poor peripheral perfusion, the amount of urea rebound can be greatly increased due to nonremoval of urea from these poorly perfused peripheral tissues during dialysis.

The method of obtaining the postdialysis blood sample is quite important; if access recirculation is present, contamination of the inlet blood sample with dialyzed outlet blood can occur, yielding erroneously low plasma urea nitrogen values. One method of obtaining the sample is described in Table 6-2.

a. Urea nitrogen. The methods described in Chapters 2 and 6 can be used to estimate a predicted Kt/V and urea reduction ratio. If the plasma urea nitrogen value has fallen to a lesser extent, possible causes include partial clotting of the dialyzer, an error in setting of the blood flow rate, and recirculation at the vascular access site.

b. Potassium. The change in the plasma potassium level as a result of dialysis is difficult to predict because of concomitant shifting of potassium into cells due to correction of acidosis or to cellular uptake of glucose.

c. Postdialysis potassium rebound. In acute patients, it is best to sample blood for potassium at least 1 hour after the end of dialysis.

SELECTED READINGS

Assouad M, et al. Biocompatibility of dialyzer membranes is important in the outcome of acute renal failure. *J Am Soc Nephrol* 1996;7:1437(Abstr).

Dellanna F, et al. Safety of hemodialysis machines: surveilance of the venous blood return. *J Am Soc Nephrol* 1995;6:486(Abstr).

Emmett M, Hootkins RE, Fine KD, et al. Effect of three laxatives and a cation exchange resin on fecal sodium and potassium excretion. *Gastroenterology* 1995;108:752–760.

Evanson JA, et al. Measurement of the delivery of dialysis in acute renal failure. *Kidney Int* 1999;55:1501–1508.

Gardiner GW. Kayexalate (sodium polystyrene sulphonate) in sorbitol associated with intestinal necrosis in uremic patients. *Can J Gastroenterol* 1997;11:573–577).

Gastaldello et al. Comparison of cellulose diacetate and polysulfone membranes in the outcome of acute renal failure: a prospective, randomized study. *Nephrol Dial Transplant* 2000;15:224–230.

Hakim RM et al. Use of biocompatible membranes improves outcome and recovery from acute renal failure. *J Am Soc Nephrol* 1996;3:367a (abst.).

Himmelfarb J, et al. A multicenter comparison of dialysis membranes in the treatment of acute renal failure requiring dialysis. *J Am Soc Nephrol* 1998;9:257–266.

Jorres A, et al. Haemodialysis-membrane biocompatibility and mortality of patients with dialysis-dependent acute renal failure: a prospective, randomised multicentre trial. International Multicentre Study Group. *Lancet* 1999;354:1337–1341.

Kelleher SP, et al. Effect of hemorrhagic reduction in blood pressure on recovery from acute renal failure. *Kidney Int* 1987;31:725.

Ketchersid TL, Van Stone JC. Dialysate potassium. *Semin Dial* 1991;4:46.

Kurtal H, von Herrath D, Schaefer K. Is the choice of membrane important for patients with acute renal failure requiring hemodialysis? *Artif Organs* 1995;19:391–394.

Lo AJ, et al. Urea disequilibrium contributes to underdialysis in the intensive care unit. *J Am Soc Nephrol* 1997;8:287A.

Madias NE, Levey AS, Metabolic alkalosis due to absorption of "nonabsorbable" antacids. *Am J Med* 1983;74:155–158.

Marshall MR, et al. Effect of sustained low efficiency dialysis (SLED) on urea generation rate (UGR) in intensive care unit (ICU) patients with acute renal failure (ARF). *J Am Soc Nephrol* 1999;10:293A (Abstr).

Nappi SE, et al. QTc dispersion increases during hemodialysis with low-calcium dialysate. *Kidney Int* 2000;57:2117–2122.

Parnes EL, Shapiro WB. Anaphylactoid reactions in hemodialysis patients treated with the AN69 dialyzer. *Kidney Int* 1991;40:1148.

Roy PS, Danziger RS. Dialysate magnesium concentration predicts the occurrence of intradialytic hypotension. *J Am Soc Nephrol* 1996;7:1496(Abstr).

Schiffl H, et al. Biocompatible membranes in acute renal failure: prospective case-controlled study. *Lancet* 1994;344:570–572.

Schiffl H, et al. Dose of intermittent hemodialysis (IHD) and outcome of acute renal failure (ART): a prospective randomized study. *J Am Soc Nephrol* 1997;8:290A(Abstr).

Sweet SJ, McCarthy S, Springfield R, Callahan T. Hemolytic reactions mechanically induced by kinked hemodialysis lines. *Am J Kidney Dis* 1996;27:262–266.

van der Sande FM, et al. Effect of dialysate calcium concentrations in intradialytic blood pressure course in cardiac-compromised patients. *Am J Kidney Dis* 1998;32:125–131.

Ward RA, et al. Hemodialysate composition and intradialytic metabolic, acid–base and potassium changes. *Kidney Int* 1987;32:129.

Yu AW, et al. Raising plasma phosphorus levels by phosphorus-enriched, bicarbonate-containing dialysate in hemodialysis patients. *Artif Organs* 1992;16:414.

6

Chronic Hemodialysis Prescription: A Urea Kinetic Approach

John T. Daugirdas and Carl M. Kjellstrand

I. Prescribing and monitoring "adequate" dialysis.
Please review Chapter 2 at this time. Many concepts developed in Chapter 2 will be only briefly touched on here.

   A. Urea as a marker solute. Uremic toxicity is due to both small and large molecular weight solutes, although removal of small molecular weight toxins is of greater importance. For this reason, the amount of dialysis prescribed is based on small-toxin removal as represented by removal of urea (MW 60).

   B. Urea removal versus plasma urea level. Both urea removal and plasma urea level should be monitored when checking dialysis adequacy, although monitoring of urea removal is more important. If urea removal is inadequate, then dialysis is inadequate, regardless of the plasma urea level. A low plasma urea level, on the other hand, does not necessarily reflect adequate dialysis. Urea is only slightly toxic, and its plasma level depends not only on the rate of urea removal but also on the rate of urea generation. The generation rate of urea is linked to the protein nitrogen appearance rate because most protein nitrogen is excreted as urea. A low predialysis or time-averaged plasma urea level may be found in patients in whom urea removal is inadequate but in whom the urea generation rate is also low (e.g., due to poor protein intake).

   C. Measures of urea removal. These are the urea reduction ratio (URR), the single-pool Kt/V (spKt/V), and the equilibrated Kt/V (eKt/V) (see Chapter 2).

   D. Urea-based standards of urea removal for thrice-weekly dialysis

   1. National Kidney Foundation Dialysis Outcomes Quality Initiative (DOQI) hemodialysis adequacy guidelines. The only hemodialysis adequacy standard based on outcomes data is for patients being dialyzed using a thrice-weekly schedule. In large cross-sectional studies, mortality increases when amounts of dialysis lower than spKt/V of 1.2 are delivered (Owen et al, 1993; Held et al, 1996). Accordingly, the current dialysis adequacy standard in the United States, the set of DOQI guidelines, recommends keeping spKt/V at greater than 1.2 (Table 6-1). Another popular standard is to keep a minimum URR of 65%. However, the relation between the URR and spKt/V is mediated by the relative weight change during a dialysis session, as explained in Chapter 2 and illustrated in Fig. A-2.

   2. Larger amount of dialysis. Whether or not larger amounts of dialysis delivered using a thrice-weekly schedule

Table 6-1. DOQI hemodialysis adequacy guidelines

R_x: Frequency of dialysis, 3 times weekly
Target delivered spKt/V: ≥1.2–1.3[a]
Target delivered URR· >65%[a]

Initial dialysis session length (t)
1. Use Fig. A-6 (males) or Fig. A-7 (females) to estimate V, or use modeled V if available
2. Use nomogram in Fig. A-1 to estimate dialyzer urea clearance (K) from KoA and Q_B.
3. Input desired Kt/V.
4. Estimated K and V are now known. Solve for t algebraically.

[a] More may be better, based on 10- to 20-sec slow-flow postdialysis SUN sample.
DOQI, Dialysis Outcomes Quality Initiative Study; SUN, serum urea nitrogen; URR, urea reduction ratio.

are beneficial is a subject of controversy and the object of the ongoing multicenter U.S. National Institutes of Health (NIH)–sponsored HEMO study. In this study, mortality is being compared in patients dialyzed to an approximate URR of 67% (standard arm, equivalent to spKt/V of about 1.3 and equilibrated eKt/V of about 1.1), and in patients dialyzed to an approximate URR of 75% (high-dose arm, equivalent to spKt/V of 1.65, double-pool eKt/V of about 1.45). If results from the HEMO study are positive, the currently recommended minimal dose of dialysis for a thrice-weekly schedule may have to be revised upward.

3. Effect of race and sex. A recent cross-sectional study has suggested that the relationship between URR and mortality differs in African American versus Caucasian patients, and may also be affected by sex (Owen et al, 1998). However, an analysis by the US Renal Data Systems (USRDS) could not confirm these findings (Wolfe et al, 2000).

4. Optimal dialysis dose in a patient who has lost body mass. Assume a patient begins with a body mass of 100 kg and then loses 50% of body weight. If we estimate that the urea distribution volume is 55% of body weight, this patient's V will fall from 55 to 27.5 L. Assume that one cause of this precipitous fall in body weight was underdialysis, and assume that the initial spKt/V as only 0.7 Kt/V unit. Now that the patient has "shrunk," if the initial dose of dialysis ($K \times t$) is continued, Kt/V will have doubled from 0.7 to 1.4 (because V will have been halved), and 1.4 is a seemingly respectable dose that meets all DOQI targets. In the DOQI peritoneal dialysis adequacy guidelines, there is a provision to increase dialysis dose in malnourished patients by the ratio of the current weight to the ideal body weight. It is logical to apply a similar correction for hemodialysis patients.

5. Equilibrated Kt/V. The DOQI guidelines do not address *equilibrated Kt/V* (eKt/V) targets, but eKt/V generally is about 0.2 Kt/V unit lower than spKt/V (see Chapter 2); hence, by inference, DOQI guidelines would suggest keeping eKt/V

> 1.0. Measuring or computing eKt/V may be important for smaller patients being dialyzed rapidly, in whom urea rebound may be increased, and in whom the eKt/V– spKt/V difference may be far greater than 0.2.

6. DOQI guidelines regarding treatment Kt/V and residual renal function. DOQI guidelines mandate use of a minimum treatment spKt/V of 1.2 (i.e., excluding any adjustment of Kt/V for K_{ru}; many urea modeling programs make this adjustment if asked). However, the DOQI guidelines limit themselves to patients in whom residual renal function is modest (glomerular filtration rate, or GFR, less than 5.0 mL per minute). The DOQI guidelines reflect common practice in the United States, which is to start patients on full-dose hemodialysis from the outset, regardless of the level of residual renal urea clearance. There are several reasons for this:

a. Dialysis patients often resist any attempt to increase the dialysis session length. As residual renal function falls, dialysis session length and/or frequency would have to be increased. One fear is that a progressively lengthening dialysis prescription would be hard for the patient to accept and might also lead to difficulties in scheduling.

b. Difficulty in collecting and measuring residual urea clearance. Unless this would be done frequently, an undocumented decrease could lead to a substantial period of underdialysis. There is substantial variation in measurement.

c. Another issue is regulatory. In the United States, dialysis adequacy is highly regulated, and the urea reduction ratio URR is used as a quality assurance tool that is seen as a prime "opportunity for improvement." Patients with residual renal urea clearance in whom treatment URR is reduced would then have apparently "inadequate" URR values.

d. Methods of adjusting hemodialysis dose for residual renal function. There are no outcome-based data to justify reduction of hemodialysis dose for patients with substantial levels of K_{ru}. However, DOQI guidelines recommend initiating dialysis when the weekly Kt/V-urea falls to below 2.0 (see Chapter 2). In the DOQI peritoneal dialysis adequacy guidelines, it is assumed that often the peritoneal dialysis prescription will be reduced initially, with a goal of maintaining total weekly Kt/V-urea at 2.0. For hemodialysis, the issue of dialysis dose for patients with substantial K_{ru} (GFR greater than 5 mL per minute, which is approximately a weekly Kt/V-urea of 0.8–1.0) remains unresolved.

The methods of prescribing "equivalent" doses of hemodialysis in patients with considerable residual renal function (e.g., GFR greater than 5.0 mL per minute) are complex and not yet tested experimentally. Gotch has recommended one approach based on the idea of keeping the mean predialysis peak urea level constant across a number of different regimens. Discussion of this method is beyond the scope of this book, but a nomogram by Gotch from the DOQI peritoneal dialysis adequacy guidelines is reproduced in Appendix A (Fig. A-4). A calculator for this purpose can be found in the "Web References" at the end of this chapter.

E. Writing the initial prescription: background and rough guidelines

1.   The dialysis dose: $K \times t$. A dialysis prescription involves only two main components: K, the dialyzer clearance, and t, the dialysis session length. K, in turn, depends on the dialyzer size used, the blood flow rate, and the dialysate flow rate, as discussed in detail in Chapter 2.

$$\left.\begin{array}{l} \text{Dialyzer } KoA \\ \text{Blood flow rate} \\ \text{Dialysate flow rate} \end{array}\right\} K$$

a. K usually ranges from 200 to 260 mL per minute. For adult patients, given that dialyzer KoA values, blood flow rate, and dialysate flow rate are usually within fairly narrow ranges, K (corrected for blood water and flow reduction due to prepump pressure as per Table A-1) will usually be 230 ± 30 mL per minute. As a rule of thumb, if one uses a high-efficiency (KoA 800) dialyzer and rapid (450 mL per minute) blood flow rate, and a dialysate flow rate of 500 mL per minute, K will be about 260 mL per minute. Increase dialysate flow rate to 800 mL per minute, and K will go up to about 290 mL per minute. One needs to connect a second dialyzer in series or in parallel to get any clinically meaningful increase in clearance beyond this level. On the other hand, in a patient with a venous catheter access, effective blood flow of 300–350 mL per minute, and a modest ($KoA = 600$) dialyzer, with Q_D of 500 mL per minute, K will be about 200 mL per minute.

If we assume that K will be 250 mL per minute, for dialysis session lengths of 3 and 4 hours, $K \times t$ will be $250 \times 180 = 45,000$, and $250 \times 240 = 60,000$ mL, respectively, or 45 and 60 L.

2.   Adjusting $K \times t$ for patient size: the Kt/V. This is done by dividing $K \times t$ by the patient's urea distribution volume, which is approximately 55% of body weight, but which can be more accurately estimated from a nomogram (Figs. A-6 and A-7) or from an anthropometric equation (e.g, Watson equations, Table A-2).

Assume that we have a clearance of 250 mL per minute and session lengths of 3 and 4 hours. How large a patient could we dialyze and still meet DOQI guidelines? Remember that the guidelines suggest using a prescribed $(K \times t)/V$ of 1.3 to ensure that the delivered dose averages 1.2.

For the 3-hour session, we are predicting 45 L of $K \times t$. If $(K \times t) = 45$, and $(K \times t)/V$ is 1.3, then V must be $45/1.3 = 35$ L. A patient who has a V of 35 L would have a weight of about $35/0.55$ (assuming $V = 55\%$ of body weight), or 62 kg. This means that if we can reliably deliver a K of 250 mL per minute, most patients up to 62 kg could be dialyzed for 3 hours and still meet DOQI guidelines. For the 4-hour session, we are delivering 60 L of $K \times t$, and if we want a Kt/V of 1.3 prescribed, V must be $60/1.3 = 46$ L, corresponding to a weight of about 84 kg. From this analysis, it is clear that as long as a blood flow rate of 450 mL per minute and a dialyzer with a *KoA* of about 800 mL per minute are used, patients weighing 62–84 kg can be dialyzed for 3–4 hours and often still meet DOQI guidelines.

   3. Prescribing based on URR. Although DOQI does not recommend following the URR, one can prescribe dialysis to achieve a given URR as well. The first step is to convert URR to sp*Kt*/*V*. One needs to use Fig. A-2, and one needs to know the patient's usual weight loss during dialysis (UF) relative to his or her postdialysis weight (UF/*W*). Figure A-2 is in terms of UF/*W*, with lines for values of 0, 0.03, 0.06, and 0.09. For example, if the usual weight loss is 3 kg in a 50-kg patient, UF/*W* is 3/50 = 0.06. If the URR target is 70%, with a UF/*W* of 0.06, the target sp*Kt*/*V* will be about 1.5. If, however, the UF/*W* is zero, to achieve a URR of 70%, sp*Kt*/*V* needs to be lower, only 1.3. Go to Fig. A-2. Find 0.70 on the vertical axis. Move to the right to intersect with the UF/*W* line = 0. Drop down to the horizontal axis. You will see that the *Kt*/*V* value is 1.3. Now repeat the maneuver, but go rightward from 0.70 on the vertical axis until you intersect with the UF/*W* line = 0.06 and drop down to the horizontal axis. Now you will find that the corresponding *Kt*/*V* is 1.5.

F. The initial prescription for a specific patient to achieve a desired sp*Kt*/*V*:
   1. General strategy:

Step 1: Estimate the patient's *V*
Step 2: Multiply *V* by the desired *Kt*/*V* to get the required *K* × *t*
Step 3: Compute required *K* for a given *t*, or the required *t* for a given *K*

   a. Step 1. Estimate V. This is best done from anthropometric equations incorporating height, weight, age, and gender as devised by Watson (Table A-2). If the patient is African American, add 2 kg to the Watson value for V_{ant}. Alternatively, one can use the Hume–Weyers equations or the nomogram derived from them (Table A-2, Figs. A-6 and A-7). Assume that, in this case, the estimated *V* is 40 L.
   b. Step 2. Compute the required *K* × *t*. If the desired *Kt*/*V* is 1.5 and estimated *V* is 40 L, then the required *K* × *t* is 1.5 times the volume for *V*, or 1.5 × 40 = 60 L.
   c. Step 3. Compute the required *t* or *K*. The required *K* × *t* can be achieved with a variety of different combinations of *K* (which depends on *KoA*, Q_B, and Q_D) and *t*. A variety of urea modeling programs are available that will do a computer simulation of various scenarios, and come up with many possible combinations of *K* (from *KoA,* Q_B, and Q_D) and *t*. Internet-based calculators can be accessed via the web references cited at the end of this chapter.
   2. Given a desired session length *t*, how to compute required *K* (Q_B, *KoA,* Q_D). One approach is to input a session length *t* and then ask: What kind of dialyzer, blood flow rate, and dialysate flow rate would I then need to achieve the required *K* × *t*? Again, simple algebra is sufficient. From the previous example:

Desired sp*Kt*/*V* = 1.5; V_{ant} = 40 L, K × t = 60 L

First, convert $K \times t$ to milliliters to get 60,000 mL. If the desired session length is 4 hours, or 240 minutes:

Desired t = 240 min

Desired $K = (K \times t)/t$ = 60,000/240 – 250 mL/min

Now we know that the patient needs a combination of KoA, Q_B, and Q_D that will result in a dialyzer clearance of 250 mL per minute. How does one now choose KoA, Q_B, and Q_D? A simple way is to select the most rapid value of Q_B that can be reliably and consistently delivered. Assume in this patient that a blood pump speed of 400 mL per minute will be possible. One can then go to the K-KoA-Q_B nomogram (Fig. A-1) to find the approximate dialyzer KoA value that will be required to achieve a K of 250 mL per minute at a blood flow rate of 400 mL per minute.

To find the required dialyzer KoA, find 400 (which is Q_B) on the horizontal axis, then go up until you find 250 (desired K) on the vertical axis. At this point, you are on a KoA line of about 900, so a dialyzer with a KoA value of at least 900 mL per minute will be needed. If such a high-efficiency dialyzer is not available, one will need to dialyze longer than 4 hours. One way of avoiding the need to go to a longer session length might be to use a dialysate flow rate of 800 mL per minute. Figure A-1 is set up for Q_D = 500 mL per minute. One would need a separate nomogram for Q_D = 800, and all of the KoA lines would be moved upward a bit. At blood flow rates over 400 mL/min, use of an 800 mL per minute dialysate flow rate will result in an increase in clearance of about 10% over what is reported in Fig. A-1. One can do detailed computation of expected clearance using the equations in Table A-1.

3.   Given an actual blood flow rate (Q_B), how to compute required session length given two possible choices of dialyzers. A common situation occurs when the maximum blood flow rate that can be reliably delivered is known. Often one has a choice between using a larger (more expensive) or a smaller (slightly cheaper) dialyzer. Let us assume that one is constrained to using a dialysate flow rate of 500 mL per minute. What would the dialysis session length then need to be to achieve a target spKt/V of 1.5? Let us assume that we are prescribing for the same patient, with an estimated V of 40 L, which means that $K \times t$ again must be 60 L, or 60,000 mL. Assume that the projected blood flow rate is 450 mL per minute. Of the two dialyzers available, we look up their KoA (maximum clearance) values and find they are 800 mL per minute for the big one and 600 mL per minute for the smaller one. So how long do we need to dialyze this patient with each of the two dialyzers?

a.   Step 1: From Fig. A-1 (which we can use because Q_D = 500 mL per minute), find the K corresponding to Q_B of 450 mL per minute (x-axis value) for each of the two dialyzers. K will be the value on the vertical axis that corresponds to the intersection of the 800- and 600-KoA lines with a perpendicular rising from the horizontal axis (Q_B) at a point representing 450 mL per minute. We find that the K values are about 250 and 220 mL per minute for the big ($KoA = 800$) and smaller ($KoA = 600$) dialyzers, respectively.

b.   Step 2: We know that sp$Kt/V = 1.5$ and $V_{ant} = 40$ L, forcing $K \times t$ to be 60 L, or 60,000 mL. By algebra:

$$600 - KoA \text{ dialyzer}, K = 220: t = \frac{(K \times t)}{K} = \frac{60,000}{220} = 273 \text{ min}$$

$$800 - KoA \text{ dialyzer}, K = 250: t = \frac{(K \times t)}{K} = \frac{60,000}{250} = 240 \text{ min}$$

Our calculations, thus, suggest that we will need to dialyze for ½ hour longer using the smaller ($KoA = 600$) dialyzer.

4.   How weight change during dialysis affects the dialysis prescription. In patients who have large weight gains, one will need a higher Kt/V to get a given URR than in patients with minimal weight gain (see Fig. A-2). We already have discussed above that to get a URR of 70%, one needs to prescribe a Kt/V of only 1.3 if no fluid is removed, but that one needs a Kt/V of 1.5 if the weight loss during dialysis (UF/W) is usually about 6% (0.06 UF/W line in Fig. A-2).

G.   Checking the delivered dose of dialysis. What was discussed above was how to prescribe an initial dose of dialysis. Now one must monitor the delivered dose of dialysis, on a monthly basis, according to DOQI guidelines, by drawing a predialysis and postdialysis blood urea nitrogen (BUN). The pre- and post-BUN values are used to compute the URR, which then is combined with information concerning UF/W and with some other adjustments to compute the delivered spKt/V.

1.   Methods of computing spKt/V from the pre- and post-BUN.

a.   Nomogram method. One uses Fig A-2 as described before. Assume that a URR of 0.70 or 70% is measured. Depending on whether 0, 3, or 6% of the body weight was removed during the dialysis treatment, the delivered spKt/V for that treatment was 1.3, 1.4, or 1.5.

b.   More exact methods. The standard method recommended by the DOQI guidelines is a urea kinetic modeling

---

Table 6-2.   Guidelines for obtaining the postdialysis plasma urea nitrogen sample

Principles

The effect of access recirculation will reverse quickly. When blood flow is slowed to 50–100 mL/min, the inflow urea concentration will rise in about 10–20 sec (depending on the amount of dead space in the arterial line; usually about 10 mL).

Method

1. Slow the blood pump to 50–100 mL/min for 10–20 sec.
2. Stop the pump.
3. Draw a sample, either from the arterial blood line sampling port or from the tubing attached to the arterial needle.

program. The basic principles of how such programs work are described in Chapter 2. These programs are available commercially, and one is available on the internet (see "Web References"). An alternative method that is approved by DOQI is to use the following equation (Daugirdas, 1996):

$$\text{sp}Kt/V = -\ln(R - 0.008 \times t) + (4 - 3.5 \times R) \times 0.55 \times \text{UF}/V_{ant}$$

where R is $(1 - \text{URR})$, or simply post-BUN/pre-BUN, t is the session length in hours, $-\ln$ is the negative natural logarithm, UF is the weight loss in kilograms, and V_{ant} is the anthropometric urea distribution volume in liters. V_{ant} can be computed using the Watson equations as discussed above, the Hume–Weyers nomogram in Appendix A, or simply estimated as $0.55 \times$ postdialysis weight W. In the last instance, $0.55 \times \text{UF}/V$ simplifies to UF/W. (See Chapter 2 for a more complete discussion of this formula.)

   2.   Importance of drawing the postdialysis blood correctly. Variations in drawing of blood samples can cause major differences in the computed value for URR and hence spKt/V. This matter is of such importance that it was the subject of three separate DOQI guidelines.

   a.   Predialysis sample. Dilution and a spuriously low value can result if the sample is drawn from a needle that has been flushed with saline or heparin prior to the sample draw. A spuriously low value also can result if the predialysis sample is drawn after dialysis has been started.

   b.   Postdialysis sample (Table 6-2). The key issue is to avoid a spuriously low sample due to dilution secondary to access recirculation. The strategy is to slow the pump to 50–100 mL per minute for 10–20 seconds prior to sampling. Once the pump speed is slowed, access recirculation almost always ceases because the demand (50–100 mL per minute) will then be less than the access flow rate. After the 10- to 20-second period, the pump can be stopped and blood drawn either from the sampling port or from the line attached to the arterial needle.

   3.   *Caveat:* Some centers stop the pump, return the blood, and then draw the blood sample from the arterial line. This method may not protect against a spuriously low post-SUN due to access recirculation. When the pump is stopped, if access recirculation is present, the blood in the tubing attached to the arterial needles (dead space about 2.5–3.0 mL) will be diluted. After blood has been returned, if a syringe is simply attached to this tubing and a sample taken, diluted blood remaining in the tubing set will lower the post-SUN.

   One potential problem with any slow-flow method is when access recirculation is due not to poor access flow but to inadvertent reversal of the dialysis needles (e.g., when the venous needle is placed upstream to the arterial needle). In this case, access recirculation is reduced, but not eliminated, by slow-flow method.

H.   Adjusting the initial dialysis prescription. When patients are put on a particular dialysis prescription, even when there are no apparent changes in therapy, the delivered

Table 6-3.   Reasons why the URR-based delivered single-pool Kt/V (spKt/V) may be different than prescribed Kt/V

Reasons why delivered Kt/V may be less than prescribed (in this case modeled V will be increased).

Patient's V greater than initial estimate (initial R_x only).

Actual blood flow less than that marked on the blood pump (very common when prepump negative pressure is high).

Blood flow temporarily lowered (symptoms or other reasons).

Actual dialysis session length shorter than prescribed.

Dialyzer KoA less than expected (manufacturer specifications incorrect, decreased due to reuse, etc.).

Access recirculation or inadvertent needle reversal (when post-dialysis SUN is drawn properly using a slow-flow period prior to the draw).

Rebound (use of delayed postdialysis SUN to compute spKt/V and V).

Reasons why delivered Kt/V may be greater than prescribed (in this case, modeled V will be decreased).

Patient's V less than initial estimate (initial R_x only) or recent, severe weight loss.

Postdialysis serum urea nitrogen specimen artifactually low:

Access recirculation or inadvertent needle reversal, and post-dialysis blood contaminated with dialyzer outlet blood (slow-flow period not used).

Specimen drawn from dialyzer outlet blood line.

Session length was longer than the time recorded.

Recent correction of access recirculation or inadvertent needle reversal.

SUN, serum urea nitrogen.

spKt/V derived from the measured URR often will vary considerably from month to month. The reasons are not completely clear, but laboratory error in measuring the SUN values in the samples, possible variations in how the postdialysis blood is drawn and variations in actual session length, time-averaged blood flow rate, and dialyzer clearance may all have a role. For this reason, DOQI–Health Care Finance Administration (HCFA) performance measures recommend averaging the spKt/V value from three monthly treatments to determine whether or not the standard minimum spKt/V of 1.2 is being delivered.

Example: For the above patient, with a target Kt/V of 1.5, one might get URR values that, based on Fig. A-2, convert to the following spKt/V values:

Mo	spKt/V
Jan	1.40
Feb	1.35
Mar	1.54
Apr	1.30

The average of these values is 1.40. Although this is well within DOQI targets for dialysis adequacy, if one wishes to achieve the original spKt/V goal of 1.5, one needs to increase the numerator $(K \times t)$ in Kt/V by a factor of 1.5/1.4, or 1.07 (7%).

One now has a choice in that either the K or the t term can be increased by 7% (or each one can be increased so that their product increases by 7%). A simple way is to increase dialysis session length (the t term in $K \times t$) by 7%. This would mean adding 17 minutes to a 4-hour treatment (1.07 × 240 = 257 min). Another option is to try to increase the K term by going to a higher blood flow rate, a larger dialyzer, or increasing the dialysate flow rate. However, it is often difficult to increase the blood flow rate further or to change to a dialyzer large enough to increase K by 7%. The easiest maneuver is to increase dialysate flow rate to 800 mL per minute, which typically results in about a 10% increase in clearance (Leypoldt et al, 1997) as long as the blood flow rate is > 400 mL/min. So in this particular patient, appropriate changes in prescription would be to add 17 minutes to the dialysis session length or to increase the dialysate flow rate to 800 mL per minute.

1. The concept of modeled V. In this patient, with an anthropometric estimate for V of 40 L, the Kt/V target undershot by 7%. One of the advantages of using spKt/V over the URR is that one can take the value of spKt/V computed from the URR, UF, and W, and then use it to compute a kinetically modeled patient urea distribution volume V. How is this done?

Step 1: Compute spKt/V from the URR, session length (t), and UF/W.

Step 2: Input values for K and t.

Step 3: Using algebra, if Kt/V is known, and if K and t are known, one can compute V.

In this patient, the delivered spKt/V now averages 1.40. Since the $(K \times t)$ term is 60 L, modeled V is 60/1.40 = 43 L.

If we are using a urea kinetics program, the program reasons as follows: It was told that V was 40 L, and it computed a value of K from the entered values for dialyzer KoA, Qb, and Qd. It also assumes that the value of t is correct. Based on what it was told, the computer continues to assume that $K \times t$ is 60 L. But now the computer finds that $K \times t/V$, (which it computes from the monthly URR and UF/W and other adjustments) is 1.4 instead of the prescribed 1.5. The only way that the computer can maintain its sanity is to reason that the patient's urea volume is actually somewhat larger than it was told, i.e., 43 L instead of 40 L. With a 43 L value for V, the computer takes $K \times t = 60$ L, divides by 43 L instead of 40 L, and finds that $(K \times t/V$ is now 60/43 = 1.4, which is equal to the spKt/V being computed from the URR. The computer then reports this volume as a modeled (single pool) urea volume, or Vsp.

After all, our initial estimate of a 40 L V in this patient (Vant) was based only on our patient's height, weight, age, and sex. We do know that Vant often deviates from the modeled urea distribution volume. Vsp will vary from treatment from treatment, but an average modeled V is more accurate than an anthropometric estimate (Vant), and is best used for any further prescription changes.

2.   Changing the prescription based on V. Above, we discussed changing the prescription based on $spKt/V$. $spKt/V$ was 1.4 instead of 1.5, so the conclusion was that $K \times t$ needed to be increased by a ratio of 1.5 : 1.4, or by 7%. Another way is to now use the modeled V. The initial prescribed $K \times t$ was computed using a V_{ant} of 40 L. Now we know that the mean V is probably closer to 43 L. So if we write a new prescription, to keep $spKt/V$ at 1.5, we find we need to increase $K \times t$ by a ratio of 43 to 40 L, or by a factor of 1.07 or 7%. It is plain that the two methods of making prescription changes are identical. Therefore, every month one should not only compute a $spKt/V$; one should also sequentially follow the V.

3.   V is a fictitious quantity. It is important to recognize that V is a tool that is used to assess dialysis adequacy. It does not always reflect the true urea distribution volume. Computers are not very smart in the sense that they use only the information given to them. For example, if the URR and hence $spKt/V$ suddenly decrease due to a batch of bad dialyzers, all the computer knows is that the $spKt/V$ has suddenly fallen, but it is not told that the dialyzer clearance (K) has changed. Also, the session length (t) has not changed. How, then, can the computer explain the sudden decrease in $spKt/V$? All it can think of is (a) $(K \times t)/V$ is down; (b) $(K \times t)$ is unchanged. The only way the computer can explain this scenario is to assert that the patient's urea distribution volume (V) must have increased. Actually, the true urea distribution volume changes only rarely. This point is amplified in some of the examples discussed below.

4.   An equilibrated postdialysis SUN sample should not be used to compute V. As discussed in Chapter 2, eKt/V will be about 0.2 unit lower than $spKt/V$. If one takes a pre-SUN sample in the usual fashion, followed by a post-SUN sample 30 minutes after dialysis, one can use these two numbers to compute eKt/V directly (Chapter 2). However, now you have a Kt/V value that is lower by about 15%–20%. If you now ask the computer to compute a V, the computer will tell you that the only way this 15%–20% reduction in Kt/V could have occurred is if the patient has somehow increased in size. Accordingly, the use of a post-SUN sample will result in a 15%–20% overestimation of V.

5.   Monitoring modeled V in individual patients. After the initial 3–6 months of dialysis, one can take the average value for V and use it as a quality assurance tool. However, to do this, one needs to first understand that the value for V can vary markedly from session to session.

Example 1. In our original patient, the prescription $(K \times t)$ is now increased by 7% based on the new value for V of 43 L. The $spKt/V$ and V values (computed from the URR and from the UF/W) for the ensuing 5 months are as follows:

Mo	spKt/V	V_{sp}
May	1.5	43
Jun	1.43	45
Jul	1.7	38
Aug	1.8	36
Sep	1.1	58

What should be done at this point? The usual coefficient of variation for V (standard error as a percentage of the mean) is about 10%. This means that the 95% confidence limits for V extend out by 20% from either side of the mean. In the example above, a transient increase in the value for V was found in September due to an unexpectedly low value for the spKt/V. Twenty percent (2 SD) of 43 is about 9, so the V of 58 L is more than 2 SD away from the previous mean value of 43 L.

Step 1: Review the dialysis run sheet for the September treatment. The low spKt/V and the apparent rise in V most probably reflect a unrecorded decrease in K or t. Was the treatment shortened? Was the blood flow rate reduced during all or part of the treatment? Did the dialysate concentrate run out? Were there problems with access during the treatment? If the answer to these questions is no, it can be assumed that the aberrant result was most likely due to measurement error.

Step 2: The prescription should not be changed at this point. One move suggested by the DOQI guidelines is to obtain one or more additional pre-/post-SUN measurements to determine if the low spKt/V value was a fluke or something about which to be concerned. In this case, as the September spKt/V measure is still 1.1, which is close to the minimum DOQI guideline of 1.2, one could justify waiting for the next regular monthly blood draw.

Caveat: If, on the other hand, the spKt/V value for September were 0.7 instead of 1.1, and if no obvious shortening of the session length or problems with the treatment were found, a repeat post-/pre-SUN should be drawn during a subsequent dialysis. A repeat spKt/V is then calculated, and if the repeat value is still low, some major problem exists in delivering either the prescribed K or t. The most likely explanation that would cause a decrease of spKt/V of this magnitude would be the development of severe access recirculation or upstream placement of the venous dialysis needle (needle reversal).

Example 2 (sustained rise in V, associated with a fall in spKt/V). Suppose that in the same patient the following results were obtained (prescribed spKt/V = 1.5, average V = 43 L) for October and November:

Mo	spKt/V	V
May	1.5	43
Jun	1.43	45
Jul	1.7	38
Aug	1.8	36
Sep	1.1	58
Oct	1.2	54
Nov	1.15	56

In this case, it appears in retrospect that the September increase in V was a sustained event. The mean V for September, October, and November is now 55 L, a 28% increase over the previous value of 43 L. What could account for such a phenomenon? It is highly unlikely that the patient's true V increased, and this possibility can be quickly excluded by checking the patient's serial weights.

So something happened in September that caused $K \times t$ to decrease by about 28%. This is where the sleuthing begins (Table 6-3) and the initial evaluation should start at the dialysis run sheet.

Step 1: Check the dialysis run sheet:

a. Was the full session length delivered?
b. Was the prescribed blood flow rate delivered for the entire treatment?

Step 2: Check for access recirculation or needle placement. Again, if explanations a and/or b above are accepted, they must together account for an almost 30% reduction in therapy from the prescribed values. A key potential culprit whenever V increases is access recirculation due either to access flow problems or to upstream venous needle placement. If there is no obvious major decrease in t or K, then the presence of access recirculation should be evaluated using methods described in Chapter 3, and flow direction in the access (to check for reversal of needle placement) should be evaluated.

Step 3: Make sure that there has been no change in how the pre- and post-BUN blood samples are being drawn. For example, a delay in drawing the pre-BUN sample will lower URR and spKt/V. If there is marked delay in drawing the post-BUN sample, some rebound will occur. Then one will be measuring eKt/V instead of spKt/V. eKt/V on average is about 0.2 unit lower than s Kt/V, so this may be a potential explanation.

Step 4: See if there might be problems with delivered blood flow rate. The dialysis machine blood pump might be miscalibrated. The roller pump may not be completely occluding the blood line, reducing stroke volume. If one is using a small (e.g., 16-gauge) needle with a high blood flow rate, there might be a high negative prepump pressure causing collapse of the blood tubing segment and reduced stroke volume leading to reduced blood flow rate during dialysis.

Step 5: Ensure that the machine is delivering the proper dialysate flow rate.

Step 6: Check dialyzer clearance and reuse procedure. These are discussed in Chapter 8. Briefly, if the fill volume of the dialyzer falls by more than 20%, the dialyzer should be discarded. Also, one may simply have a bad batch of dialyzers (unlikely in this age of quality control).

Example 3 (sustained fall in V). Suppose that in another patient we have a sustained increase in spKt/V, causing a decrease in apparent V:

Mo	spKt/V	V
Jul	1.2	54
Aug	1.15	56

Sep	1.35	48
Oct	1.18	55
Nov	1.5	43
Dec	1.43	45
Jan	1.5	43
Feb	1.43	45
Mar	1.7	38
Apr	1.47	43

Here we have a patient whose V was initially about 54 L, and then, sometime around November, the V appeared to decrease suddenly by about 11 L to 44 L. What could cause this (Table 6-3)?

Step 1: The first possibility to rule out is a true decrease in V, which, unfortunately, can occur either because of better removal of chronic overhydration, or because of loss of lean body mass due to intercurrent illness. The first step, then, is to check the patient's weight to exclude this possibility.

Step 2: Review the dialysis run sheets. Again, if the patient's weight is unchanged, the true V probably has not decreased. Rather, the $K \times t$ must have increased in some manner somewhere around October. The goal is to explain how this could have occurred. One needs to compare the run sheets before and after October. It is possible that a pre-existing problem in delivering the entire session length or prescribed blood flow rate that was active prior to October was corrected in October and the months that followed.

Step 3: Access recirculation/needle placement. If there was a change in access in October, then this might have resulted in cessation of access recirculation, or perhaps prior to October the needles were reversed, and in October the problem was found and corrected.

Step 4: Check to see if there was a systematic change in how the blood samples were collected. This is unlikely, of course. One pernicious problem occurs when a slow-flow technique is not used. Consider the following scenario: This patient always had access recirculation (or upstream venous needle placement). However, prior to October, the postdialysis sample was drawn using a proper slow-flow method. However, in October a new technician arrived, who drew the post samples after simply stopping the blood pump, without any antecedent slow-flow period to clear the blood line of recirculated blood. This would result in a sudden, unexplained drop in the postdialysis SUN, which would translate to an apparent, factitious rise in the URR and spKt/V, with a concomitant fall in V_d.

Step 5: A previously existing delivered blood flow or dialysate flow problem may have been corrected. Perhaps prior to October, problem with blood pump calibration, occlusion, or reduced stroke volume secondary to use of a small needle were corrected; or perhaps a malfunctioning dialysate pump was fixed.

A troubleshooting guide is presented in Table 6-3. See also the DOQI hemodialysis guidelines for a more detailed approach.

6.   Monitoring changes in V_d for the entire unit as a quality assurance tool. Whereas large fluctuations in V

can occur in individual patients, averaging the modeled V for the entire unit is useful as a quality assurance tool and can identify several problems associated with dialysis delivery. Here a small change in V for the unit over time can often be detected. It is useful to compute both an anthropometric V (V_{ant}) and the modeled V for each patient, and to follow the ratio of the two. Unit wide, V_d/V_{ant} should average close to 0.90–1.0. A ratio greater than 1 suggests that one or both components of $K \times t$ are being overestimated.

a. Correction of V_d to a double-pool V (V_{dp}). (This is an advanced topic not needed for routine clinical use.) As described in Chapter 2, there is an inherent error in computing V_d due to urea rebound. The magnitude of this error depends on the URR. It is zero when the URR is about 67%. V_d increases slightly at high values of URR, and falls markedly at very low values for URR (such as may be seen in a daily dialysis program, with URR values of 50%). One can use a simple formula to convert V_d to V_{dp}, which then gives a value that is independent of URR. For quality assurance purposes, when looking at modeled/anthropometric ratios of V, it is best to first convert V_d to V_{dp}, and follow the V_{dp}/V_{ant} ratio. This will eliminate any effect of a unit-wide change in URR over time on the ratio of modeled to anthropometric V.

I. Inability to reach the desired spKt/V. Patients in whom it is difficult to reach an spKt/V of at least 1.2 fall into three categories: (a) patients with poor access, resulting in either limitation of blood flow and/or access recirculation; (b) very large patients; and (c) patients with frequent hypotension, angina, or other side effects, resulting in frequent reductions in blood flow during dialysis.

1. Access problems. When access is the problem, it should be fixed, if possible. If the access cannot be improved, the dialysis session length can often be increased to compensate for the reduced clearance, especially in smaller patients. The problem becomes patient acceptance of the increased session length.

2. Very large patients. Assume the patient has an anthropometric volume of 60 L. The best dialyzers available have a KoA in the 800– to 1,000–mL per minute range. Using a 900 mL per minute KoA dialyzer and a blood flow rate of 450 mL per minute, one can use Fig. A-1 to get an estimated K of about 260 mL per minute, which can be increased to 290 mL per minute by using a dialysate flow rate of 800 mL per minute. Now, to achieve a prescribed spKt/V of 1.3 according to DOQI guidelines, $K \times t$ needs to be $1.3 \times 60 = 78$ L, or 78,000 mL. Dividing by the maximum K value of 290, one gets 78,000/290 = 270 min, or 4.5 hours. So even under the best circumstances (a K of 290 minutes is difficult to deliver consistently), such large patients need to be dialyzed longer than 4 hours.

a. Simultaneous use of two dialyzers. Although not yet supported officially by dialyzer manufacturers or machines, in such a patient, one can add a second dialyzer downstream to the first, connecting them both in series.

Parallel connection of two dialyzers also has been described. In the case of a serial connection, the *KoA* values of the two dialyzers are additive, giving a *KoA* value for the combination of about 1,600 mL per minute. Use of a second dialyzer will result in an additional 20%–40% increase in *K*, allowing a proportional shortening of the treatment time. In the case above, use of two dialyzers would allow shortening of the treatment time to below 4 hours. Great care must be taken to ensure that a proper rinsing procedure is used when two dialyzers are used, as it may be more difficult to remove residual processing material from the dialyzer fibers. Use of two dialyzers in series or in parallel is not specifically approved by the U.S. Food and Drug Administration, although to the best of our knowledge it is not forbidden, and the method is being done routinely in some dialysis units.

It should be pointed out that the benefits of using a second dialyzer depend on the extraction percentage in the first dialyzer. At slow blood flow rates, a large dialyzer easily removes 90% of urea. A second dialyzer will then remove 90% of what is left, so the overall increase is only 9%. At more rapid blood flow rates, the extraction ratio (see Chapter 2) is only 60%. The second dialyzer then removes 60% of the remaining 40% or an additional 24%, and the increase in clearance is 84/60, or 1.4, or 40%. Therefore, for patients in whom maximum achievable blood flow rate is severely curtailed due to access problems, the use of a second dialyzer to increase clearance is not very effective.

b. Therapy four times per week. Using techniques pioneered by Gotch in the peritoneal dialysis adequacy DOQI guidelines (see below), one can compute a kinetically equivalent four-times-a-week prescription for large patients that is equivalent to a DOQI-approved three-times-a-week prescription (e.g., delivered Kt/V more than 1.2). This method of writing equivalent prescriptions is described below in the twice-weekly therapy section, but this is an advanced topic.

3. Patients with intradialytic symptoms. There is concern among some practitioners that use of a high blood flow rate might result in increased intradialytic symptoms. Many dialysis technicians will reduce the blood flow rate at the first occurrence of cramps, hypotension, angina, or other symptoms. Reduction of blood flow rate is not logical in a setting where bicarbonate dialysate is being used and where the ultrafiltration rate is being volumetrically controlled and therefore is independent of the blood flow rate. There is no documented proof that reduction of blood flow rate (assuming bicarbonate dialysis and volumetric ultrafiltration control) has any benefit. Because reduction of the blood flow rate can result in underdialysis, it should be avoided as much as possible. In such patients, symptoms are usually due to an excessively high ultrafiltration rate. The dialysis session length should be increased to the maximum extent possible, which will also help to ensure that adequate dialysis is taking place.

J. Problems associated with a high blood flow rate

1. Need for special needles/blood tubing sets. Sixteen-gauge needles are adequate for blood flow rates of up to

350 mL per minute. With higher blood flow rates, one should use 15-gauge needles or, even better, 14-gauge needles with ultrathin walls. In addition, short blood tubing lines should be used. Many physicians prefer to use smaller needles in fistulas, either indefinitely or during the early maturation phase only.

    a. High negative prepump pressures. When high blood flow rates are used, especially when using a small arterial needle, a high negative pressure can develop in the blood tubing segment between the arterial needle and the roller pump. When this prepump pressure exceeds –200 mm Hg, the tubing walls begin to flatten, causing the pump to deliver less blood flow than is indicated on the dial. The falloff in flow is usually about 5% at –200 mm Hg prepump pressure, and 12% at –300 mm Hg pressure, although it may be higher with certain tubing sets.

    –250 mm Hg is the usual limit for prepump vacuum to avoid hemolysis and other problems.

  2. High venous pressure. The pressure in the venous blood lines is a function of blood flow rate. Normally, a high venous pressure will not reduce the ability of the blood pump to deliver the calibrated blood flow. In machines without volumetric ultrafiltration control, the high pressure in the blood compartment of the dialyzer will drive a large amount of "spontaneous ultrafiltration," and this can result in patient dehydration.

  3. Increased access recirculation. Many peripheral accesses deliver extracorporeal blood flow rates of 600 mL per minute or greater. However, in a patient with poor vessels or a partially stenosed access, it may be difficult to obtain an extracorporeal blood flow rate of even 300 mL per minute. Some fistulas work for an extended period of time with low fistula flow rates. As the blood pump demands more flow than the access can deliver, a large amount of access recirculation may occur, reducing the expected amount of dialysis.

K. Urea-based standards of urea removal for twice-weekly dialysis. A twice-weekly dialysis schedule should be used primarily for smaller patients who have substantial residual renal function (e.g., residual urea clearance greater than 5.0 mL per minute). Because residual renal function in hemodialysis patients falls quickly, a twice-weekly schedule should be thought of primarily as a transitional treatment strategy. In most dialysis units, very few patients are following a twice-weekly schedule (Hanson et al, 1999).

All outcomes data concerning Kt/V have been obtained for dialysis three times weekly. There is no clinically derived information about dialysis twice weekly. In preliminary data (Hanson et al, 1999), patients following a twice-weekly schedule had increased survival, probably because of selection bias. Some such patients may have substantial residual renal function, the extent of which is not always recorded in the U.S. national databases.

L. Urea-based standards of urea removal for 6 ×/week (daily) dialysis

1. **Nocturnal hemodialysis.** Currently, there are two forms of "daily" (actually six times per week) dialysis. One is nocturnal dialysis, which is given while the patient sleeps. This is described by Pierratos et al (1999). The amount of dialysis given is so large, even on a per-treatment basis, that any form of adequacy measurement becomes moot. For such long (8–10 hours) nocturnal treatments, the effect of urea generation on the URR becomes very important, and the URR can no longer be used to estimate Kt/V. Furthermore, the second-generation Daugirdas equation described earlier in this chapter should not be used either to estimated spKt/V in this setting, as it has not been validated for such long treatment times.

2. **Short daily dialysis schedules.** This typically entails giving 1.5- to 2.5-hour treatments six times per week. There are several issues that can be encountered from a prescription and monitoring setting.

   a. **Therapy target.** There are no outcomes-based data that point to an optimal dialysis prescription for daily hemodialysis. A single-pool Kt/V (spKt/V) of 1.2 in a 3×/week schedule is equivalent to a single-pool Kt/V of about 0.53 when using a 6×/week schedule (see Fig. A-8) according to Gotch's mean peak SUN approach (discussed in Chapter 2 and in Gotch et al, 1998), but this amount of dialysis would result in a higher time-averaged SUN during the 6×/week schedule than with the 3×/week schedule. To keep time-averaged SUN the same with the 6×/week schedule, the daily treatment spKt/V needs to be about 0.65.

   b. **Rebound.** There are no published rebound data using a short daily hemodialysis schedule. However, from the regional blood flow model, one can predict that rebound for such short sessions should average about 0.15 Kt/V unit (Daugirdas JT, unpublished observations).

   c. **Effect of URR on V.** As alluded to above and in Chapter 2, single-pool urea modeling correctly estimates V when the URR is about 67%. When the URR is low, as in daily dialysis, V will typically be only 70% to 80% of the anthropometric volume. This is just a mathematical curiosity but should be taken into account when computing an initial target prescription and when comparing V to V_{ant} for quality assurance purposes.

II. Computing and monitoring the normalized protein nitrogen appearance rate (nPNA). This is described in Chapters 2 and 23.

III. Dialyzer

   A. Membrane material

   1. **Theoretical considerations.** The types of dialyzer membranes available and their complement activating ability are described in Chapter 3. With regard to membranes, there are two issues: biocompatibility and flux.

      a. **Biocompatibility.** In theory, membranes that activate complement and cause complement fragment release are not desirable because complement activation can increase neutrophil superoxide production. In a reuse situation, when bleach is not used, unsubstituted cellulose membranes become coated with blood proteins during the first use. During subsequent uses, the amount of complement activation is greatly reduced.

b.   Flux. Synthetic membranes tend to be more "open"; that is, many of them have a higher permeability to large molecular weight solutes and have increased clearance of molecules, in the 1,000–15,000 MW range, including β_2-microglobulin. However, one can buy synthetic membranes with low-flux characteristics, and one can buy high-flux membranes made of unsubstituted cellulose or of cellulose di- or triacetate. The increased removal of "middle molecules" associated with use of high-flux membranes may or may not be of clinical benefit.

c.   Back-filtration. There are potential disadvantages to the use of high-flux membranes. They are very permeable to water and require use of expensive dialysis machines with volumetric ultrafiltration control circuitry. Some of these dialysis machines are difficult to disinfect properly due to the complexity of their fluid paths. If not cleaned well between uses, such machines have been associated with pyrogen reactions during dialysis. In many centers, water used to make dialysis solution contains high levels of bacteria and pyrogens. With high-flux membranes, there can be increased back flux of pyrogenic material from dialysis solution to blood (due to the lower pressure difference between blood and dialysate compartment and due to the openness of the membrane).

2.   Clinical reasons for choosing one type of membrane over another

a.   Intradialytic symptoms. Recent well-controlled studies report no difference in intradialytic symptoms among various membranes, whether or not they activate complement. The theoretical disadvantages of back-filtration are difficult to demonstrate clinically, and the occurrence of pyrogen reactions due to use of high-flux dialysis membranes is an uncommon problem.

(1)   Dialyzer reactions. Dialyzer reactions due to the membrane, sterilants, contaminated dialysis solution, or other chemicals in the dialysis circuit can be an important clinical problem (see Chapter 7). However, a consistent advantage of any one membrane type with regard to intradialytic symptoms has not been demonstrated.

b.   Morbidity and mortality.

(1)   Biocompatibility issues. A number of nonrandomized studies have suggested that morbidity and mortality may be higher in patients dialyzed with unsubstituted cellulose membranes. The reasons are unclear but may be related to a higher incidence of infections. Controlled studies are urgently required in this area. The use of unsubstituted cellulose membranes is decreasing rapidly, and we may never know the definitive answer to this question.

(2)   Flux issues. A separate question is whether or not use of high-flux dialysis is beneficial. For example, when comparing high-flux vs. low-flux biocompatible membranes, does use of a high-flux membrane improve outcome? This question is being addressed by the ongoing NIH HEMO trial (Depner et al, 1999).

(3) Back-filtration issues. One recent report has found increased plasma levels of C-reactive protein, an acute-phase reactant, when high-flux dialysis is done in a setting where substantial back-filtration is allowed to occur (Panichi et al, 1998).

High C-reactive protein levels are a marker for increased mortality in dialysis patients, but this certainly does not mean that mortality is higher with dialyzers in which back-filtration occurs. In fact, cross-sectional evidence suggests an improved survival with high-flux dialyzers (Hakim et al, 1996).

c. Amyloidosis. Whether use of a high-flux membrane improves β_2-microglobulin–associated disease is a controversial topic that is discussed in detail in Chapter 37.

B. Water permeability (K_{Uf}). The choice of a dialyzer based on its water permeability proceeds along lines similar to those detailed for acute dialysis in Chapter 5. If an ultrafiltration controller is available, one may (and should) use a dialyzer with a high water permeability (K_{Uf} greater than 6.0). If an ultrafiltration controller is not available, then a dialyzer with a lower K_{Uf} should be used. Use of a dialyzer with a relatively low K_{Uf} necessitates use of a higher transmembrane pressure (TMP) to effect removal of the required amount of excessive fluid. This minimizes the effect of variations in the TMP on the fluid removal rate. As a rule of thumb, when an ultrafiltration controller is unavailable, the in vivo dialyzer K_{Uf} (mL per hour per mm Hg) should be about four times the desired fluid removal rate in liters per hour.

C. Mode of sterilization. The three common methods of sterilizing new dialyzers are exposure to ethylene oxide gas, γ-irradiation, and steam. Anaphylactic reactions due to ethylene oxide used to be a major problem. They are less so now that dialysis companies are paying more attention to adequately degassing their dialyzers before sale. Use of γ-irradiated or steam-sterilized dialyzers largely avoids this problem.

IV. Fluid removal orders

A. Concept of "dry weight." The so-called dry weight is the postdialysis weight at which all or most excess body fluid has been removed. If the dry weight is set too high, the patient will remain in a fluid-overloaded state at the end of the dialysis session. Fluid ingestion during the interdialysis interval might then result in edema or pulmonary congestion. If the dry weight is set too low, the patient may suffer frequent hypotensive episodes during the latter part of the dialysis session. Patients who have been ultrafiltered to below their dry weight often experience malaise, a washed-out feeling, cramps, and dizziness after dialysis.

In practice, the dry weight of each patient must be determined on a trial-and-error basis. The dry weight often changes periodically (e.g., due to seasonal variations in the amount of body fat) and therefore should be reevaluated at least every 2 weeks. A progressive decrease in the dry weight can be a clue to an underlying nutritional disturbance or disease process.

When setting the ultrafiltration rate, allow for the 0.2 L that the patient will receive at the end of dialysis during the blood return procedure. Also, compensate for any fluid ingestion or parenteral fluid administration during the treatment session.

1. Frequent resetting of the dry weight. A common error in dialysis units is failure to reevaluate the dry weight often enough. If a patient then loses nonfluid weight, dialysis down to the previously set dry weight can result in overhydration and a preventable hospitalization for fluid overload.

B. Fluid removal rate. After the total amount of fluid to be removed has been calculated, the TMP is set to remove this volume at a constant rate during the treatment session (see Chapter 3 for the method of calculating the TMP). On machines with an ultrafiltration controller, the total amount of fluid to be removed is dialed in.

There is some interest in using a nonconstant fluid removal rate during a dialysis session. In one approach, the fluid removal rate is increased during the initial 1–2 hours of dialysis and reduced towards the end of dialysis (Donauer et al, 2000). The dialysis solution sodium level also may be increased during the initial phase of dialysis to help maintain the blood volume osmotically. The benefits of this approach remain controversial.

V. Dialysis solutions (Table 6-4)

A. Flow rate. The standard dialysis solution flow rate is 500 mL per minute. When the blood flow rate is high (e.g., greater than 400 mL per minute) and when a high-*KoA* dialyzer is used, increasing the dialysis solution flow rate to 800 mL per minute will increase dialyzer clearance (K) by about 10%.

B. Composition

1. Bicarbonate concentration. Bicarbonate dialysis solution is the fluid of choice, and use of acetate-based dialysate is now considered obsolete in most countries.

The concentration of base should be adjusted to achieve a predialysis plasma bicarbonate concentration of 20–23 mEq per L. There has been some interest in increasing dialysis solu-

---

Table 6-4. Dialysis solution orders

Flow rate:
   500 mL/min when dialyzers with *KoA* <700 are used
   800 mL/min when dialyzer *KoA* >700 and when blood flow rate
      is >400 mL/min (this will increase clearance, K, by about 10%)
Base:
   Bicarbonate (35 mEq/L) plus acetate (4 mEq/L)
Electrolytes and dextrose
Potassium = 2.0 mEq/L (3.0 mEq/L for patients taking digitalis)
Sodium = 135–145 mEq/L
Dextrose = 200 mg/dL
Calcium = 2.5–3.5 mEq/L
Magnesium = 0.5–1.0 mEq/L

tion bicarbonate level, or giving supplementary oral bicarbonate to increase the predialysis HCO_3 level. A definite clinical benefit of raising predialysis HCO_3 beyond 20–23 has not been shown. Metabolic alkalosis may result post dialysis in such patients, with theoretical increased risk of calcium–phosphorus precipitation, and of cardiac arrhythmia should alkalemia due to sudden hyperventilation supervene.

2. Potassium. The usual dialysis solution potassium level is 2.0 mEq per L unless the patient's usual predialysis plasma potassium concentration is less than 4.5 or unless the patient is receiving digitalis. In the latter two instances, the dialysis solution potassium level should usually be 3.0 mEq per L. Should the interdialytic serum potassium levels be high because of the use of this 3 mEq per L dialysis solution, chronic administration of sodium polystyrene sulfonate resin may be required. Malnourished patients may have low predialysis serum potassium levels.

3. Sodium. The usual dialysis solution sodium level is between 135 and 145 mEq per L. Levels above 140 mEq per L are associated with increased thirst and weight gain between dialyses, but the extra fluid often can be removed easily during dialysis due to the beneficial effect of a high-sodium dialysis solution on blood pressure during the dialysis treatment. Dialysis solution sodium levels lower than 135 mEq per L predispose to hypotension and cramps.

Recent evidence suggests that patients may have individual "set points" for sodium (Keen et al, 1997). In patients with a low sodium set point, a lower dialysis sodium level can logically be used, which should minimize postdialysis thirst and weight gain.

4. Dextrose. It is routine to add dextrose (200 mg per dL) to dialysis solutions for all patients. The presence of dextrose may reduce the incidence of hypoglycemia during dialysis.

5. Calcium. Dialysis solution calcium levels normally range from 2.5 to 3.5 mEq per L. The usual level in patients taking calcium-containing phosphorus binders is 2.5 mEq per L, but the level may have to be adjusted upward or downward depending on clinical response and parathyroid hormone status. In patients taking the newer resin-based phosphate binders, which do not contain calcium, the dialysis solution calcium level may need to be increased towards 3.5 mEq per L to avoid negative calcium balance.

6. Magnesium. The usual dialysis solution magnesium level is 0.5–1.0 mEq per L.

C. Temperature. The dialysate temperature should be set as low as possible without engendering patient discomfort, generally in the range of 34.5–36.5°C.

VI. Anticoagulation orders. See Chapter 9.

VII. Standing orders for complications. Complications are discussed in depth in Chapter 7. Frequently occurring complications, such as hypotension, cramps, restlessness, nausea, vomiting, itching, and chest pain, can be managed with a set of standing orders (Table 6-5). However, symptoms during dialysis may be the result of a more serious disease process that can require immediate diagnosis and specific treatment (see Chapter 7).

Table 6-5. Management of complications[a]

Hypotension and cramps
  Reduce ultrafiltration rate
  Place patient in Trendelenburg position
  Normal saline administration: 100–500 mL, *or*
  Hypertonic (23.4%) saline administration: 10–20 mL over
    3–5 min, *or*
  Hypertonic (50%) glucose administration: 50 mL, *or*
  Increase dialysis solution sodium concentration

Chest pain
  Nasal oxygen at 3 L/min
  Reduce blood flow rate?
  Set ultrafiltration rate to zero (esp. when UF controller is not
    being used)
  Treat hypotension promptly
  Sublingual nitroglycerin if not hypotensive and pain suggests
    angina

Itching
  Diphenhydramine hydrochloride 25 mg PO or IV
  Cyproheptadine hydrochloride 4 mg PO

Nausea and vomiting
  Reduce ultrafiltration rate
  Reduce blood flow rate only if acetate dialysis solution is being used
  Prochlorperazine 10 mg PO or 2.5 mg IV (increases risk of hypo-
    tension)

Pain
  Acetaminophen 650 mg PO

---

[a] Hypotension, chest pain, and other symptoms may be manifestations of more
severe conditions requiring immediate diagnosis and specific treatment. See
Chapter 7 for a full discussion of complications during dialysis.

VIII. Patient monitoring
A. Prior to and during the treatment session
1. Prior to dialysis
a. Weight. The predialysis weight should be compared
with the patient's last postdialysis weight and with the target dry weight to obtain some idea of interdialysis weight
gain. A large interdialysis weight gain, especially when coupled with symptoms of orthopnea or dyspnea, should prompt
a complete cardiovascular examination and reassessment of
the target dry weight (it may be too high). Patients should
strive to keep their interdialysis weight gain below 1.0 kg
per day. They also need to be counseled about limiting
sodium rather than fluid intake, as the water intake generally follows that of salt. Excessive thirst may be due to a
high dialysis solution sodium level or to high plasma renin
activity, and may be mitigated by use of an angiotensin-
converting enzyme inhibitor, although evidence for this is

controversial. Complaints of a washed-out feeling or of persistent muscle cramps after dialysis suggest that the target dry weight is too low.

b.   Blood pressure. Predialysis hypertension is often volume-related. However, in many patients, hypertension appears to be renin-mediated or due to some other unknown factor(s). In these patients, blood pressure can increase during dialysis despite fluid removal. In one report, even volume-resistant hypertensive patients benefited from further fluid removal (Fishbane et al, 1996).

Patients with hypertension are routinely counseled to withhold their blood pressure medication on the day of dialysis to limit the incidence of dialysis hypotension. This is not absolutely necessary, especially for patients who will be dialyzed in the afternoon.

c.   Temperature. The patient's temperature should be measured. The presence of a fever prior to dialysis is a serious finding and should be investigated diligently. The manifestations of infection in a dialysis patient may be subtle. On the other hand, a rise in body temperature of about 0.5°C during dialysis is normal and not necessarily a sign of infection or pyrogen reaction.

d.   Access site. Whether or not fever is present, the vascular access site should always be examined for signs of infection before each dialysis.

2.   During the dialysis session. Blood pressure and pulse rate are usually measured every 30 to 60 minutes. Any complaints of dizziness or of a washed-out feeling are suggestive of hypotension and should prompt immediate measurement of the blood pressure. Symptoms of hypotension may be quite subtle, and patients sometimes remain asymptomatic until the blood pressure has fallen to dangerously low levels.

B.   Laboratory tests (predialysis values)

1.   Serum urea nitrogen. This should be measured monthly as part of the URR. Predialysis values greater than 110 mg per dL or less than 60 mg per dL were associated with increased mortality risk (in patients being dialyzed to a mean Kt/V of about 1.0). Values below 60 mg per dL are common now that spKt/V targets have been increased.

The predialysis urea nitrogen can be measured prior to the first treatment of the week or prior to the midweek session. A urea kinetic modeling program can then be used, along with determination of residual renal urea clearance, to compute spKt/V, V, and nPNA.

2.   Serum albumin. The predialysis serum albumin level should be measured every 3 months. The serum albumin concentration is an important indicator of nutritional state. A low serum albumin level is a very strong predictor of subsequent illness or death in dialysis patients. The increased mortality risk begins at serum albumin levels less than 4.0 g per dL. Patients with serum albumin levels less than 3.0 g per dL are at high risk of morbid events, and every effort should be made to find the cause of the low albumin value and correct it. The optimum serum albumin level is more than 4.0 g per dL, but setting a single target is difficult because the range of normal values depends on the assay method used. Specifically, two methods commonly used, involving bromcresol purple or bromcresol green, give levels that differ by about 0.4 g per dL.

3.   Serum creatinine. The predialysis serum creatinine level is measured monthly. The usual mean value in hemodialysis patients is 12–15 mg per dL, with a common range of 8–20 mg per dL. Paradoxically, in dialysis patients, high serum creatinine levels are associated with a low risk of mortality (Lowrie and Lew, 1990), probably because the serum creatinine value is an indicator of muscle mass and nutritional status.

The serum creatinine and urea nitrogen levels should be examined in tandem. If parallel changes in both occur, then alteration in the dialysis prescription or degree of residual renal function should be suspected. If the serum creatinine level remains constant but a marked change occurs in the serum urea nitrogen value, the change in the latter is most likely due to altered dietary protein intake or altered catabolic rate of endogenous body proteins.

4.   Serum cholesterol. The serum cholesterol level is an indicator of nutritional status. A predialysis value of 200–250 mg per dL is associated with the lowest mortality risk in dialysis patients. Low serum cholesterol values, especially less than 150 mg per dL, are associated with an elevated mortality risk in dialysis patients, probably because they reflect poor nutritional status.

5.   Serum potassium. Dialysis patients with a predialysis serum potassium level of 5.0–5.5 mEq per L have the lowest mortality risk. The mortality risk increases greatly for values over 6.5 and under 3.5 mEq per L.

6.   Serum phosphorus. Measure monthly. The value associated with the lowest mortality is 5–7 mg per dL. Mortality rates increase sharply for values over 9.0 and under 3.0 mg per dL.

7.   Serum calcium. Measure monthly (more often when changing the dose of vitamin D). The lowest mortality is associated with values of 9–12 mg per dL. Mortality rates increase markedly at values over 12 mg per dL and under 7 mg per dL. The target value should be at the upper limit of the normal range.

8.   Serum alkaline phosphatase. Measure every 3 months. High values are a sign of hyperparathyroidism or liver disease. Lowest mortality is for values less than 100 units per L (normal being 30–115 units per L). Mortality doubles for values over 150 units per L.

9.   Serum bicarbonate. Measure monthly. Lowest mortality for values between 20 and 22.5 mEq per L. Mortality increases for both lower and higher values. Marked increases in mortality are noted when the predialysis value is under 15 mEq per L. Predialysis acidosis can be corrected by administration of alkali between dialyses.

10.   Hematocrit. The optimal predialysis hematocrit level is not known but is at least 33%, according to DOQI guidelines, and 33%–36% is the current target range. Spontaneously high hematocrit levels (without erythropoietin therapy) may be a sign of polycystic kidney disease, acquired renal cystic disease, hydronephrosis, or renal carcinoma.

Serum ferritin levels, iron levels, and iron binding capacity, as well as erythrocyte indexes, should be checked every 3 months.

11. Serum aminotransferase values are usually checked monthly. High values may unmask silent liver disease, especially hepatitis or hemosiderosis. The blood should be screened for the presence of hepatitis B surface antigen and for hepatitis C (see Chapter 28).

12. Serum parathyroid hormone levels and serum aluminum concentrations should be measured as needed, whenever the possibility of hyperparathyroidism or aluminum intoxication is suspected.

SELECTED READINGS

Daugirdas JT. Simplified equations for monitoring Kt/V, PCRn, eKt/V, and ePCRn. *Adv Ren Replace Ther* 1995;2(4):295–304.

Depner T, et al. Lessons from the Hemodialysis (HEMO) study: an improved measure of the actual hemodialysis dose. *Am J Kidney Dis* 1999;33:142.

Donauer J, et al. Ultrafiltration profiling and measurement of relative blood volume as strategies to reduce hemodialysis-related side effects. *Am J Kidney Dis* 2000;36:115–123.

Fishbane S, et al. Role of volume overload in dialysis-refractory hypertension. *Am J Kidney Dis* 1996;28:257.

Gotch F. The current place of urea kinetic modelling with respect to different dialysis modalities. *Nephrol Dial Transplant* 1998;13:10–14

Hanson JA, et al. Prescription of twice-weekly hemodialysis in the USA. *Am J Nephrol* 1999;19:625–633.

Hakim RM, et al. Effect of the dialysis membrane on mortality of chronic hemodialysis patients. *Kidney Int* 1996;50:566–570.

Held PJ, et al. The dose of hemodialysis and patient mortality. *Kidney Int* 1996;50(2):550–556.

Joseph R, et al. Comparison of methods for measuring albumin in peritoneal dialysis and hemodialysis patients. *Am J Kidney Dis* 1996;27(4):566–572.

Keen M, et al. Plasma sodium (CpNa) "set point": relationship to interdialytic weight gain (IWG) and mean arterial pressure (MAP) in hemodialysis patients (HDP). *J Am Soc Nephrol* 1997;8:241A (abst).

Kjellstrand CM (guest ed.). Daily dialysis symposium. *Semin Dial* 1999;12:403.

Leypoldt JK, et al. Hemodialyzer mass transfer–area coefficients for urea increase at high dialysate flow rates. The Hemodialysis (HEMO) study. *Kidney Int* 1997;51(6):2013–2017.

Lowrie EG, Lew NL. Death risk in hemodialysis patients: the predictive value of commonly measured variables and an evaluation of death rate differences between facilities. *Am J Kidney Dis* 1990;15:458–482.

National Kidney Foundation. NKF–DOQI clinical practice guidelines for hemodialysis adequacy. *Am J Kidney Dis* 1997;30(3 Suppl 2):S15–S66, S67–S136.

Owen WF Jr, et al. The urea reduction ratio and serum albumin concentration as predictors of mortality in patients undergoing hemodialysis. *N Engl J Med* 1993;329(14):1001–1006.

Owen WF Jr. et al. Dose of hemodialysis and survival: differences by race and sex. *JAMA* 1998;280:1764–1768.

Panichi V, et al. Plasma C-reactive protein is linked to back filtration associated interleukin-6 production. *ASAIO J* 1998;44:M415–M417.

Pierratos A. Nocturnal home   haemodialysis: an update on a 5-year experience. *Nephrol Dial Transplant* 1999;14:2835.

Wolfe RA, et al. Body size, dose of hemodialysis, and mortality. *Am J Kidney Dis* 2000;35:80–88.

Web References

NKF-DOQI guidelines for hemodialysis adequacy: http://www.kidney.org

NKF-DOQI guidelines for peritoneal dialysis adequacy: http://www.kidney.org

Urea kinetics calculators: http://www.hdcn.com/calc.htm

7

Complications During Hemodialysis

Harold Bregman, John T. Daugirdas, and Todd S. Ing

I. **Common complications.** The most common complications during hemodialysis are, in descending order of frequency, hypotension (20%–30% of dialyses), cramps (5%–20%), nausea and vomiting (5%–15%), headache (5%), chest pain (2%–5%), back pain (2%–5%), itching (5%), and fever and chills (less than 1%).

A. **Hypotension** (Table 7-1)

1. **Common causes**

a. **Hypotension related to excessive or unduly rapid decreases in the blood volume.** Hypotension during dialysis is a very common event and is primarily a reflection of the large amount of fluid relative to the plasma volume that is removed during an average dialysis session. Maintenance of blood volume during dialysis depends on rapid refilling of the blood compartment from surrounding tissue spaces. A decrease in the blood volume results in decreased cardiac filling, which, in turn, causes reduced cardiac output and, ultimately, hypotension.

(1) **Therapeutic implications.**

(a) **Use an ultrafiltration controller.** Ideally, the rate of fluid removal should be constant throughout the dialysis session. When an ultrafiltration control device is not used, the fluid removal rate can fluctuate considerably as the pressure across the dialyzer membrane varies. Transiently rapid rates of fluid removal can then occur, causing acute contraction of the blood volume and hypotension.

The best prevention is to use a dialysis machine with an ultrafiltration control device. If such a machine is not available, then one should use a dialyzer membrane that is not very permeable to water, so that the unavoidable fluctuations in the transmembrane pressure during dialysis will translate to small changes in the fluid removal rate.

(b) **Avoid large interdialytic weight gain or short treatment.** As the total amount of fluid that needs to be removed per session increases and session length is reduced, the required rate of fluid removal rises. To avoid the necessity for rapid ultrafiltration rates, patients should be counseled to limit their salt intake and hence their interdialysis weight gain (e.g., to less than 1 kg per day). Paradoxically, in cross-sectional studies, patients with high interdialytic weight gains have a better outcome than patients with low interdialytic weight gains. The reason for this is most likely nutritional in that persons with good appetites ingest-

Table 7-1. Causes of hypotension during dialysis

Common causes

1. Related to excessive decreases in blood volume
   a. Fluctuations in the ultrafiltration rate
   b. High ultrafiltration rate (to treat a large interdialytic weight gain)
   c. Target dry weight set too low
   d. Dialysis solution sodium level too low
2. Related to lack of vasoconstriction
   a. Acetate-containing dialysis solution
   b. Dialysis solution too warm
   c. Food ingestion (splanchnic vasodilatation)
   d. Tissue ischemia (adenosine-mediated, aggravated by low hematocrit)
   e. Autonomic neuropathy (e.g., diabetic)
   f. Antihypertensive medications
3. Related to cardiac factors
   a. Cardiac output unusually dependent on cardiac filling
      (i) Diastolic dysfunction due to left ventricular hypertrophy, ischemic heart disease, or other conditions
   b. Failure to increase cardiac rate
      (i) Ingestion of β-blockers
      (ii) Uremic autonomic neuropathy
      (iii) Aging
   c. Inability to increase cardiac output for other reasons
      (i) Poor myocardial contractility due to age, hypertension, atherosclerosis, myocardial calcification, valve disease, amyloidosis, etc.

Uncommon causes

1. Pericardial tamponade
2. Myocardial infarction
3. Occult hemorrhage
4. Septicemia
5. Arrhythmia
6. Dialyzer reaction
7. Hemolysis
8. Air embolism

ing large amounts of food will also demonstrate large interdialytic weight gains. However, it is our belief that moderate sodium restriction and avoidance of high-sodium dialysate can be safely used to reduce interdialytic weight gain, as long as food intake is not curtailed as a result of the dietary salt restriction.

(2) Avoid excessive ultrafiltration below the patient's "dry weight." As the patient's dry weight is approached, the rate at which the blood compartment refills from surrounding tissue spaces is diminished. Some patients gain little or no weight between dialysis treatments. Attempts to remove fluid from patients when excess fluid is absent result in hypotension both during and after dialysis, associated with cramps, dizziness, malaise, and a washed-out feeling.

On the other hand, sometimes staff will be excessively cautious in attempting to ultrafilter hypotension-prone patients, leading to hypertension and fluid overload. Use of an intradialytic hematocrit monitor may be helpful in these circumstances, as a "flat-line" hematocrit response (e.g., lack of an increase during dialysis) despite fluid removal suggests fluid overload.

(3) Use an inappropriate dialysis solution sodium level. When the dialysis solution sodium level is less than that of plasma, the blood returning from the dialyzer is hypotonic with respect to the fluid in the surrounding tissue spaces. To maintain osmotic equilibrium, water leaves the blood compartment, causing an acute reduction in the blood volume. This effect is most pronounced during the early part of dialysis, when the plasma sodium level is falling most abruptly.

The problem can be avoided by using a dialysis solution with a sodium level that is equal to or greater than the plasma value. If a "low-sodium" dialysis solution (dialysis solution sodium level less than the plasma sodium level by more than 4 mEq per L) must be used, then the ultrafiltration rate should be reduced during the early part of dialysis to compensate for the osmotic reduction in blood volume.

Recent evidence by Keen et al, (1997) suggests that patients have individual sodium set points and drink water during the interdialytic interval until this set point is restored. If confirmed, this evidence militates against a one-size-fits-all strategy for setting dialysate sodium level. Higher dialysate sodium levels may be necessary for those patients with high serum sodium set points, whereas use of high dialysate sodium levels in patients with low set points may lead to greater interdialytic water ingestion and interdialytic weight gains.

Blood volume also can be "protected" during dialysis by using a high dialysate sodium level initially and then reducing dialysate sodium over time (sodium gradient dialysis). Despite a large number of papers, there is no consensus that sodium gradient dialysis protects against intradialytic hypotension. If the time-averaged dialysate sodium level is increased with sodium gradient technique, interdialytic weight gain and blood pressure usually are increased (Sang et al, 1997).

Another approach to monitoring blood volume during dialysis is to use a hematocrit monitor. It has been suggested that a patient-specific "crash crit" can be identified, and ultrafiltration can be adjusted to avoid approaching this value. However, as with sodium gradient dialysis, definitive evidence of benefit of hematocrit monitoring in regard to preventing hypotension is not available. The use of hematocrit monitoring has been suggested to be useful in preventing intradialytic symptoms (Steuer et al, 1996).

b. Hypotension related to lack of vasoconstriction. Blood volume depletion causes a state in which cardiac output is limited by cardiac filling. Any minor decrease in peripheral vascular resistance or decrease in cardiac filling can precipitate hypotension because the cardiac output cannot increase in a compensatory manner. Under conditions of decreased cardiac filling, increases in heart rate have little effect on cardiac output.

More than 80% of the total blood volume is in veins; therefore, changes in venous capacity can cause decreased cardiac filling, decreased cardiac output, and hypotension. The splanchnic and cutaneous blood flow beds have the greatest ability to change their capacity. Most of the change in venous capacity is believed to be due to passive stretching of the veins from pressure transmitted distally from the arterioles. Thus, a decreased arteriolar resistance will cause increased transmission of arterial pressure to veins. The veins will distend and sequester an increased amount of blood. This is not important in euvolemic patients given a vasodilator because cardiac filling is more than adequate. However, with hypovolemia, the increased blood sequestration can result in hypotension. The degree of arteriolar constriction, or total peripheral resistance (TPR), is also important because TPR will determine the blood pressure for any level of cardiac output (Daugirdas, 1991).

(1) Therapeutic implications

(a) Lower dialysate temperature. Dialysis solution temperature is normally kept at about 37°C. Dialysis patients often are slightly hypothermic. For reasons that are not completely clear, the body temperature often increases slightly during a dialysis session. Core heating is a powerful vasodilatory stimulus, resulting in both venous and arteriolar dilatation. Use of a cooler dialysis solution (34–36°C) can reduce the incidence of hypotension during dialysis, presumably by preventing temperature-induced vasodilatation. As a practical point, however, patients dialyzed against cool dialysis solution often feel uncomfortably cold and shiver. A blood temperature module, available in Europe but not in the United States, allows for more precise control of thermal balance during the dialysis treatment.

(b) Avoid intradialytic food ingestion in hypotension-prone patients. Food ingestion during hemodialysis can cause an accentuated fall in blood pressure. Food ingestion causes decreased constriction of resistance vessels in certain vascular beds, especially the splanchnic bed. There is both a fall in TPR and probably an increase in splanchnic venous capacity (Barakat et al, 1993). The "food effect" on blood pressure probably lasts at least 2 hours. Patients who are prone to hypotension during dialysis may be wise to avoid eating just before or during a dialysis session.

(c) Minimize tissue ischemia during dialysis. During any type of hypotensive stress, the resulting tissue ischemia causes release of adenosine. Adenosine blocks release of norepinephrine from sympathetic nerve terminals and also has intrinsic vasodilator properties. In this sense, severe hypotension can amplify itself in that hypotension → ischemia → adenosine release → impaired norepinephrine release → vasodilatation → hypotension. This may be one reason for the clinical observation that patients with low hematocrit levels (e.g., less than 20%–25%) are very susceptible to dialysis hypotension (Sherman et al, 1986).

Use of adenosine-receptor blockers to prevent dialysis hypotension is experimental (Shinzato et al, 1992). Since the advent of erythropoietin, there should be few patients with levels of anemia severe enough to cause hypotension. However, in an acute dialysis setting, refractory dialytic hypotension in a severely anemic patient sometimes responds to transfusion sufficient to raise the predialysis hematocrit to the region of 30%.

(2)   Consider use of midodrine in refractory cases. Autonomic neuropathy is especially common in diabetic patients. In such patients, arteriolar vasoconstriction in response to volume depletion is impaired. As a result, there is decreased ability to maintain blood pressure when the cardiac output falls. In hypotension-prone patients, even those without autonomic neuropathy, there often is a decreased plasma norepinephrine response during hypotension. Midodrine, an orally acting α-adrenergic agonist, given 10 mg orally 30 minutes before a dialysis session, has been shown to limit intradialytic hypotension in several studies and is apparently safe over an 8-month period (Cruz et al, 1999). However, midodrine may not be more effective than use of low-temperature dialysate, and the results of low temperature dialysis and midodrine are not additive.

(3)   Antihypertensive medication (see Chapter 26).
c.   Hypotension related to cardiac factors
(1)   Diastolic dysfunction and left ventricular outflow tract obstruction. A stiff, hypertrophied heart cannot maintain its output in response to minor reductions in filling pressure. Left ventricular hypertrophy and diastolic dysfunction are both common in dialysis patients. Dialysis patients also may have asymmetrical ventricular hypertrophy and impairment of left ventricular outflow, increasing susceptibility to reductions in cardiac filling (Straumann et al, 1998).

(2)   Heart rate and contractility. When cardiac output is not limited by cardiac filling, it can increase via increased heart rate and contractility to compensate for a fall in TPR. Although most dialysis hypotension is associated with decreased cardiac filling, this is not the case in all situations. In some patients, there may be a fall in TPR (due to temperature effects, food ingestion, or tissue ischemia) but no fall in cardiac filling. Normally, this decrease in TPR could be compensated for by increased cardiac output mediated by increased heart rate or contractility. When cardiac compensatory mechanisms are impaired, small decreases in TPR may result in hypotension.

(a)   Therapeutic implications. A dialysate calcium concentration of 1.75 mM has been shown to improve maintenance of intradialytic blood pressure versus a low calcium dialysate of 1.25 mM, especially in patients with cardiac disease (van der Sande et al, 1998). The mechanism is increased cardiac contractility.

2. Unusual causes of hypotension during dialysis. Rarely, hypotension during dialysis may be a sign of an underlying, serious event (Table 7-1).

3. Dialyzer membranes and hypotension. A tremendous amount of speculation has been put forth to the effect that cellulosic membranes, by activating complement and a number of cytokine systems, might be associated with more dialysis hypotension than synthetic membranes. There is no evidence to support these contentions. Several good studies, several of them double-blinded, suggest no difference among membranes with regard to intradialytic hypotension.

4. Detection of hypotension. Most patients complain of feeling dizzy, light-headed, or nauseated when hypotension occurs. Some experience muscle cramps. Others may experience very subtle symptoms, which may be recognizable only to dialysis staff familiar with the patient (e.g., lack of alertness, darkening of vision, and so forth). In some patients, there are no symptoms whatsoever until the blood pressure falls to extremely low (and dangerous) levels. For this reason, blood pressure must be monitored on a regular basis throughout the hemodialysis session. Whether this is done hourly, or half-hourly, or on a more frequent basis depends on the individual case.

5. Management. Management of the acute hypotensive episode is straightforward. The patient should be placed in the Trendelenburg position (if respiratory status allows this). A bolus of 0.9% saline (100 mL or more, as necessary) should be rapidly administered through the venous blood line. The ultrafiltration rate should be reduced to as near zero as possible. The patient should then be observed carefully. Ultrafiltration can be resumed (at a slower rate, initially) once vital signs have stabilized.

As an alternative to 0.9% saline, hypertonic saline, glucose, mannitol, or albumin solutions can be used to treat the hypotensive episode. Unless cramps are also present, use of hypertonic solutions appears to offer no benefit over 0.9% saline. Nasal oxygen administration may also be of benefit during hypotensive episodes by virtue of helping to improve or maintain myocardial performance, as well as by limiting tissue ischemia and adenosine release.

a. Slowing the blood flow rate. In the past, part of initial therapy for dialysis hypotension was to slow the blood flow rate, a practice developed at a time when plate dialyzers and acetate dialysis solution were in use. There are four potential reasons to lower the blood flow rate in the management of hypotension:

(1) When plate dialyzers are used, reduction of the blood flow rate (along with reduction of dialysate negative pressure) reduces pressure in the blood compartment of the dialyzer. The plates come closer together, shrinking the dialyzer blood compartment somewhat and thus reducing the total volume of the extracorporeal circuit. This factor is of dubious clinical importance; no one has ever shown a difference in number of hypotensive episodes between parallel-plate and hollow-fiber dialyzers.

(2)   When acetate dialysis solution was used, reduction of blood flow rate reduced the transfer of vasodilatory acetate to the patient.

(3)   High blood flows engender a high pressure in the blood compartment of the dialyzer. In machines without an ultrafiltration controller, unless a correspondingly high pressure can be developed in the dialysate compartment, a high obligatory ultrafiltration results. When an ultrafiltration controller is not used, slowing the blood flow rate reduces the amount of ultrafiltration.

(4)   At very rapid blood flow rates and at a low cardiac output, one might envision a "steal" effect by the extracorporeal circuit, with increased net access flow and diversion of blood from systemic tissue beds. However, such a steal has never been documented. The usual access blood flow rate is 1,000 mL per minute It is difficult to understand how altering the flow of a parallel circuit within the access would affect net access flow or cardiac output.

  b.   Today, in almost all centers, dialysis is performed using hollow-fiber dialyzers, in which filling volume is independent of blood flow rate, and almost all centers in the United States and western Europe (with a few exceptions) use bicarbonate dialysis solution. Volumetric ultrafiltration controllers are commonly used, which allow for reduction of the ultrafiltration rate to zero despite a continued high blood flow rate. In these circumstances, three of the four reasons for reducing blood flow rate when hypotension occurs no longer apply, and whether or not a steal effect occurs is unknown.

At present, reduction of the blood flow rate to manage hypotension during dialysis should not be done initially unless the hypotension is severe or the patient is not responding to other treatment measures (stopping ultrafiltration and/or infusion of volume expander). One common cause of underdialysis is reduction in solute removal due to repeated slowing of the blood flow rate to manage recurring hypotensive episodes.

  6.   Prevention. A useful strategy to help prevent hypotension during dialysis is given in Table 7-2.

B.   Muscle cramps

  1.   Etiology. The pathogenesis of muscle cramps during dialysis is unknown. The three most important predisposing factors are (a) hypotension, (b) the patient's being below dry weight, and (c) use of low sodium dialysis solution.

    a.   Hypotension. Muscle cramps most commonly occur in association with hypotension, although cramps often persist after seemingly adequate blood pressure has been restored. In a minority of patients, cramps during dialysis will occur without any antecedent fall in blood pressure.

    b.   Patient below dry weight. Severe and prolonged cramps beginning during the latter part of dialysis and

**Table 7-2.   Strategy to help
prevent hypotension during dialysis**

1. Use a dialysis machine with an ultrafiltration controller whenever possible.
2. Counsel patient to limit salt intake, which will result in a lower interdialytic weight gain, ideally <1 kg/d.
3. Do not ultrafilter to below patient's dry weight.
4. Keep dialysis solution sodium level at or above the plasma level or use sodium gradient dialysis (controversial).
5. Give daily dose of antihypertensive medications after, not before, dialysis.
6. Use bicarbonate-containing dialysis solution.
7. In selected patients, try lowering the dialysis solution temperature to 34–36°C.
8. Ensure that hematocrit is >33% prior to dialysis.
9. Do not give food or glucose orally during dialysis to hypotension-prone patients.
10. Consider use of a blood volume monitor.
11. Consider use of α-adrenergic agonists (midodrine) prior to dialysis.

persisting for many hours after dialysis can occur when the patient has been dehydrated to below dry weight.

c.   Use of low-sodium dialysis solution. Acute lowering of the plasma sodium concentration will result in constriction of the blood vessels in an isolated muscle preparation. For this reason (and possibly others), the use of low-sodium dialysis solution has been associated with a high incidence of muscle cramps.

d.   Chronic leg cramps. In some patients, leg cramps are a chronic condition, occurring during the interdialytic interval. The cause is unknown, and leg cramps also occur in a nondialysis setting.

2.   Management. When hypotension and muscle cramps occur concomitantly, hypotension may respond to treatment with 0.9% saline; however, the muscle cramps may persist. Muscle-bed blood vessels can be dilated by hypertonic solutions. Perhaps for this reason, administration of hypertonic saline or glucose (see Table 6-5) is very effective in the acute management of muscle cramps. Such hypertonic solutions will also act to transfer water osmotically into the blood compartment from the surrounding tissues, helping to maintain the blood volume. Because the sodium load associated with hypertonic saline administration can result in postdialysis thirst, hypertonic glucose administration is preferred for treatment of cramps in nondiabetic patients.

3.   Prevention. Prevention of hypotensive episodes will eliminate the majority of episodes of cramping. Increasing the dialysis solution sodium level to 145 mEq per L or higher may also be of benefit. Such high sodium levels may increase postdialysis thirst and interdialytic weight gain. However, the extra fluid gained can usually be removed asymptomatically with high-sodium dialysis, probably because the high-sodium dialysis solution acts osmotically to maintain the blood volume during dialysis (due to accelerating refilling from tissue fluid).

a. Strategies of decreasing sodium dialysis sometimes can be useful to treat patients with refractory intradialytic cramps.

(1) Start out with a sodium level of 150–155 mEq per L and program in a linear decrease to 135–140 mEq per L by the end of the treatment. Some centers finish up with 135 mEq per L for the final 30–60 minutes of dialysis. Although there are no controlled studies, it is most logical to combine a decreasing sodium strategy with one of decreasing ultrafiltration rate, removing the bulk of the excess fluid during the first one-half to two-thirds of the dialysis treatment. Not all dialysis machines are capable of a programmable ultrafiltration rate.

b. **Vitamin E and quinine.** Vitamin E 400 IU at bedtime has been shown to be effective for chronic leg cramps (Roca et al, 1992). Quinine 325 mg at bedtime also was effective. A recent well-controlled study of hydroquinine 300 mg per day in nondialysis patients confirmed the usefulness of quinine in treating leg cramps (Jansen et al, 1997).

In 1994, the Food and Drug Administration, concerned about the high incidence of reports of health problems due to use of quinine, including thrombotic thrombocytopenic purpura, prohibited non-prescription (over-the-counter) marketing of quinine for leg cramps and instructed manufacturers to stop labeling prescription quinine for this use.

c. **Carnitine.** One carefully controlled, double-blinded study of carnitine supplementation of dialysis patients found that carnitine-supplemented patients had fewer muscle cramps during dialysis (Ahmad et al, 1990).

d. **Other drugs.** Another useful drug is oxazepam 5–10 mg, given 2 hours prior to dialysis. The mechanism whereby oxazepam helps prevent muscle cramping during dialysis is unknown.

e. **Stretching exercises.** A program of stretching exercises targeted at the affected muscle groups may also be useful.

C. **Restless legs syndrome.** This can be a difficult problem to treat and is associated with increased nocturnal leg movements. This disorder, as well as its treatment, is described in Chapter 38.

D. **Nausea and vomiting**

1. **Etiology.** Nausea or vomiting occurs in up to 10% of routine dialysis treatments. The cause is multifactorial. Most episodes in stable patients are probably related to hypotension. Nausea or vomiting also can be an early manifestation of the so-called disequilibrium syndrome described in II.A. Both type A and type B varieties of dialyzer reactions can cause nausea and vomiting. Non-dialysis causes must always be considered when nausea and vomiting occur outside of the dialysis setting, as discussed in Chapter 34. For example, hypercalcemia may manifest as (primarily interdialytic) nausea and vomiting, and should be looked for when no other explanation is at hand.

2. Management. The first step is to treat any associated hypotension. If nausea persists, an antiemetic (see Table 6-5) can be administered.

3. Prevention. Avoidance of hypotension during dialysis is of prime importance. In some patients, reduction of the blood flow rate by 30% during the initial hour of dialysis may be of benefit. However, the treatment time must then be lengthened accordingly.

E. Headache

1. Etiology. Headache is a common symptom during dialysis, and its cause is largely unknown. It may be a subtle manifestation of the disequilibrium syndrome (see II.A). In patients who are coffee drinkers, headache may be a manifestation of caffeine withdrawal as the blood caffeine concentration is acutely reduced during the dialysis treatment.

2. Management. Acetaminophen can be given during dialysis, as in Table 6-5.

3. Prevention. As for nausea and vomiting, a reduction in the blood flow rate during the early part of the dialysis treatment can be tried. Decreasing sodium dialysis also may be helpful.

F. Chest pain and back pain. Mild chest pain (often associated with mild back pain) occurs in 1%–4% of dialysis treatments. The cause is unknown. There is no specific management or prevention strategy other than switching to a different variety of dialyzer membrane (whether this change helps is controversial). The occurrence of angina during dialysis is common, and angina, as well as numerous other potential causes of chest pain (e.g., hemolysis), must be considered in the differential diagnosis. The management and prevention of angina is discussed in Chapter 33.

G. Itching. Itching is a common problem in dialysis patients, and is sometimes worse during the dialysis session. Itching appearing only during the treatment, especially if accompanied by other minor allergic symptoms, may be a manifestation of low-grade hypersensitivity to dialyzer or blood circuit components. More often than not, however, itching is simply present chronically, and is noticed in the course of the treatment while the patient is forced to sit still for a prolonged period of time.

Standard symptomatic treatment using antihistamines is described in Table 6-5. Topical capsaicin cream has been shown to be effective in one randomized, albeit unconfirmed trial (Tarng et al, 1996). Odansetron and naltrexone have failed to help in randomized trials.

Chronically, general moisturizing and lubrication of the skin using emollients is recommended. Ultraviolet light therapy, especially UVB light, may be of help (Blachley et al, 1985). Pruritus often is found in patients with elevated serum calcium × serum phosphorus products, and control of serum phosphorus and evaluation of the parathyroid glands are indicated. Whether uremic pruritus is helped by an increased dose of dialysis, use of a high flux dialyzer membrane, oral activated charcoal, or erythropoietin, remain questions for further investigation. There have been reports that each of these therapies is of benefit.

H. Fever and chills. See Chapter 28.

II. Less common but serious complications. These include disequilibrium syndrome, hypersensitivity reactions, arrhythmia, cardiac tamponade, intracranial bleeding, seizures, hemolysis, and air embolism.

A.   Disequilibrium syndrome

1.   **Definition.** The disequilibrium syndrome is a set of systemic and neurologic symptoms often associated with characteristic electroencephalographic findings that can occur either during or following dialysis. Early manifestations include nausea, vomiting, restlessness, and headache. More serious manifestations include seizures, obtundation, and coma.

2.   **Etiology.** The cause of the disequilibrium syndrome is controversial. Most believe it to be related to an acute increase in brain water content. When the plasma solute level is rapidly lowered during dialysis, the plasma become hypotonic with respect to the brain cells, and water shifts from the plasma into brain tissue. Others incriminate acute changes in the pH of the cerebrospinal fluid during dialysis as the cause of this disorder.

The disequilibrium syndrome was a much larger problem two or more decades ago, when acutely uremic patients with very high serum urea nitrogen values were commonly subjected to prolonged dialysis. However, milder forms of the syndrome may still occur in long-term dialysis patients, manifesting as nausea, vomiting, or headache. The full-blown disequilibrium syndrome, including coma and/or seizures, can still be precipitated when an acutely uremic patient is dialyzed too energetically.

3.   **Management**

   a.   **Mild disequilibrium.** Symptoms of nausea, vomiting, restlessness, and headache are nonspecific; when they occur, it is difficult to be certain that they are due to disequilibrium. Treatment is symptomatic. If mild symptoms of disequilibrium develop in an acutely uremic patient during dialysis, the blood flow rate should be reduced to decrease the efficiency of solute removal and pH change, and consideration should be given to terminating the dialysis session earlier than planned. Hypertonic sodium chloride or glucose solutions can be administered as for treatment of muscle cramps.

   b.   **Severe disequilibrium.** If seizures, obtundation, or coma occur in the course of a dialysis session, dialysis should be stopped. The differential diagnosis of severe disequilibrium syndrome should be considered (see Chapter 39). Treatment of seizures is discussed in Chapter 39. The management of coma is supportive. The airway should be controlled and the patient ventilated if necessary. Intravenous mannitol may be of benefit. If coma is due to disequilibrium, then the patient should improve within 24 hours.

4.   **Prevention**

   a.   **In an acute dialysis setting.** When planning dialysis for an acutely uremic patient, one should not prescribe an overly aggressive treatment session (see Chapter 5). The target reduction in the plasma urea nitrogen level should initially be limited to about 30%. Use of a low-sodium dialysis solution (dialysis solution sodium concentration more than several milliequivalents per liter lower than the plasma sodium level) may exacerbate cerebral edema and should be avoided if possible. In hypernatremic patients, one should not attempt to correct the plasma sodium concentration and the uremia at the same time. It is safest to dialyze a hypernatremic patient initially with a dialysis solution sodium value close to the hypernatremic plasma level and then to correct the hypernatremia slowly postdialysis by administering 5% dextrose or 5% dextrose in 0.45% saline.

   b. In a chronic dialysis setting. The incidence of disequilibrium syndrome can be minimized by use of a dialysis solution sodium concentration of at least 140 mEq per L and by using a dialysis solution that contains at least 200 mg per dL of glucose. The use of decreasing sodium dialysis solution for patients with these complaints has been advocated, with the idea that the initial rise in plasma sodium level that occurs counteracts the initial rapid removal of urea and other solutes from plasma. There is substantial evidence that use of sodium gradient dialysis reduces the incidence of disequilibrium-type intradialytic symptoms.

B. Dialyzer reactions. This is a broad group of events that includes both anaphylactic and less well-defined adverse reactions of unknown cause. In the past, many of these reactions were grouped under the term "first-use" syndrome because they presented much more often when new (as opposed to reused) dialyzers were employed. However, similar reactions occur with reused dialyzers, and we now discuss them under the more general category used here. There appear to be two varieties (Table 7-3) an anaphylactic type (type A) and a nonspecific type (type B). The occurrence of type B reactions appears to have diminished considerably during the past several years.

   1. Type A (anaphylactic type)
   a. Manifestations. When a full-blown, severe reaction occurs, the manifestations are those of anaphylaxis. Dyspnea, a sense of impending doom, and a feeling of warmth at the fistula site or throughout the body are common presenting symptoms. Cardiac arrest and even death may supervene. Milder cases may present only with itching, urticaria, cough, sneezing, coryza, or watery eyes. Gastrointestinal manifestations, such as abdominal cramping or diarrhea, may also occur. Patients with a history of atopy and/or with eosinophilia are prone to develop these reactions.

   Symptoms usually begin during the first few minutes of dialysis, but onset may occasionally be delayed for up to 30 minutes or more.

   b. Etiology
   (1) Ethylene oxide. Initially, about two-thirds of patients with type A (anaphylactic) reactions were found to have elevated serum titers of immunoglobulin E (IgE) antibodies to ethylene oxide–altered protein. Ethylene oxide was used to sterilize almost all hollow-fiber dialyzers in the late 1980s, and it tended to accumulate in the potting compound used to anchor the hollow fibers, hampering efforts to remove it by degassing prior to sale. Ethylene oxide hypersensitivity reactions were observed exclusively during first use of dialyzers, often after less

Table 7-3. Dialyzer reactions

Factor	Type A	Type B
Incidence	As high as 5/100,000 dialyzers sold	was 3–5/100 dialyses; uncommon now
Onset	First 20–30 min of dialysis, usually first 5 min	First 60 min of dialysis
Manifestations	Dyspnea Burning, heat sensation Angioedema Urticaria, itching Rhinorrhea, lacrimation Abdominal cramping	Back pain or chest pain
Severity	Moderate or severe	Usually mild
Cause	Ethylene oxide ACE inhibitors Bradykinin (AN69) Acetate Contaminated dialysate Heparin Some factor (unknown) associated with reuse Azide Latex allergy ? Complement activation	? Complement activation
Treatment	Stop dialysis immediately Do not return blood Epinephrine, antihistamines, steroids	Continue dialysis No specific treatment
Prevention	Depends on cause In all cases, **rinse the dialyzer well** immediately prior to use Change suspected ETO-sensitized patients to a gamma- or steam-sterilized dialyzer Stop ACE inhibitor therapy in affected patients If the reaction occurred while using the AN69 membrane, use a different membrane.	Put patient on a reuse program without bleach if using an unsubstituted cellulose membrane (membrane is coated with protein, reducing complement activation)

ACE, angiotensin-converting enzyme; ETO, ethylene oxide.

than adequate rinsing. Most of the initial reactions were reported in dialyzers made of unsubstituted cellulose. Current thinking is that the membrane itself plays no role in ethylene oxide hypersensitivity reactions. Recently, manufacturers have taken great pains to remove most residual ethylene oxide from dialyzers, and some have changed the composition of the potting compounds to reduce absorption of ethylene oxide during sterilization. Today ethylene oxide reactions are uncommon.

(2) **AN69-associated reactions.** These were initially reported in patients dialyzed with the AN69 membrane and also taking angiotensin-converting enzyme (ACE) inhibitors. The reactions are thought to be mediated by the bradykinin system. The negatively charged AN69 membrane activates the bradykinin system, and the effects are magnified because of ACE inhibition (ACE also participates in bradykinin inactivation). In sheep, where the reactions occur reproducibly, reactions and laboratory evidence of kinin production were both abolished by pretreating with the bradykinin β_2 receptor antagonist icatibant (Krieter et al, 1998).

(i) **AN69 versus other polyacrylonitrile (PAN) membranes.** The AN69 membrane is a copolymer of PAN and sodium methallyl sulfonate. Dialyzer membranes made of PAN with other copolymers also are available. It is unclear to what extent ACE inhibitor–associated reactions occur with other PAN-based membranes or with other non–PAN-based membranes.

(3) **Contaminated dialysis solution.** Type A dialyzer reactions have occurred when high-flux dialyzers have been used with bicarbonate-containing dialysis solution (Bigazzi et al, 1990). The treatment is usually better and more frequent cleaning and sterilization of dialysis machines between uses to reduce dialysis solution bacterial colony counts.

(4) **Reuse.** Clusters of anaphylactic-type dialyzer reactions have occurred in a reuse setting. Sometimes the problem can be linked to bacterial or endotoxin contamination of the water utilized in the reuse procedure, but in many cases the cause is unknown. Both formaldehyde and glutaraldehyde can cause allergic reactions in nondialysis settings, but reuse dialyzer reactions have not been linked to these sterilants. Ingestion of ACE inhibitors may amplify such reactions or increase their incidence (Pegues et al, 1992).

(5) **Heparin.** Heparin has occasionally been associated with allergic reactions, including urticaria, nasal congestion, wheezing, and even anaphylaxis (Gervin, 1975). When a patient seems to be allergic to a variety of different dialyzers regardless of the sterilization mode, and dialysate contamination also has been reasonably excluded, a trial of heparin-free dialysis or citrate anticoagulation should be considered.

(6) **Others.** Clinically indistinguishable reactions have occurred for a variety of other reasons. In one case,

residual azide in an ultrafilter used to pretreat dialysis water was implicated. Several other reports implicate acetate (acetate causes adenosine release when metabolized; adenosine can exacerbate bronchoconstriction). Failure to remove sterilant from dialyzers in a reuse setting can result in anaphylactoid reactions, although true IgE reactions to formaldehyde apparently do not occur.

With the use of universal precautions, patient's exposure to latex from use of gloves or other items is increased, and latex allergy should be part of the differential diagnosis.

(7) Complement fragment release. Acute increases in pulmonary artery pressure have been documented in both animals and humans during dialysis with unsubstituted cellulose membranes. However, there is no definitive proof that complement activation causes type A dialyzer reactions.

c. Management. It is safest to stop dialysis immediately, clamp the blood lines, and discard the dialyzer and blood lines without returning the contained blood. Immediate cardiorespiratory support may be required. According to the severity of the reaction, treatment with intravenous antihistamines, steroids, and epinephrine can be given.

d. Prevention. For all patients, proper rinsing of dialyzers prior to use is important to eliminate residual ethylene oxide and other putative allergens. In a patient with a history of type A reaction to an ethylene oxide–sterilized dialyzer, further use of dialyzers sterilized with this agent should be avoided. A large number of γ-irradiated and steam-sterilized dialyzers are now available (see Table 3-1). Most blood lines are still being sterilized with ethylene oxide. The necessity of using non–ethylene oxide–sterilized blood lines when switching to a γ-irradiated dialyzer has not been established. For patients whose mild type A symptoms persist following a switch to equipment free of ethylene oxide, predialysis administration of antihistamines may be of benefit. Placing the patient on a reuse program and subjecting even new dialyzers to the reuse procedure prior to first use may be of benefit due to enhanced washout of potential noxious substances or allergens from new dialyzers.

Until more information is available about the reactions associated with the AN69 membrane, some believe that AN69 use should be avoided in patients taking ACE inhibitors. One preliminary report suggests that rinsing AN69 and PAN-DX membranes with alkaline (pH 8.0) phosphate-buffered saline minimizes both enhanced bradykinin and nitric oxide synthase production normally associated with use of these membranes (Coppo et al, 1997).

2. Nonspecific type B dialyzer reactions

a. Symptoms. The principal manifestations of a type B reaction are chest pain, which may or may not be accompanied by back pain. Symptom onset may be within several minutes of starting dialysis but may be delayed for up to 1 hour or more. Typically type B reactions are less severe than type A reactions, and generally dialysis can be continued.

   b.   Etiology. The cause is unknown. Complement activation has been suggested to be a culprit, but its etiologic
role in the development of these symptoms has never been
proved. Initially it was reported that chest and back pain
occurred less frequently with reused dialyzers (reprocessed
without bleach) than with new dialyzers. This is now controversial (see Chapter 8). If reuse is beneficial with respect
to these symptoms, it is not known if the effects are due to
protein coating of the membrane (resulting in increased biocompatibility) from previous uses of the dialyzer or to washout of potentially toxic substances from the dialyzer during
previous uses and reprocessing procedures. The incidence of
type B reactions has declined in the United States.
   Other causes of chest and back pain must be excluded, and
the diagnosis of a type B dialyzer reaction is one of exclusion.
In particular, subclinical hemolysis must be ruled out. A syndrome of acute respiratory distress associated with heparin-
induced thrombocytopenia has been described (Popov et al,
1997), which may superficially resemble a type B dialyzer
reaction.
   c.   Management. Management is supportive. Nasal oxygen should be given. Myocardial ischemia should be considered, and angina pectoris, if suspected, can be treated as discussed in Chapter 33. Dialysis can usually be continued, as
symptoms invariably abate after the first hour.
   d.   Prevention. One solution is to place the patient on a
reuse program. Subjecting new dialyzers to the reuse washing and sterilization procedure may have some benefit,
although this is controversial. A different dialyzer membrane can be tried.
C.   Arrhythmia. Arrhythmias during dialysis are especially
common in patients receiving digitalis. Prevention and management are discussed in Chapter 33.
D.   Cardiac tamponade. Unexpected or recurrent hypotension during dialysis can be a sign of pericardial effusion or impending cardiac tamponade (see Chapter 33).
E.   Intracranial bleeding. Underlying vascular disease and
hypertension combined with heparin administration can sometimes result in the occurrence of intracranial, subarachnoid, or
subdural bleeding during the dialysis session (see Chapter 39).
F.   Seizures. Children, patients with high predialysis plasma
urea nitrogen levels, and patients with severe hypertension are
the most susceptible to seizures during dialysis. Seizure activity can be one manifestation of the disequilibrium syndrome.
Seizures are more fully discussed in Chapter 39.
G.   Hemolysis. Acute hemolysis during dialysis may be a medical emergency.
   1.   Manifestations
      a.   Symptoms. The symptoms of hemolysis are back
pain, tightness in the chest, and shortness of breath.
      b.   Signs. A dramatic deepening of skin pigmentation has
recently been described (Seukeran et al, 1997). Common
are a port-wine appearance of blood in the venous blood
line, a pink discoloration of the plasma in centrifuged blood
samples, and a marked fall in the hematocrit.

c. **Consequences of hemolysis.** If massive hemolysis is not detected early, then hyperkalemia can result due to release of potassium from the hemolyzed erythrocytes, leading to muscle weakness, electrocardiographic abnormalities, and, ultimately, cardiac arrest.

2. Etiology. Acute hemolysis has been reported in two primary settings: (a) an obstruction or narrowing in the blood line, catheter, or needle, and (b) a problem with the dialysis solution.

a. **Blood line obstruction/narrowing.** Blood line kinks may be present in the arterial blood line (Sweet et al, 1996). An epidemic of hemolysis also has been reported due to manufacturing defects in the link between the dialyzer outlet blood line and the venous air trap chamber (CDC, 1998). Hemolysis (usually subclinical) may also appear when blood flow rate is high and the dialysis or catheter needle holes are relatively small (De Wachter et al, 1997).

b. **Problems with dialysis solution.** These are:

   (1) Overheated dialysis solution

   (2) Hypotonic dialysis solution (insufficient concentrate-to-water ratio)

   (3) Dialysis solution contaminated with:

      (a) Formaldehyde

      (b) Bleach

      (c) Chloramine (from city water supply)

      (d) Copper (from copper piping)

      (e) Nitrates (from water supply)

3. Management. The blood pump should be stopped immediately and the blood lines clamped. The hemolyzed blood has a very high potassium content and should not be reinfused. One should be prepared to treat the resultant hyperkalemia and possible drop in hematocrit. The patient should be observed carefully and hospitalization should be considered. Delayed hemolysis of injured erythrocytes may continue for some time after the dialysis session. Severe hyperkalemia may occur and this may require additional dialysis or other measures (e.g., administration of an Na/K ion exchange resin by mouth or rectum) to control.

4. Prevention. Unless the problem is an obstruction in the blood path or faulty roller pump causing excessive blood trauma, the cause of the hemolysis must be assumed to be in the dialysis solution, and samples of dialysis solution must be investigated to determine the cause.

H. Air embolism. Air embolism is a potential catastrophe that can lead to death unless detected and treated quickly.

1. Manifestations

a. **Symptoms.** These depend to an extent on the position of the patient. In seated patients, infused air tends to migrate into the cerebral venous system without entering the heart, causing obstruction to cerebral venous return, with loss of consciousness, convulsions, and even death. In recumbent patients, the air tends to enter the heart, generate foam in the right ventricle, and pass into the lungs. At this point, dyspnea, cough, and chest tightness can be expected. Further passage of air across the pulmonary cap-

illary bed into the left ventricle can result in air embolization to the arteries of the brain and heart, with acute neurologic and cardiac dysfunction.

   b.   Signs. Foam is often seen in the venous blood line of
the dialyzer. If air has gone into the heart, a peculiar churn-
ing sound may be heard on auscultation.

   2.   Etiology. The predisposing factors and possible sites of
air entry have been discussed in Chapter 3. The most common sites of air entry are the arterial needle, the prepump
arterial tubing segment, and an inadvertently opened end of
a central venous catheter.

   3.   Management. The first step is to clamp the venous
blood line and stop the blood pump. The patient is immediately placed in a recumbent position on the left side with the
chest and head tilted downward. Further treatment includes
cardiorespiratory support, including administration of 100%
oxygen by mask or endotracheal tube. Aspiration of air from
the ventricle with a percutaneously inserted needle can be
attempted.

   4.   Prevention. See Chapters 3 and 5.

**III.   Dialysis-associated neutropenia and complement
activation.** As discussed in Chapter 3, dialyzer membranes made
of unsubstituted cellulose have on their surface many exposed
hydroxyl groups. The latter can activate the complement cascade
in blood flowing through the dialyzer. The liberated complement
fragments cause circulating blood neutrophils to migrate to the
lungs where they localize next to blood vessel walls, resulting in
neutropenia. After 30–60 minutes of dialysis, the circulating neutrophil count again rises to normal or even supranormal levels.

   Cellulose membranes in which the hydroxyl groups have been
chemically "covered" by either acetate (to form cellulose acetate)
or a tertiary amino group (Hemophan) activate complement to a
much lesser extent and cause less neutropenia. Most synthetic
membranes (polysulfone, polycarbonate, polymethylmethacrylate)
cause little complement activation or neutropenia. PAN activates
complement but then adsorbs the complement fragments, obviating most of their secondary effects.

   A.   Clinical importance

   1.   Symptoms. Whether complement activation and
neutropenia during dialysis are responsible for intradialytic
symptoms (i.e., hypotension, nausea, chest pain, back pain)
remains a matter of controversy, although the majority of
patients can be asymptomatically dialyzed using membranes
of unsubstituted cellulose.

   2.   Renal injury. Complement activation causes activation of leukocytes with increased generation of superoxide. In
a rat model of ischemic renal failure, complement infusion
or exposure to a complement-activating membrane causes
sequestration of neutrophils in glomeruli and delay of recovery of renal function. The trials concerning use of complement-
activating membranes for acute dialysis are discussed in
Chapter 5.

   **3.   Chronic effects of dialysis using complement-
activating membranes on the immune system.** Membranes of unsubstituted cellulose have deleterious effects on

the immune system that persist over the subsequent inter-dialytic interval. However, there are no definitive studies link-ing use of unsubstituted cellulose membranes to an adverse outcome. One randomized trial (Parker et al, 1996) suggesting an adverse effect of complement-activating membrane use on patient dry weight and serum albumin value was not con-firmed by a larger, multicenter randomized trial (Locatelli et al, 1996).

   4.   Hypoxemia. See Section IV.

   5.   Interference with complete blood count determi-nation. Because the white blood cell count may be transiently reduced by 50%–80% during dialysis with a cellulose mem-brane, all blood counts done for diagnostic purposes should be drawn predialysis.

IV.   Dialysis-associated hypoxemia

   A.   Definition and clinical importance. During hemodial-ysis, the arterial blood PO_2 drops by 5–30 mm Hg. The fall in PO_2 is of no clinical significance in the routine patient but may be deleterious in a patient with severe preexisting pulmonary or cardiac disease.

   B.   Etiology. There are several possible reasons for the drop in PO_2 during dialysis.

      1.   Hypoventilation. Studies have shown that hypoven-tilation can almost always be implicated. Two mechanisms for hypoventilation during dialysis have been proposed:

         a.   Acetate-containing dialysis solution. Hypocap-nia due to loss of carbon dioxide in the dialyzer. Acetate-containing dialysis solution is in gas equilibrium with room air, the PCO_2 of which is less than 1 mm Hg. During dialysis against an acetate-containing dialysis solution, blood passing through the dialyzer loses carbon dioxide to the dialysis solution, resulting in hypocapnia. The patient hypoventilates slightly, maintaining blood PCO_2 close to the baseline value.

         Bicarbonate-containing dialysis solution has an elevated PCO_2, due to the special way in which bicarbonate-containing dialysis solution is made. For this reason, dialysis against a bicarbonate bath does not result in hypocapnia.

         b.   Bicarbonate-containing dialysis solution: alka-losis. When a bicarbonate-containing dialysis solution is used, especially when the dialysis solution bicarbonate level is high (greater than 35 mEq per L), prompt transfer of bicarbonate from dialysis solution to the blood can result in metabolic alkalosis. Metabolic alkalosis is a well-known cause of hypoventilation and hypoxemia.

      2.   Intrapulmonary diffusion block. As noted above, dialysis using unsubstituted cellulose membranes causes sequestration of neutrophils in the lung. Some studies have suggested that the alveolar-to-arterial oxygen gradient is increased very early during dialysis, presumably due to neu-trophil embolization into the pulmonary capillaries. This con-cept is controversial, and absence of hypoxemia during dial-ysis when the patient is on mechanical ventilation (Huang et al, 1998) suggests that a such a diffusion block is of little importance.

C. Management. Nasal oxygen administration is sufficient treatment in almost all instances. In patients with carbon dioxide retention, delivery of oxygen by Venturi mask may be more appropriate.

D. Prevention. Prevention of hypoxemia includes oxygen administration. In high-risk patients, one might consider avoiding dialyzer membranes made of unsubstituted cellulose and using a bicarbonate-containing dialysis solution with a bicarbonate concentration low enough to avoid alkalemia.

SELECTED READINGS

Ahmad S, et al. Multicenter trial of L-carnitine in maintenance hemodialysis patients. II. Clinical and biochemical effects. *Kidney Int* 1990;38:912–918.

Barakat MM, et al. Hemodynamic effects of intradialytic food ingestion and the effects of caffeine. *J Am Soc Nephrol* 1993;3:1813.

Bigazzi R, et al. Highly-permeable membranes and hypersensitivity-like reactions: role of dialysis fluid contamination. *Blood Purif* 1990;8:190.

Blachley JD, et al. Uremic pruritus: skin divalent ion content and response to ultraviolet phototherapy. *Am J Kidney Dis* 1985 May; 5(5):237–241.

Canzanello VJ, Burkart JM. Hemodialysis-associated muscle cramps. *Semin Dial* 1992;5:299.

Centers for Disease Control and Prevention (CDC). Multistate outbreak of hemolysis in hemodialysis patients. *JAMA* 1998;280:1299.

Coppo R, et al. pH of the washing solutions for dialysis filters and generation of vasodilatory mediators (bradykinin and nitric oxide): Role in first use syndrome. *J Am Soc Nephrol* (abstr) 1997;8:231A.

Cruz DN, et al. Midodrine and cool dialysate are effective therapies for symptomatic intradialytic hypotension. *Am J Kidney Dis* 1999; 33:920–926.

Daugirdas JT. Dialysis hypotension: a hemodynamic analysis. *Kidney Int* 1991;39:233.

Daugirdas JT, Ing TS. First-use reactions during hemodialysis: a definition of subtypes. *Kidney Int* 1988;24:S37.

De Wachter DS, et al. Blood trauma in plastic haemodialysis cannula. *Int J Artif Organs* 1997;20:366–370.

Gervin AS. Complications of heparin therapy. *Surg Gynecol Obstet* 1975;140:789–796.

Huang CC, et al. Oxygen, arterial blood gases and ventilation are unchanged during dialysis in patients receiving pressure support ventilation. *Respir Med* 1998;92:534.

Jansen PH, et al. Randomised controlled trial of hydroquinine in muscle cramps. *Lancet* 1997;349:528.

Keen M, et al. Plasma sodium setpoint: Relationship to interdialytic weight gain and mean arterial pressure in hemodialysis patients. *J Am Soc Nephrol* (abstr) 1997;8:241A.

Krieter DH, et al. Anaphylactoid reactions during hemodialysis in sheep are ACE inhibitor dose-dependent and mediated by bradykinin. *Kidney Int* 1998;53:1026–1035.

Lemke H-D, et al. Hypersensitivity reactions during haemodialysis: role of complement fragments and ethylene oxide antibodies. *Nephrol Dial Transplant* 1990;5:264.

Locatelli F, et al. Effects of different membranes and dialysis technologies on patient treatment tolerance and nutritional parameters. The Italian Cooperative Dialysis Study Group. *Kidney Int* 1996;50:1293–1302.

Mendelsohn DC, et al. Chronic mannitol accumulation in hemodialysis patients. *J Am Soc Nephrol* 1992;3:379(abst).

Ornt DB. Volumetric control of ultrafiltration reduces the rate of hypotension on hemodialysis. *J Am Soc Nephrol* 1992;3:384(abst).

Parker TF 3rd, et al. Effect of the membrane biocompatibility on nutritional parameters in chronic hemodialysis patients. *Kidney Int* 1996; 49:551–556.

Parnes EL, Shapiro WB. Anaphylactoid reactions in hemodialysis patients treated with the AN69 dialyzer. *Kidney Int* 1991;40:1148.

Pegues DA, et al. Anaphylactoid reactions associated with reuse of hollow-fiber hemodialyzers and ACE inhibitors. *Kidney Int* 1992; 42:1232.

Poldermans D, et al. Cardiac evaluation in hypotension-prone and hypotension-resistant dialysis patients. *Kidney Int* 1999;56: 1905–1911.

Popov D, et al. Pseudopulmonary embolism: acute respiratory distress in the syndrome of heparin-induced thrombocytopenia. *Am J Kidney Dis* 1997;29:449–452.

Robertson KE, Mueller BA. Uremic pruritus. *Am J Health Syst Pharm* 1996;53:2159–2170; quiz 2215–2216. Review.

Roca AO, et al. Dialysis leg cramps. Efficacy of quinine versus vitamin E. *ASAIO J* 1992;38:M481.

Sang GL, et al. Sodium ramping in hemodialysis: a study of beneficial and adverse effects. *Am J Kidney Dis* 1997;29:669.

Seukeran D, et al. Sudden deepening of pigmentation during haemodialysis due to severe haemolysis. *Br J Dermatol* 1997;137:997–999.

Sherman RA, et al. The effect of red cell transfusion on hemodialysis-related hypotension. *Am J Kidney Dis* 1988;11:33–35.

Shinzato T, et al. Relationship between dialysis induced hypotension and adenosine released by ischemic tissue. *ASAIO J* 1992;38:M286.

Silver SM, et al. Dialysis disequilibrium syndrome (DDS) in the rat: role of the "reverse urea effect." *Kidney Int* 1992;42:161.

Steuer RR, et al. Reducing symptoms during hemodialysis by continuously monitoring the hematocrit. *Am J Kidney Dis* 1996; 27:525.

Straumann E, et al. Symmetric and asymmetric left ventricular hypertrophy in patients with end-stage renal failure on long-term hemodialysis. *Clin Cardiol* 1998;21:672–678.

Sweet SJ. Hemolytic reactions mechanically induced by kinked hemodialysis lines. *Am J Kidney Dis* 1996;27:262.

Tarng DC, et al. Hemodialysis-related pruritus: a double-blind, placebo-controlled, crossover study of capsaicin 0.025% cream. *Nephron* 1996;72(4):617–622.

van der Sande FM, et al. Effect of dialysate calcium concentration on intradialytic blood pressure course in cardiac-compromised patients. *Am J Kidney Dis* 1998;32:125.

8

Dialyzer Reuse

Allen M. Kaufman and Nathan W. Levin

After a dialyzer is used, it can be rinsed free of blood, chemically cleaned, disinfected, and reused. Dialyzer reuse is a safe and effective practice in the United States that is applied in the treatment of approximately 80% of U.S. hemodialysis patients (Held, 1997). Most reuse is performed utilizing hollow-fiber dialyzers. The average number of times that a dialyzer is reused varies from unit to unit, although many programs average more than 10 reuses per dialyzer.

I. Reprocessing technique. The major steps in dialyzer reprocessing are rinsing, cleaning, measurement of dialyzer performance, disinfection/sterilization, and germicide removal (Table 8-1 and 8-2).

A. Rinsing and reverse ultrafiltration. To maintain the patency of fibers and to minimize clotting after dialysis, blood should be returned with heparinized saline. Removal of residual blood can be accomplished by reverse ultrafiltration with dialysate while still at the dialysis station. Once the dialyzer has been removed from the machine, a pressurized rinse of both the blood and dialysate compartments should begin with minimal delay. If a delay is unavoidable, the dialyzers should be refrigerated.

B. Cleaning

1. Bleach. Sodium hypochlorite (bleach), diluted to 1% or less, dissolves proteinaceous deposits that may occlude fibers. Bleach increases albumin losses in high-flux cellulose triacetate (CT 190) and polysulfone–polyvinylpyrrolidone (F80B) dialyzers. Albumin losses are generally not clinically significant unless bleach is used on high-flux membranes with exceptionally high water permeability (see III.B, "Clinical concerns"). However, bleach can result in an increase in the ultrafiltration coefficient and overt membrane damage in cellulosic membranes, especially when used in high concentrations, at an elevated temperature or for prolonged exposure time (Pizziconi, 1990).

2. Other cleaning agents. Hydrogen peroxide (3% or less) and peracetic acid/hydrogen peroxide/acetic acid mixtures (available in the United States as Renalin) are commonly used. These agents may not completely remove proteins deposited on the dialyzer membrane. For this reason, the ultrafiltration coefficient may become reduced in dialyzers cleaned with this agent (Berkseth, 1984).

C. Tests of dialyzer performance. These check the integrity of the membrane and its clearance and ultrafiltration properties. The tests may be done manually or using automated techniques.

1. Pressure test for leaks. A blood path integrity test works by generating a transmembrane pressure gradient

Table 8-1. Characteristics of several automated dialyzer reprocessing devices

Feature	Mesa Medical Echo	Renal Systems Renatron II	Seratronics DRS-4
Pressure test	Yes	Yes	Yes
Fiber bundle volume test	Yes	Yes	Yes
Ultrafiltration rate test	No	No	Yes
Stations	Single station	Modular (6 units can be combined)	Multistation (4)
			Water
Cleaning agents	Hydrogen peroxide	Renalin	Hydrogen peroxide
	Sodium hypochlorite		Sodium hypochlorite
	Peracetic acid		Peracetic acid
Germicides	Multiple	Renalin	Multiple
Computerized database management	No	Yes	Yes
Water requirements			
Input pressure (psi)	40–100	20–55	30–80
Peak flow (L/min)	1.5	6	1.5–2.3
Water volume (L/dialyzer)	6–9	13–19	6–9
Processing time	8–30 min/dialyzer	8–10 min/dialyzer	35 min/4 dialyzers

Table 8-2. Typical manual reprocessing procedure for hollow-fiber dialyzers

1. **Rinsing.** The blood compartment is rinsed with water of AAMI quality at 15–20 psi until the effluent is clear. Clots in the dialyzer header are removed. The dialysate compartment is then rinsed.
2. **Cleaning.** Cleaning is facilitated by reverse ultrafiltration from the dialysate to the blood compartment. A dialysate port is connected to a water source at 15–20 psi, and a closed Hansen connector is placed on the other dialysate port. Reverse ultrafiltration continues until the effluent from the blood compartment is clear (3–10 min).

    Cleaning compounds may be instilled via gravity feed or by vacuum. These chemicals are then promptly removed by rinsing at 15–20 psi. Tests on the blood compartment effluent should be performed to standardize the rinse time necessary to remove the cleaning compound.
3. **Testing and disinfecting.** Fiber bundle volume is measured by displacing the water in the blood compartment with air. A filtered bulb utilizing a 0.45-µm transducer or a filtered compressed air source can be used to force blood compartment water into a graduated cylinder. If the fiber bundle volume is less than 80% of the original priming volume, the dialyzer is discarded.
4. Additional procedures such as a pressure-holding integrity test or an ultrafiltration rate test can be performed at this time.
5. When all tests have been passed, the dialysate and blood compartments are filled with germicide, the disinfection times are recorded on the dialyzer label, and the dialyzer is stored for an appropriate period of time.

AAMI, Association for the Advancement of Medical Instrumentation.

across the membrane and observing for a pressure fall in either the blood or the dialysate compartment. The gradient may be produced by instilling pressurized air or nitrogen into the blood side of the dialyzer or by producing a vacuum in the dialysate side. Only minimal amounts of air can leak through an intact wetted membrane; damaged fibers usually rupture when a transmembrane pressure gradient is applied. Leak tests also screen for defects in the dialyzer O-rings, potting compound, and end-caps.

    2. Blood compartment volume. This test indirectly measures changes in membrane clearance for small molecules, such as urea. The blood compartment volume (total cell volume, TCV) is measured by purging the filled blood compartment (header volume and fiber volume) with air and measuring the volume of obtained fluid. Every dialyzer should be processed before the first use in order to obtain a dialyzer-specific baseline TCV. The change in TCV is then followed after each reuse. A reduction in TCV of 20% corresponds to 10% reduction in urea clearance, the maximum decrease acceptable for continued use (Gotch, 1986). Meaningful tests of TCV cannot be done in plate dialyzers because their blood

compartment volume changes with the amount of transmembrane pressure applied. In a given patient, repeated failure to reach a target number of reuses because of TCV test
failures suggests excessive clot formation during dialysis and
should prompt a review of the heparin prescription.

   3.   In vitro K_{Uf}. The dialyzer ultrafiltration coefficient
(K_{Uf}; described in Chapter 2) is another indirect measure of
membrane mass transfer properties because a change in the
K_{Uf} reflects changes in membrane resistance, as well as surface area. The in vitro K_{Uf} can be measured by determining
the volume of water passing through the membrane at a
given pressure and temperature. However, changes in this
parameter do not have a clinical impact when used with
machines with ultrafiltration control.

D.   Disinfection/sterilization. Once cleaned, the dialyzer
must undergo a physical or chemical process that renders all living organisms inactive. High-level disinfection differs from sterilization in that the former may not destroy spores. High-level
disinfection is all that current standards require. Sterilization as
defined legally is not easily accomplished in a dialysis facility.

   1.   Germicides. Germicides are generally instilled in both
blood and dialysate compartments for 24 hours. Peracetic acid/
hydrogen peroxide/acetic acid mixtures (54.1%), formaldehyde
(37.2%), and glutaraldehyde (Diacide) (8.8%) are the most common germicides used. Formaldehyde vapor is effective in disinfecting fibers that do not come in direct contact with the liquid formaldehyde. Renalin offers the advantage of qualifying
as a sterilant with the limitations mentioned above. Heated citric acid (Levin et al, 1995) or the original method with heated
water (Kaufman, 1992) are nonnoxious chemical alternatives
to disinfection.

   2.   Documenting the presence of germicide. The presence of germicide must be ensured through procedural controls,
ideally verified in every dialyzer prior to use. When formaldehyde is the germicide used, an indicator substance, such an
FD&C blue dye no. 1, can be added to the concentrated stock
solution. When dilute (batch) solutions are made and instilled
in the dialyzer, their light blue color indicates that formaldehyde is present. This method avoids the need to test each dialyzer individually for presence of germicide on a routine basis.
However, daily verification that the concentration of formaldehyde in the batch solution is adequate is still required, as are
periodic spot checks of dialyzers for formaldehyde presence
and concentration. The usual concentration of formaldehyde is
4% when disinfection is performed at room temperature for
24 hours. A 2% solution should not be used at room temperature because some types of mycobacteria have been shown to
survive 2% formaldehyde exposure for 24 hours. However,
even 1% solutions of formaldehyde may have excellent germi-
cidal efficacy when dialyzers are incubated at 40°C for 24 hours
(Hakim et al, 1985).

   3.   Germicide removal. Germicide removal is accomplished by either automated or manual techniques. The basic
maneuvers include initial flushing of the blood compartment,
followed by flushing of the dialysate compartment. Removal

(by diffusion) of formaldehyde can be accomplished by circulating saline through the blood compartment while coursing heated dialysate through the dialysate compartment in a single-pass fashion for 15 minutes.

Air must be removed from the arterial line before flushing in order to avoid introduction of air into the blood compartment. Trapped air in the fibers or dialysate compartment may retard the effectiveness of germicide removal techniques. In addition, the dialyzer should be rotated at intervals during flushing to release trapped air in the dialysate compartment.

The blood circuit should be checked for residual germicide immediately prior to use by two individuals. Residual formaldehyde can be checked with modified Schiff's reagent and should be within the currently acceptable levels of 5 ppm. Residual levels of other germicides can be checked with specific manufacturer–recommended test kits.

4.   Heat sterilization. Germicide-free reprocessing utilizing high temperature to achieve sterilization obviates many of the concerns related to the use of chemicals to process dialyzers. In the original technique, the dialyzers are cleaned and tested in the usual manner, reverse-osmosis water is instilled, and the dialyzers are heated in a 105°C convection oven for 20 hours (Kaufman, 1992). An additional integrity test at the bedside is required prior to use. In a subsequent technique, 1.5% citric acid solution allows for heating at 95°C at 20 hours to achieve identical disinfection and to limit structural damage to the dialyzer (Levin et al, 1995). At present, polysulfone is the only membrane material that has proved sufficiently heat-resistant for clinical use. In addition, potting compounds must meet certain design specifications for use under these conditions. In the case of heat methodology that utilizes a convection oven, appropriate temperature is assured by a continuous temperature recorder and by heat-sensitive labels.

5.   Final inspection. Dialyzers should not be used if they have an abnormal or unaesthetic appearance (e.g., if there is an overall brownish or blackish discoloration, if there are clots in the header, or if bands of clotted fibers are present).

II.   Automated versus manual systems. Several types of automated machines are now manufactured; some provide the ability to process multiple dialyzers simultaneously. With automated methods, the cleansing cycles are highly reproducible and a variety of quality control tests measuring fiber bundle volume, ultrafiltration coefficient, and pressure holding are built in. Dialyzer labels can also be automatically printed. Computerized analysis of records and results are available with some of the systems. A summary of commonly used automated systems is presented in Table 8-1.

Although the use of automated systems now predominates, manual reprocessing of dialyzers is still performed with success in some dialysis units. The core steps and some technical details of a manual method of reprocessing is presented in Table 8-2.

III.   Clinical issues. When reprocessing is performed in accordance with accepted standards and practices (AAMI, 1995), the risks of the procedure are negligible. The incidences of sepsis and hepatitis B infection are not different in patients treated with reused dialyzers from those treated with new dialyzers (Alter et al,

1990). There are no reports of transmission of HIV infection related to dialyzer reuse.

A. Clinical benefits (Table 8-3)

   1. Wider use of costlier dialyzers. It is now well established that mortality in dialysis patients decreases as the amount of dialysis given is increased above substandard levels (Table 8-3). Large patients and patients who resist longer dialysis session lengths usually can be adequately dialyzed only when high-efficiency (high-KoA) dialyzers are used (see Chapter 3). For a given dialysis session length and blood flow rate, use of a high-efficiency dialyzer results in more dialysis for every patient. Furthermore, evidence is accumulating that use of a high-flux synthetic membrane may confer an additional beneficial effect on survival (see Chapter 6). High-efficiency dialyzers, as well as high-flux synthetic dialyzers, can be widely offered only by those units practicing reuse.

   2. First-use reactions. In the past, anaphylactic reactions occurred less frequently with reprocessed dialyzers than with new dialyzers. Most likely, this was the result of removal of residual amounts of ethylene oxide or other substances used during manufacture (Daugirdas and Ing, 1988). Milder, more common forms of "first-use syndrome" associated with cellulosic (Cuprophan) dialyzers may occur less frequently or are milder with reuse (Bok et al, 1980). It has been advocated that new dialyzers be reprocessed prior to clinical use. With this "preprocessing," the incidence of anaphylactic reactions during first use may be reduced, as may the incidence of symptoms during the first use (Charoenpanich et al, 1987).

   3. Complement activation. With unsubstituted cellulose dialyzers, reuse lessens the degree of membrane-induced

---

Table 8-3. Advantages and disadvantages of dialyzer reuse

Advantages

Allows more widespread use of costlier dialyzer (e.g., high-KoA, high-flux, synthetic membrane with their attendant benefits)

Reduced exposure to residual industrial chemicals used in the manufacture of new dialyzers

Reduced incidence of intradialytic symptoms (controversial)

Enhanced dialyzer biocompatibility/reduced immune system activation (with unsubstituted cellulose membranes and when bleach is not used)

Reduction in treatment cost

Disadvantages

Potential for exposure of patient and personnel to chemicals

Potential for bacterial/endotoxin contamination of dialyzer

Potential for loss of dialyzer mass transfer (clearance) and ultrafiltration capacity

Potential for transmission of an infectious agent from one dialyzer to another during the reprocessing procedure

Potential loss of β_2-microglobulin clearance with certain reuse techniques.

activation of complement and the resulting transient leukopenia (Hakim and Lowrie, 1980). This may be the result of protein coating of the membrane during its first clinical use. The benefit disappears if bleach is used in the reprocessing method because bleach acts to remove or alter the protein coat from the membrane (Pizziconi et al, 1984). Nonreused cellulosic dialyzers can cause chronic suppression of several aspects of the immune system (Zaoui et al, 1991). These adverse immune effects may occur to a lesser extent in a reuse situation.

B.   Clinical concerns: formaldehyde. Anti-N-like antibodies, which can be produced when residual dialyzer formaldehye levels are high, have been associated with hemolysis and with early transplant failure. Formation of these antibodies does not usually occur at currently recommended residual formaldehyde levels (Crosson et al, 1976), although one group has reported their development even when dialyzers were rinsed to the point that effluent formaldehyde levels were always below 2–3 ppm (Vanholder et al, 1988).

1.   Acute reactions. Immediate burning at the fistula site may indicate that formaldehyde has been improperly removed from the dialyzer. Under these circumstances, the dialysis should be stopped immediately, the venous blood line clamped, and the dialyzer contents checked for formaldehyde. Dialysis should continue with a new dialyzer.

2.   Itching. In some studies, itching during dialysis has improved after switching from formaldehyde to alternative disinfecting agents.

3.   Morbidity and mortality. A reduction in mortality rates has been suggested in programs that reuse dialyzers using formaldehyde reprocessing (Held et al, 1987). On the other hand, an association between the use of peracetic acid/hydrogen peroxide/acetic acid mixture or glutaraldehyde and increased death rate has been reported (Held et al, 1994; Feldman et al, 1996). In Held's study, increased mortality was associated only with manual reprocessing of dialyzers using peracetic acid/hydrogen peroxide/acetic acid as a sterilant. A direct causative link between these germicides and increased patient mortality remains to be established. The U.S. Food and Drug Administration (FDA) response has been to instruct dialysis units to review their manual and automated procedures carefully and ensure that manufacturing instructions be followed meticulously. No increased mortality was found when dialyzers were reprocessed with formaldehyde.

4.   Potential bacterial/pyrogen contamination. Bacteremia and pyrogen reactions can result from improperly processed dialyzers. Clusters of pyrogen reactions occur slightly more often in centers that reuse dialyzers. In general, the source of such problems are generally the water used to rinse and clean the dialyzers and to prepare the germicides used for disinfection. Scrupulous attention to water treatment is required.

5.   Potential of anaphylactoid reactions with use of peracetic acid/hydrogen peroxide/acetic acid reuse agents and angiotensin-converting enzyme (ACE) inhibitors. An outbreak of anaphylactoid reactions to reused dialyzers occurred in patients dialyzed with cuprammonium cellulose, cellulose acetate, and polysulfone dialyzers reprocessed with peracetic acid/hydrogen peroxide/acetic acid. Most were being treated with ACE inhibitors (Pegues et al, 1992). Reuse of dialyzers with oxidizing agents, such as peracetic acid/hydrogen peroxide/acetic acid, can produce a strong negative charge on the protein coated membrane and thereby activate factor XII, kininogen, kallikrein, and, subsequently, bradykinin. ACE inhibitor–induced inhibition of bradykinin degradation may potentiate the reaction. Similar reactions have been described with the use of polyacrylonitrile membrane and attributed to membrane-induced bradykinin generation (Verresen et al, 1994). In another small case series, reactions in patients taking ACE inhibitors began when bleach was added to the reuse procedure and ceased when use of bleach was discontinued (Schmitter and Sweet, 1993).

6. Potential transmission of infectious agents. Of greatest concern are hepatitis B virus and the human immunodeficiency virus (HIV). The potential inadvertent spillage of blood at the time that the dialyzer is reprocessed poses the theoretical risk of exposure of both staff and other patients to these viruses. However, bleach and germicides inactivate both the hepatitis B virus and HIV. For added safety, patients with sepsis or with acute hepatitis should not reuse dialyzers. Patients who are hepatitis B surface antigen–positive should not participate in a reuse program unless their dialyzers are reprocessed using a separate machine or manually in a separate area. According to current Centers for Disease Control and Prevention (CDC) recommendations, patients with HIV may continue on a reuse program. The epidemiology of hepatitis C virus in the dialysis setting is under investigation. Currently, the CDC does not object to dialyzer reuse in patients infected with hepatitis C.

7. Potential for decreased dialyzer performance.

a. Urea clearance. A reused hollow-fiber dialyzer ultimately becomes less efficient as a portion of its capillaries become plugged with protein or clot from previous uses. However, as long as the fiber bundle volume is at least 80% of the baseline value, urea clearance remains clinically acceptable (Gotch, 1986).

1. Heparin dosing. With reuse of dialyzers, reusability of dialyzers will deteriorate quickly unless adequate heparin anticoagulation is given. One group has reported increased numbers of reuses with individual targeted heparin dosing (Ouseph et al, 2000).

2. Bicarbonate dialysate containing citric acid. Bicarbonate dialysate containing a small amount of citrate has been reported to result in increased urea clearance in a reuse setting (Ahmed et al, 2000). The mechanism of how this occurs is not known, but may be related to calcium chelation by citrate coming in from the dialysate at the membrane boundary layer, with perhaps reduced activation of clotting or protein deposition.

b. β_2-Microglobulin clearance. Protein deposits adsorbed by the membrane or convectively transported to the membrane surface and not removed by the reuse process may reduce the ultrafiltration rate and larger molecule clearance (Pizziconi, 1990). The clearance of β_2-microglobulin (b2M, molecular weight 11,815) is negligible by low-flux dialyzers and does not change in a clinically significant way with reuse. High-flux dialyzer performance with respect to b2M clearance may be altered dramatically by reuse, depending on the type of membrane and type of reuse procedure (Cheung, 1999). In the current National Institutes of Health Hemodialysis Study (HEMO), use of peracetic acid/hydrogen peroxide/acetic acid (which normally is used without a bleach cycle) reduced b2M clearance by 65% between the first use and reuse 15 in cellulose triacetate (CT 190) dialyzers. On the other hand, there was no significant effect observed on b2M clearance when polysulfone (F80B) dialyzers were reused in the same fashion. The use of bleach with either formaldehyde or glutaraldehyde increased b2M clearance by 10% through reuse 20. The effectiveness of bleach to increase b2M clearance was also noted with CT 190 dialyzers when peracetic acid/hydrogen peroxide/acetic acid was selected for reuse. Heated citric acid increased b2M clearance by 41% in polysulfone (F80B) dialyzers. Thus, the effects of reuse on dialyzer flux is highly dependent on the dialyzer membrane property and the reuse method. Of most concern is the rapid falloff in b2M clearance when high-flux cellulose dialyzers are reused with peracetic acid/hydrogen peroxide/acetic acid without a bleach cycle.

   8. Albumin loss. Some dialyzers exposed to bleach during reuse procedures may undergo an increase in permeability to albumin that correlates with the number of reuses. Non–high-flux membranes do not increase albumin losses in a clinically significant manner. However, when polysulfone dialyzers with very high water permeability (e.g., more than 60 mL per hour per mm Hg in vivo) are reused with methods that use bleach, losses of albumin can be substantial, particularly as the number of reuses increases to greater than 20 (Kaplan et al, 1995). On the other hand, high-flux membranes of lesser water permeability (F80B, CT 190) exposed to bleach develop only limited albumin losses, with 1–2 g per dialysis reported over 20 reuses (Gotch et al, 1994). Albumin losses in high-flux polysulfone dialyzers reprocessed with peracetic acid or heat are negligible (Gotch et al, 1994). Thus, the effects of reuse on albumin losses, as noted for b2M, cannot be simply described. A full understanding requires knowledge of the type of dialyzer membrane and the reuse method.

IV. Other issues
  A. Medicolegal aspects
   1. U.S. laws. Federal regulations pertaining to dialyzer reprocessing follow, with some additions (Reuse of hemodialyzers, AAMI, 1995). Clinical practice guidelines are also discussed in the National Kidney Foundation's Dialysis Outcomes Quality Initiative (DOQI).
   2. Manufacturer single-use recommendation. Because of the widespread practice of reusing dialyzers labeled for single use only, the FDA has developed guidelines that allow manufactures to label their dialyzers for multiple use, recommend

an appropriate reuse method, and provide performance data of dialyzers over 15 reuses (FDA, October 6, 1995). Dialyzer manufacturers may choose to continue to label their dialyzers for single use only. At present, Althin, Baxter, Fresenius, and Terumo are developing multiple-use dialyzer labeling.

   3. Reuse of other dialysis disposables. Health Care Finance Administration regulations do not allow reuse of transducer protectors. Guidelines for the reuse of blood tubing have been published (Reuse of hemodialyzers, AAMI, 1995). However, blood tubing reuse is permitted only when the manufacturer has developed a specific protocol that has been accepted by the FDA (via premarket notification, section 501[k] of the provision of the Food, Drug and Cosmetic Act).

   4. Informed consent. Programs differ in the way that they define the patient's role in the decision to use reprocessed dialyzers. There are no federal requirements as to whether informed consent is needed, although commonly it is obtained. Patients should be fully apprised of the potential advantages and disadvantages of reuse. Given appropriate interaction with their physicians and the dialysis staff, most patients will cooperate with a recommendation for reuse. Once a patient has agreed to participate in a reuse program, it is recommended that he or she take an active role in the process. For example, federal guidelines recommend that the patient participate in the final checks for proper labeling of the reprocessed dialyzer just before its use.

B. Cost. Although a reuse program requires increased staff and expenditure for supplies and equipment, reuse is cost-effective. This is particularly true when high-efficiency or high-flux dialyzers (that are more expensive than conventional dialyzers) are prescribed. At current prices, the use of high-efficiency membranes with high ultrafiltration coefficients (high-flux membranes) is not economically feasible under the current (U.S.) reimbursement schedules unless the dialyzers are reused.

C. Quality assurance. For safe and successful reuse of dialyzers, a quality assurance program must be in place that systematically ensures the implementation and effectiveness of the reuse policies and procedures. Audits of the program should be carried out on a regular basis by individuals not directly performing the reprocessing procedures.

   1. Record keeping. Records must be kept in a way that allows for identification of the individual completing each step in the reuse process. Documentation of all aspects of present and past reuse of a patient's individual dialyzers should be retrievable. Each patient's dialyzer is individually labeled with a unique identifier and with information related to the use number. A log is kept of all incoming materials used in the reuse process. A log is also kept of the weekly test results of the disinfectant stock for proper concentration. A percentage of the program's reused dialyzers are cultured weekly for bacteria and checked for proper disinfectant concentration. All equipment performance is monitored regularly. If dialyzers are incubated during disinfection, 24-hour temperature-recording devices are utilized to ensure consistent temperatures. A carefully monitored preventive maintenance program minimizes malfunction of equipment employed in the reuse process. Detailed files are kept for possible adverse clinical events related to reprocessed dialyzers.

D. Personnel and physical plant considerations. A comprehensive training course should be established for all personnel performing reprocessing. Competence should be verified for each item on the curriculum. The use of protective eye-wear and clothing is stressed, as is proper handling of germicide spills. Where germicides are used, the work space should be designed with air turnover at least equivalent to the clinical area with forced inward air and additional ceiling exhaust ducts. Exposure to germicides is regulated by the U.S. Occupational Health and Safety Administration (OSHA). Current (1990) maximum allowable time-weighted average (TWA) exposure for formaldehyde is 1 ppm and for short-term exposure is 3 ppm. Maximum exposure limits for hydrogen peroxide is 1 ppm TWA and for glutaraldehyde is 0.2 ppm. There are no current OSHA exposure limits for peracetic acid.

E. Reuse water. Water purity is of crucial importance in the reuse process (Bland and Favero, 1995). It is preferable that reuse water be treated by reverse osmosis. Water used to prepare germicides should be tested weekly and have a bacterial colony count of less than 200 colony-forming units per mL, an endotoxin concentration (determined by limulus amebocyte lysate assay) of less than 2 endotoxin units per mL. Particularly with high-flux treatment, some authors believe that the currently accepted standards for water are too liberal and that only sterile, pyrogen-free water should be used (Henderson, 1993). For any system, however, special attention should be paid to the occurrence of pyrogenic reactions, particularly in clusters. In general, this should prompt immediate checks of the water system for bacteria and endotoxins, as well as a review of quality control procedures.

V. Patient monitoring. Measurements such as fiber bundle volume are only one aspect of the process of ensuring dialyzer performance. Careful evaluation of the patient's treatment and course is the primary validation of dialyzer performance. If conventional fluid removal systems are used, unexplained deviation from the ultrafiltration rate, as evidenced by unanticipated deviation of the postdialysis weight, may indicate altered dialyzer water permeability. However, this is not relevant in modern machines using ultrafiltration control. An unusual rise in predialysis plasma urea or creatinine concentration or a general deterioration of the patient's clinical condition may indicate reduced dialyzer solute permeability. Validation of the effectiveness of treatment by approaches such as urea kinetic modeling is also fundamental to the quality assurance process. Comparison of kinetically determined volume of total-body water with previous kinetically established values or demographically determined values serves as a useful screen for a number of technical problems including inadequate dialyzer clearance as a result of poor reprocessing technique. However, kinetic measurements are generally performed monthly and may not identify a problem in a timely manner. The advent of on-line clearance will provide immediate and direct information of dialyzer performance (Steil et al, 1993; Garred et al, 1993).

SUGGESTED READINGS

Ahmad S, et al. Dialysate made from dry chemicals using citric acid increases dialysis dose. *Am J Kidney Dis* 2000;35:493–499.

Alter MJ, et al. National surveillance of dialysis-associated diseases in the United States, 1988. *Trans Am Soc Artif Intern Organs* 1990; 26:107.

Association for the Advancement of Medical Instrumentation. *AAMI standards and recommended practices*. Vol. 3. *Dialysis*. Arlington, VA: 1995.

Berkseth R, et al. Paracetic acid for reuse of hemodialyzers. Clinical studies. *Trans Am Soc Artif Intern Organs* 1984;30:270–275.

Bland LA, Favero MS. Microbiological and endotoxin considerations in hemodialyzer reprocessing. In: AAMI, ed. *AAMI standards and recommended practices*. Vol. 3. *Dialysis*. Arlington, VA: Association for the Advancement of Medical Instrumentation, 1995:293.

Bok DV, et al. Effect of multiple use of dialyzers on intradialytic symptoms. *Proc Clin Dial Transplant Forum* 1980;10:92.

Charoenpanich R, et al. Effect of first and subsequent use of hemodialyzers on patient well being. *Artif Organs* 1987;11:123.

Cheung A, et al. Effects of hemodialyzer use on clearances of urea and beta-2 microglobulin. The Hemodialysis (HEMO) Study Group. *J Am Soc Nephrol* 1999;10:117–127.

Crosson JT, et al. A clinical study of anti-NDP in the sera of patients in a large repetitive hemodialysis program. *Kidney Int* 1976;10:463.

Daugirdas JT, Ing TS. First-use reactions during hemodialysis: a definition of subtypes. *Kidney Int* 1988;33(Suppl 2A):S37.

Feldman HI, et al. Effect of dialyzer reuse on survival of patients treated with hemodialysis. *JAMA* 1996;276:620.

Food and Drug Administration. Center for Devices and Radiological Health. Office of Device Evaluation. *Guidance for hemodialyzer reuse labeling*. October 6, 1995.

Garred LJ, et al. Urea kinetic modeling with a prototype urea sensor in the spent dialysate stream. *ASAIO J* 1993;39:M337.

Gotch FA, et al. Effects of reuse with peracetic acid, heat and bleach on polysulfone dialyzers. *J Am Soc Nephrol* 1994;5:415(abstr).

Gotch FA. Solute and water transport and sterilant removal in reused dialyzers. In: Deane N, et al, eds. *Guide to reprocessing of hemodialyzers*. Boston: Martinus Nijhoff, 1986:39.

Hakim RM, Lowrie EG. Effect of dialyzer reuse on leukopenia, hypoxemia and total hemolytic complement system. *Trans Am Soc Artif Intern Organs* 1980;26:159.

Hakim RM, Friedrich RA, Lowrie EG. Formaldehyde kinetics in reused dialyzers. *Kidney Int* 1985;28:936.

Held PJ, Pauly MV, Diamond L. Survival analysis of patients undergoing dialysis. *JAMA* 1987;257:645–650.

Held PJ, et al. Analysis of the association of dialyzer reuse practices and patient outcomes. *Am J Kidney Dis* 1994;23L:692–708.

Held PJ, et al. Excerpts from United States Renal Data System 1997 annual data report. *Am J Kidney Dis* 1997;30 (2 Suppl 1):S178–S186.

Henderson L. Should hemodialysis fluid be sterile? *Semin Dial* 1993;6:26–27.

Kaplan AA, et al. Dialysate protein losses with bleach processed polysulfone dialyzers. *Kidney Int* 1995;47:573–578.

Kaufman AM, et al. Clinical experience with heat sterilization for reprocessing dialyzers. *ASAIO J* 1992;38:M338–M340.

Levin NW, et al. The use of heated citric acid for dialyzer reprocessing. *J Am Soc Nephrol* 1995;6:1578–1585.

Miles AM, Friedman EA. Dialyzer reuse—techniques and controversy. In: Jacobs C, et al, eds. *Replacement of renal function by dialysis.* Boston: Kluwer Academic, 1996:454–471.

National Kidney Foundation. Revised standards of reuse of hemodialyzers. *Am J Kidney Dis* 1984;3:466.

National Kidney Foundation. Dialysis Outcomes Quality Initiative (DOQI). *Clinical practice guidelines for hemodialysis adequacy: hemodialyzer reprocessing and reuse. Am J Kidney Dis* 1997;30 (3 suppl 2):S15–S66.

Ouseph R, et al. Improved dialyzer reuse after use of a population pharmacodynamic model to determine heparin doses. *Am J Kidney Dis* 2000;35:89–94.

Pegues DA, et al. Anaphylactoid reactions associated with reuse of hollow fiber hemodialyzers and ACE inhibitors. *Kidney Int* 1992; 42:1232–1237.

Pizziconi VB. Performance and integrity testing in reprocessed dialyzers: a QC update. In: AAMI, ed. *AAMI standards and recommended practices.* Vol 3. *Dialysis.* Arlington, VA: 1990:176.

Pizziconi VB, et al. Factors affecting complement activation and neutropenia during dialysis using cuprophane membranes. *ASAIO J* 1984;7(2):64.

Pollak V, et al. Repeated use of dialyzers is safe: long-term observations on morbidity and mortality in patients with end-stage renal disease. *Nephron* 1986;42:217.

Reuse of hemodialyzers. In: AAMI, ed. *AAMI standards and recommended practices.* Vol. 3. *Dialysis.* Arlington, VA: 1993:85–118.

Schmitter L, Sweet S. Anaphylactic reactions with the additions of hypochlorite to reuse in patients maintained on reprocessed polysulfone hemodialyzers and ACE inhibitors. Paper presented at the annual meeting of the American Society for Artificial Internal Organs, New Orleans, April 1998.

Steil H, et al. In vivo verification of an automated noninvasive system for real time *Kt* evaluation. *ASAIO J* 1993;39:M348–M352.

Task Force on Reuse of Dialyzers. Council on Dialysis. National Kidney Foundation. National Kidney Foundation report on dialyzer reuse. *Am J Kidney Dis* 1997;30:859–871.

Vanholder R, et al. Development of anti-N-like antibodies during formaldehyde reuse in spite of adequate predialysis rinsing. *Am J Kidney Dis* 1988;11:477–480.

Verresen L, et al. Bradykinin is a mediator of anaphylactoid reactions during hemodialysis with AN69 membranes. *Kidney Int* 1994;45: 1497–1503.

Zaoui P, Green W, Hakim M. Hemodialysis with cuprophane membrane modulates interleukin-2 receptor expression. *Kidney Int* 1991;39:1020.

Internet References

American Association for the Advancement of Medical Instrumentation (AAMI) (http://www.aami.org/)

Reuse: recent literature and links. (http://www.hdcn.com/hd/reuse)

9

Anticoagulation

Joachim Hertel, Dawn M. Keep,
and Ralph J. Caruana

I. Blood clotting in the extracorporeal circuit. The patient's blood is exposed to intravenous cannulas, tubing, drip chambers, headers, potting compound, and dialysis membranes during the dialysis procedure. These surfaces exhibit a variable degree of thrombogenicity and may initiate clotting of blood, especially in conjunction with exposure of blood to air in drip chambers. The resulting thrombus formation may be significant enough to cause occlusion and malfunction of the extracorporeal circuit. Clot formation in the extracorporeal circuit begins with coating of the surfaces by plasma proteins, followed by platelet adherence and aggregation, thromboxane A_2 generation, and activation of the intrinsic coagulation cascade, leading to thrombin formation and fibrin deposition. Factors favoring clotting are listed in Table 9-1.

Anticoagulation with heparin, one of the key developments that has made hemodialysis possible to this day, is the standard method for preventing thrombosis in the extracorporeal circuit. Heparin is an anionic sulfated mucopolysaccharide of variable molecular weight extracted commercially from cow lung or pig intestine. Heparin bonds to circulating antithrombin III, which then complexes with serine proteases of coagulation factors I, IX, XI, and XII, resulting in rapid inactivation of these factors. The platelet aggregation and activation stimulated by heparin is counterbalanced by interference with binding and activation of coagulation factors at the platelet membrane.

The half-life of heparin in normal individuals and dialysis patients is 30–120 minutes and is prolonged by dissociation of heparin from antithrombin III complexes or by dissociation from protamine sulfate when this agent is used to reverse the effect of heparin.

Undesired side effects of heparin include pruritus, allergy, osteoporosis, hyperlipidemia, thrombocytopenia, and excessive bleeding. Heparin sensitivity varies from patient to patient and over time in a given patient. Alternative anticoagulation methods or anticoagulation-free methods have been developed for patients in whom the use of heparin causes excessive adverse effects.

II. Assessing coagulation during dialysis

A. Visual inspection. Signs of extracorporeal circuit clotting are listed in Table 9-2. Visualization of the circuit can be best accomplished by rinsing the system with saline solution while occluding the blood inlet temporarily. An undesired effect of utilizing this method to visualize the circuit may be that a clot that had formed in the T-piece can be propelled into the arterial header and cause clotting of dialyzer fibers. During intermittent hemodialysis treatments this may not contribute very much to dialyzer clotting. During continuous treatments,

**Table 9-1. Factors favoring clotting
of the extracorporeal circuit**

Low blood flow
High hematocrit
High ultrafiltration rate
Dialysis access recirculation
Intradialytic blood and blood product transfusion
Intradialytic lipid infusion
Use of drip chambers (air exposure, foam formation, turbulence)

such as continuous arteriovenous hemofiltration (CAVH) or continuous venovenous hemofiltration (CVVH), repeated clot propulsion into the dialyzer header can cause significant clotting and ultrafiltration loss. We therefore prevent clot formation in the T-piece of continuous-modality circuits by using them as the access site for continuous heparin infusion and periodically switching to saline flushes using a three-way stopcock.

B. Extracorporeal circuit pressures. Arterial and venous pressure readings may change as a result of clotting in the extracorporeal circuit depending on the location of thrombus formation. An advantage of using blood lines with a postpump arterial pressure monitor is that the difference between the postpump and venous pressure readings can serve as an indicator of the location of the clotting. An increased pressure difference is seen when there is significant clot formation in the arterial blood chamber or when the clotting is confined to the dialyzer itself (increased postpump pressure, decreased venous pressure). If the clotting is occurring in or distal to the venous blood chamber, then the postpump and venous pressure readings are increased in tandem. If the clotting is extensive, then the rise in pressure readings will be precipitous. A clotted or malpositioned venous needle also results in increased pressure readings.

C. Dialyzer appearance after dialysis. The presence of a few clotted fibers is not unusual, and the headers often collect small blood clots or whitish deposits (especially in patients with hyperlipidemia). More significant dialyzer clotting should be recorded by the dialysis staff to serve as a clinical parameter for

Table 9-2. Signs of clotting in the extracorporeal circuit

Extremely dark blood

Shadows or black streaks in the dialyzer

Foaming with subsequent clot formation in drip chambers and
venous trap

Rapid filling of transducer monitors with blood

"Tetering" (blood in the postdialyzer venous line segment that is
unable to continue into the venous chamber but falls back into the
line segment)

Presence of clots at the arterial-side header

adjustment of heparin dosing. It is useful to classify the amount of clotting based on the visually estimated percentage of clotted fibers in order to standardize documentation (e.g., less than 10% of fibers clotted, grade 1; less than 50% clotted, grade 2; more than 50% clotted, grade 3).

D. Measurement of residual dialyzer volume. In units practicing dialyzer reuse, automated or manual methods are used to determine the clotting-associated fiber loss during each treatment. This is done by comparing the predialysis and post-dialysis fiber bundle volumes. Dialyzers suitable for reuse characteristically have less than 1% fiber loss over each of the first 5–10 reuses.

E. Clotting time tests. Blood for clotting studies should be drawn from the arterial blood line, proximal to any heparin infusion site, to reflect the clotting status of the patient rather than that of the extracorporeal circuit.

   1. Whole-blood partial thromboplastin time (WBPTT). The WBPTT test accelerates the clotting process by addition of 0.2 mL of actin FS reagent (Thrombofax) to 0.4 mL of blood. The mixture is set in a heating block at 37°C for 30 seconds and then tilted every 5 seconds until a clot forms. The prolongation of the WBPTT is linearly related to the blood heparin concentration (in the range applicable to dialysis).

   2. Activated clotting time (ACT). The ACT test is similar to the WBPTT test but uses siliceous earth to accelerate the clotting process. ACT is less reproducible than WBPTT, especially at low blood heparin levels. Devices that automatically tilt the tube and detect clot formation facilitate standardization and reproducibility of both WBPTT and ACT.

   3. Lee–White clotting time (LWCT). The Lee–White test is performed by adding 0.4 mL of blood to a glass tube and inverting the tube every 30 seconds until the blood clots. Usually, the blood is kept at room temperature. Disadvantages of the LWCT test include the long period of time required before clotting occurs and the relatively poor standardization and reproducibility of the test. LWCT is the least desirable method of monitoring clotting during hemodialysis.

   4. Variability in clotting times among different dialysis centers. A number of target clotting times during dialysis are listed in Table 9-3. The values given may not be appropriate for all dialysis centers because baseline clotting times (off heparin) will vary among different units, depending on techniques and reagents used. Each dialysis center should establish its own range of normal values. If the range of normal is different from that listed in Table 9-3, then the target clotting times may also need adjustment.

III. Anticoagulation techniques
   A. Routine heparin
      1. Target clotting times. Heparin can usually be given liberally during dialysis without fear of precipitating a bleeding episode in patients who do not exhibit an abnormal bleeding risk. The effect of two routine heparin regimens on clotting time is shown in Fig. 9-1. The goal is to maintain WBPTT or ACT at the baseline value plus 80% during most of the dialysis

Table 9-3.   Target clotting times during dialysis

Test	Reagent	Baseline value	Routine heparin Desired range During dialysis	Routine heparin Desired range At end of dialysis	Tight heparin Desired range During dialysis	Tight heparin Desired range At end of dialysis
WBPTT	Actin FS	60–85 sec	+80% (120–140)	+40% (85–105)	+40% (85–105)	+40% (85–105)
ACT[a]	Siliceous earth	120–150 sec	+80% (200–250)	+40% (170–190)	+40% (170–190)	+40% (170–190)
LWCT[b]	None	4–8 min	20–30	9–16	9–16	9–16

WBPTT, whole blood partial thromboplastin time; ACT, activated clotting time; LWCT, Lee-White clotting time.

[a] There are various methods of performing the ACT, and the baseline value with some methods is much lower, e.g., 90–120 seconds.

[b] Baseline values of the LWCT vary greatly depending on how the test is performed.

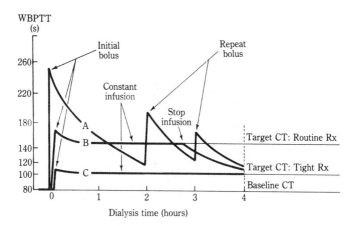

Figure 9-1.   Effect of various heparin regimens on clotting time as reflected by the whole-blood partial thromboplastin time (WBPTT). CT, clotting time using the WBPTT test; A, routine regimen, repeated-bolus method; B, routine regimen, constant-infusion method; C, tight regimen, constant-infusion method.

session. However, at the end of the session, the clotting time should be shorter (baseline plus 40% for WBPTT or ACT) to minimize the risk of bleeding from the access site after withdrawal of the access needles.

In patients with a baseline WBPTT or ACT that is prolonged out of the normal range, further prolongation of the clotting time to baseline plus 80% during dialysis may be associated with bleeding and is not necessary. For this reason, the target WBPTT or ACT during dialysis generally should not exceed 180% of the average baseline value of the patients in the dialysis center.

The target clotting times using the Lee–White test are also listed in Table 9-3. With LWCT, in contrast to WBPTT or ACT, the target clotting times during dialysis are considerably greater than baseline plus 80%, and the target LWCT values at the end of the session are greater than baseline plus 40%.

2.   Routine heparin prescriptions. There are two basic techniques of administering routine heparin. In one method, a heparin bolus is followed by a constant heparin infusion. In the second, a heparin bolus is followed by repeated bolus doses as necessary. For the purpose of discussion, we present a typical prescription in each category.

Rₓ: Routine heparin, constant-infusion method

   a.   Administer the initial bolus dose (e.g., 2,000 units).

   b.   Wait 3–5 minutes to allow heparin dispersion before initiating dialysis and heparin infusion into the arterial blood line (e.g., at a rate of 1,200 units per hour).

   c.   Monitor clotting time (WBPTT, ACT, or LWCT) every hour. Adjust the heparin infusion rate to keep:

(1) WBPTT or ACT at baseline plus 80%, but not more than 180% of the average baseline value for patients in the dialysis center, or

(2) LWCT at 20–30 minutes.

d. Stop the heparin infusion 1 hour before the end of dialysis.

Rx: Routine heparin, repeated-bolus method

a. Administer the initial bolus dose (e.g., 4,000 units).

b. Monitor clotting times every hour if:

(1) WBPTT or ACT is less than baseline plus 50%, or

(2) LWCT is less than 20 minutes

c. Then give an additional 1,000- to 2,000-unit bolus dose and repeat the clotting time in 30 minutes.

3. With the constant-infusion method, the initial bolus dose of heparin is lower (2,000 units) than with the repeated-bolus method (4,000 units) because with constant heparin infusion the initial bolus dose is required to prolong ACT or WBPTT to only baseline plus 80% (see curve B in Fig. 9-1. On the other hand, with the repeated-bolus technique the initial bolus dose is designed to prolong the clotting time initially to well above the baseline-plus-80% value (see curve A in Fig. 9-1).

a. Indications for altering the suggested initial bolus heparin dose

(1) **Increasing the dose.** An initial bolus dose of 2,000 units of heparin (constant-infusion method) will not increase WBPTT to baseline plus 80% in all patients; the dose required to achieve a baseline-plus-80% prolongation can range from 500 to 4,000 units, depending on the sensitivity to heparin of the individual patient and on the potency of the heparin preparation being used. WBPTT or ACT can be checked 3 minutes after the initial 2,000 units has been given; if the prolongation of the clotting time is insufficient, a second bolus dose can be promptly administered. The prolongation of WBPTT or ACT will be directly proportional to the amount of heparin given (e.g., if the initial heparin bolus has prolonged the WBPTT by 40 seconds, then a supplementary dose of half the initial amount will increase the WBPTT by an additional 20 seconds).

(2) **Reducing the dose**

(a) **Prolongation of baseline bleeding and clotting times.** With both the constant-infusion and repeated-bolus techniques, the initial bolus dose of heparin should be reduced in extremely uremic patients in whom uremia-induced platelet and endothelial cell dysfunction may have prolonged the bleeding time, and in all patients in whom the baseline clotting time (off heparin) is prolonged.

(b) **Repeated-bolus method, short-session dialysis.** When using the repeated bolus technique, the initial suggested heparin dose of 4,000 units may need to be reduced in patients who are to be dialyzed for a short period (e.g., 2 hours). If the bolus dose anticoagulates the patient excessively, then the clotting time may still be markedly prolonged at the end of dialysis, resulting in bleeding from the access site when the needles are removed.

(3)   Effect of body weight on the size of the heparin dose. In adult patients weighing between 50 and 90 kg, the sensitivity to heparin does not appear to be related to body weight. Within this population, there is no reason to modify the suggested heparin doses because of body weight.

b.   Determination and adjustment of the heparin infusion rate. The "average" heparin infusion rate required to maintain WBPTT or ACT at baseline plus 80% is 1,200 units per hour, but the infusion rate can range from 500 to 3,000 units per hour. The required infusion rate is based on both the patient sensitivity to heparin and the heparin half-life. Once a steady state has been reached, the infusion rate is directly proportional to prolongation of WBPTT or ACT. Hence, if an infusion rate of 1,200 units per hour is causing a 60-second prolongation of WBPTT, then an infusion rate of 1,800 units per hour will effect an overall prolongation of 90 seconds, and a rate of 600 units per hour will effect an overall prolongation of 30 seconds.

(1)   Importance of being at steady state. It is difficult to adjust the heparin infusion rate if the patient's clotting times are changing (if the patient has not reached steady state). This is especially a problem when the initial bolus dose of heparin was incorrect and resulted in an initial WBPTT or ACT value that was much longer or shorter than the baseline-plus-80% value.

c.   When to terminate the heparin infusion. The heparin half-life in dialysis patients averages 50 minutes but ranges from 30 minutes to 2 hours. Because the prolongation in WBPTT is directly proportional to the plasma heparin level, if one knows the current prolongation of WBPTT then one can predict the prolongation in WBPTT at any time (assuming no further heparin is administered) based on the heparin half-life in that patient. For example, assume that in a given patient the heparin half-life is 1 hour. If the current prolongation in WBPTT is 60 seconds (e.g., current WBPTT 135 seconds, baseline 75 seconds), in 1 hour the plasma heparin level will have decreased by 50%, at which time the prolongation in WBPTT will be only 30 seconds. Similarly, after an additional hour, the prolongation in WBPTT will be only 15 seconds.

The exact calculation of the time at which to stop a heparin infusion based on the heparin half-life can be found in Gotch and Keen (1991). For a patient with an average heparin half-life of 1 hour, if the heparin infusion during dialysis is prolonging WBPTT or ACT to the required baseline-plus-80% value, stopping heparin administration approximately 1 hour prior to the end of dialysis will result in the desired WBPTT or ACT value of baseline plus 40% at termination of the session.

3.   Effectiveness of routine heparinization. At heparin blood levels of 0.2 unit per mL, the risk of significant dialyzer clotting is generally less than 5%. Systemic heparinization can permit multiple reuses of dialyzers and is the gold standard for anticoagulation efficacy.

4. Evaluation of clotting during routine heparinization. A small incidence of inadvertent clotting of the extracorporeal system is expected and generally does not necessitate a change in heparin prescription. When clotting occurs it is useful to evaluate the likely cause. Often the underlying cause may be correctable (e.g., access revision). Operator-induced errors, as listed in Table 9-4, must be considered and managed through education. Recurrent clotting warrants individual reevaluation and adjustments in heparin dosing.

5. Bleeding complications of routine heparinization. The risk of increased bleeding due to systemic anticoagulation is 25%–50% in high-risk patients with bleeding gastrointestinal lesions (gastritis, peptic ulcer, angiodysplasia), recent surgery, pericarditis, or diabetic retinopathy. De novo bleeding can involve the central nervous system, retroperitoneum, and mediastinum. The tendency to bleed is potentiated by uremia-associated defects in platelet function and possibly by endothelial abnormalities.

B. Tight heparin

1. General comments. Tight heparinization schemes are recommended for patients who are at slight risk for bleeding. When using WBPTT or ACT to monitor therapy, the target clotting time (see Table 9-3 and curve C in Fig. 9-1) is equal to the baseline value plus 40%. Target clotting times using the Lee–White method are given in Table 9-3. Again, in some patients, the baseline WBPTT or ACT values will be prolonged beyond the normal range, and the target WBPTT or ACT value should not be more than 140% of the average baseline value for patients in the dialysis unit.

Table 9-4.   Technical or operator-induced factors (resulting in clotting)

Dialyzer priming
Retained air in dialyzer (due to inadequate priming or poor priming technique)
Lack or inadequate priming of heparin infusion line

Heparin administration
Incorrect heparin pump setting for constant infusion
Incorrect loading dose
Delayed starting of heparin pump
Failure to release heparin line clamp
Insufficient time lapse after loading dose for systemic heparinization to occur

Vascular access
Inadequate blood flow due to needle/catheter positioning or clotting
Excessive access recirculation due to needle/tourniquet position
Frequent interruption of blood flow due to inadequate delivery or machine alarm conditions

In the tight heparin technique, when it is desired to estimate the patient sensitivity to heparin (see below), the initial heparin dose is best administered to the patient via the venous access tubing and flushed in with saline (rather than being infused into the arterial blood line).

2. The tight heparin prescription. A bolus dose followed by a constant infusion of heparin is the best technique for administering a tight heparin prescription because constant infusion avoids the rising and falling clotting times that are inevitable with repeated-bolus therapy. A repeated-bolus method (1,000 units loading dose followed by bolus doses of 500 units as needed to keep the WBPTT or ACT above baseline plus 25%) can be used when machines with a heparin pump are not available. A typical tight heparin prescription is as follows:

R$_x$: Tight heparin, constant-infusion method

   a.   Obtain baseline clotting time (WBPTT or ACT).
   b.   Initial bolus dose = 750 units.
   c.   Recheck WBPTT or ACT after 3 minutes.
   d.   Administer a supplemental bolus dose if needed to prolong WBPTT or ACT to a value of baseline plus 40%.
   e.   Start dialysis and heparin infusion at a rate of 600 units per hour.
   f.   Monitor clotting times every 30 minutes.
   g.   Adjust the heparin infusion rate to keep WBPTT or ACT at baseline plus 40% (but not longer than 140% of the average baseline value of patients in the unit).
   h.   Continue heparin infusion until the end of the dialysis session.

   a.   Determination of the optimum initial bolus dose. Depending on the heparin sensitivity of the patient and the actual potency of the heparin preparation used, the initial dose required to achieve a 40% prolongation of the baseline WBPTT or ACT value can range from 300 to 2,000 units. For this reason, when administering the "usual" 750-unit dose to an unknown patient, it is wise to wait and recheck the WBPTT or ACT 3 minutes after having administered the bolus dose. When drawing the blood for these clotting studies, great care must be taken to avoid contamination of the sample with residual heparin or saline in the vascular access tubing. If the clotting time is insufficiently prolonged by the initial 750-unit bolus dose, then a supplementary bolus dose should be administered. For example, if an initial bolus dose of 750 units prolonged WBPTT by 20 seconds, then an additional 375 units will prolong WBPTT by an additional 10 seconds.

   b.   Adjusting the heparin infusion rate. For a tight heparin prescription, the average infusion rate required to maintain WBPTT or ACT at baseline plus 40% will be approximately 600 units per hour but can range from 200 to 2,000 units per hour. If the initial bolus dose of 750 units resulted in a prolongation of WBPTT that was much smaller or larger than expected, the first estimate for the proper infusion rate (600 units per hour) should be revised accordingly.

Example

If the initial dose of 750 units prolongs WBPTT by only 20 seconds instead of the required 30 seconds, the correct step is to give an additional 375-unit bolus and then start the heparin infusion at a rate of 1,200 units per hour instead of the usual 600 units per hour. If, on the other hand, the initial 750 units prolongs the WBPTT by 60 seconds instead of the required 30 seconds, one should start dialysis and not start the heparin infusion, checking the clotting times periodically. Once WBPTT has fallen to the required 30 seconds above initial value (baseline plus 40%), the infusion should be started but at the reduced rate of 300 units per hour.

Whether or not the heparin sensitivity is close to the expected value, the initial estimated infusion rates may need to be increased or decreased due to different heparin half-lives in different patients. The adjustment should be made based on close monitoring of the clotting time. For methods to calculate the heparin infusion rate and half-life directly, see Gotch and Keen (1991).

C. Heparin-associated complications. Apart from bleeding, complications of note are increase in blood lipids, thrombocytopenia, and the potential for hypoaldosteronism and exacerbation of hyperkalemia.

    1. Lipids. Heparin activates lipoprotein lipase, and in this way can increase the serum triglyceride concentration. Lower levels of HDL cholesterol also are associated with heparin use. Both lipid abnormalities are improved when using low molecular weight heparin (LMWH) (Elisaf et al, 1997).

    2. Thrombocytopenia, heparin-associated antibody formation. There are two types of heparin-associated thrombocytopenia (HAT). In type 1 HAT, the reduction in platelet count occurs in a time- and dose-dependent manner, and responds to reduction in heparin dose. In type 2 HAT, there is agglutination of platelets and paradoxical arterial and/or venous thrombosis. Type 2 HAT, which is attributable to development of immunoglobulin G (IgG) antibodies against the heparin–platelet factor 4 complex, is more commonly induced with bovine versus porcine heparin. Given the frequency of HAT in the nondialysis population, it is surprising that it is not encountered more often in a dialysis setting. Diagnosis of type 2 HAT is by an abnormal platelet aggregation test or by even more sensitive enzyme-linked immunosorbent assay (ELISA) using bound platelet factor 4 complexed with heparin.

    Whereas use of LMWHs alleviates heparin-associated lipid abnormalities, their application to the management of type 2 HAT is problematic, as there often is cross-reactivity of the heparin–platelet factor 4 antibodies with the LMWHs. Cross-reactivity is lowest with the synthetic heparinoid danaproid; however, ideally prostacyclin or regional citrate anticoagulation is a better alternative if heparin-free dialysis (without a heparin pre-rinse) cannot be performed (Davenport, 1998).

    3. Pruritus. Heparin can cause local itching when injected subcutaneously, and it has been speculated that heparin may be the cause of itching and other allergic reactions during dialysis. On the other hand, LMWH has been used to treat the itching associated with lichen planus, on the basis of inhibition of T-lymphocyte heparinase activity (Hodak et al, 1998). There is no evidence that removal of heparin from the extracorporeal circuit reliably improves uremic pruritus.

   1.   Hyperkalemia. Heparin-associated hyperkalemia, attributable to heparin-induced suppression of aldosterone synthesis, has been well-described. In oliguric dialysis patients, it has been speculated that aldosterone may still aid potassium excretion via a gastrointestinal mechanism, and there is evidence that treatment with fludrocortisone often is an effective treatment for hyperkalemia in dialysis patients. However, use of fludrocortisone is risky in dialysis patients because the drug has a considerable glucocorticoid activity. There is one report suggesting that changing from heparin to LMWH may improve the aldosterone/plasma renin activity ratio and result in slight improvement of hyperkalemia in dialysis patients (Hottelart et al, 1998).

D.   Heparin-free dialysis
   1.   General comments. Heparin-free dialysis is the method of choice in patients who are actively bleeding, who are at high risk of bleeding, or in whom the use of heparin is contraindicated (e.g., persons with heparin-induced thrombocytopenia). The frequent saline flushing makes heparin-free dialysis work-intensive for the dialysis staff, but its low association with dialyzer clotting is rendering tight heparin regimens obsolete. The indications for heparin-free dialysis are listed in Table 9-5. Because of its simplicity and safety, many centers now use heparin-free dialysis routinely for most dialysis performed in acutely ill patients.
   2.   The heparin-free prescription. There are a variety of techniques, but all are similar to the one given below:
   R_x: **Heparin-free dialysis**
      a.   Heparin rinse. (Avoid if heparin-associated thrombocytopenia is present. Rinse extracorporeal circuit with saline containing 3,000 units of heparin per L, so that heparin can coat extracorporeal surfaces and dialyzer

Table 9-5.   Anticoagulation strategy: indications for heparin-free dialysis

Pericarditis (tight heparin acceptable if bleeding risk deemed low)
Recent surgery, with bleeding complications or risk. Especially:
   Vascular and cardiac surgery
   Eye surgery (retinal and cataract)
   Renal transplant
   Brain surgery
Coagulopathy
Thrombocytopenia
Intracerebral hemorrhage
Active bleeding
Routine use for dialysis of acutely ill patients by many centers

membrane to mitigate the thrombogenic response). To prevent systemic heparin administration to the patient, allow the heparin-containing priming fluid to drain by filling the extracorporeal circuit with either the patient's blood or unheparinized saline at the outset of dialysis.

   b.   High blood flow rate. Set the blood flow rate as high as possible (e.g., 400–500 mL per minute if tolerated). If a high blood flow rate is contraindicated due to the risk of disequilibrium (e.g., small patient, very high predialysis plasma urea nitrogen level), consider using a small surface area dialyzer and/or slowing the dialysate flow rate. Generally, double-lumen hemodialysis catheters can deliver sufficiently high blood flows to be effective.

   c.   Periodic saline rinse. Rinse the dialyzer rapidly with 100–250 mL of saline while occluding the blood inlet line every 30 minutes. The frequency of the flushes can be increased or decreased as needed. The use of volumetric control is desirable for the accurate removal of volumes of ultrafiltrate equal to those of the administered saline rinses. The purpose of the periodic rinsing is to allow inspection of a hollow-fiber dialyzer for evidence of clotting and to allow for timely discontinuation of treatment or changing of the dialyzer. Also, periodic saline rinsing may on its own reduce the propensity for dialyzer clotting or interfere with clot formation.

   d.   Different dialyzer design or material. If clotting occurs then blood loss is greater with parallel-plate dialyzers due to their higher blood compartment volumes compared with those of hollow-fiber dialyzers. There is no solid evidence to suggest that any one type of membrane material is superior for heparin-free dialysis.

   e.   Risk of clotting. Using the above method of heparin-free dialysis, complete clotting of the dialyzer occurs in approximately 5% of cases—an acceptable risk that more than balances the danger of bleeding associated with heparin administration to high-risk patients. The risk of subsequent clotting can be reduced by increasing the frequency of flushes, limiting duration of dialyzer use, maximizing the blood flow rates, and avoiding blood product transfusion or lipid administration during the treatment.

E.   Regional citrate anticoagulation. An alternative to heparin-free dialysis is to anticoagulate the blood in the extracorporeal circuit by lowering its ionized calcium concentration (calcium is required for the coagulation process). The extracorporeal blood ionized calcium level is lowered by infusing trisodium citrate (which complexes calcium) into the arterial blood line and by using a dialysis solution containing no calcium. It would be very dangerous to return blood with a very low ionized calcium concentration to the patient. Thus, the process is reversed by infusion of calcium chloride into the dialyzer blood outlet line. About one-third of the infused citrate is dialyzed away and the remaining two-thirds is quickly metabolized by the patient.

The advantages of regional citrate anticoagulation over heparin-free dialysis are (a) the blood flow rate does not have to be high and (b) clotting almost never occurs. The principal disadvantages are the requirement for two infusions (one of citrate and one of calcium) and the requirement for monitoring the blood calcium level. Because citrate metabolism generates bicarbonate, use of this method results in a greater than usual increment in the plasma bicarbonate value. Hence, regional citrate anticoagulation should be used with extreme caution in patients who are at risk for alkalemia. When citrate anticoagulation is to be used on a long-term basis, the dialysate bicarbonate level must be reduced (e.g., to 25 mEq per L) if metabolic alkalosis is to be avoided (van der Meulen et al, 1992). Chronic citrate use may result in aluminum overload (contamination from glass container).

1. Method. The technique described below (provided through the courtesy of Dr. John C. Van Stone) has been validated only for dialysis using two blood access lines. The method has not been tested using single blood pathway dialysis.

a. Solutions. Trisodium citrate for intravenous use is available from American Bentley, Inc. (Irvine, CA) or from Haemonetics Corporation (Braintree, MA). The citrate is packaged in 30-mL vials containing 46.7% citrate (1.6 mol per L). A stock solution (132 mmol per L) is made by diluting three 30-mL vials into 1 L of 5% D/W. Calcium chloride is obtained in 10% vials, 10 mL per vial. Five 10-mL vials (50 mL) are diluted with 100 mL of 0.9% saline (final concentration 3.33% or 467 mEq of calcium per liter). The citrate solution is administered into the arterial blood line and the calcium solution into the venous blood line using volumetric intravenous infusion pumps. Because the infusions may be opposed by pressures in the blood lines, intravenous infusion pumps that actually pump the solution, rather than those that deliver solution based on gravity drip, must be used.

b. Dialyzer and dialysis solution. Any dialyzer can be used, but water permeability should be sufficient to allow easy removal of the extra 300 mL per hour of fluid that will be administered with the citrate and calcium infusions. The dialysis solution will usually be bicarbonate-buffered given that the method is used primarily in unstable, intensive-care–bound patients. A zero calcium dialysis solution must be used.

c. Sample prescription. The initial infusion rates of citrate and calcium described below are based on a blood flow rate of 200 mL per minute. If lower or higher blood flow rates are used, the infusion rates listed should be altered accordingly.

(1) Obtain baseline clotting studies (WBPTT or ACT) and plasma total calcium level.

(2) Initiate dialysis solution flow.

(3) Initiate the citrate infusion into the arterial blood line at a starting rate of 270 mL per hour. Start the blood flow at the same time. Increase blood flow rapidly to 200 mL per minute. At a blood flow rate of 200 mL per minute, this citrate infusion rate will result in a citrate concentration of 3.0 mmol per L in the blood entering the dialyzer.

(4) Immediately start the calcium chloride infusion into the venous blood line at a rate of 30 mL per hour. At a blood flow rate of 200 mL per minute, this calcium infusion rate will result in an increase of about 1.2 mEq per L of calcium in the blood leaving the dialyzer.

(5) Check the patient's plasma total calcium level (sampling from the arterial blood line) 30 minutes after starting dialysis and then as needed. Adjust the calcium infusion rate to keep the plasma total calcium level within the normal range (the usual infusion rate of the calcium solution ranges from 24 to 42 mL per hour, average = 30–36 mL per hour).

(6) Check the clotting time (WBPTT or ACT) periodically in the arterial blood line, downstream to the citrate infusion (reflects citrate effect). WBPTT or ACT downstream to the citrate infusion should be prolonged by approximately 100%. If prolongation of the clotting time here is less than 100%, increase the rate of citrate infusion (up to about 420 mL per hour). If the prolongation of WBPTT or ACT here is greater than 100%, consider reducing the citrate infusion rate, although this is not always necessary. WBPTT or ACT should not change during dialysis.

(7) If the dialyzer goes into the bypass mode due to some problem with the dialysis solution (the dialysis solution will then be shunted around the dialyzer directly to drain), the effect of the zero calcium dialysis solution will cease to occur. In this case, shut off the calcium infusion and reduce the citrate infusion rate by 50% until the flow of dialysis solution is restored. This method has not been tested to be suitable for extended operation in the bypass mode or for procedures in which dialysis solution is not used, such as isolated ultrafiltration.

(8) At the end of dialysis, stop the citrate and calcium infusions simultaneously, and return the blood in the usual fashion.

F. Anticoagulation for continuous renal replacement therapies. The same methods as described above for hemodialysis can also be used for continuous renal replacement therapies with the caveat that patients treated with continuous therapies generally are more prone to bleeding complications as they often have multiorgan failure (see Chapter 10).

IV. Newer anticoagulation techniques

A. LMWH. LMWH fractions (molecular weight = 4,000–6,000 daltons) are obtained by chemical degradation or sieving of crude heparin (molecular weight = 2000–25,000 daltons). LMWH inhibits factor Xa, factor XIIa, and kallikrein but causes so little inhibition of thrombin and factors IX and XI that partial thromboplastin time and thrombin time are minimally prolonged, thus decreasing bleeding risks.

Hemodialysis using LMWH as the sole anticoagulant has been shown in some long-term studies to be safe and effective.

LMWH's longer half-life permits anticoagulation with a single dose at the start of dialysis though split dosing may be superior.

LMWH is now commercially available in the United States but is not widely used because it is more expensive, and it is not yet FDA- approved for hemodialysis. Activity and dosing of LMWH is generally expressed in anti–factor Xa Institute Choay units (aXaICU). For a 4-hour dialysis treatment, a single standard dose of 10,000 or 15,000 aXaIC U or an adjusted dose of 125–250 aXaIC U/kg has been successful in providing adequate anticoagulation for hemodialysis with little or no prolongation of APTT.

Potential benefits of LMWH, as discussed in Section III.C., above, include an improved lipid profile and possibly some amelioration of hyperkalemia.

B.   Prostanoids. Natural and synthetic vasodilator prostaglandins (PGI_2, PGE_2; epoprostenol, iloprost) are potent inhibitors of platelet aggregation and have been used successfully for anticoagulation in short- and long-term dialysis. At the dosages employed, these agents are somewhat less effective than giving full heparinization. Side effects include hypotension, flushing, nausea, vomiting, and headaches. Prostanoids are not yet commercially available in the United States.

C.   Other antiplatelet agents. Aspirin, nonsteroidal antiinflammatory agents, sulfinpyrazone, and ticlopidine are incapable of maintaining suitable anticoagulation in the extracorporeal circuit when administered alone. However, their antiplatelet effects can counteract heparin-induced platelet factor 4 release. Because platelet factor 4 has heparin-neutralizing effects, these agents may be heparin-sparing.

D.   Protease inhibitors [nafamostat mesylate (FUT-175a), gabexate mesylate]. These synthetic protease inhibitors affect both the coagulation/fibrinolysis cascades and platelet aggregation. Preliminary work suggests that protease inhibitors can adequately anticoagulate the extracorporeal circuit and reduce bleeding complications. Further clinical trials are needed to assess the ultimate utility of these agents in clinical dialysis.

E.   Hirudin. Hirudin is a polypeptide thrombin inhibitor produced by the peripharyngeal glands of the medicinal leech *(Hirudo medicinalis)*. Hirudin blocks both thrombin-induced fibrinogen clotting and thrombin-induced platelet aggregation. Unlike heparin, hirudin does not require endogenous cofactors such as antithrombin III and does not cause platelet stimulation or aggregation, which can result in thrombocytopenia or thrombosis. Small short-term studies in humans have demonstrated that it can provide adequate anticoagulation for hemodialysis.

F.   Extracorporeal device modification. Heparinase-coated cartridges capable of removing heparin infused into the extracorporeal circuit have been developed. Similarly, successful coating of elements of the extracorporeal circuit with biologically active heparin and development of nonthrombogenic membranes, such as polyacrylonitrile/polyethylene oxide, have been reported. Adequate clinical trials of these devices have not yet been performed.

SELECTED READINGS

Caruana RJ, et al. Heparin-free dialysis: comparative data and results in high-risk patients. *Kidney Int* 1987;31:1351.

Caruana RJ, et al. A controlled study of heparin versus epoprostenol sodium (prostacyclin) as the sole anticoagulant for chronic hemodialysis. *Blood Purif* 1991;9:296.

Davenport A. Management of heparin-induced thrombocytopenia during continuous renal replacement therapy. *Am J Kidney Dis* 1998;32:E3.

Elisaf MS, et al. Effects of conventional vs. low-molecular-weight heparin on lipid profile in hemodialysis patients. *Am J Nephrol* 1997; 17:153.

Flanigan MJ, et al. Regional hemodialysis anticoagulation: hypertonic trisodium citrate or citrate dextrose-A. *Am J Kidney Dis* 1996;27:519.

Gotch FA, Keen ML. Care of the patient on hemodialysis. In: Cogan MG, Garovoy MR, eds. *Introduction to dialysis*, 2nd ed. New York: Churchill Livingstone, 1991.

Hirsh J. Heparin. *N Engl J Med* 1991;324:156.

Hodak E, et al. Low-dose low-molecular-weight heparin (enoxaparin) is beneficial in lichen planus: a preliminary report. *J Am Acad Dermatol* 1998;38(4):564–568.

Hottelart C, et al. Heparin-induced hyperkalemia in chronic hemodialysis patients: comparison of low molecular weight and unfractionated heparin. *Artif Organs* 1998;22:614.

Janssen MJFM, et al. Citrate compared to low molecular weight heparin anticoagulation in chronic hemodialysis patients. *Kidney Int* 1996;49:806.

Lai KN, et al. Use of low-dose low molecular weight heparin in hemodialysis. *Am J Kidney Dis* 1996;28:721.

Mehta RL. Anticoagulation strategies for continuous renal replacement tharapies: what works? *Am J Kidney Dis* 1996;28(Suppl 3):S8.

Ouseph R, et al. Improved dialyzer reuse after use of a population pharmacodynamic model to determine heparin doses. *Am J Kidney Dis* 2000;35:89–94.

Sagedal S, et al. A single dose of dalteparin prevents clotting during hemodialysis. *Nephrol Dial Transplant* 1999;14:1943–1947.

Schwab SJ, et al. Hemodialysis without anticoagulation. One year prospective trial in hospitalized patients at risk for bleeding. *Am J Med* 1987;83:405.

Van der Meulen J, et al. Citrate anticoagulation and dialysate with reduced buffer content in chronic hemodialysis. *Clin Nephrol* 1992; 37:36.

Van Wyck V, et al. A comparison between the use of recombinant hirudin and heparin during hemodialysis. *Kidney Int* 1995;48:1338.

Wallis DE, et al. Failure of early heparin cessation as treatment for heparin-induced thrombocytopenia. *Am J Med* 2000;106:629–635.

Ward DM. The approach to anticoagulation in patients treated with extracorporeal therapy in the intensive care unit. *Adv Ren Replace Ther* 1997;4:160.

Ward RA. Heparinization for routine hemodialysis. *Adv Ren Replacement Ther* 1995;2:362.

Whole blood coagulation analyzers. *Health Devices* 1997;26:296–332.

Yamamoto S, et al. Heparin-induced thrombocytopenia in hemodialysis patients. *Am J Kidney Dis* 1996;28:82.

Yang C, Wu T, Huang C. Low molecular weight heparin reduces triglyceride, VLDL, and cholesterol/HDL levels in hyperlipidemic diabetic patients on hemodialysis. *Am J Nephrol* 1998;18:384.

Internet References

Anticoagulants during dialysis: internet links (http://www.hdcn.com/hd/hepa)

10

Slow Continuous Therapies

Miles H. Sigler, Brendan P. Teehan,
John T. Daugirdas, and Todd S. Ing

I. General principles. The popularity of "slow continuous therapies" for the treatment of critically ill patients with renal failure is increasing. The techniques most commonly used are slow continuous hemodialysis and hemodiafiltration. Slow continuous hemofiltration and slow continuous ultrafiltration also are commonly used.

A. Nomenclature. In this chapter, we abbreviate as follows (hyphens are added here for clarity but will not be used subsequently): Slow continuous hemodialysis is shown as C-HD when discussed without regard to vascular access, or as CAV-HD and CVV-HD when use of an arteriovenous (AV) or venovenous access (VV) is emphasized. Similarly, slow continuous hemodiafiltration is abbreviated as C-HDF, CAV-HDF, and CVV-HDF. Slow continuous hemofiltration is C-H, CAV-H and CVV-H. Slow continuous ultrafiltration is abbreviated as SCUF.

B. What are the differences among CHD, CH, and CHDF? Each of these procedures involves slow, continuous passage of blood, taken from either an arterial or a venous source, through a filter.

1. Continuous hemodialysis (CHD). In CHD, dialysis solution is passed through the dialysate compartment of the filter continuously and at a slow rate. In CHD, diffusion is the primary method of solute removal. The amount of fluid that must be ultrafiltered across the membrane is low (3–6 L per day). A typical setup for CHD is using a venous access shown in Fig. 10-1.

2. Continuous hemofiltration (CH). In CH, dialysis solution is not used. Instead, a large volume (about 25–50 L per day) of replacement fluid is infused into either the inflow or the outflow blood line (predilution or postdilution mode, respectively). With CH the volume of fluid that needs to be ultrafiltered across the membrane (on the order of 30–55 L per day, representing replacement fluid plus removal of excess fluid) is much higher than with CHD, where the ultrafiltered fluid volume is on the order of 3–6 L per day. A typical circuit for CH is shown in Fig. 10-2.

3. Continuous hemodiafiltration (CHDF). This is simply a combination of CHD and CH. Dialysis solution is used, and replacement fluid is also infused into either the inflow or the outflow blood line. The daily volume of fluid that is ultrafiltered across the membrane is high, but not as high as with CH, as the volume of replacement fluid used in CHDF (typically about 20 L per day) is lower than with CH.

4. Slow continuous ultrafiltration (SCUF). Neither dialysis solution nor replacement fluid is used. Setup is

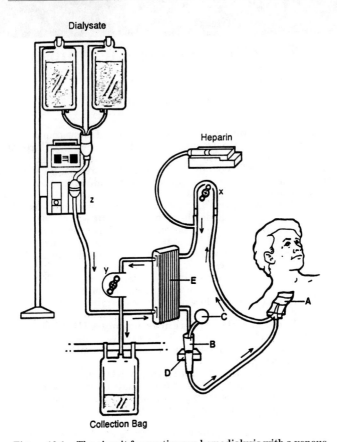

Figure 10-1.   The circuit for continuous hemodialysis with a venous access (CVVHD). A: Double-lumen central vein access (internal jugular or femoral vein access is preferred). B: Venous air trap. C: Venous pressure monitor. D: Air detector. E: Hemodialyzer. X, roller blood pump; Y, dialysate outflow pump. Although pumps X and Y are shown separately, they often are mounted together and electronically synchronized. Z, dialysate inflow pump. (Reproduced with permission from: Sigler M, Teehan B. In: Nissenson AR, Fine RN, eds. *Dialysis therapy*, 2nd ed. London: Hanley and Belfus, 1993.)

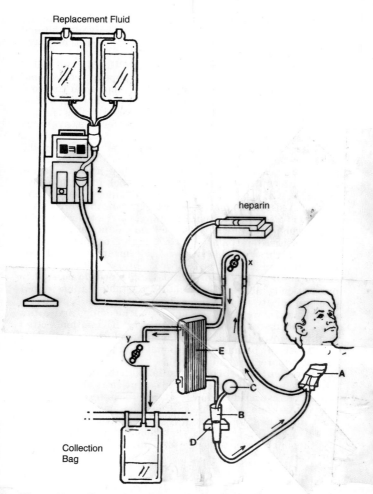

Figure 10-2. Circuit for continuous hemofiltration using a pumped venous access (CVVH). A two-pump method is illustrated, with one pump used to control the rate of replacement fluid infusion and the other the rate of ultrafiltration. In this case, replacement fluid is infused into the filter inlet blood line (predilution mode). A third pump is used to infuse heparin. Modified from: Sigler M, Teehan B. In: Nissenson AR, Fine RN, eds. *Dialysis therapy,* 2nd ed. London: Hanley and Belfus, 1993.)

similar to that shown in Fig. 10-1 for CHD, but without the dialysis solution being part of the setup. Daily ultrafiltered fluid volume across the membrane is low (3–6 L per day), similar to CHD.

C.   Trends in use of CHD, CHDF, and CH. CHD and CHDF are now used more often than CH. The pumped, "venovenous" access approach has almost completely supplanted the non-pumped "arteriovenous" method, for reasons that will be discussed below. All of the techniques described in this chapter are still used, depending on regional preference, available equipment, and clinical circumstances.

II.   Clinical indications. The potential advantages of the slow continuous procedures are listed in Table 10-1.

A.   Lower rate of fluid removal. When hemodialysis is applied intermittently, 3–4 times per week in an intensive care unit (ICU) setting, the total fluid gained plus any pre-existing excess fluid must be removed episodically, during a 3- to 4-hour treatment session. Assuming (very conservatively) a daily weight gain due to positive fluid balance of 2.1 L, or a weekly positive fluid balance of $7 \times 2.1 = 14.7$, or approximately 15 L, with thrice-weekly dialysis, this means that 5 L per treatment would need to be removed. This is a difficult task in a stable chronic renal failure patient, and a near impossibility in a critically ill, hemodynamically unstable patient, often with precipitating comorbid conditions such as septicemia, myocardial infarction, gastrointestinal bleeding, and acute respiratory distress syndrome. Moreover, ICU patients often require removal of much larger amounts of excess fluid than the 2 L per day because of additional fluid infused with medications or parenteral nutrition.

B.   Excellent control of azotemia. With the slow continuous therapies, especially when dialysis solution is used (CHD or CHDF), one can easily achieve daily urea clearances of 30–55 L per day. Assuming a patient urea distribution volume of 40 L, this translates into a daily $(K \times t)/V$ of 0.75 (30/40) to 1.4 (55/40). Many ICU patients are catabolic and require removal of large amounts of urea to control azotemia.

Table 10-1.   Advantages of slow continuous therapies in treatment of intensive care patients

1. Hemodynamically well tolerated; minimal change in plasma osmolality.
2. Better control of azotemia and electrolyte and acid–base balance; corrects abnormalities as they evolve; steady-state chemistries.
3. Highly effective in removing fluid (postsurgery, pulmonary edema, acute respiratory distress syndrome).
4. Facilitates administration of parenteral nutrition and obligatory intravenous medications (i.e., pressor, inotropic drugs) by creating unlimited "space" by virtue of continuous ultrafiltration.
5. Recent efforts to make procedure user-friendly.

C. Caveats

1. The comparison standard, intermittent hemodialysis, is evolving. Despite the seemingly obvious advantages of slow continuous therapies, there has been no evidence from randomized trials that use of continuous, as opposed to intermittent, renal replacement therapy offers a survival advantage in the acute renal failure setting. In fact, two randomized trials that attempted to study this question failed to show a survival advantage for continuous therapies (Mehta et al, 1996; Sandy et al, 1998). Also, with the increasing popularity of daily (6 times per week) hemodialysis for ICU patients, some of the advantages of continuous therapies with regard to a reduced rate of fluid removal and amount of delivered clearance become diminished.

2. **Training and equipment costs.** The use of continuous procedures requires an effort on the part of nursing staff in the ICU to become familiar with the procedures. In units with high staff turnover rates, and in units where continuous therapies are done infrequently, use of intermittent hemodialysis or peritoneal dialysis regimens may be a more practical option. However, in high-volume units, where continuous therapies are a common part of the dialysis armamentarium, use of such therapies will greatly aid in the fluid, solute, and nutritional management of the most challenging patients.

III. Differences among CHD, CHDF, and CH in clearance of small and large molecular weight solutes

A. Urea clearance with CHD and CHDF. In CHD and CHDF, once the blood flow rate is 100–150 mL/min or more, clearance of urea and other small molecules is determined primarily by the dialysis solution flow rate. As outflow dialysate is 90% or more saturated with urea (except when filters begin to clot or when very high dialysate flow rates are used), urea clearance can be estimated simply by the total daily filter outflow volume (which includes dialysis solution used, replacement fluid infused plus any excess fluid removed). The standard dialysis solution inflow rate is now about 25–50 L per day. Thus, taking into account an additional 5 L per day for excess fluid removal, it is easy to achieve urea clearances with CHD on the order of 30–55 L per day (20–38 mL per minute). With CHDF, the replacement fluid infused will add to the clearance as a comparable amount of fluid is removed by the filter. This is automatically taken into consideration if one starts the clearance computation from the total daily outflow volume.

Assuming a urea volume of distribution of 40 L for an average-size patient, the daily Kt/V with CHD can be computed. Assume a clearance of 40 L per day. This is the $(K \times t)$ term of Kt/V. To compute Kt/V, we divide $(K \times t)$ by V (40 L in this case) to get 40/40 or a Kt/V of about 1.0 per day or 7.0 per week. This compares favorably with the Kt/V delivered by thrice-weekly intermittent hemodialysis (usually 3.6 per week). Clearance can easily be increased further, either by increasing dialysis solution flow rate or by adding a filtration component with infusion of replacement fluid. Furthermore, with CHD or CHDF, urea removal is further enhanced (relative to intermittent hemodialysis) because urea clearance is operating continuously while the plasma urea concentration is at a steady-state level.

B.   Urea clearance with continuous hemofiltration. CH is a purely convection-based blood cleansing technique. As blood flows through the hemofilter, a transmembrane pressure gradient between the blood compartment and the ultrafiltrate compartment causes plasma water to be filtered across the highly permeable membrane. As the water crosses the membrane, it convects small and large molecules across the membrane and thus leads to their removal from the blood. The ultrafiltrate is replaced by a balanced electrolyte solution infused into either the inflow (predilution) or the outflow (postdilution) line of the hemofilter. Typically about 25–50 L of replacement fluid is infused per day. The filter outflow or "drainage fluid" is nearly 100% saturated with urea when postdilution mode is used. At high replacement fluid infusion rates the blood flow rate needs to be increased from the usual 100–150 mL per min to prevent excessive hemoconcentration (and resultant clotting) in the filter. When replacement fluid is given in predilution mode, the drainage fluid will not be 100% saturated, because levels of waste products in the blood entering the filter will be diluted. For example, a replacement fluid infusion rate of 35 L per day is equivalent to 24 mL per min. If the blood flow rate is 140 mL per min, the dilution or desaturation will be $24/164 = 15\%$ (when replacement fluid is infused downstream to the blood pump). Assuming that 35 L per day of replacement fluid is used and that 5 L per day of excess fluid is removed, daily "drainage volume," to borrow a term from the peritoneal dialysis literature, will typically be about 40 L per day, and daily Kt/V with CH will be about $40/40 = 1.0$.

1.   Solute removal with CH versus CHD. On a milliliter for milliliter basis (plasma ultrafiltrate out versus dialysate out), CH is more efficient than CHD as a means for solute removal. With CHD, the dialysate is almost completely saturated with urea (at dialysate solution flow rates below 50 L per day and when clotting is not occurring). However, outflow dialysate is not completely saturated with higher molecular weight substances (because these move slowly in solution and thus have a lower diffusive transfer across the dialyzer membrane). With CH, the plasma ultrafiltrate is almost completely saturated with both low and middle molecular weight solutes (because the convective removal rates of small and larger molecular weight solutes are similar) and, hence, is more efficient if one considers larger molecules, such as inulin and vitamin B_{12}. However, the theoretical advantage of CH is not practically realizable, as it is very difficult to ultrafilter more than about 25 L from patients using CH techniques. Fluid balance becomes very critical, as the replacement fluid infusion rate is high. Any slowing of the blood flow rate will result in transient hemoconcentration in the hemofilter, with attendant risk of clotting. On the other hand, it is easy to perform CHD using dialysis solution flow rates of 50 L per day. For this reason, in daily practice, plasma urea clearance with CH is often less than that with CHD.

IV. Vascular access

A. Venovenous blood access. The circuitry for CVVHD (which from the point of view of the blood pathway is identical for CHD, CHDF, CH, and SCUF) is pictured in Fig. 10-1. Vascular access is obtained using a dual-lumen cannula inserted into a large (internal jugular or femoral) vein. As discussed in Chapter 4, the subclavian vein can be used but is not the site of first choice.

   1. Technique of venous catheter insertion. See Chapter 4. Use of a single venous access using a double-lumen catheter is associated with less morbidity. There may be blood recirculation with dual-lumen catheters and to minimize this problem, femoral dual-lumen catheters should be 24 cm long. The low blood flow rates used in the continuous therapies make recirculation less problematic than in intermittent hemodialysis.

B. AV blood access. In CAVHD, this also applies to AV access for the patient's arterial pressure, rather than a pump, is used to propel blood through the extracorporeal circuit. By far the most common arterial site used is the femoral artery.

   1. Technique. Prior to femoral artery cannulation, Doppler audible foot pulses should be present and there should be no vascular bruits over the femoral artery. Using commercially available kits (Medcomp or Vas-Cath), the femoral artery is entered 2 cm below the inguinal ligament using the percutaneous Seldinger technique. A special 8F catheter mounted on a dilator is inserted over the guide wire into the femoral artery. The catheter designed for CAVHD has a single hole at its end and no side holes. Thus, if the catheter tip is inadvertently placed outside of the artery, there will be little or no blood return. The femoral vein is cannulated in the same manner. The arterial and venous catheters are securely sewn in place and povidone iodine dressing applied. We avoid transparent dressings because they trap moisture and create conditions conducive to exit site infection.

   2. Precautions. The cannulated leg must be constantly monitored for signs of ischemia or atheroembolism. The patient must remain in bed as long as the femoral artery catheter is in place. The rate of hemorrhage associated with femoral arterial cannulation is about 5%–6%.

   3. Results. Spontaneous arterial blood flows of 90–150 mL per minute are routinely obtained in patients with mean arterial pressures of 80 mm Hg or more. Patients with lower mean arterial pressures sometimes deliver adequate blood flows as well.

C. Venovenous versus arteriovenous blood access. Use of a venovenous access avoids risks associated with arterial cannulation (distal arterio-occlusive and atheroembolic complications and bleeding). The patient can sit in a chair during treatment with a venovenous access, whereas with femoral arterial cannulation, continuous bed rest is mandatory. With venovenous access, the risk of a large local hematoma on removal of an arterial access catheter is avoided. Use of a roller pump with venovenous access assures a relatively rapid, constant blood flow rate. Pumped blood flow may enhance dialyzer performance and may reduce the likelihood of clotting, as clotting may occur with an AV access due to temporary slowing of blood flow in the extracorporeal circuit.

The disadvantages of a pumped venovenous extracorporeal blood circuit relate to the possibility of inadvertent disconnection of the lines, leading to hemorrhage or air embolism with continued pump operation. Use of dedicated equipment for CVV-based therapies with proper fail-safe monitors and alarm devices minimizes but does not eliminate the risk of potentially fatal hemorrhage or air embolism. Lines are longer with pumped venovenous systems, thus predisposing to more line clotting. Risks associated with cannulation of central veins are described in Chapter 4, and include exit site and catheter-induced bacteremia, and central vein thrombosis and stenosis. Risks are increased when the catheter is left in place longer than 5 days.

Although arterial cannulation avoids the need for blood pumps, the above-mentioned risks of arterial cannulation have caused us and others to abandon arterial cannulation in favor of the pumped venovenous approach.

V. Hemofilters and Dialyzers (Table 10-2)

A. Nomenclature. The terms "hemofilter" and "dialyzer" are used interchangeably in this chapter. Hemofilters initially had only one outlet in the housing, making use of dialysis solution impossible. Subsequently, a second port was added. Currently, most hemofilters/dialyzers can be used to perform either CH, CHD, or CHDF, with certain limitations as detailed below.

B. Choosing a dialyzer or hemofilter. The choice of a hemofilter or hemodialyzer depends somewhat on whether CHD, CHDF, or CH is being contemplated.

1. A water permeability coefficient (K_{Uf}) of at least 12 mL per hour per mm Hg required for CH when using a nonpumped system. For CH, where all small-molecule clearance will need to come from fluid ultrafiltered across the membrane, a high ultrafiltration rate is required, and a high membrane water permeability is a must.

2. Dialyzer diffusivity important when CHD or CHDF is to be used. If a diffusive method of solute transport is to be used (CHD or CHDF), then the layout of the membrane–dialysate interface in the filter becomes important. Some of the early devices designed primarily for CH had excellent water permeability and convective solute clearance, but had poor diffusive clearance when used for CHD; there was poor optimization of contact between dialysis solution and all parts of the membrane in these filters.

All of the dialyzers in Table 10-2, with the exception of the polyamide filters, allow urea in the blood compartment of the filter to equilibrate promptly with dialysate. Contrary to regular hemodialysis, with CHD, because of the low blood flow rates used there is no advantage in terms of clearance to use a large, high-efficiency dialyzer. The risk of clotting in large dialyzers may be increased, as they have been designed for much higher blood flow rates than those used in CHD, and flow velocity through each fiber will be relatively decreased.

Table 10-2. Current hemofilters/hemodialyzers suitable for slow continuous hemofiltration or slow continuous hemodialysis

Type	Source	Brand	Membrane	Surface Area (m²)	K_{UF} mL/h/ mm Hg	Priming Vol. (mL)	Cost (List)
HF[a]	Renal Systems	Renaflo IIHF-700[c,d]	Polysulfone	0.71	15.0	53	80.00[f]
HF[a]	Renal Systems	Renaflo IIHF-400[c,d]	Polysulfone	0.30	4.8	28	70.00[f]
HF[a]	Fresenius	Ultraflux AV 400[c,d]	Polysulfone	0.70		48	64.95[f]
HF[a]	Fresenius	Ultraflux AV 600[c,d]	Polysulfone	1.35		90	74.95[f]
HF[a]	Fresenius	F-5[c]	Polysulfone	0.90	4.2	63	37.95[f]
HF[a]	Fresenius	F-6[c,d]	Polysulfone	1.2	5.5	63	39.95[f]
HF[a]	Fresenius	F-8[c,d]	Polysulfone	1.8	7.5	120	43.95[f]
HF[a]	Fresenius	F-40[c,d]	Polysulfone	0.65	20	44	42.95[f]
HF[a]	Hospal (CGH)	Multiflow 60[c,d]	AN69	0.60	15[e]	47	100.00[g]
PP[b]	Hospal (CGH)	Hemospal[c,d]	AN69	0.43	13[e]	60	114.00[g]
HF[a]	Gambro	FH66[c]	Polyamide	0.60	14–15	43	80.00[f]
HF[a]	Gambro	FH88[c]	Polyamide	2.0		137	90.00[f]

continued

Table 10-2. *Continued*

Type	Source	Brand	Membrane	Surface Area (m²)	K_{UF} mL/h/ mm Hg	Priming Vol. (mL)	Cost (List)
PP[b]	Gambro	Lundia 1C-5H[d]	Cuprophane	1.1	7.4	120	13.50[f]
HF[a]	Baxter	CA210[c,d]	Cellulose acetate	2.1	10.1	133	97.58[f]
HF[a]	Asahi	PAN-50[c,d]	Polyacrylo-nitrile	0.5	15	50	31.00[f]
HF[a]	Amicon	D10	Polysulfone	0.2		15	
HF[a]	Amicon	D20	Polysulfone	0.25	7.2	38	86.00[f]
HF[a]	Amicon	D30	Polysulfone	0.60	8.5	58	98.00[f]

[a] Hollow fiber.
[b] Parallel plate.
[c] Suitable for slow hemofiltration, particularly with a pump.
[d] Suitable for slow continuous hemodialysis.
[e] In vitro, blood, TMP 25 to 100 mm Hg.
[f] Cost of filter only in U. S. dollars.
[g] Cost of complete kit including lines.
TMP, transmembrane pressure.
From Sigler MH, Manns M. *Semin Dial* 1996;9(2):98–106.

VI.   Dialysis and replacement solutions

A.   Methods of preparation. Commercially prepared sterile dialysis solutions packaged in 5-L bags are most commonly used for CHD and CHDF.

   1.   Composition. Table 10-3A lists the concentrations of solutes in some commercially available solutions used for CHD.

   a.   Sodium. The sodium concentration of some commercial solutions is only 130–132 mEq per L. To these solutions, 2 mL of hypertonic (23%) sodium chloride (4 mEq per mL) should be added to each liter to raise the sodium concentration to approximately 140 mEq per L. When citrate anticoagulation is used (see Section E., below), dialysis solution concentration should be 117 mEq/L. This is made by starting with a 5 L bag containing 0.45% saline, and then adding sufficient 23% sodium chloride to raise the sodium level to 117.

   b.   Alkali

   (1)   Lactate. In the United States, all of the commercially available dialysis-replacement solutions for continuous therapy contain lactate as the bicarbonate-forming base. The fluid must contain enough bicarbonate or bicarbonate equivalents (including organic anions such as lactate) to replace bicarbonate lost to dialysis bath, treat preexisting acidosis, and buffer ongoing acid generation. Available lactate concentrations range from 28 to 49 mEq per L.

   (2)   Bicarbonate. Preliminary studies suggest that bicarbonate-buffered replacement fluid is associated with a 25%–50% reduction in the urea appearance rate as compared with a lactate-buffered solution (Olbricht et al, 1992). There is concern that lactate-buffered solutions may cause an increase in blood lactate levels and may affect hemodynamics and acid–base status. This concern is controversial but is acknowledged in patients with severe liver disease. In cases of severe lactic acidosis and in the face of coexisting severe liver disease, we avoid using lactate-buffered dialysis solution and instead use bicarbonate as the buffer base.

   When bicarbonate-containing solutions are not readily available, acetate-containing Ringer's solution can be used advantageously. In the CH setting at least, acetate does not seem to have adverse hemodynamic effects, probably because the amount of acetate infused per unit time is much lower than that absorbed during conventional hemodialysis.

   (a) One can prepare sterile dialysis/replacement fluid manually to achieve solutions containing 30–35 mEq per L bicarbonate (Tables 10-3B and 10-3C). Bicarbonate is in equilibrium with carbonic acid, which breaks down to CO_2 and H_2O; therefore, bicarbonate solutions are unstable. Bicarbonate also forms insoluble salts when in solution with calcium and magnesium. Therefore, bicarbonate based dialysis/replacement solutions should be prepared just before use, as described in Tables 10-3B and 10-3C.

Table 10-3A. Composition of lactated Ringer's solution (used for CHD and CH), peritoneal dialysis fluid (used for CHD), and hemofiltration fluid (used for CHD and CH)

Component	Lactated Ringer's Solution	Peritoneal Dialysis Fluid[a]	Hemodiafiltration Fluid[b]
Glucose	—	1,360 mg/dL	100 mg/dL
Na^+	130 mEq/L	132 mEq/L	140 mEq/L
K^+	4 mEq/L	—	2 mEq/L
Cl^-	109 mEq/L	96 mEq/L	117 mEq/L
Ca^{2+}	2.7 mEq/L	3.5 mEq/L	3.5 mEq/L
Mg^{2+}	—	0.5 mEq/L	1.5 mEq/L
Lactate	28 mEq/L	40 mEq/L	30 mEq/L

[a] 1.5% Dianeal, Baxter Healthcare Corp., Renal Division, McGaw Park, IL.
[b] Premixed dialysate for hemodiafiltration, Baxter Healthcare Corp., Renal Division, McGaw Park, IL.
CHD, slow continuous hemodialysis; CH, continuous hemofiltration.

Table 10-3B. Saline-based, bicarbonate-containing solutions for slow continuous therapies

Single-bag formulation[a]
    1 L 0.45% saline + 35 mL 8.4% $NaHCO_3$ (35 mEq)
      + 10 mL 23% NaCl (40 mEq)
      + 2 mL 10% $CaCl_2$ (2.8 mEq)
Two-bag formulation[b]
    Solution A: 1 L 0.9% saline + 5 mL 10% $CaCl_2$ (7 mEq)
    Solution B: 1 L 0.45% saline + 75 mL 8.4% $NaHCO_3$ (75 mEq)

[a] Dialysis fluid or replacement fluid
[b] Replacement fluid only. Alternate solution A with solution B. Mixing the two will cause precipitation of calcium carbonate.

    (i) Single-bag method. Dialysis or replacement solution containing bicarbonate and no lactate is made by adding (usually this is done by the hospital pharmacy service) $NaHCO_3$ and some additional NaCl to 0.45% NaCl obtained commercially (Tables 10-3B and 10-3C). A small amount of $CaCl_2$ is added as well, and magnesium is given parenterally as needed.
    (ii) Two-bag method (Tables 10-3B and 10-3C). Bags of 0.9% saline with added calcium are alternated with bags of 0.45% saline with added bicarbonate.
   (b) Machine method. One can also prepare bicarbonate-containing dialysis solution for CHD by ultrafiltering dialysis solution prepared by a standard dialysis machine across two dialyzers connected in series (to remove bacteria) and storing the solution in a 15 L sterile drainage bag from a peritoneal dialysis cycler. Such solutions should be used promptly after preparation (see Leblanc et al, 1995).
   c. Glucose. Different dialysis solution dextrose concentrations are available, ranging from 0.10% glucose in commercial hemodiafiltration fluid to 1.5%–4.25% in peritoneal dialysis fluids adapted for use with continuous extracorpo-

Table 10-3C. Composition of solutions listed in Table 10-3B.

Component	One-bag Formulation[a]	Two-bag Formulation
Volume	1.05 L	2.08 L
Na^+	145 mEq/L	147 mEq/L
Cl^-	114 mEq/L	114 mEq/L
HCO_3^-	33 mEq/L	36 mEq/L
Ca^{2+}	2.7 mEq/L	3.4 mEq/L
Mg^{2+}	—	—

[a] Can also be used as dialysis fluid.

real therapies. Use of high-glucose–containing fluids results in an uptake of 1,300–2,400 glucose-derived kilocalories per day from the dialysis solution. Because of the rapid dissipation of the dialysate–blood glucose concentration gradient, increasing the concentration of glucose to 4.25% in the dialysis solution does not result in much increased osmotic removal of fluid from the blood compartment of the dialyzer. However, use of a high dialysis solution glucose concentration may result in hyperglycemia and necessitate use of an insulin drip to control blood glucose levels.

    2.   **Sterility.** Sterile dialysis solution is used because filtration of dialysate into blood can occur (this has not been convincingly demonstrated in plate dialyzers).

B. **Predilution versus postdilution mode of replacement fluid infusion (for CH and CHDF).** Replacement fluid can be infused either into the arterial blood line leading to the hemofilter (predilution) or into the venous blood line leaving the hemofilter (postdilution). The standard method is postdilution. However, when using postdilution at high fluid removal rates (more than 25 L per day), the blood in the hemofilter can become concentrated as its water is rapidly removed, leading to difficulty in obtaining adequate ultrafiltration and to increased resistance in the blood flow pathway (which can lead to poor blood flow and clotting). As a rule of thumb, in postdilution mode, the ultrafiltration rate should not exceed 20% of the blood flow rate. The problem can be solved by increasing the blood flow rate to 150 to 200 mL per minute, or by diluting the blood with replacement fluid before it reaches the hemofilter (predilution). The disadvantage of predilution is that the ultrafiltrate in the hemofilter is generated from blood diluted with replacement fluid and therefore contains a lower concentration of waste products. However, the loss of efficiency is not great because at the usual flow rates the urea concentration of ultrafiltrate obtained from the blood and replacement fluid mixture will be 80%–90% of the corresponding plasma value.

    We recommend using predilution whenever it is desirable to remove more than 25 L per day. Predilution is also performed if the baseline blood viscosity is relatively elevated (e.g., if the hematocrit is greater than 35%). However, postdilution mode has been used with replacement rates of greater than 60 L per day, when a blood flow rate of up to 240 mL per minute was maintained (Ronco et al, 2000).

C. **Temperature of dialysis solution/replacement fluid.** In many configurations of slow continuous therapy, dialysis solution and replacement fluid are infused at room temperature. This is a departure from conventional dialysis, where dialysis solution is warmed, and use of room temperature fluid results in heat subtraction from the patient. It has been speculated that this cooling may be potentially deleterious to patients in terms of ability to ward off or resolve infections. At present, there are no data to support or refute this interesting hypothesis. Many newer continuous therapy machines include a provision for warming the dialysis solution or replacement fluid during use.

VII. **Prescribing and delivering the appropriate clearance to achieve a given level of blood urea nitrogen (BUN).**

Adequacy or dose of dialysis for acutely ill patients in an ICU setting has not been defined. The nephrologist decides what is an acceptable level of azotemia based on clinical experience.

A. Empiric dosing. In the absence of dose–response data, and with suggestions that urea may not be an ideal uremic marker in the acute renal failure setting, it is reasonable to at least initially offer a relatively standard prescription to adult patients of usual size. One such standardized approach would be to use 1.5 L per hour of inflow dialysis solution with a CHD approach. If one is a believer in the importance of removal of molecules larger than urea, one can use a CHDF approach and divide up the same 36 L per day of fluid using 24 L per day of dialysis solution and 12 L of intravenous replacement fluid. (Peritoneal dialysis solution has not been approved by the Food and Drug Administration for use as a replacement fluid, and commercially available hemodiafiltration fluid should be used in such an instance.) Removal of replacement fluid by ultrafiltration across the membrane will increase convective removal of larger molecular weight solutes.

After factoring in removal of 4 L per day excess fluid, either of these approaches should result in a daily urea clearance of about 40 L per day. In hypercatabolic patients, this amount of urea removal will be insufficient to maintain a SUN in the 40- to 60-mg/dL range, and the dialysis solution inflow rate can be increased to as high as 70 L per day to maintain the SUN in the range of 40–60 mg per dL. In patients with low rates of urea generation (e.g., those who are not eating and who are not hypercatabolic and patients with impaired urea synthesis, such as those patients with liver disease), provision of 40 L per day of clearance by continuous therapy may result in steady-state urea nitrogen levels that are substantially lower than 40–60 mg per dL. Of course, residual renal function, if present, can also result in relatively low SUN levels. Our approach, even in patients with relatively low SUN levels, is to maintain 40 L per day solute (urea) clearance as a minimum, under the assumption that not all uremic toxins are represented by urea. One large, prospective, randomized study using CH found that, for a 70 kg patient, increasing the daily ultrafiltrate volume from 36 L per day to about 60 L per day resulted in a substantial reduction in mortality (Ronco et al, 2000).

B. Kinetic dosing based on urea. A more targeted dosing strategy can be used, based on maintaining a target level of SUN. However, it should be kept in mind that such a strategy may not be ideal for all patients. The biggest risk is undertreatment of patients with a low urea generation rate.

Dosing can be estimated using six steps.

1. Estimate or measure the patient's urea generation rate.
2. Decide on the desired level of SUN.
3. Calculate the total rate of urea clearance necessary to keep the SUN at the desired level for the urea generation rate that was estimated or measured in step 1.
4. Measure residual renal urea clearance. Subtract this from the total required urea clearance to obtain the required extracorporeal urea clearance.

5. Calculate the required drainage fluid volume. Set this equal to the required extracorporeal urea clearance, assuming a 100% saturation. Exceptions: With predilution CH or with CHD when using a very rapid dialysis solution inflow rate (more than 2 L per hour), the urea saturation of the drainage fluid may be substantially less than 100%. In such cases, the required "drainage volume" should be increased appropriately.

6. Calculate the required dialysis solution/replacement fluid inflow rate. This is simply equal to the required drainage volume minus the expected removal volume/day of excess fluid.

Problem: A 60-kg male patient (height 5 ft 8 in., or 170 cm) has a SUN of 40 mg per dL on day 1 and 65 mg per dL on day 2. A 24-hour urine collection from day 1 to day 2 contains 5 g of urea nitrogen. On day 2, weight increased to 64 kg. Estimated edema fluid on day 1 is 8 kg and 12 kg on day 2. Calculate the clearance necessary to maintain the SUN at 40 mg per dl.

Solution:
  1. Estimate total-body water at day 1 and day 2.

  a.   Initial total-body water: Initial weight is 60 kg with 8 kg estimated edema fluid. Total-body water therefore is $8 L + (0.55 \times 52) = 8 L + 28.6 L = 36.6 L$ (we are estimating total-body water as 55% of the "nonedematous" weight of 52 kg).

  b.   Final total-body water: Final weight is 64 kg, or 4 kg higher, all of which is water, so final total-body water is $36.6 + 4 = 40.6 L$.

  2. Estimate initial and final total-body urea nitrogen:

  **a.   **Initial and final SUN levels are 40 mg per dL and 65 mg per dL, respectively.

  **b.   **Total-body urea nitrogen at time $1 = 36.6 \times 400$ mg per $L = 14.6$ g.

  **c.   **Total-body nitrogen at time $2 = 650$ mg per $L \times 40.6$ L $= 26.4$ g.

  **d.   **Change in total-body urea nitrogen content from time 1 to time 2 is 26.4 g $- 14.6$ g $= 11.75$ g urea nitrogen.

  **e.   **This 12-g change in urea nitrogen now needs to be corrected to a daily basis. If time 1 and time 2 are 24 hours apart, then the change in body urea nitrogen content is 12 g per day.

  3. Assume that measurements were taken 24 hours apart. Then the change in body urea nitrogen content was 12 g per day. However, the patient also had losses of urea nitrogen during this period. Urinary urea nitrogen loss during the 24-hour observation period was measured to be 5 g per day.

  4. Urea nitrogen generation rate equals that component that caused the increase in serum concentration (12 g per day), plus the component reflected by loss of 5 g per day in the urine, or $12 + 5 = 17$ g per day.

  5. Calculate a clearance necessary to maintain the SUN at some arbitrary desired level. If we assume (without evidence) that a SUN of 40 mg per dL is an acceptable level in critically ill patients with acute renal failure and an elevated protein

catabolic rate, we can compute a clearance that will achieve such a serum level given a urea nitrogen generation rate of 17 g per day:

Urea N removal = clearance $(K_D) \times$ serum level

Urea N removal = $K_D \times 0.40$ g/L

At steady state, urea generation = removal, so $K_D \times 0.40$ (removal) must equal 17 g per day (generation). Now we can solve for K_D:

$K_D = (17 \text{ g/day})/(0.4 \text{ g/L}) = 43 \text{ L/day}$

6.   Determine dialysate inflow rate. So total urea clearance (extracorporeal plus residual renal) must be 43 L per day. If we neglect the renal component, which may be unstable, then we can set the desired extracorporeal clearance equal to total clearance. Then we must plan for a required extracorporeal drainage volume of 43 L per day. Inflow rate of dialysate and/or replacement fluid must equal drainage volume minus excess fluid removal. For example, if we need to remove 3 L of fluid per day to offset hyperalimentation and fluid given with medications, subtract 3 L from 43 L in the example to obtain a required dialysate inflow rate of 40 L per day.

7.   Adjust for residual renal function. This patient actually had a urea clearance of about 10 L per day (about 7 mL per minute), so we can subtract this from the required dialysate inflow rate and use only 30 L per day of dialysis solution rather than 40 L per day.

There are graphical methods that simplify these calculations. Thus, if one knows the urea generation rate and sets a goal steady-state SUN, the required clearance can be read from a graph as created by L. J. Garred and shown in Fig. 10-3. In the present example, 17 g/day = 17,000 mg/1440 min = 12 mg/min of urea nitrogen generation. To use the nomogram in Fig. 10-3, one starts with the desired SUN level on the vertical axis (40 mg/dl) and then one extends a horizontal line to the right until it intersects with the middle of the space between the curved lines representing g = 15 mg per min and g = 10 mg per min. Finally one drops from this point to the horizontal axis to find the required drainage volume flow rate; in this case, about 1.8 L per hour, or 43 L per day.

VIII.   Equipment for slow continuous therapies
  A.   Equipment for pumped venovenous access. A blood pump is required whenever venous access is used. New equipment is being developed by different manufacturers. At present, at least four different setups are available from various manufacturers.

  1.   Prisma system from CGH Medical, Inc. (Lakewood, CO). This consists of four integrated pumps (blood, dialysate, effluent, and replacement solution), three weighing devices (dialysate, effluent, and substitution fluid), and an anticoagulant syringe. When the blood pump stops (because of a pressure alarm, for example), all of the other pumps stop. The circuitry is diagramed in Fig. 10-4. In the circuit, there are four pressure-sensing pods. The sensors and pressure pods make

STEADY STATE SUN AS A FUNCTION OF G AND K

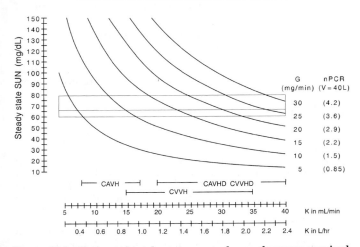

Figure 10-3.   **Estimated total extracorporeal urea clearance required to attain various steady-state serum levels of urea nitrogen. Clearance, on the bottom, is read from the intersection of the urea generation level (G) and the steady-state goal SUN. [From: Garred LJ. Syllabus of the second international conference on CRRT (San Diego, CA, Feb. 9, 1997), p. 7.]**

possible noninvasive pressure monitoring of the access line, filter, return line, and effluent line. There are no blood–air interfaces in the blood line, a feature that may decrease clotting. Control of ultrafiltration and net patient fluid removal is achieved using an integrated control panel with touch screen, which regulates the dialysis solution, effluent, and replacement pump speeds. Filter clotting, fluid balance errors, air detection in the circuit, blood leaks, and changes in pressure are monitored with appropriate alarms.

2.   Use of a modified "2008H" machine from Fresenius, Inc. (Lexington, MA). Theoretically, many standard dialysis machines can be used for slow continuous therapy, although maintenance of a low bacterial colony count in the dialysis solution circuit is a theoretical problem.

Use of a modified Fresenius machine for CHD (run in a 24-hour per day continuous fashion) was reported by Amerling (1998). The machine was altered to permit delivery of a dialysis solution flow rate of 100 mL per minute, and 4 mEq per L potassium was added to the dialysis solution. Blood lines and dialyzers were replaced every 24 hours. Another option called SLED (sustained low efficiency dialysis) treatment mode wherein dialysis using conventional equipment is done for 6–12 hours per day, using low blood and dialysis solution flow rates, with a rest period every night (see also Kuman et al, 2000).

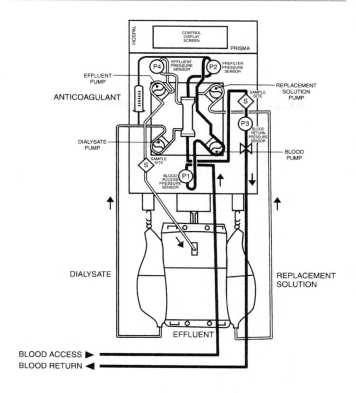

PRE-DILUTION

Figure 10-4. Prisma machine for continuous therapy (CGH Medical). Predilution mode setup is shown. The Prisma machine consists of four pumps (blood, dialysate, effluent, and replacement fluid), three weighing devices (dialysate, effluent, replacement fluid), and an anticoagulant syringe pump. S, sample site; P1, blood access pressure sensor; P2, prefilter pressure sensor; P3, blood return pressure sensor; P4, effluent pressure sensor.

    3. BSM-22 system from CGH Medical. The BSM-22 system consists of two coordinated roller pumps. The blood pump has a pre-pump safety shutoff that senses prepump negative pressure and turns off the blood pump if an excessive vacuum is present. The venous return line traverses an air detector and venous pressure monitor that, if alarmed, will clamp the venous return line and stop the blood pump. A second pump, linked to the blood pump, is applied to the dialysate outflow line and functions as a dialysate outflow pump. A third pump, independent of the BSM-22 or BM-11, is applied to the dialysis solution inflow line. When using the BSM-22 pumps for blood and dialysate outflow, this separate pump is usually an IMED Gemini PC-II (I-Med Corporation, San Diego, CA) used for dialysis solution inflow. The latter pump has an air detector and can infuse up to 2 L per hour or 48 L per day (33.3 mL per minute).

4. BM-11 blood monitor pump and Flo-Gard 6300 pump from Baxter Heathcare (Deerfield, IL). The former is a single blood pump only, which requires the assistance of two additional pumps, one for dialysis solution inflow and one for dialysate outflow for CHD. The Baxter Flo-Gard 6300 dual-channel volumetric infusion pump can be used for dialysis: one channel pumps dialysate into the dialyzer and the second pumps dialysate out, at flow rates that differ as necessary to control overall fluid balance. Each pumping head or channel is capable of flow rates of up to 1,999 mL per hour.

B. Equipment for AV access. The principles are the same as for continuous therapy using a venous access, except, of course, that a blood pump is not required.

C. Setting the ultrafiltration rate

1. Automated systems. With many of the above equipment configurations, the ultrafiltration rate is simply "dialed in," and the machine achieves this as the difference between the drainage fluid outflow rate and the dialysis or replacement solution inflow rate.

2. More primitive "two- or three-pump" systems. With some of the earlier equipment, one needs to manually adjust rates of the dialysate compartment outflow pump and the pump infusing either dialysis solution or replacement fluid.

For example, if the dialysis solution inflow rate is 900 mL/minute, and a ultrafiltration rate of 300 mL per minute is desired, one simply sets the dialysate outflow pump rate at 1,200 mL per minute.

The two-pump method is suitable for ultrafiltration rates of up to 10–20 L per day. Both the replacement fluid rate and the ultrafiltration rate are dialed in using intravenous infusion pumps. We prefer peristaltic pumps that use "fingers" that slide along the tubing to pump the fluid, as opposed to those using pistons. The latter work intermittently, causing transiently high negative pressures that can lead to rupture of hollow-fiber hemofilters. If a piston-type pump is to be used, then a parallel-plate hemofilter should be employed because the plates, by lateral movement, can compensate for sudden pressure changes within the hemofilter.

3. Gravity method (CHD only). An alternative to pumping dialysate outflow is to allow the dialysate to flow out by gravity into the collection bag, which is placed about 40 cm below the level of the dialyzer. The net ultrafiltration rate can be varied by manipulating the vertical distance between the dialyzer and the outflow bag. All air needs to be removed from the tubing between the dialyzer and outflow bag for the siphon effect to work properly. This system is too insensitive to be used with CH, as even small errors in the difference between replacement fluid inflow rate and drainage fluid outflow rate can rapidly cause severe volume overload or dehydration.

When used with CH, the gravity method is suitable for ultrafiltration rates of up to 10 L per day only. The amount of negative pressure that can be generated by gravity is usually not sufficient to support higher ultrafiltration rates.

4.   Suction method (predilution CH only). The ultrafiltrate port is connected directly to the drainage bag, but suction is applied through a T-tube in the line. The ultrafiltration rate is adjusted by changing the amount of suction. Replacement fluid is metered in the usual fashion by an intravenous infusion pump. The replacement rate is usually ordered in terms of the output during the preceding hour.

5.   Stopping ultrafiltration (CH only). When earlier systems are used, ultrafiltration during CH can be stopped at any time by simply clamping the line that drains the ultrafiltrate compartment of the hemofilter.

6.   Interpreting spontaneous changes in the amount of ultrafiltrate (CH only): Clotting, inadequate blood flow, or excessive concentration of blood in the hemofilter (with post-dilution) can lead to formation of less ultrafiltrate than the amount dialed in on the pump leading to the drainage bag. One should periodically check the drainage volume against the volume dialed in, and any discrepancies should be promptly investigated.

7.   Problems with some of the older equipment for continuous therapy

a.   When three pumps are used but only two are electronically or mechanically coupled. With systems where the blood pump is coupled to the dialysate (or replacement fluid outflow) pump, but the dialysis or replacement solution inflow pump operates independently, if the blood pump shuts off for some reason, the coupled dialysate/replacement fluid outflow pump stops automatically, as well. This can be problematical because the independently operating dialysis/replacement solution inflow pump will not shut off automatically. In a dialysis situation, this can build up pressure in the dialysate compartment and cause back-filtration of the dialysate into the blood compartment. In the case of parallel-plate dialyzers, the increased pressure in the dialysate compartment will collapse the blood path. With either CHD or CH, if the inflow pump continues to operate when the outflow pump is stopped, massive fluid overload can eventually develop. For this reason, input/output balances need to be tracked meticulously, and the inflow pump must be shut off manually, if necessary, whenever the outflow pump is stopped.

b.   Errors in ultrafiltration rate with paired dialysate pumps. Small errors in the dialysate inflow and outflow pumps can combine to generate a large error in the net amount of fluid removed from the patient. The output of many pumps is affected by the amount of negative or positive pressure present in the pump inflow and outflow lines. One should always monitor the patient's weight on a daily basis and compare the fluid removal rates as estimated from pump settings with actual weight loss. An alternative is to weigh the dialysis solution bags prior to infusion and compare this to the weight of the drainage bags.

D.   Priming and setup. Strict sterile precautions are used. The lines used for the BSM-22 pump system are available from the manufacturer (Cobe-Gambro-Hospal). With suitable adapters, these lines (along with their pump segments and venous return line with air trap and pressure monitoring lines) can be used for all of the dialyzers listed in Table 10-2. Heparinized saline (2,000 units per L) is used to prime the lines and the dialyzers according to detailed instructions that accompany the kits. Approximately 2 L of heparinized saline is used in the rinsing and priming process. An alternative way to rinse and prime is to mount the lines and dialyzer on a standard dialysis machine and proceed as for routine hemodialysis. After the blood side and dialysate side are primed (the dialysate side being primed with bicarbonate dialysate), the lines are clamped and removed, and the primed dialyzer and lines are reinserted onto the BSM-22 system.

   1.   Positioning the hemofilter. The position of the hemofilter is important to assure adequate blood flow when an arterial access and a pumpless blood circuit is used. The hemofilter should be located slightly below heart level. The device can be attached to the patient's extremity or can be loosely fixed with tape and safety pins to the bed sheets close to the vascular access site. The hemofilter and blood lines should be positioned in such a way as to be constantly visible to the nursing staff. It is best to use Luer lock–type fittings to avoid potential line separation and bleeding. With a pumped venous access, the vertical positioning of the filter is of no importance.

E.   Anticoagulation. Anticoagulation is similar for all of the slow continuous therapies. Clotting in the extracorporeal circuit is the single most difficult technical problem with these procedures. Prolonged anticoagulation is required, which increases the risk of bleeding. On the other hand, insufficient anticoagulation results in premature clotting and ineffective therapy.

   1.   Heparin. After attachment of the primed hemofilter or dialyzer, if baseline clotting times are not elevated, 2,000 units of heparin is injected into the arterial blood line, the clamps are removed, and blood flow allowed to begin. With a parallel-plate hemofilter, one of the ultrafiltrate ports may have to be unclamped as blood flow is started to permit adequate expansion of the blood compartment as the filter fills with blood. Immediately, a constant infusion of heparin (at a rate of 500 units per hour) is begun via an intravenous infusion pump into the arterial line. Heparin therapy is monitored as per Table 10-4.

   2.   Heparin-free method. In patients with liver disease, in postoperative patients, in patients with active or recent bleeding, or in patients with heparin-induced thrombocytopenia, CVVHD can be performed without heparin, although the filter will clot periodically and need to be changed at more frequent intervals. If acute bleeding occurs while CVVHD with heparin is being performed, the procedure can be continued even after heparin administration has been stopped.

   When heparin is not given, a "clotting strategy" can be used. The dialysis solution inflow rate is increased by 20% to 40%. The higher dialysate flow rate will compensate for the antici-

Table 10-4. Heparin protocol for continuous therapies

1. *Initial therapy:* Heparin in priming and rinsing solution as described in text. At start of procedure, give 2,000–5,000 IU heparin in arterial line. Start 500–1,000 IU/h constant infusion.
2. *Monitoring:* PTT measured at the arterial and venous blood lines every 6 h.
   Maintain arterial PTT 40–45 sec
   Maintain venous PTT >65 sec
   If arterial PTT >45 sec, decrease heparin by 100 IU/hr
   If venous PTT <65 sec, increase heparin by 100 IU/hr, but only if arterial PTT <45 sec
   If arterial PTT <40 sec, increase heparin by 200 IU/hr

PTT, partial thromboplastin time.

pated loss of clearance as the unheparinized dialyzer slowly clots. When no heparin is used in patients without coagulation disturbances, the dialyzers will usually clot within 8 hours. A sign of early clotting is a reduction to less than 0.8 in the ratio of dialysate to serum urea nitrogen levels. When the ratio is less than 0.6, clotting is imminent.

   3. Regional anticoagulation with heparin. A method of regional heparin administration for slow continuous therapy has been described (Kaplan and Petrillo, 1987). The technique involves neutralization of infused heparin by administration of protamine into the venous blood line.

   4. Regional citrate anticoagulation (Fig. 10-5). Regional citrate anticoagulation is a new method of anticoagulating the extracorporeal circuit during CHD. It is applicable to patients with heparin-induced thrombocytopenia, and it may be associated with a lower bleeding risk than the use of heparin. Filter life is prolonged when using this technique, in comparison with that when heparin is employed (Mehta et al, 2000).

   The rationale behind citrate anticoagulation, as well as the risks associated with decreased plasma ionized calcium levels, have been described in Chapter 9.

   Figure 10-5 depicts one method of regional citrate anticoagulation. Citrate (4% trisodium citrate, which contains 140 mmol per L citrate and 420 mEq per L sodium) is infused into the dialyzer blood inlet at a rate of about 180 mL per hour, depending on blood flow rate, to maintain the activated clotting time (ACT) in the venous blood line at 180–220 seconds. Instead of the ACT, one can target the postfilter ionized calcium level, aiming at 0.25 to 0.30 mmol per L (0.50 to 0.60 mEq per L). Citrate infusion should be performed cautiously in small patients or in patients with possible hepatic dysfunction (who may not be able to metabolize citrate quickly).

   A special dialysis solution (Fig. 10-5) is prepared that is low in sodium (to offset the hypertonic sodium citrate infusion) and does not contain calcium or base (no bicarbonate and no lactate). Calcium is infused via a separate central venous access using a solution of 20 mL of 10% calcium chloride added to 250 mL of 0.9% saline infused at 40 mL per hour. Calcium

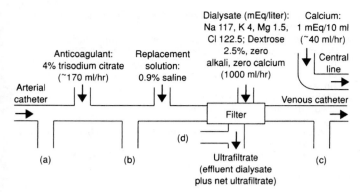

Figure 10-5.   Circuit diagram for citrate CAV-HD. Sampling ports are marked (a) peripheral, (b) prefilter, (c) postfilter, and (d) ultrafiltrate. (Reproduced with permission from: Mehta R, et al. Regional citrate anticoagulation for continuous arteriovenous hemodialysis in critically ill patients. *Kidney Int* 1990;38:976.)

replacement infusion rate is adjusted to keep a peripheral serum ionized calcium level of 1.13 to 1.20 mmol per L. For additional details about this method, see Mehta et al (1990) and the "Internet References" at the end of this chapter.

5.   Monitoring. A sustained reduction in the volume of ultrafiltrate to less than 150–200 mL per hour not attributable to blood pressure fall is suggestive of clotting in the filter or the line. Check the FUN/SUN ratio where FUN is the filtrate urea nitrogen level. If less than 0.6, clotting is eminent. Ionized calcium is monitored in citrate anticoagulation.

6. Signs of **markedly reduced blood** flow include:

Darkening of the blood in the extracorporeal circuit,
Coolness of blood in the venous blood line, and
Separation of erythrocytes and plasma in the extracorporeal circuit.

7.   Diagnosis and treatment. To diagnose and treat a decreasing ultrafiltration rate, the following steps can be performed:

a.   With the arterial blood line clamped proximally, carefully inject 30–50 mL of 0.9% saline into the hemofilter via one of the blood line infusion ports, being careful not to dislodge any clots from the venous end of the hemofilter (stop immediately if any resistance to injection is encountered). If the hemofilter is clotted, then clots may now be visible in transparent parts of the hemofilter.

b.   Unclamp the arterial line and observe the rate at which blood refills the hemofilter and venous line. A partially clotted hemofilter should be replaced. If clotting is not apparent but the rate of refilling is slow, then check the lines for kinking and verify the patency of the access site.

F. Electrolyte imbalances. With CHD, as long as dialysis solution contains an appropriate quantity of electrolytes, electrolyte imbalances should be infrequent. With CH, monitoring and replacing sodium, calcium, and magnesium is important because of the large amount of ultrafiltrate removed. All intravenous fluids, including parenteral nutrition solutions and replacement fluids, should contain close to 140 mEq per L sodium (unless a low sodium solution is being used with citrate anticoagulation). Adequate replacement of calcium, magnesium, potassium, and bicarbonate (given back as bicarbonate, lactate, or acetate) is also of key importance. Phosphate clearance with continuous renal replacement therapies is high, and intravenous phosphate replacement is usually required after several days of therapy.

G. Compensating for dialytic removal of therapeutic drugs. Because of the high 24-hour cumulative clearances with CHD, there is substantial incidental removal of therapeutic drugs (antibiotics and pressors) and nutrient substances, such as crystalline amino acids in parenteral nutrition solutions. Table 10-5 lists the approximate dosage adjustments for antibiotics in renal failure patients being treated with CHD. Antibiotic blood levels, if available, should be obtained because it is difficult to predict what the combined diffusive and convective clearances will be. The doses in Table 10-5 may need to adjusted upwards when the drainage volume is greater than 30 L per day.

Total amino acids are removed in the amount of 12 g per 24 hours at dialysate flow rates of 1 L per hour and when standard parenteral nutrition solutions are infused at a rate of 60–100 mL per hour. The amount of pressor drugs removed during CHD does not appear to be clinically important, and pressor infusion rates are usually adjusted to maintain a given hemodynamic response.

H. Compensating for removal of therapeutic drugs by CH. The ultrafiltrate removed by CH also may contain any drugs present in the patient's plasma. The removal of drugs using the purely convection-based therapies (CVVH and CAVH) depends

Table 10-5. Approximate dosage adjustments of antibiotics in patients with acute renal failure while receiving CHD[a]

Cefuroxime	500–700 mg q 12 h
Ceftazidime	1 g q 24 h
Tobramycin	Loading dose followed by 60–80 mg/24h
Gentamicin	Loading dose then 80–100 mg/24h
Ciprofloxacin	200 mg q 8 h
Vancomycin	1 g q 48 h

[a] For a 70-kg patient. Blood levels should also be determined, if possible.
Modified from Davis SP, Brown EA, Knox WJ, et al. Pharmacokinetic studies in patients with acute renal failure treated by continuous arteriovenous hemodialysis. In: Abstracts of the 1990 Interscience Conference on Antimicrobial Agents, p 213, 1990.

on the sieving coefficient, the degree of protein binding, and the ultrafiltration rate. These variables are listed in the literature (Golper, 1993). The steady-state arterial concentration is determined at the time midway between maintenance doses after the lapse of at least three half-lives. The amount removed then is the steady-state concentration multiplied by the unbound fraction, multiplied by the filtration rate, Q_F. The calculated amount removed in 24 hours is then readministered each day.

Table 10-6 outlines the practical doses of commonly used drugs to be used in CH at ultrafiltration rates of 20–30 mL per minute (29–43 L per day). The CH procedure can be thought of as an extra kidney, the glomerular filtrate rate (GFR) of which will depend on the ultrafiltrate volume. Each 10 L per day of ultrafiltrate volume is equivalent to about 7 mL per minute of GFR (7.0 mL per minute × 1,440 minutes per day = 10.08 L per day). Thus, when prescribing drugs to otherwise anuric patients receiving CH, one should write the drug dose as for a patient with a GFR of 7 mL per minute for every 10 L of ultrafiltrate volume.

IX.   Slow continuous ultrafiltration (SCUF) and isolated ultrafiltration (IU)

A.   SCUF is achieved using the circuitry described in Fig. 10-1, omitting dialysis solution. IU is achieved using standard dialysis equipment as shown in Fig. 10-6. IU can be performed prior to dialysis, after dialysis, or independently of dialysis. In patients with renal failure, IU is most often performed just prior to hemodialysis.

B.   Procedure for IU. Almost all dialysis machines will perform IU and will also allow the desired ultrafiltration rate to be dialed in. One method of doing this is shown in Fig. 10-6. Dialysis solution is routed around the dialyzer using the bypass pathway. Negative pressure is generated in the dialysis solution in the usual fashion and is transmitted to the dialysate compartment of the dialyzer, promoting ultrafiltration. Various machines accomplish IU by different methods, but the principle is always the same: dialysis solution is not circulated through the dialyzer, and a negative pressure is generated in the ultrafiltrate compartment, effecting ultrafiltration.

C.   Clinical application. The clinical role for IU can best be illustrated by several examples:

Example 1. A chronic hemodialysis patient has gained 4 kg since his last treatment 3 days ago. He presents with ankle edema and pulmonary congestion.

R_x:

Perform IU for one hour prior to dialysis. Remove 2.0 kg of fluid during this hour at constant rate. Then perform 4 hours of hemodialysis, removing the remaining 2.0 kg over the 4 hours.

Example 2. A patient has a serum urea nitrogen level of 50 mg per dL and a serum creatinine level of 4.3 mg per dL. He is in marked respiratory distress, with pulmonary congestion, and has a large amount of peripheral edema. The patient has not responded to large doses of furosemide. He has a functioning AV fistula in place but has not yet begun maintenance hemodialysis.

R_x:

Perform IU for 2 hours. Remove 3 L over 2 hours.

Table 10-6. Drug dosage during CH (Q_F = 20-30 mL/min); medians of (n) paired pharmacokinetic and predictive evaluations. Expressed as mg/24h/70 kg BW

Drug	(n)	Normal dosage [mg/day]	Dosage from kinetics [mg/day]	Dosage from predictions [mg/day]	Practical dosage [mg]
Amikacin	(4)	1,050[a]	280	273	250 qd–bid
Netilmicin	(11)	420[b]	139	136	100–150 qd
Tobramycin	(10)	350[b]	115	107	100 qd
Vancomycin	(10)	2,000[b]	645	653	500 qd–bid
Teicoplanin	(8)	400[b]	300	290	300 qd
Ceftazidim	(11)	6,000[b]	1,675	1,622	1,000 bid
Cefotaxime	(13)	12,000[b]	3,235	3,380	2,000 bid
Ceftriaxone	(6)	4,000[b]	1,357	1,457	2,000 qd
Ciprofloxacin	(9)	400[b]	98	167	200 qd
Imipenem	(10)	4,000[b]	1,754	1,614	500 tid–qid
Metronidazol	(7)	2,100[b]	1,376	1,860	500 tid–qid
Piperacillin	(17)	24,000[b]	10,271	9,737	4,000 tid
Digitoxin	(9)	0.065	0.05	0.06	0.05 qd
Digoxin	(9)	0.29[b]	0.07	0.10	0.10 qd
Phenobarbital	(8)	233	330	480	100 bid–qid
Phenytoin	(2)	524	453	364	250 qd–bid
Theophylline	(12)	720	889	745	600–900 qd

[a] p < 0.05.
[b] p < 0.01; paired Wilcoxon-rank test
From Kroh et al. *Semin Dial* 1996;9:161–165.

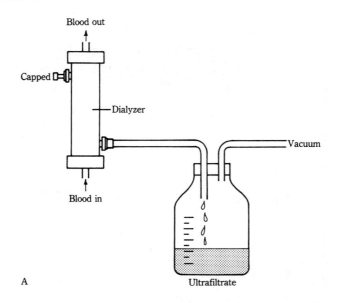

A

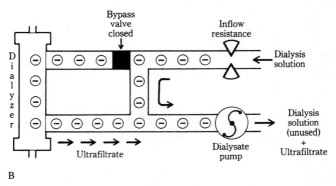

B

Figure 10-6.   Circuit for isolated ultrafiltration. (A) Manual method (now virtually obsolete). (B) One method using a dialysis machine. Circled dash, region of negative pressure.

D. Advantages and disadvantages of IU versus conventional hemodialysis. The principal advantage of IU is that fluid removal is better tolerated than with conventional hemodialysis. IU has no advantage over SCUF in terms of fluid removal; in fact, fluid removal with IU is less well tolerated than with SCUF because with IU the desired amount must be removed much more rapidly.

In the past 5 years, the definition of conventional hemodialysis has changed such that today IU may no longer be a superior method of fluid removal. Some studies have suggested that poor tolerance to fluid removal during older forms of conventional hemodialysis may have been due to use of acetate-containing dialysis solution, excessively warmed dialysis solution, and solutions containing an inappropriately low sodium concentration (e.g., 5–10 mEq per L below that of plasma). If these factors are avoided (i.e., if a bicarbonate-containing, high-sodium, slightly cooled dialysis solution is used), then the previous superiority of IU in terms of hemodynamic stability may no longer be apparent.

The disadvantage of removing fluid in renal failure patients using a combination of IU and hemodialysis is that waste product removal is minimal during IU. For this reason, the subsequent hemodialysis session length should not be shortened, and thus the total treatment time for the IU–hemodialysis combination must be prolonged.

At present, for renal failure patients, the IU–hemodialysis combination is still useful when a bicarbonate-containing dialysis solution is not available, when limited flexibility is present regarding the choice of dialysis solution sodium level, and when a machine that permits volumetric control of the ultrafiltration rate during dialysis cannot be used. For fluid-overloaded patients who do not yet require hemodialysis (as in the patient in Example 2, above), solute removal is unnecessary and IU remains the procedure of choice. In the past, an additional use for IU was to remove excess fluid from dialysis patients with refractory ascites (see Chapter 34). It is notoriously difficult to remove excess fluid from these patients during hemodialysis. However, the benefits of IU in the management of dialysis ascites were established when conventional hemodialysis was not as refined as it has become. With carefully tailored hemodialysis using a high-sodium, slightly cooled, bicarbonate-containing dialysis solution, and with precise control of the ultrafiltration rate, hemodialysis may be equally effective.

E. Complications

   1. Hypotension. Despite the relatively good tolerance to fluid removal with IU, hypotension can still occur if the ultrafiltration rate is excessive. If overt edema is present, then hypotension is rare at ultrafiltration rates less than 1.5–2.0 L per hour (for a 70-kg patient). It is best not to exceed an ultrafiltration rate of 30 mL per kg per hour.

   2. Hyperkalemia. A rebound hyperkalemia has been reported after intensive IU, perhaps due to exit of intracellular potassium into the extracellular fluid. Although the existence of this complication is controversial, any possible hyperkalemia with IU can best be avoided by routinely following IU with several hours of hemodialysis.

3. Other. Because dialysis equipment is used, many of the complications of hemodialysis, such as anaphylactic reactions, air embolism, and so forth, can occur with IU as well.

X. Intermittent maintenance hemofiltration. Intermittent hemofiltration has been used as a complete substitute for maintenance hemodialysis. Hemofiltration treatments are given three times per week using highly permeable hemofilters. Usually, 25–30 L of ultrafiltrate is removed per session, coupled with infusing the appropriate amount of sterile replacement fluid.

The theoretical advantage of intermittent maintenance hemofiltration is a higher removal rate of larger molecular weight substances, which are removed poorly by dialysis (as discussed in Chapter 2); large molecular weight substances may also be important uremic toxins. However, it has been difficult to demonstrate unequivocally that maintenance intermittent hemofiltration is superior to maintenance hemodialysis. The requirement for large volumes of sterile replacement fluid, the need for an accurate mechanism to control fluid balance, and, undoubtedly, the increased monetary cost have combined to limit greatly the popularity of maintenance hemofiltration therapy in the United States.

XI. Hemodiafiltration. Hemodiafiltration is a combination of intermittent hemofiltration with simultaneous hemodialysis. Clearance of large molecules, such as β_2- microglobulin is markedly enhanced. To date, the clinical advantage of maintenance hemodiafiltration over hemodialysis have not been convincingly demonstrated. Hemodiafiltration is not widely practiced in the United States, and its description is beyond the scope of this book.

XII. Continuous renal replacement therapy pointers for certain subgroups of patients

  A. Hepatic failure and acute renal failure (method of Davenport)

    1. Patients with liver failure are at risk for developing cerebral edema, which is also associated with difficulty in maintaining cerebral autoregulation of blood flow. When renal failure develops, control of cerebral edema is problematic. Davenport and co-workers (1996) have used CH and CHD to cope with the increased intracranial pressure and cerebral edema.

    2. CH and CHD systems using the new generation of continuous machines with tight volumetric control and biocompatible membranes, such as polysulfone or polyacrylonitrile, must be used.

    3. Anticoagulation

        a. If possible, no anticoagulation is preferred. Use predilution to extend filter life.

        b. Rinse the membrane and circuit with heparin or heparin/albumin solution; use no additional anticoagulant.

  B. Sepsis and multiorgan failure

    1. Multiple organ dysfunction syndrome occurs as a result of an outpouring of proinflammatory (tumor necrosis factor β, thromboxane B_2, platelet activating factor) and anti-inflammatory mediators (interleukin-10). This response is provoked by gram-negative bacteria endotoxins, gram-positive bacteria, viruses, splanchnic ischemia, and trauma.

Many of these septic mediators are found in the filtrate of septic patients or adsorbed to the filter membrane, suggesting that CH has the ability to remove septic mediators from the circulation. In experimental shock, high-volume hemofiltration has a beneficial effect. However, there are no adequate clinical trials that support the use of continuous high-volume hemofiltration. There is debate as to whether such clinical trials should be attempted. Also, inflammatory mediators could be generated by blood–membrane interaction. Further prospective randomized control studies are necessary before high-volume CH can be recommended as a treatment in sepsis and multiorgan failure. Many centers will treat septic patients with CHDF instead of CHD to increase removal of potential sepsis-mediating molecules while retaining the efficiency associated with use of dialysis. Simultaneous use of 1 L per hour dialysis solution and 1 L per hour replacement solution is one example of a CHDF approach for such patients.

C. Infants and children. Details of these procedures are beyond the scope of this article but are reviewed by Zobel and colleagues (see selected readings).

SELECTED READINGS

Amerling R, et al. CVVHD with modified Fresenius 20084 dialysis machines: initial experience. *J Am Soc Nephrol* 1998;9:116A(abstr).

Boereboom FT, et al. Vancomycin clearance during continuous venovenous hemofiltration in critically ill patients. *Intens Care Med* 1999;25:1100–1104.

Canaud B, et al. Ultrafiltration in congestive heart failure. *Am J Kidney Dis* 1996;28(3):S67–S73.

Clark WR, et al. Extracorporeal therapy requirements for patients with acute renal failure. *J Am Soc Nephrol* 1997;8:804–812.

Davenport MA. Continuous renal replacement therapy in patients with hepatic and acute renal failure. *Am J Kidney Dis* 1996(Suppl 3);28(5):S62–S66.

Golper TA. Drug removal during continuous renal replacement therapy. *Dial Transplant* 1993;22:185–212.

Grootendorst AF, et al. The role of continuous renal replacement therapy in sepsis and multiorgan failure. *Am J Kidney Dis* 1996(Suppl 3); 28(5):S50–S57.

Heering P, et al. The use of different buffers during continuous hemofiltration in critically ill patients with acute renal failure. *Intens Care Med* 1999;25:1244–1245.

Ing TS, et al. Continuous arteriovenous hemodialysis. *Int J Artif Organs* 1985;8:117.

Kaplan AA, Petrillo R. Regional heparinization for continuous arteriovenous hemofiltration (CAVH). *Trans Am Soc Artif Organs* 1987; 33:312.

Keller F, et al. Individualized drug dosage in patients treated with continuous hemofiltration. *Kidney Int Suppl* 1999;72:S29–31.

Kuman VA, et al. Extended daily dialysis: a new approach to renal replacement for acute renal failure in the intensive care unit. *Am J Kidney Dis* 2000;36:294–300.

Kutsogiannis DJ, et al. Regional citrate anticoagulation in continuous venovenous hemodiafiltration. *Am J Kidney Dis* 2000;35:802–811.

Leblanc M, et al. Bicarbonate dialysate for continuous renal replacement therapy in intensive care unit patients with acute renal failure. *Am J Kidney Dis* 1995;26:910–917.

Lee W. Acute liver failure. *Am J Med* 1994;96:3S–9S.

Mehta R, et al. Regional citrate anticoagulation for continuous arteriovenous hemodialysis in critically ill patients. *Kidney Int* 1990;38: 976–981.

Mehta R, et al. Continuous versus intermittent dialysis for acute renal failure (ARF) in the ICU: results from a randomized multicenter trial. *J Am Soc Nephrol* 1996;7:1457A (abstr).

Mehta R, et al for the ARF Collaborative Study Group. Citrate anticoagulation for continuous renal replacement therapy: an update. *J Am Soc Nephrol* 2000;12:in press (abst.).

Mehta RL, et al, eds. Proceedings of the international conference on continuous renal replacement theray. *Am J Kidney Dis* 1996 (Suppl 3);28(5).

Mehta RL, ed. A symposium on practical issues in the use of continuous renal replacement therapies. *Semin Dial* 1996;9(2):79–215.

Olbricht CJ, et al. Effect of lactate and bicarbonate buffered solutions on urea generation rate in continuous hemofiltration. *Int Soc Blood Purif* 1992;0:48(abst).

Reeves JH, et al. A controlled trial of low-molecular-weight heparin (dalteparin) versus unfractionated heparin as anticoagulant during continuous venovenous hemodialysis with filtration. *Crit Care Med* 1999;10:2224–2226.

Ronco C, et al. Effects of different doses in continuous venovenous hemofiltration on outcomes of acute renal failure: a prospective randomized trial. *Lancet* 2000;356:26–30.

Ronco C. Continuous renal replacement therapies: evolution towards a new era. *Semin Dial* 1996;9(2):215–221.

Sandy D, et al. A randomized, stratified, dose equivalent comparison of continuous venovenous hemodialysis, CVVHD, vs. intermittent hemodialysis support in ICU acute renal failure patients. *J Am Soc Nephrol* 1998;9:225A (abstr).

Sigler MH, Teehan BP. Continuous renal replacement therapy. In: Nissenson et al, eds. *Clinical dialysis,* 3rd ed. Norwalk, CT: Appleton & Lange, 1995:907–926.

Zobel G, Ring E, Rodl S. Continuous renal replacement therapy in critically ill pediatric patients. *Am J Kidney Dis* 1996(Suppl 3); 28(5):S28–S34.

Plasmapheresis

Nuhad Ismail, Roxana Neyra,
and Raymond M. Hakim

Therapeutic apheresis refers to an extracorporeal procedure in which blood separator technology is used to remove abnormal blood cells and plasma constituents. The terms **plasmapheresis, leukapheresis,** and **erythrocytapheresis** describe the specific blood element that is removed. In plasmapheresis, or therapeutic plasma exchange (TPE), large quantities of plasma are removed from a patient and replaced with fresh frozen plasma (FFP), albumin solution, and/or saline.

I. Rationale. There are several mechanisms by which plasmapheresis exerts its beneficial effects (Table 11-1). Its major mode of action is rapid depletion of specific disease-associated factors. Examples of these factors include pathogenic autoantibodies [e.g., anti–glomerular basement membrane antibody (anti-GMB), antibody to myelin sheath], immune complexes, cryoglobulins, myeloma light chains, thrombotic factors, cholesterol-containing lipoproteins, and other putative toxic mediators. The basic premise of treatment is that removal of these substances allows for reversal of the pathologic process related to their presence. There also is evidence that plasmapheresis contributes to immune modulation by processes other than mechanical removal of antibodies or other intravascular compounds. For example, splenic clearance of autologous heat-inactivated red blood cells improves after plasmapheresis, an indication that this procedure may deblock the reticuloendothelial system and improve the endogenous clearance of antibodies or immune complexes. Another specific effect of plasmapheresis is its ability to remove other high molecular weight proteins that may participate in the inflammatory process (intact complement C3, C4, activated complement products, fibrinogen, and possibly cytokines). Several other theoretical effects of TPE on immune function have been proposed, including immunomodulatory actions such as alterations in idiotypic/anti-idiotypic antibody balance, a shift in the antibody-to-antigen ratio to more soluble forms of immune complexes (facilitating their clearance), and stimulation of lymphocyte clones to enhance cytotoxic therapy. Therapeutic plasma exchange also allows the infusion of normal plasma, which may replace a deficient plasma component, and may be the principal mechanism of action of TPE in thrombotic thrombocytopenic purpura.

II. Principles of treatment

A. Because of the immunologic nature of most diseases treated by plasmapheresis, therapy should almost always include concomitant immunosuppression (i.e., in most diseases, TPE should not be the sole modality of treatment). Adjunct drug protocols usually include high doses of corticosteroids and cytotoxic agents, such as cyclophosphamide. These agents would be expected to reduce the rate of resynthesis of pathologic antibodies (e.g.,

Table 11-1. **Possible mechanisms of action of therapeutic plasma exchange**

Removal of abnormal circulating factor
  Antibody (anti-GBM disease, myasthenia gravis,
    Guillain–Barré syndrome)
  Monoclonal protein (Waldenstrom's macroglobulinemia,
    myeloma protein)
  Circulating immune complexes (cryoglobulinemia, SLE)
  Alloantibody (Rh alloimmunization in pregnancy)
  Toxic factor (TTP/HUS, FSGS)
Replenishment of specific plasma factor
  TTP
Other effects on immune system
  Improvement in function of reticuloendothelial system
  Removal of inflammatory mediators (cytokines, complement)
  Shift in antibody-to-antigen ratio, resulting in more soluble
    forms of immune complexes
  Stimulation of lymphocyte clones to enhance cytotoxic therapy

GBM, glomerular basement membrane; SLE, systemic lupus erythematosus; TTP, thrombotic thrombocytopenic puapura; HUS, hemolytic uremic syndrome. FSGS, focal segmental glomerulosclerosis.

immunoglobulin G [IgG]), and to further modulate cell-mediated immunity, which may contribute to many of these disorders.

  B. Diseases that respond to plasmapheresis are best treated early to halt the inflammatory response that often contributes to disease progression. For example, plasmapheresis of anti-GBM disease is most effective if therapy is initiated when serum creatinine is less than 5 mg per dL.

  C. Pharmacokinetics of immunoglobulin removal

    1. As the most important rationale for TPE is removal of pathogenic autoantibodies, knowledge of the kinetics of immunoglobulin removal as it relates to TPE is fundamental. Results of experiments in which isotopically labeled immunoglobulins have been infused into humans have demonstrated three fundamental concepts: (a) immunoglobulins have relatively long half-lives ($t_{1/2}$), approaching 21 days for IgG and 5 days for immunoglobulin M [IgM]. The plasma $t_{1/2}$ will determine how quickly the plasma level of the pathogen will rebound and *how often* subsequent plasmapheresis sessions will have to be performed. (b) Immunoglobulins have a substantial extravascular distribution. The distribution volumes of various immunoglobulins and their half-lives are shown in Table 11-2. The extent of intravascular versus extravascular distribution will determine *how effectively* they can be removed in the course of a single plasmapheresis session. For example, the extravascular distribution of IgG is approximately 50%, whereas that of IgM is 20%; therefore, depletion of IgM occurs more quickly than that of IgG (Fig. 11-1). This distinction is also probably accounted for by the substantial differences in the molecular weights (160,000 for IgG and 900,000 for IgM) of these immunoglobulins. (c) Immunoglobulins exhibit an

Table 11-2. Distribution volumes of immunoglobulins

Substance	Molecular Weight	% Intra-vascular	Half-life (d)	Normal Serum Conc. (mg/dL)
Albumin	69,000	40	19	3,500–4,500
IgG	180,000	50	21	640–1430
IgA	150,000	50	6	30–300
IgM	900,000	80	5	60–350
LDL-cholesterol (β-lipoprotein)	1,300,000	100	3–5	140–200

IgG, immunoglobulin G; IgA, immunoglobulin A; immunoglobulin M; LDL, low-density lipoprotein.

intravascular-to-extravascular equilibration that is approximately 1%–2% per hour, whereas extravascular-to-intravascular equilibration may be somewhat faster because it is governed by the rate of lymphatic flow.

The importance of these three concepts to clinical application of TPE is dual. First, considering the relatively long $t_{1/2}$ of immunoglobulins, the use of immunosuppressive agents that decrease antibody production cannot be expected to lower the levels of a pathogenic autoantibody for at least several weeks, even if production is completely blocked. This is the basic rationale for their removal by extracorporeal means. Second, since the extravascular-to-intravascular equilibration is relatively slow, the kinetics of immunoglobulin removal by plasma exchange can be calculated by using first-order kinetics governing removal rates from a single compartment (the intravascular space).

2. The macromolecule reduction ratio and V_e/EPV.
In Chapter 2, the relationship between urea reduction ratio

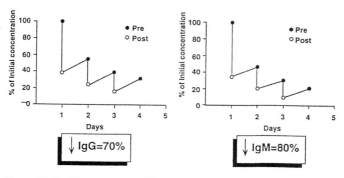

Figure 11-1. Percentage decline in pretreatment serum concentrations for immunoglobulin G (IgG) and immunoglobulin M (IgM) after three days of plasmapheresis (one plasma volume exchanged each day).

(URR) and Kt/V was described, as depicted in Fig. 2-6. A similar relationship holds for removal of immunoglobulins by TPE.

The kinetics of immunoglobulin removal by TPE follows an exponential relationship:

$$C_t = C_0 e^{-Ve/EPV}$$

where C_0 is the initial plasma concentration of the macromolecule in question, C_t is its concentration at time t, V_e is the volume of plasma exchanged at time t, and EPV is the estimated plasma volume, which, while smaller than the volume of distribution of many of these macromolecules, functions as the volume from which they are removed, given the slow rate of equilibration between the extravascular and intravascular compartments. The macromolecule reduction ratio (MRR), expressed as a percentage, is $100 \times (1 - C_t/C_0)$, so MRR = $100 \times (1 - e^{-Ve/EPV})$. If we plug in numbers for V_e from 1,400 mL to 8,400 mL (Table 11-3), and if we assume that a patient's EPV is 2,800 mL, we will get values of V_e/EPV from 0.5 to 3.0. TPE using these V_e/EPV ratios will result in values for the MRR (Table 11-3) ranging from 39% (when EPV/V_e = 0.5) to 95% (when EPV/V_e = 3.0). Note that for EPV/V_e = 1.0, the MRR is 63%. This is exactly the number seen for URR in hemodialysis when Kt/V = 1.0 (see Fig. 2-6, dotted line assuming generation is zero and no volume change). EPV/V_e is similar to Kt/V because the quantity $K \times t$ is the volume of plasma that has been cleared of urea during an extracorporeal treatment, and this is very similar to the V_e, the volume cleared or exchanged during TPE. The V term in Kt/V is the volume of distribution of urea, similar in concept to (although of course much larger than) the EPV, the volume from which macromolecules are removed during TPE.

The relationship between MRR and V_e/EPV implies that the largest decrease (MRR) occurs with the removal of the first plasma volume; removal of subsequent plasma volumes becomes less effective in decreasing the concentration of the substance. This is shown in Table 11-3. As can be seen,

Table 11-3.   Relationship between plasma volume removed and concentration of substance

Portion of Plasma Volume[a] Exchanged (Ve/EPV)	Volume Exchanged (Ve, ml)	Immunoglobulin or Other Substance Removed (MRR, %)
0.5	1,400	39
1.0	2,800	63
1.5	4,200	78
2.0	5,600	86
2.5	7,000	92
3.0	8,400	95

[a] Plasma volume = 2,800 mL in a 70-kg patient, assuming hematocrit = 45%.
Ve, volume of plasma exchanged; EPV, estimated plasma volume; MRR, macromolecule reduction ratio.

although the removal of the first plasma volume leads to an initial 63% reduction (approximately) of the intravascular concentration of the substance, the exchange of the second plasma volume leads only to an additional 23% reduction (86% versus 63%), whereas the third plasma volume exchange leads only to a further 9% reduction (95% versus 86%). **For this reason, usually one, and at most two, plasma volume equivalents (V_e/EPV) are exchanged during a plasmapheresis session.**

Subsequent to the removal of the macromolecule in question, there is a reaccumulation of its concentration in the vascular space from two sources: (a) lymphatic drainage into the vascular space, with a concentration of macromolecules that reflects its presence in the extravascular (primarily interstitial) space, as well as from diffusion of the macromolecule across capillaries from the interstitial to the intravascular space, and (b) endogenous synthesis. Endogenous synthesis has been documented in Goodpasture's syndrome, in which the anti-GBM antibodies will be predictably lowered by a given plasma exchange treatment, but intertreatment increases in serum levels are too rapid to be compatible with simple reequilibration from extravascular stores.

Thus, over the course of the 24–36 hours following a plasmapheresis treatment, the intravascular concentration of the macromolecule in question would rise from approximately 35% of basal levels, to approximately 60%–65% of basal concentration. A second plasma exchange of one plasma volume would then reduce the plasma macromolecule concentration to 20%–25% of the original concentration, only to be followed by a gradual reaccumulation over the subsequent 24 hours to 38% of the original concentration as shown in Fig. 11-2. At the time of the fourth or fifth TPE, the concentration of the

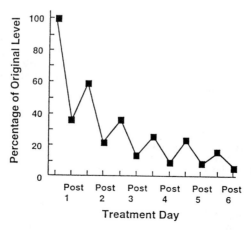

Figure 11-2.   Plasma levels of IgG before and after plasmapheresis.

macromolecule would be oscillating between 10% of basal levels at the end of the procedure to 20%–25% of basal levels before the next procedure. At this range of concentration, the efficiency of plasmapheresis is greatly reduced, and further plasma exchange is generally unwarranted.

3.   Pharmacokinetic basis for TPE prescriptions. Based on these concepts, a rational approach to prescribing TPE is generally to recommend one plasma volume exchange daily for 5 consecutive days at intervals of 24 hours to allow for adequate lymphatic drainage into the vascular space. Clearly, the rate of accumulation and the frequency of TPE should also be targeted to the specific macromolecule that is pathogenic, if this is known. For example, whereas the half-life of IgG is approximately 17 days, that of IgM and immunoglobulin A (IgA) is much shorter (5–7 days). Therefore, if the macromolecule in question is IgM, there may be a role for a more extended period of TPE because the endogenous synthesis rate is expected to be higher for IgM than for IgG. If the substance to be removed is measurable by reliable quantitative means (such as with specific autoantibody), then the treatment schedule should be designed to achieve a significant reduction of that substance based on kinetic considerations. If treatments are performed without identification of the offending agent, then the physician remains dependent on empirical treatment regimens.

4.   Estimation of plasma volume. An estimate of the plasma volume is required to arrive at an appropriate plasmapheresis prescription. For this purpose, there are several nomograms and equations using height, weight, and hematocrit (Hct). These have been incorporated into newer versions of the plasmapheresis equipment. A useful rule of thumb is to consider plasma volume to be approximately 35–40 mL per kg of body weight, with the lower number (35 mL per kg) applicable to patients with normal Hct values and 40 mL per kg applicable to patients with Hct values that are less than normal. For example, in a 70-kg patient with a normal Hct (45%), plasma volume (PV) would be $70 \times 40 = 2,800$ mL.

Predicted blood volume equations have been derived by curve-fitting techniques using subjects' height (cm) and body weight (kg) compared with actual blood volumes measured by isotope (iodine-131 albumin) dilution techniques: $PV = (1 - Hct)$ $(b + cW)$ where W = lean body weight, $b = 1,530$ for males, 864 for females and $c = 41$ for males, 47.2 for females.

Kaplan (1992) uses a simplified method for predicting the estimated plasma volume:

$$EPV = [0.065 \times weight\ (kg)] \times (1 - Hct)$$

III.   Technical considerations. Until recently, most TPE was performed with centrifugation devices used for blood banking procedures. These devices offer the advantage for selective cell removal (cytopheresis) but are often associated with thrombocytopenia. TPE also can be performed with highly permeable filters (hollow-fiber devices, similar to hollow-fiber dialyzers but with large pore sizes) and standard dialysis equipment, a technique often referred to as membrane plasma separation (MPS). MPS is being utilized with increasing frequency and often is more efficient than the centrifugation method. The advantages and disadvantages of each technique are summarized in Table 11-4.

A. Centrifugal plasma separation. In centrifugation, blood cells are separated by gravity, based on the different densities of the various components. At present, there are two types of centrifugation methods: intermittent and continuous. Currently available centrifugal intermittent-flow cell separators are the Haemonetics Model 30, Model V50, PEX, and Ultralite (Haemonetics, Braintree, MA). Continuous-flow devices include Cobe 2997 (Cobe Laboratories; Lakewood, CO), Spectra, Fenwal, CS 300, and Fresenius AS104. The V50, AS104, CS3000, and Spectra models require no operator monitoring or intervention except in the changing of bags. The Haemonetics Model 30 requires continuous operator monitoring and/or intervention, whereas the Cobe 2997 and PEX require some operator monitoring intervention in addition to changing of bags.

1. Intermittent-flow separation. In this technique, multiple aliquots (125–375 mL) of blood are sequentially withdrawn, processed, and reinfused. After withdrawal, the withdrawn aliquot is anticoagulated and centrifuged at high speed until the plasma fraction has layered out. The plasma layer is then discarded, and the red blood cells (RBCs), white blood cells (WBCs), and platelets are returned to the patient along with the replacement fluid. Subsequent aliquots are then withdrawn and processed in the same fashion until the required volume of plasma has been exchanged.

Table 11-4. Comparison of membrane apheresis and centrifugal devices

	Advantages	Disadvantages
Membrane apheresis	No loss of cellular elements	Removal of substances limited by sieving coefficient of membrane
	No requirements for citrate	Requires high blood flows (>50 mL/min)
	Can be adapted for cascade filtration	Often requires central vein catheter
		Limited to plasmapheresis
Centrifugal devices	More efficient removal of all plasma components	Loss of cellular elements of blood
	Can be adapted for cytopheresis	Uses citrate for anticoagulation: hypocalcemia, arrhythmias, hypotension
		Expensive

The Haemonetics Model 30 system (Fig. 11-3) is the most commonly used and consists of a disposable bowl assembly that is available in a variety of sizes (125, 250, and 375 mL). The bowl has two parts: a stationary inner core and a rotating outer shell. Blood (taken from an antecubital or other large vein) is anticoagulated and pumped to the bottom of the bowl, where it is distributed peripherally by centrifugal forces due to rotation of the bowl assembly. The major components of blood separate according to their density: RBCs move to the outside of the bowl; plasma, the lightest component, remains

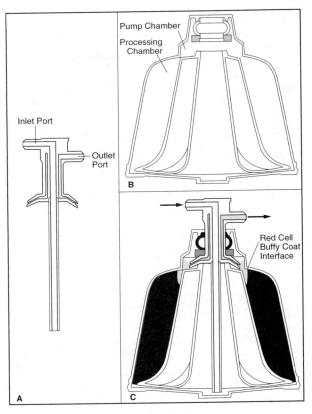

Figure 11-3.   Haemonetics rotating bowl of plasma separation. The two subassemblies are shown. The port assembly (A) remains stationary and provides the inlet and outlet ports. The bowl (B) rotates at about 4,800 rpm. (C) The bowl after it has been filled with blood. At the point shown, the periphery of the bowl is filled with red cells, and most of the plasma, which remains in the center, has already been removed through the strategically placed outlet port. (From Haemonetics Model 30 Blood Processor Operator Manual, Haemonetics Corporation, Braintree, MA, 1982.)

at the center, where it overflows and is collected through an appropriately placed outlet port; platelets and WBCs localize between the red cell and plasma layers. Any one of these components can be collected, discarded, or reinfused.

    2. Continuous-flow separation. In the continuous method, blood is withdrawn, centrifuged, and separated, and the packed volume is returned to the patient in a continuous mode, (rather than in batches) using a hoop-shaped annulus that has sampling ports for the collection of plasma, RBCs, WBCs, and platelets.

    3. Intermittent versus continuous flow. With the intermittent systems, only a single-needle vascular access is required. However, the extracorporeal blood volume is substantial (125–375 mL). The continuous-flow system requires two venous accesses, but the extracorporeal circuit volume is significantly lower (80 mL), making the continuous system more suitable for treatment of children and patients with severe anemia. Processing time with the continuous-flow system is usually faster than with the intermittent system. For example, the average time required to perform a one-PV ($V_e/EPV = 1.0$) exchange with the intermittent system is more than 4 hours, whereas it takes only 1.5 hours with the continuous system.

B. MPS. Plasma separators use membranes with a molecular weight cutoff of about 3 million, generally sufficient to allow passage of immune complexes (MW ≈ 1 million). They can be manufactured in either a hollow-fiber or parallel-plate configuration. An example of a hollow-fiber plasma separator is the Plasma-Flo made by Asahi (Apheresis Technologies, Palm Harbor, FL). This uses a cellulose diacetate membrane, with an inside fiber diameter of 340 μm, a surface area of 0.5 m^2, and a pore size of 0.2 μm. The membrane allows plasma only to pass, as the pores are small enough to hold back the formed elements of the blood. The membrane has a sieving coefficient (ratio of concentration in filtrate to blood) between 0.8 and 0.9 for albumin, IgG, IgA, IgM, C3, C4, fibrinogen, cholesterol, and triglycerides [at a blood flow rate of 100 mL per minute and a transmembrane pressure (TMP) of 40 mm Hg]. The Asahi plasma flow filter can be used with many dialysis machines (Fig. 11-4) in the ultrafiltration, dialysis bypass mode (as would be used for hemoperfusion); however, some dialysis machines, such as the Cobe 3 (Cobe Laboratories; Lakewood, CO) or Hospal dialysis machines, currently are incompatible with many plasmapheresis tubings. With the Asahi Plasma-Flo separator, the manufacturer recommends treatment with a double-track roller pump, which allows the simultaneous removal and replacement of equivalent volumes of plasma and replacement fluid, thus reducing the risk of hypotension or volume overload.

    Some membrane-based plasmapheresis devices are configured as flat sheets of membranes instead of hollow fibers. The TPE Cobe Centry plasma separator (Cobe Laboratories, Lakewood, CO) is one example. The membrane used is made of clear polyvinyl chloride, with a 0.13 m^2 surface area and 0.6 μm pore size. The Cobe TPE system requires a dedicated plasmapheresis machine.

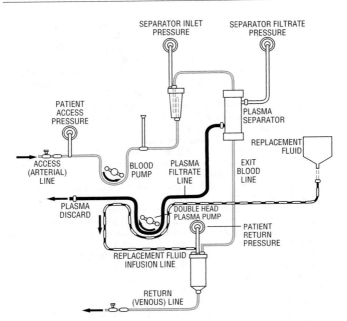

Figure 11-4.   Circuitry for the Asahi hollow-fiber membrane plasma separator, showing the dual-track pump of plasma removal and replacement fluid. (From Asahi Plasma-Flo plasma separator product literature, Apheresis Technologies, Palm Harbor, FL, 1991.)

MPS must be performed at low TMP (less than 500 mm Hg) to avoid hemolysis. With hollow-fiber devices, the blood flow rate should exceed 50 mL per minute to avoid clotting. The ideal blood flow rate (Q_B) is usually 100–150 mL per minute. When the blood flow rate is 100 mL per minute, a plasma removal rate of 30–50 mL per minute can be expected. Thus, the average time required to perform a typical membrane filtration ($V_e = 2,800$ mL) is less than 2 hours (40 mL per minute × 60 minutes = 2,400 mL per hour). As shown in Fig. 11-5, the plasma removal rate is linearly related to Q_B and also depends on Hct and to a lesser extent on TMP.

C.   Comparison of MPS and centrifugation devices. Compared with centrifugal devices, MPS has several advantages. For example, equipment requirements are relatively minimal, and only a blood pump and pressure monitors are required. MPS can thus be performed by using standard hemodialysis delivery equipment, and patients with acute renal failure who require hemodialysis and plasmapheresis can receive both treatments sequentially using the same dialysis machine. MPS is less costly in that it does not require an initial capital investment of approximately $40,000 for a centrifugation device. However, MPS and centrifugation are roughly comparable in terms of cost per treat-

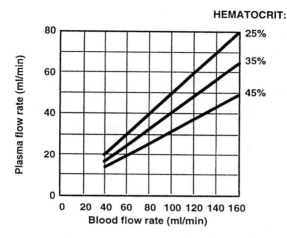

HEMATOCRIT:

Figure 11-5. Relationship between blood flow rate and plasma filtration rate with the Cobe TPE flat-plate membrane plasma separator. This device automatically adjusts transmembrane pressure, which is not operator-controllable. (From Physician Information About the Cobe TPE System, Cobe Laboratories, Lakewood, CO, 1989.)

ment (approximately $200 plus $250–$500 for blood products per treatment). On the other hand, removal of white cells or platelets is possible only with centrifugation devices, and such devices may be more effective for removing very large macromolecules, such as IgM.

IV. Vascular access. For the centrifuge device systems, Q_B in the range of 40–50 mL per minute is required. This can sometimes be obtained from a large peripheral vein (antecubital vein). On the contrary, a central venous access is indicated when using MPS because a blood flow rate between 100 and 150 mL per minute is required for the successful and efficient operation of the filtration system. The best approach is the use of a large-bore, dual-lumen catheter similar to the ones used for dialysis and especially dedicated for apheresis. The majority of intravascular devices available for nondialysis use, such as Swan–Ganz catheters and triple-lumen catheters, almost never provide adequate blood flow for plasmapheresis, although they may be suitable for blood return.

Citrate infusion (see later) causes an acute reduction in the plasma ionized calcium level, which can have a local effect on the cardiac conduction system and generate life-threatening arrhythmia, particularly when blood is returned centrally. Use of the femoral vein is preferable to the subclavian or internal jugular vein to decrease the risk of arrhythmias arising from return of hypocalcemic blood close to the arterioventricular node of the heart. Although the presence of a catheter in the femoral vein limits the patient's mobility, it is a safer alternative to the subclavian or internal jugular vein, and in many patients treated with TPE, mobility may not be possible and treatment is of short duration.

Cardiac rhythm should be monitored, and blood-warming devices should be used, especially if processed blood is returned centrally.

When the nature of the disease requires chronic therapeutic plasma exchange (e.g., hypercholesterolemia, cryoglobulinemia), the creation of a permanent access is preferred. Patients may undergo placement of a central catheter for long-term use, such as the Broviac Hickman catheter, or long-term access may be achieved using an arteriovenous fistula or polytetrafluoroethylene graft.

V. Anticoagulation. Anticoagulation is mandatory for plasmapheresis procedures whether by MPS devices or by centrifugal devices. Citrate solutions and heparin may be used in either type of device. In general, filtration devices use heparin, whereas centrifugal machines mostly operate with citrate.

A. Heparin. Heparin sensitivity and half-life vary greatly in patients, and individual adjustment of dosage is necessary. For most patients, heparin can be used at an initial loading dose of 50 units per kg, followed by an infusion rate of 1,000 units per hour. Frequent monitoring (half-hour) of the activated clotting time (ACT) to maintain an ACT of 180–220 seconds is desirable (1.5–2.0 times normal). Heparin doses may need to be increased in patients with low Hct (increased volume of distribution) and when the plasma filtration rate is high (a high plasma filtration rate results in increased net removal of heparin, which has a sieving coefficient of 1.0).

B. Citrate. Acid citrate dextrose (ACD) is used as the anticoagulation solution for most therapeutic plasma exchange procedures. Citrate chelates calcium, which is a necessary cofactor in the coagulation cascade, and this inhibits thrombus formation and platelet aggregation. ACD comes in two standard formulations. Formula A (ACD-A) contains 2.2 g per dL of sodium citrate and 0.73 g per dL of citric acid. Formula B (ACD-B) contains 1.32 g per dL of sodium citrate and 0.44 g per dL of citric acid. ACD-B is commonly used for the Haemonetics centrifugal system, and ACD-A is used for the Cobe centrifugal and membrane (TPE) systems. Citrate solutions (ACD-A) can be infused into the blood access at a ratio of citrate to blood of 1 : 15–1 : 25. The higher citrate flow ratios (1 : 10–1 : 15) tend to be used for the continuous centrifugal flow system (except when FFP, which contains citrate, is used as a replacement fluid). Lower citrate flow ratios (1 : 15–1 : 25) are recommended for membrane therapeutic plasma exchange.

Although bleeding disorders are not common with citrate, hypocalcemia commonly occurs (60%–70% of the overall complications during TPE). Therefore, symptoms and signs of hypocalcemia must be carefully watched for (perioral and/or acral paresthesias; some patients may experience shivering, lightheadedness, twitching, tremors, and, rarely, continuous muscular contractions that result in involuntary carpopedal spasm). If hypocalcemia becomes more severe, symptoms can progress to frank tetany with spasm in other muscle groups, including life-threatening laryngospasm. Grand mal seizures have been reported. These symptoms and signs may be accentuated by alkalosis due to hyperventilation. Reductions of ionized calcium values also lengthen the plateau phase of myocardial depolarization, manifested electrocardiographically by prolongation of the QT interval. Very high citrate levels, with corresponding low ionized calcium, lead to depressed myocardial contractility, which, though very rare, can provoke fatal arrhythmias in apheresis patients.

1. **Prevention of hypocalcemia during citrate anticoagulation.** The following measures can be considered:

a. **Limiting the rate of citrate delivery to the patient.** The rate of citrate infusion must not exceed the capacity of the body to metabolize citrate rapidly. The ability to metabolize citrate varies from patient to patient. Because the amount of citrate infused will be proportional to the blood flow rate, very high blood flow rates should not be used in small patients. When ACD-A is being infused in a 1:10, 1:15, or 1:25 volumetric dilution with blood, the blood flow rates should not exceed 60, 100, or 150 mL per minute, respectively, for an average-sized patient. In smaller patients, the maximum blood flow rate will be even less. The maximum recommended blood flow rate can be estimated in milliliters per minute as a proportion of body weight depending on the ACD-A/blood ratio being used:

ACD-A/ blood ratio	Maximum blood flow rate (mL/min)
1:10	1.2 × body weight (kg)
1:15	2.0 × body weight (kg)
1:25	3.0 × body weight (kg)

For example, when using an ACD-A/blood dilution ratio of 1:15 in a 30-kg patient, the maximum recommended blood flow rate would be $2 \times 30 = 60$ mL per minute. One of the systems, the Cobe Spectra (Cobe Laboratories, Lakewood, CO), estimates the patient's blood volume by a nomogram. It then automatically sets the blood flow rate to limit the rate at which citrate is being infused.

Patients with liver disease may have an impaired ability to metabolize citrate, and in these patients, citrate infusion should be performed with great caution. FFP contains up to 14% citrate by volume. In cases where FFP, instead of albumin, is being used as the replacement fluid, the citrate reinfusion rate should be lowered even further.

b. **Providing additional calcium to the patient during the plasmapheresis procedure.** Calcium can be given either orally or intravenously. One can, for example, give orally 500-mg tablets of calcium carbonate every 30 minutes. Another approach is to infuse calcium gluconate 10% continuously intravenously, in a proportion of 10 mL of the calcium gluconate solution per liter of return fluid (Weinstein, 1996). In addition to these measures, intravenous boluses of calcium (10 mL of 10% $CaCl_2$ infused over 15–30 minutes) can be given whenever symptoms of hypocalcemia become manifest.

2. **Alkalosis during citrate infusion.** There is the danger of developing metabolic alkalosis because citrate is metabolized to bicarbonate. In patients with liver disease, who may have impaired ability for citrate metabolism, acid–base status during plasmapheresis using citrate anticoagulation should be monitored with special care.

VI.   Replacement solution. The selection of the type and amount of replacement fluids is an important consideration in the prescription of plasmapheresis. The diversity of disease and patient conditions makes the elaboration of uniform suggestions for replacement fluid difficult. Nevertheless, certain guidelines are useful, and they can be modified by the specific conditions encountered.

In most plasmapheresis procedures, replacement by colloidal agents is essential to maintain hemodynamic stability. In practice, this is limited to albumin, generally in the form of an isonatric 5% solution, or to plasma in the form of FFP. The advantages and disadvantages of each are outlined in Table 11-5.

A.   FFP as replacement solution. FFP has the advantage of being similar in composition to the filtrate being removed from the patient but is associated with side effects, such as allergic reactions. Urticaria and hives, which may be severe, are frequently present with the use of FFP. Rarely, anaphylactic reactions result in a form of noncardiogenic pulmonary edema caused by passive transfusion of leukoagglutinins. Another cause of anaphylaxis is infusion of IgA-containing FFP to a patient with selective IgA deficiency. Because FFP may contain appreciable amounts of anti-A and anti-B isoagglutinins, ABO compatibility between donor and recipient is necessary. As noted above, FFP contains citrate, and use of FFP increases the risk of citrate-mediated hypocalcemic reactions. Also, there is a small but measurable incidence of transmission via FFP of hepatitis B (0.0005% per unit), hepatitis C (0.03% per unit), and HIV (0.0004% per unit). Although these infectious risks are now much smaller with predonation and postdonation testing, it should be kept in mind that with each plasmapheresis treatment where 3 L of plasma are replaced with FFP, the 3 L of

Table 11-5.   Choice of replacement solution

Solution	Advantage	Disadvantages
Albumin	No risk of hepatitis Stored at room temperature Allergic reactions are rare No concern about ABO blood group Depletes inflammation mediators	Expensive No coagulation factors No immunoglobulins
Fresh frozen plasma	Coagulation factors Immunoglobulins "Beneficial" factors Complement	Risk of hepatitis, HIV transmission Allergic reactions Hemolytic reactions Must be thawed Must be ABO-compatible Citrate load

replacement FFP is made up of 10–15 units of plasma coming from an equal number of donors.

Use of FFP as the replacement fluid makes measurement of the efficacy of plasmapheresis more difficult in certain patients (e.g., one cannot simply follow serum levels of IgG and other immunoglobulins). Also, FFP may replenish some factors removed during plasmapheresis that could participate in the inflammatory process.

At present, the specific indications for replacing some or all of the removed plasma with FFP during plasma exchange are (a) thrombotic thrombocytopenic purpura–hemolytic uremic syndrome (TTP/HUS), (b) preexisting defect in hemostasis and/or low pretreatment serum fibrinogen level (less than 125 mg per dL), and (c) risk of cholinesterase depletion.

With regard to TTP/HUS, there is a rationale for using FFP as the sole replacement fluid because infusion of FFP by itself may be therapeutic and because in the presence of thrombocytopenia the risk of bleeding as a consequence of minor perturbations in the coagulation factors may be higher.

In general, because plasmapheresis also depletes coagulation factors, replacement by albumin and crystalloids alone may deplete these factors and place the patient at increased risk of bleeding. This is not likely to occur after one or two plasma exchanges, particularly if they are performed more than a day apart, because the half-life for most clotting factors is approximately 24–36 hours. Nevertheless, we recommend measurement of prothrombin time (PT) and partial thromboplastin time (PTT) before the third and subsequent procedures. If the PT and PTT are more than 1.5 times longer than control samples, we recommend infusion of at least 2 or 3 units of FFP as part of the replacement solution.

B. Albumin as replacement fluid. Because of the above concerns with the use of FFP, we recommend albumin as the initial replacement solution. Albumin, at a concentration of 5 g per dL in 0.9% saline, can be replaced in volume equal to that of the removed filtrate. With modern equipment this can be done simultaneously and at the same rate as plasma removal. However, because a substantial proportion of the albumin that is infused early during the procedure is exchanged during the course of plasmapheresis procedure, a more economical approach (when exchange volume is equal to one plasma volume and in the absence of hypoalbuminemia) is to replace the initial 20%–30% of the removed plasma volume with crystalloid, such as normal saline or Ringer's lactate, and then substitute the balance with 5% albumin. This method would result in a final concentration of albumin in the vascular space of approximately 3.5 g per dL, sufficient to maintain oncotic pressure and avoid hypotension.

Purified human serum albumin (HSA) solutions do not transmit viral diseases because of prolonged heat treatment during processing and have become a favored replacement fluid in TPE. A pitfall in the routine use of albumin is its cost and the lack of clotting factors. It has an excellent overall safety record. The incidence of adverse reactions of any kind has been estimated to be 1 in 6,600 infusions. Severe, potentially life-threatening reactions occur in approximately 1 of every 30,000 infusions. When preparing 5% albumin solution from more concentrated solutions, 0.9% saline (with addition of supplementary electrolytes as needed) must be used as the diluent; use of water as a diluent has resulted in severe hyponatremia and hemolysis (Steinmuller et al., 1998).

The amount of fluid replacement given depends on the patient's volume status. The replacement volume can be adjusted, either manually or automatically, from 100% of the removed volume to less than 85%. Use of lower replacement volumes is generally not recommended, since this may contract the intravascular volume and result in hemodynamic instability.

VII.   Complications. The side effects observed in plasma exchange are generally not severe and can be managed easily if they are anticipated. The main side effects are listed in Table 11-6.

Complications range from 4% to 25%, with an average of 10%. Minimal reactions occur in about 5% of treatments and are characterized by urticaria, paresthesias, nausea, dizziness, and leg cramps. Moderate reactions (5%–10% of treatments) include hypotension, chest pain, and ventricular ectopy. All are usually brief and without sequelae. Severe events occur in less than 3% of treatments and are mainly related to anaphylactoid reactions associated by FFP administration. The estimated mortality rate associated with plasmapheresis is 3–6 per 10,000 procedures. The majority of deaths include anaphylaxis associated with FFP replacement, pulmonary embolism, and vascular perforation. The most important complications are discussed below and are summarized in Table 11-6. Citrate reactions have been reviewed extensively above in the anticoagulation section. Strategies for avoidance and management of these complications are summarized in Table 11-7.

Table 11-6.   Complications of plasmapheresis

Related to vascular access
>   Hematoma
>   Pneumothorax
>   Retroperitoneal bleed

Related to the procedure
>   Hypotension from externalization of blood in the extracorporeal circuit
>   Hypotension due to decreased intravascular oncotic pressure
>   Bleeding from reduction in plasma levels of coagulation factors
>   Edema formation due to decreased intravascular oncotic pressure
>   Loss of cellular elements (platelets)
>   Hypersensitivity reactions

Related to anticoagulation
>   Bleeding, especially with heparin
>   Hypocalcemic symptoms (with citrate)
>>   Arrhythmias
>>   Hypotension
>>   Numbness and tingling of extremities
>   Metabolic alkalosis from citrate

Table 11-7. Strategies to avoid complications during plasmapheresis

Complication	Management
Hypocalcemia	Prophylactic infusion of 10% $CaCl_2$ during treatment.
Hemorrhage	Two units of fresh frozen plasma at the end of the session.
Thrombocytopenia	Consider membrane plasma separation.
Volume-related hypotension	Consider continuous-flow separation with matched input and output.
Infection post apheresis	Infusion of intravenous immunoglobulin (100–400 mg/kg)
Hypokalemia	Ensure a potassium concentration of 4 mmol/L in the replacement solution.
Membrane biocompatibility	Change membrane or consider centrifugal method of plasma separation.
Hypothermia	Warm replacement fluids.
ACE inhibitors	Discontinue ACE inhibitor therapy 24–48 hr before treatments.
Sensitivity to replacement fluids	Consider diagnostic evaluation (anti–IgA antibody, anti–ethylene oxide antibody, anti–human serum albumin antibody, endotoxin assay, and bacterial cultures of replacement fluid, etc.). Consider using starch-based fluids. Premedication regimen for sensitized individuals: (a) prednisone 50 mg orally 13 hr, 7 hr, and 1 hr before treatment; (b) diphenhydramine 50 mg orally 1 hr before treatment; and (c) ephedrine 25 mg orally 1 hr before treatment.

ACE, angiotensin converting enzyme; IgA, immunoglobulin A.
Modified from Mokrzycki MH, Kaplan, AA. Therapeutic plasma exchange: complications and management. *Am J Kidney Dis* 1994;23:817.

A.   Hemodynamic complications. Hypotension (2% overall incidence) is due mainly to intravascular volume depletion which may be exaggerated by the large (250–375 mL) volume of blood externalized in the extracorporeal circuit of centrifugal-type cell separators. Other causes include vasovagal episodes, use of hypo-oncotic fluid replacement, delayed or inadequate volume replacement, anaphylaxis, cardiac arrhythmia, and cardiovascular collapse.

B.   Hematologic complications. Hemorrhagic episodes are rare. Bleeding post insertion of femoral catheter, bleeding from a previous catheter site, hematemesis, and epistaxis have been described.

After a single plasma exchange, the serum fibrinogen level typically falls by 80%, and prothrombin and many other clotting factor levels also fall by about 50%–70%. The PTT usually increases by 100%. Recovery of plasma levels of coagulation factors is biphasic, characterized by a rapid initial increase up to 4 hours postapheresis and followed by a slower increase 4–24 hours post exchange. Twenty-four hours after treatment, fibrinogen levels are approximately 50% and antithrombin-III levels are 85% of initial levels; both require 48–72 hours for complete recovery. One day following treatment, the prothrombin level is 75% and factor X is 30% of the original level; by this time, all other coagulation factors will have completely recovered to normal values. When multiple treatments are performed over a short period, the depletion in clotting factors is more pronounced and may require several days for spontaneous recovery. As stated before, when multiple closely spaced treatments are given, it is advisable to replace 2 units of FFP at the end of each treatment.

C.   Angiotensin-converting enzyme (ACE) inhibitors. Anaphylactic or atypical anaphylactoid reactions have been reported in patients taking ACE inhibitors during hemodialysis, low-density lipoprotein (LDL) affinity apheresis, and staphylococcal protein A affinity apheresis. These reactions have been related to negatively charged membranes or filters. Experimental evidence has shown that this reaction is not related to the extracorporeal circulation alone. It is speculated that the fragments of prekallikrein-activating factor present in human albumin leads to endogenous bradykinin release. The severity of the reactions depends on different variables, including drug type and lot of albumin (which may contain different concentrations of the prekallikrein-activating factor). Ideally, therefore, short-acting ACE inhibitors should be held for 24 hours, and long-acting ACE for 48 hours, prior to plasma exchange.

D.   Infection. The true incidence of infection in TPE is controversial. Studies have not clearly shown a significantly higher occurrence of opportunistic infections among patients treated with immunosuppression and therapeutic plasma exchange than with immunosuppressive therapy alone. However, if a severe infection develops in the immediate post–plasma exchange period, a reasonable approach would be a single infusion of immunoglobulins (100–400 mg per kg intravenously).

E.   Electrolyte, vitamin, and drug removal
    1.   Hypokalemia. When the replacement solution is albumin in saline, there could be a 25% reduction in serum potas-

sium levels in the immediate post-apheresis period. The risk of hypokalemia can be reduced by adding 4 mmol of potassium to each liter of replacement solution.

2. Metabolic alkalosis. This may result from infusion of large amounts of citrate.

3. Vitamins. Levels of vitamin B_{12}, B_6, A, C, and E diminish immediately (24%–48%) after treatment and return to baseline values in 24 hours.

4. Drugs. In general, drugs that are significantly cleared by plasma exchange are the ones that have small volumes of distribution and extensive protein binding. Evidence shows that supplemental dosing of prednisone, digoxin, cyclosporine, ceftriaxone, ceftazidime, valproic acid, and phenobarbital is not necessary after plasma exchange. In contrast, the dosages of salicylates, azathioprine, and tobramycin should be supplemented. The many reports of phenytoin clearance are conflicting; thus, it is necessary to carefully monitor unbound drug levels. Therefore, we generally recommend that **all scheduled medications be given immediately after the procedure.**

VIII. Indications for plasmapheresis. In this section, emphasis will be placed on a few diseases in which plasmapheresis has been shown to have a clear benefit, either as primary or adjunctive therapy (categories I and II). Category I indications are those for which TPE is standard and acceptable, but this does not imply that it is mandatory in all situations. Evidence is usually derived from controlled and well-designed clinical trials. Category II indications are those for which TPE is generally accepted; however, it is considered to be supplemental to other more definitive treatments rather than serving as primary therapy. Table 11-8 lists diseases for which plasmapheresis is definitely indicated as well as diseases in which plasmapheresis has been used as adjunctive treatment.

A. Indications for emergency plasmapheresis. Life-threatening or organ-threatening situations that may require emergency plasmapheresis include:

1. Anti-GBM disease and/or pulmonary hemorrhage in Goodpasture's syndrome.

2. Hyperviscosity syndrome with signs and symptoms suggesting impending stroke or loss of vision.

3. Microangiopathic thrombocytopenia (TTP/HUS).

4. Presence of very high factor VIII inhibitor levels in patients requiring urgent surgery. The purpose of plasmapheresis is to reduce the risk of intrasurgical and postsurgical bleeding complications.

5. Respiratory insufficiency in Guillain–Barré syndrome.

6. Myasthenia gravis with respiratory distress not responding to medication.

7. Acute poisoning with certain mushrooms or with other strongly protein-bound poisons, such as parathion or paraquat, depending on the severity of the intoxication.

IX. Treatment strategies. General orders for plasmapheresis are listed in Table 11-9. The following sections describe plasmapheresis treatment prescriptions in selected diseases.

A. Anti-GBM disease

1. In patients with severe disease [oliguria requiring dialysis, serum creatinine value greater than 600 μmol per L

Table 11-8.   Indications for plasmapheresis[a]

Goodpasture's syndrome (anti-GBM disease)
TTP/HUS
Cryoglobulinemia
Hyperviscosity syndrome
Myeloma cast nephropathy
Acute demyelinating polyneuropathy (Guillain–Barré)
Homozygous familial hypercholesterolemia (selective adsorption)
Myasthenia gravis crisis
Chronic inflammatory demyelinating polyneuropathy
Eaton–Lambert myasthenic syndrome
Posttransfusion purpura
Refsum's disease
Cutaneous lymphoma (photopheresis)
HIV-related syndromes (polyneuropathy, hyperviscosity, TTP)
Coagulation factor inhibitors
Rapidly progressive glomerulonephritis (without anti-GBM)
Paraproteinemic peripheral neuropathy
Systemic vasculitis associated with ANCA
ABO-incompatible marrow transplant
SLE (in particular SLE cerebritis)
Bullous pemphigoid
Pemphigus vulgaris
Immune thrombocytopenia (*Staphylococcus* protein A adsorption)
Hemolytic disease of the newborn

[a] These conditions are considered category I or II according to the American Society for Apheresis Writing Committee and Extracorporeal Committee of the American Association of Blood Banks, 1992. See text for details.
GBM, glomerular basement membrane; TTP, thrombotic thrombocytopenic purpura; ANCA, antineutrophil cytoplasmic autoantibody; SLE, systemic lupus erythematosus; HUS, hemolytic uremic syndrome.

(6.8 mg per dL)], plasmapheresis should probably be reserved for treatment of pulmonary hemorrhage because renal function is unlikely to recover even with aggressive treatment.

   2. The frequency of plasmapheresis should be high enough to rapidly decrease the circulating level of anti-GBM antibodies; and an exchange of two plasma volumes daily for 7 consecutive days is indicated in this disease. Because of the consequences of even small titers of circulating antibody, our practice is to continue plasmapheresis for a second week on an alternate-day basis to allow the cytotoxic effects of immunosuppressive medicines to become evident. Note that serial measurements of circulating anti-GBM antibody may be positive in only 65%–70% of cases. A renal biopsy is often indicated for definitive diagnosis of any rapidly progressive renal failure. However, if the index of suspicion for the presence of the anti-GBM disease is high and the clinical situation is suggestive (rapidly rising creatinine, lung hemorrhage), and because of the time needed for renal biopsy and the necessity for being cautious about plasmapheresis for 24 hours after biopsy to reduce the risk of

Table 11-9. General orders for plasmapheresis

Calculate the plasma volume

Measure the preplasmapheresis PT, PTT, and platelets.

When feasible, measure the plasma level of the substance targeted for removal (e.g., anti-GBM antibody titer, acetylcholine receptor antibody, cryoglobulin).

Space treatments approximately 24 hr apart (variable).

For heparin anticoagulation (low bleeding risk patient): heparin 50 units/kg initially, then 1,000 units/hr. Target ACT (when baseline mean control value = 145 sec) during the procedure is about 180–220 sec. If the ACT is less than 3 min, increase the infusion rate by 500 units/hr. If the ACT is greater than 4 min, discontinue heparin infusion, continue to measure the ACT, and resume heparin infusion at a reduced rate when appropriate. Stop heparin infusion about 30 min prior to the end of the procedure.

For citrate anticoagulation, use ACD-A at 1:15 to 1:25 dilution with blood.

Use calcium infusion if necessary.

Cardiac monitor.

Administer scheduled medications only at the end of the session.[a]

Catheter care as per routine.

---

[a] Especially cyclophosphamide and azathioprine. Prednisone and prednisolone are minimally removed by TPE and supplemental dosing after TPE has been found to be unnecessary.

PT, prothrombin time; PTT, partial thromboplastin time; GBM, glomerular basement membrane; ACT, activated clotting time; ACD-A, anticoagulant citrate dextrose type A; TPE, therapeutic plasma exchange.

---

bleeding, our recommendation is to initiate plasmapheresis of large plasma volumes (two plasma volumes each day) for 2 days before biopsy and defer biopsy to a time when the level of circulating antibodies is low. Citrate anticoagulation may be particularly indicated in this case to decrease the risk of pulmonary or renal bleeding. Plasmapheresis beyond a second week may be necessary, and both clinical course as well as anti-GBM antibody titers (if available) will dictate such a need.

    3. Replace removed plasma (milliliter for milliliter) with isonatric 5% albumin. If patient is in fluid overload, reduce the amount of albumin solution infused to 85% (but not less) of the removed plasma volume.

B. TTP and HUS

    1. TTP with central nervous system and renal complications can be a fulminant and rapidly fatal disorder, and it requires the institution of plasmapheresis as soon as possible. The recommended regimen is 1.5 plasma volumes for the first three treatments followed by one plasma volume exchange thereafter The procedure is performed daily until the platelet count is normalized and hemolysis has largely ceased (as evidenced by lactate dehydrogenase level below 400

IU/L). Serum creatinine and urine output have a delayed recovery, generally improving after resolution of thrombocytopenia. Usually, 7–10 treatments are required to induce remission. Because relapse may occur in 50% of patients within a few days of stopping treatment, it is advised not to remove the vascular access catheter until the platelet count is at least 100,000 per mm^3 for 5 days without treatment. If platelet count decreases to less than 100,000 per mm^3, one can resume plasmapheresis on an every-other-day schedule for five more treatments.

   2.   Removed plasma is replaced milliliter for milliliter with FFP. It should be emphasized that the citrate present in FFP may exacerbate hypocalcemic symptoms.

   3.   In children, HUS is frequently a benign illness that often responds to supportive therapy. Although plasmapheresis is effective in shortening the duration of the illness, the difficulties of plasmapheresis in children outweigh the benefit in most cases. However, there may be a role of plasmapheresis in pediatric cases where supportive therapy does not reverse a rapidly deteriorating clinical condition.

   4.   Considering the severe prognosis (maternal and fetal) of TTP in pregnancy and the clear benefit in non-pregnant patients, TPE is also the treatment of choice for TTP during pregnancy despite the possibility of treatment-induced removal of pregnancy-maintaining hormones.

   5.   Except for mitomycin-induced TTP and cancer-associated HUS, in which plasma perfusion over staphylococcal protein A immunoadsorbent column has been found to be more effective than the conventional exchange, the general recommendation is the use of standard plasma exchange for secondary causes of TTP-HUS.

 C.   Cryoglobulinemia. Plasma exchange has been used for 20 years for the treatment of cryoglobulinemia. Although there are no randomized, controlled studies to document the efficacy of plasmapheresis in the disease, almost all of the published reports demonstrate the efficacy of plasmapheresis if the patient has overt symptoms or has progressive renal failure. Indications for TPE include (a) thrombocytopenia (platelet count less than 50,000 per mm^3) or petechiae, or both; (b) hyperviscosity syndrome; (c) cryoglobulin titer greater than 1%; (d) patient about to undergo surgery requiring hypothermia; and (e) renal insufficiency.

In general, patients are treated with immunosuppression and plasma exchange, but some investigators are concerned that this approach may have detrimental effects when cryoglobulinemia is associated with chronic hepatitis C infection.

A suggested prescription is to exchange one plasma volume three times weekly for 2–3 weeks. The replacement fluid can be isonatric 5% albumin, which must be warmed to prevent precipitation of circulating cryoglobulins. IgM antibodies may reaccumulate rapidly and may require chronic treatment once a week.

Selective removal techniques can be used to eliminate or minimize the need for replacement fluid. Double-cascade filtration, which allows separation of cryoglobulins (based on their high molecular weight), is a new technique that can substantially eliminate the need for replacement fluid, yet it is time consuming, relatively expensive, conducive to clotting, and increasingly difficult to obtain in the United States. Cryofiltration is another method that selectively removes cryoglobulins with a special filter by cooling plasma in an extracorporeal system. After removal of cryoglobulins, the remaining plasma is rewarmed and reinfused. Clinical trials are needed to determine the efficacy of these new approaches.

D.   Pauci-immune rapidly progressive (necrotizing) glomerulonephritis (RPGN). Patients usually have Wegener's granulomatosis, polyarteritis nodosa, or "renal-limited" disease. Many have antineutrophil cytoplasmic autoantibodies (ANCA) in their circulation. ANCA titers often correlate with disease activity, and ANCA seem to contribute to the pathophysiology of pauci-immune RPGN through reactivity with neutrophils, endothelial cells, and other inflammatory mechanisms. Available data indicate that 80% of these patients progress to end-stage renal disease without therapy with high-dose immunosuppression or cytotoxic drugs. The results of five randomized trials argue against a role for plasma exchange in mild forms of pauci-immune RPGN. However, Pusey et al (1991) in a randomized trial on 48 patients showed a potential benefit when plasma exchange was used as an adjunct to conventional immunosuppressive therapy in patients who were originally dialysis-dependent. These results probably reflect the efficacy of immunosuppression in controlling the inflammatory response and preservation of renal function.

Plasma exchange should be performed at least daily for 4 days for the first week, using 4-L exchanges with albumin and FFP to avoid coagulopathy. Response to therapy should be monitored with repeated assessments of urine output, serum creatinine values, and possibly ANCA titers. For those patients with positive ANCA, there is a subpopulation with IgM ANCA who might be at a particular risk for pulmonary hemorrhage. If these antibodies are pathogenic, then a centrifugal method of plasma exchange may be required because standard MPS may be relatively inefficient in removing the large IgM-containing immune complexes.

E.   Multiple myeloma and paraproteinemias. Renal failure complicates 3%–9% of cases of multiple myeloma and is associated with a poor prognosis. Renal impairment is caused by toxicity of myeloma light chains to renal tubules, although other factors can also contribute, including hypercalcemia, hyperuricemia, cryoglobulinemia, amyloidosis, light-chain deposition, hyperviscosity, infections, and chemotherapeutic agents. Serum levels of light chains and severity of renal damage are the main factors determining the recovery of renal function. Acute renal failure secondary to multiple myeloma or other paraproteinemia is a new indication for TPE. In a randomized controlled trial of 29 patients with mean pretreatment serum creatinine levels of 11 mg per dL, 13 of 15 patients treated with TPE (3–4 L of plasma exchange on 5 consecutive days) had substantial return of renal function (to a mean creatinine of 2.6 mg per dL) within

2 months, whereas improvement occurred in only 2 of 14 treated without TPE.

If chemotherapy is successful in limiting new light-chain synthesis, then a single prescription of five consecutive plasma exchanges may be sufficient to control the deleterious effects of light chains. Additional treatments may be necessary if there is continued light-chain production. Having identified a given abnormal "spike" as a light chain by immunofixation, regular monitoring by serum protein electrophoresis is an easy means to detect recurrent light-chain accumulation.

F. Lupus nephritis. Several prospective randomized controlled trials do not support a role for plasma exchange in the routine treatment of lupus nephritis. There is experimental and clinical evidence that rapid removal of circulating antibody by plasma exchange triggers a rebound B-cell clonal proliferation and enhanced antibody synthesis. Because proliferating cells have increased vulnerability to cytotoxic agents, it has been suggested that plasma exchange may be useful in patients with lupus nephritis if synchronized with pulse cyclophosphamide (with the latter administered shortly after plasma exchange).

An international trial has been designed to take advantage of this proposed mechanism. More than 170 patients enrolled from 35 centers in Europe, Canada, and the United States. Partial reporting from the study center in Germany has described a rapid beneficial response in all 14 patients undergoing the synchronized protocol, with 8 remaining off all therapy for a mean of 5.6 years. Unfortunately, 4 of 14 patients developed irreversible amenorrhea, and 1 patient developed a squamous cell carcinoma of the oropharynx within 17 months of treatment initiation. Definitive results are pending.

G. Focal segmental glomerulosclerosis (FSGS). Following renal transplantation, FSGS has an estimated recurrence of 15%–55%, with a rapid onset of proteinuria. A protein that has a molecular weight less than 100,000, which is capable of increasing glomerular permeability to albumin, has been characterized in these patients.

A recent report in which standard plasma exchange (1.5 plasma volumes with isonatric 5% albumin as replacement fluid for 3 consecutive days, then every other day up to a total of 9 treatments) was performed in patients soon after the recurrence of proteinuria. Protein excretion was reduced from 11.5 to 0.8 g per day in 6 of 9 patients. Based on these results, the authors concluded that plasma exchange is likely to be effective in the treatment of recurrent FSGS if treatment is initiated promptly after the onset of proteinuria and if there is no significant hyalinosis in the allograft biopsy.

X. Nonrenal indications of therapeutic plasma exchange
A. Acute Guillain–Barré syndrome. This entity appears to be mediated by a monophasic IgM, anti–peripheral nerve–myelin antibody, and by high-titers of IgG antiganglioside antibodies. The IgM antibody can be removed very efficiently by plasma exchange or inhibited by intravenous gamma globulin early in the course of the disorder. With plasma exchange, the antibody level is reduced to less than 20% by 2–3 weeks, whereas without plasma exchange levels do not decrease to 20%

for 3 to 9 weeks. In the United States, intravenous gamma globulin is generally reserved for situations in which plasma exchange is not available or cannot be done for several days. Van der Meche et al (1992) found four factors correlating with poorer outcomes; these factors include (a) old age, (b) time of onset of disease of 7 days or less, (c) need for ventilatory support, and (d) a decreased mean amplitude of 20% of normal or less of the compound muscle action potential after a distal stimulus. Delay in treatment may result in severe dysfunction, requiring twice as many months for recovery.

The Van der Meche study concluding that intravenous gamma globulin treatment for acute Guillain–Barré syndrome is at least as effective as plasma exchange and may be superior needs independent confirmation. An accompanying review found these results difficult to interpret because the patients treated with TPE did less well than expected. A recent comparison of the use of intravenous immunoglobulins and plasma exchange for neurologic diseases suggested that those receiving intravenous immunoglobulins may have a tendency to relapse.

Early and accurate diagnosis is crucial. Hospitalization is mandatory because disease progression is unpredictable. Respiratory function (including tidal volume, negative inspiratory force, vital capacity, oxygen saturation) and physical activity should be monitored. Should the patient become unable to walk unaided, demonstrate significant respiratory impairment, or develop bulbar insufficiency marked by loss of ability to gag or swallow, therapeutic plasma exchange should be initiated promptly.

Usually 1–1.5 plasma volumes should be exchanged within 12–24 hours of the decision to perform TPE. This should be followed by daily plasmapheresis for the first 5 days, then five additional one–plasma volume exchanges every other day. Isonatric 5 percent albumin is the recommended replacement solution. FFP has also been used and in at least one study demonstrated partially superior benefit compared with albumin. However, given the known risks and lack of clear superiority over albumin, use of FFP is not recommended in this case. Some also suggest the intravenous infusion of IgG (40 g) at the end of the treatment.

B. Myasthenia gravis. This is an autoimmune disease associated with anti–acetylcholine receptor antibodies (anti-AchR). Several uncontrolled trials suggest that TPE can induce short-term improvement, and numerous anecdotal reports describe dramatic post-treatment results. The indications for plasma exchange include (a) disease unresponsive to conventional (i.e., cholinergic and immunosuppressive) therapy; (b) episodes of acute deterioration ("myasthenic crisis"); (c) the period before and after thymectomy, when plasma exchange has been shown to diminish the period of ventilator support post surgery; and (d) the period of introduction of corticosteroid therapy, when nearly 50% of patients experience a clinical deterioration.

A reasonable initial treatment prescription is four to eight plasma exchanges over a 1- to 2-week period. Each treatment should consist of one plasma volume, which can be replaced with isonatric 5% albumin. If the patient is in the immediate prethymectomy period, a partial replacement of approximately

1 L of FFP, given toward the end of the treatment, should help reverse the expected depletion coagulopathy. Although levels of AchR antibody are unlikely to be immediately available to monitor therapy, retrospective comparison between observed and expected declines in AchR antibodies reveals an excellent correlation with calculated total IgG removal kinetics. In seriously ill patients, daily or every-other-day therapeutic plasma exchange treatments is indicated.

Improvement is generally seen in 2–4 days, but maximal benefit may not occur for several weeks after cessation of plasma exchange. Long-term remissions are not seen with plasma exchange, and concurrent drug therapy is necessary before and after exchange therapy. Chronic therapeutic plasma exchange (every 4–12 weeks) has been successfully utilized in a minority of patients.

C.   Hyperviscosity syndrome. This occurs most commonly with Waldenström's macroglobulinemia (50% of the time) and occasionally with myeloma (2% of the time) and cryoglobulinemia. Rarely do other causes of elevated serum proteins, such as benign monoclonal gammopathy and rheumatoid arthritis, cause hyperviscosity. It is produced by very high plasma concentrations of monoclonal immunoglobulins, which increase red blood cell aggregation and impede overall blood flow, leading to ischemia and dysfunction of all organ systems. Usually, symptoms do not occur until plasma viscosity is three to four times that of water. The clinical syndrome includes neurologic symptoms, a bleeding diathesis due to effects of the protein on platelets and clotting factors, retinopathy with dilatation and segmentation of retinal and conjunctival vessels, retinal hemorrhages, papilledema, hypervolemia, distention of peripheral blood vessels, increased vascular resistance, and congestive heart failure. The therapeutic approach is to reduce the plasma viscosity to normal and reverse the neurologic symptoms, stop the bleeding diathesis, reverse or stop the visual impairment, and reverse the cardiovascular effects, including hypervolemia and increased vascular resistance. Therapy includes plasma exchange as well as treatment of the primary disorder. The suggested TPE regimen includes daily one–plasma volume sessions for 2 days and continuation of daily one–plasma volume exchanges for 5 days if serum IgM levels remain above normal.

D.   Multiple sclerosis (MS). Based on the analysis of various studies, plasma exchange in combination with immunosuppressive drug therapy may be an effective therapy for MS in certain circumstances, both for chronic progressive and acute relapsing forms. Plasma exchange appears best utilized in the following settings: In acute relapsing MS when (a) conventional corticotropin or corticosteroid therapy is ineffective, (b) the attack is particularly severe, and (c) conventional therapy is contraindicated (e.g., diabetes, hypertension, pregnancy, peptic ulcer disease). TPE also may be indicated in chronic progressive MS when conventional therapy has failed to either improve or stop the progression of disease, and conventional therapy is contraindicated.

The recommended regimen has generally been to use an exchange volume between 1.0 and 1.5 plasma volumes using isonatric 5% albumin solution in saline as replacement fluid. In the acute forms, three exchanges per week for 2 weeks followed by a short course of maintenance therapy–one TPE session weekly for 6 weeks–is recommended.

E. Idiopathic (or immune) thrombocytopenic purpura (ITP). ITP results from the presence of autoantibody to platelets. The antibody is usually IgG directed against membrane glycoprotein antigens. Traditional therapy includes splenectomy or administration of steroids, immunosuppressive agents, vinca alkaloids, danazole, and intravenous immunoglobulin. Several reports describing the use of TPE have documented a rapid short-lived increase in platelet counts felt to be related to a concomitant decline in antiplatelet antibodies. However, plasma exchange needs to be combined with another therapy to produce sustained remission, especially in patients with chronic ITP. FFP is the suggested replacement solution, and it may prevent the risk of hemorrhage that these patients have. In cases of refractory ITP, a staphylococcal protein A immunoadsorbant column is capable of selective adsorption of three subclasses of IgG and may be particularly selective for immune complexes. The efficacy of this approach may be in the removal of immune complexes, infusion of anaphylatoxin-producing substances (such as activated complement), and stimulation of anti-idiotypic antibodies, since it results in removal of only 10% of protein, in contrast with regular plasma exchange.

F. Rh disease. With Rh immunization and technical advances in umbilical cord sampling and intrauterine transfusion, Rh hemolytic disease is very uncommon these days. Several reports suggest that intensive plasma exchange using up to 20 L per week can successfully lower the level of maternal antibodies directed against fetal blood antigens. Plasma exchange is used for situations in which the mother has been immunized against a blood antigen for which the father is homozygous and in which the mother has had a previous history of hydrops at or before 24–26 weeks of pregnancy. Plasma exchange should start at 10–12 weeks of gestation, when maternal–fetal transfer of IgG is beginning. Amniocentesis or fetal sampling is recommended at 18–22 weeks.

G. Coagulation factor inhibitors. The presence of coagulation factor inhibitors generates a de novo appearance of a bleeding disorder. These inhibitors are usually IgG antibodies that bind to a component of the coagulation cascade, with the most common being those with activity against factor VIII.

Therapy is directed at control of bleeding episodes and suppression of synthesis of the inhibitory antibody. The use of large doses of factor VIII, occasionally preactivated, is the best option for these patients; however, this treatment is costly, sometimes reaching $20,000 per day. Immunosuppressive agents, together with therapeutic plasma exchange, have been used to control these antibodies. The recommended regimen varies from two exchanges in a 3-week period to one plasma volume exchange daily for 5 or more days. Replacement should be made with FFP to prevent dilutional coagulopathy.

Recently, plasma exchange with an immunoadsorption device, which is a staphylococcal column that removes IgG and that is capable of regenerating its IgG binding capacity, allowing intensive plasma exchange, has been successfully utilized in association with prednisone and cyclophosphamide therapy.

H. Hypercholesterolemia. Therapeutic plasma exchange is a well-defined treatment for patients with homozygous familial hypercholesterolemia, as well as for hypercholesterolemic persons with pronounced coronary artery disease, in whom it may provide a preventative advantage. Ideally, elevated LDL cholesterol and/or lipoprotein (a) [Lp(a)] levels should be the only or at least the major risk factor, and mean interapheresis target levels of less than 100–120 mg per dL of LDL cholesterol should be achieved. Most patients can be treated satisfactorily by weekly or biweekly processing of one plasma volume; however, those with homozygous familial hypercholesterolemia need to be closely monitored in terms of posttreatment levels. Primary biliary cirrhosis can also result in severe hypercholesterolemia that leads to xanthomatous neuropathy. Repeated treatments (daily for 5 days and then weekly to maintain low plasma levels) lead to resolution of xanthomas, remission of neuropathic pain, and relief of the intractable pruritus. Plasma exchange is indicated when all conservative measures, such as physical exercise, low-cholesterol diet, and cholesterol-reducing drugs, have been unsuccessful.

Currently, there are five different lipid apheresis procedures for clinical application: unselective plasma exchange, semiselective double filtration, highly selective immunoadsorption, chemoadsorption onto dextran sulfate, and heparin-induced extracorporeal LDL precipitation (the so-called HELP system). Plasma exchange has lost popularity in the last few years due to the removal of high-density lipoproteins and immunoglobulins, and the occasional occurrence of anaphylactoid reactions to replacement solutions or disposables. Today most centers prefer immunoadsorption, which uses a Sepharose column of immobilized antibodies to apolipoprotein B (apoB) that interacts with a patient's apoB and removes the LDL cholesterol. With this method the HDL is recovered.

Recently, a new Lp(a) column was described based on immobilized anti–apo(a) antibodies. This column might be advantageous if Lp(a) is the only risk factor for a specific patient. Another device is the LDL hemoperfusor, which adsorbs LDL directly from whole blood and is currently under investigation. Preliminary reports both in vitro and ex vivo and a pilot study in 12 patients have demonstrated good efficacy and selectivity as well as an excellent biocompatibility of the system.

XI. New techniques

A. Cryofiltration. Cryoglobulins removed by conventional cell separators have caused plugging of the membranes due to their small pore size (0.2 µm). Recently, a technique that uses a cryoglobulin filter with an average pore size of 4.3 µm has been shown to be effective in removing cryoglobulins.

Blood and plasma circuits are primed with heparin and 0.9% NaCl. After passing through the cell separator, plasma is continuously cooled by being passed through heat exchange tubings placed inside a refrigeration unit at 4°C (Daido Hoxan Inc., Piscataway, NJ). Cryoglobulins are selectively filtered from plasma by the high-capacity cryofilter, also kept at 4°C. The plasma is then rewarmed to the patient's body temperature before being recombined with the packed red cell fraction. Pressure at the cryofilter is monitored throughout the procedure, and treatment is stopped when pressure reaches 300–400 mm Hg. The replacement solution is isonatric 5% albumin. Siami et al (1995) evaluated the efficacy of this system in a series of seven patients who received 10 treatments. The filter performed safely in all patients, and it was particularly effective in patients with high cryglobulin concentrations.

B. HELP apheresis (heparin-induced extracorporeal LDL precipitation). The HELP system uses a fluid phase reaction of the polyanion heparin with positively charged species such as LDL- and very low-density lipoprotein–derived apoB, Lp(a), and fibrinogen, all risk factors for cardiovascular disease. The use of a low-pH buffer increases the number of positive charges on the target proteins and thus facilitates their precipitation. The resulting coprecipitate of these substances with heparin is then filtered off and excess heparin is removed in a special adsorber containing DEAE cellulose. The risk factor–depleted plasma is then subjected to dialysis to restore physiologic pH, volume, and electrolyte conditions. On theoretical grounds, this triple risk factor removal might be an advantage of the HELP procedure. On the other hand, fibrinogen removal can be limiting in patients with poor coagulation or at risk of bleeding. Although rarely a clinical problem, risk factor removal is limited by the capacity of the precipitate filter. The system uses sterile disposables. Because the HELP system uses a dialyzer for plasma regeneration anyway, a modification in terms of a simultaneous HELP/hemodialysis procedure has also been developed for the treatment of patients with chronic renal failure and LDL-induced coronary heart disease. Several non-controlled studies suggest that this method has a high grade of efficacy.

C. Thermofiltration. This technique was initially described by Nose et al at the Cleveland Clinic. In this technique, the temperature-dependent filtration differences of different plasma components are utilized to improve the differential fractionation of LDL from HDL. During regular therapeutic plasma exchange, it was noted that temperature changes in the line systems would affect the filtration process, due to the formation of a cryogel that occluded the membrane pores. Therefore, a technique that uses plasma warming was developed, and it was found that in the temperature range between 37°C and 42°C the amount of LDL cholesterol removed was the largest, whereas the HDL removed was less than 0.1 g. This technique is considered safe, simple, and cost-effective when compared with other extracorporeal methods. However, one limitation to its use is the requirement of heating of the plasma after its separation. Several reports have established successful reduction of cholesterol using thermofiltration, and results are even better than with plasma adsorption, with the advantage of retention of albumin and HDL cholesterol.

D. Extracorporeal immunoadsorption. Extracorporeal immunoadsorption is a treatment modality based on the use of special ligands to specifically remove blood components considered pathogenic for different diseases, mainly immune complexes and lipids. Separated plasma is passed through a column containing the specific ligand for the substance to be removed, and the depleted plasma is then returned to the patient. Different substances have been used as ligands, with staphylococcal protein A being most widely used, due to its ability to selectively bind immunoglobulins. These columns also cause transient production of beneficial antibodies. Prosorba columns also stimulate the activity of natural killer cells, granulocytes, and macrophages. The main disadvantages are cost and the requirement of trained personnel to set up and monitor the procedure. One randomized trial suggested efficacy in treating refractory rheumatoid arthritis (Felson et al, 1999).

E.   Extracorporeal photopheresis. This therapy involves the extracorporeal treatment of a particular subset of cells with psoralen and ultraviolet A (PUVA). It provides marked selectivity in treating diseased cells only. Psoralens are derived from the plant *Psoralea corylifolia*. At the cellular level, psoralen binds to the pyrimidine bases of DNA. Upon exposure to UV-A light, the psoralen forms covalent bonds with the DNA. The bonds that are formed disrupt DNA replication and the viability of the affected cell, but the exact mechanism of action is unknown.

Photopheresis treatments are accomplished using the UVAR photopheresis system. One and a half hours after the patient receives 0.7 mg per kg of 8-methoxypsoralen (8-MOP) or 0.5 mg/kg of Oxsoralen Ultra, access through a peripheral vein is obtained and patients undergo a discontinuous leukapheresis procedure with exposure of removed leukocytes to UV-A radiation. During the procedure, approximately 240 mL of leukocyte-enriched blood is mixed with 300 mL of the patient's plasma and 200 mL of sterile normal saline plus approximately 10,000 units of heparin. The final buffy coat preparation contains an estimated 25%–50% of the total peripheral blood mononuclear cell compartment and has an Hct varying from 2.5% to 7%. The buffy coat is then passed as a 1-mm film through a sterile cassette surrounded by UV-A–emitting bulbs, permitting a 180-minute exposure to UV-A light, yielding an average exposure per lymphocyte of 2 J per cm^2. Following exposure of the cells to UV-A, the buffy coat is returned to the patient. The entire procedure requires approximately 3–5 hours. Recommended levels of psoralen during treatment are 100 ng per mL or above 50 ng per mL within the photopheresis buffy coat bag. Substantial intraindividual variation in psoralen absorption can occur, depending on gastric contents and disease state. Thus, measurements are taken several times to assure the maintenance of therapeutic levels of 8-MOP.

Photopheresis is currently approved in the United States for the treatment of cutaneous T-cell lymphoma (CTLC). In the initial multicenter trial, patients with erythrodermic CTLC were treated for 2 consecutive days at intervals for a total of 12 months. Highly beneficial results were obtained with few associated adverse effects.

F.   AIDS-related complex. There have been reports on a small number of patients that extracorporeal photopheresis may have a role in up-regulation of the immune system, which may be directly or indirectly related to the UV-A–psoralen interaction in cells infected with the HIV virus. Patients become culture-negative, maintain a stable CD4/CD8 ratio, and do not develop opportunistic infections. Additional studies are needed to investigate this area.

SELECTED READINGS

Bosch T. State of the art of lipid apheresis. *Artif Organs* 1996;20: 292–295.

Bouget J, et al, and The French Cooperative Group. Plasma exchange morbidity in Guillain–Barré syndrome: results from the French prospective, double-blind, randomized, multicenter study. *Crit Care Med* 1993;21:651–658.

Cole E, et al. A prospective randomized trial of plasma exchange as additive therapy in idiopathic crescentic glomerulonephritis. *Am J Kidney Dis* 1992;20(3):266–269.

Felson DT, et al. The Prosorba column for treatment of refractory rheumatoid arthritis: a randomized, double-blind, sham-controlled trial. *Arthritis Rheum* 1999;42:2153–2159.

Glockner WM, et al. Plasma exchange and immunosuppression in rapidly progressive glomerulonephritis: a controlled, multicenter study. *Clin Nephrol* 1988;29:1–8.

Guillain–Barré Study Group. Plasmapheresis and acute Guillain–Barré syndrome. *Neurology* 1985;35:1096–1104.

Hakim RM. Plasmapheresis. In: Jacobson HR, et al, eds. *The principles and practice of nephrology*, 2nd ed. St. Louis: Mosby–Year Book, 1995:713–721.

Hakim RM, et al. Successful management of thrombocytopenia, microangiopathic anemia, and acute renal failure by plasmapheresis. *Am J Kidney Dis* 1995;5:170–176.

Johnson WJ, et al. Treatment of renal failure associated with multiple myeloma: plasmapheresis, hemodialysis and chemotherapy. *Arch Intern Med* 1990;150:863–869.

Kale-Pradhan PB, Woo MH. A review of the effects of plasmapheresis on drug clearance. *Pharmacotherapy* 1997;17:684–695.

Kaplan AA. Toward the rational prescription of therapeutic plasma exchange: the kinetics of immunoglobulin removal. *Semin Dial* 1992;5:227–229.

Kaplan AA. General principles of therapeutic plasma exchange. *Semin Dial* 1995;8:294–298.

Kaplan AA. Plasma exchange for non-renal indications. *Semin Dial* 1996;9:265–275.

Kaplan AA. Plasma exchange in renal disease. *Semin Dial* 1996;9: 61–70.

Leitman SF, et al. *Guidelines for therapeutic hemapheresis*. Bethesda, MD: American Association of Blood Banks, 1992.

Lockwood CM, et al. Reversal of impaired splenic function in patients with nephritis or vasculitis (or both) by plasma exchange. *N Engl J Med* 1979;300:524–530.

Madore F, et al. Therapeutic plasma exchange in renal diseases. *J Am Soc Nephrol* 1996;7:367–386.

Martin J, et al. Plasma exchange for preeclampsia: III. Immediate peripartal utilization for selected patients with HELLP syndrome. *J Clin Apheresis* 1994;9:162–165.

Mokrzycki MH, Kaplan AA. Therapeutic plasma exchange: complications and management. *Am J Kidney Dis* 1994;23:817–827.

Montagnino G, et al. Double recurrence of FSGS after two renal transplants with complete regression after plasmapheresis and ACE inhibitors. *Transpl Int* 2000;13(2):166–168.

Nose Y, et al. Clinical thermofiltration: initial application. *Artif Organs* 1985;9:425.

Pusey CD, et al. Plasma exchange in focal necrotizing glomerulonephritis without anti-GBM antibodies. *Kidney Int* 1991;40: 757–763.

Rock GA, et al. Comparison of plasma exchange with plasma infusion in the treatment of thrombotic thrombocytopenic purpura. *N Engl J Med* 1991;325:393–397.

Siami G, et al. Cryofiltration apheresis for treatment of cryoglobulinemia associated with hepatitis C. *ASAIO J* 1995;41:M315–M318.

Steinmuller DR, et al. A dangerous error in the dilution of 25 percent albumin. *N Engl J Med* [letter] 1998;38:1226–1227.

Strauss RG. Mechanisms of adverse effects during hemapheresis. *J Clin Apheresis* 1996;11:160–164.

Tatami R, et al. Regression of coronary atherosclerosis by combined LDL-apheresis and lipid-lowering drug therapy in patients with familial hypercholesterolemia: a multicenter study. *Atherosclerosis* 1992;95:1–13.

Thornton CA, Griggs RC. Plasma exchange and intravenous immunoglobulin treatment of neuromuscular disease. *Ann Neurol* 1994;35: 260–268.

United States Centers for Disease Control. Renal insufficiency and failure associated with IGIV therapy. *Morb Mortal Weekly Rep* 1999; 48:518–521.

van der Meche FGA, Schmitz PI. A randomized trial comparing intravenous immune globulin and plasma exchange in Guillain–Barré syndrome. Dutch Guillain–Barré Study Group. *N Engl J Med* 1992; 326:1123–1129.

Weinstein R. Is there a scientific rationale for therapeutic plasma exchange or intravenous immune globulin in the treatment of acute Guillain–Barré syndrome? *J Clin Apheresis* 1995;10:150–157.

Weinstein R. Prevention of citrate reactions during therapeutic plasma exchange by constant infusion of calcium gluconate with the return fluid. *J Clin Apheresis* 1996;11:204–210.

Zucchelli P, et al. Controlled plasma exchange trial in acute renal failure due to multiple myeloma. *Kidney Int* 1988;33:1175–1180.

Use of Dialysis and Hemoperfusion in Treatment of Poisoning

James F. Winchester and Chagriya Kitiyakara

Peritoneal dialysis, hemodialysis, and hemoperfusion, particularly the latter two procedures, can be useful adjuncts in the management of drug overdose and poisoning. However, these treatments should be applied selectively in the context of a comprehensive management strategy that includes cardiorespiratory support, early gastric lavage (when indicated and safe), and administration of activated charcoal or specific antidotes (Kulig, 1992). Also, in patients with reasonably adequate renal function, forced diuresis along with alkalinization or acidification of the urine can accelerate removal of a number of drugs from the body. More than 2 million cases of toxic exposures were compiled in the 1998 annual report of the American Association of Poison Control Centers (AAPCC), which covers approximately 95% of exposures in the United States (Litovitz et al, 1999). Although the majority of cases were managed at home, 480,647 cases required treatment in health care settings and 775 patients died. During 1998, 6,680 patients were treated by alkalinization, 978 received hemodialysis, and 48 received hemoperfusion. Multiple-dose activated charcoal (MDAC) is used increasingly and has been shown to enhance the clearance of several drugs (Chyka, 1995). MDAC should be continued even if dialysis and hemoperfusion are employed.

I. Dialysis and hemoperfusion

A. Indications. Extracorporeal techniques should be considered when the conditions listed in Table 12-1 apply. Early use of dialysis or hemoperfusion can also be considered if the serum levels of a drug or poison are found to be increased to values known to be associated with death or serious tissue damage. Critical serum concentrations for several drugs are listed in Table 12-2. The information given in Tables 12-1 and 12-2 represents a set of guidelines only; the decision to institute dialysis or hemoperfusion must be made on an individual basis. In addition to treatment of systemic poisoning, hemoperfusion of blood draining a limb or organ has been used in clinical studies to enhance regional removal of anticancer drugs, such as adriamycin, to limit systemic exposure (Ku et al, 1995).

B. Choice of therapy. Peritoneal dialysis, hemodialysis, and hemoperfusion have all been used in the treatment of poisoning.

1. Peritoneal dialysis is not very effective in removing drugs from the blood, being one-eighth to one-fourth as efficient as hemodialysis. Nevertheless, when hemodialysis is difficult to institute quickly, such as in small children, a prolonged session of peritoneal dialysis can be a valuable adjunctive treatment of poisoning.

**Table 12-1.   Criteria for consideration of dialysis
or hemoperfusion in poisoning**

1. Progressive deterioration despite intensive supportive therapy
2. Severe intoxication with depression of midbrain function leading
    to hypoventilation, hypothermia, and hypotension
3. Development of complications of coma, such as pneumonia
    or septicemia, and underlying conditions predisposing to such
    complications (e.g., obstructive airway disease)
4. Impairment of normal drug excretory function in the presence
    of hepatic, cardiac, or renal insufficiency
5. Intoxication with agents with metabolic and/or delayed effects,
    e.g., methanol, ethylene glycol, and paraquat
6. Intoxication with an extractable drug or poison, which can be
    removed at a rate exceeding endogenous elimination by liver
    or kidney

2.   Hemodialysis is the therapy of choice for water-soluble
drugs, especially those of low molecular weight, which will
diffuse rapidly across the dialyzer membrane. Examples
are salicylates, ethanol, methanol, and lithium. Water-soluble
drugs that have high molecular weights, such as amphotericin B (MW 924) and vancomycin (MW 1,486), diffuse
across dialyzer membranes more slowly but can be removed
using high flux membranes. Hemodialysis is not very useful
in removing lipid-soluble drugs (e.g., glutethimide) with
large volumes of distribution (see Section **C**) or drugs with
extensive protein binding.

**Table 12-2.   Serum concentrations of common
poisons in excess of which hemodialysis
or hemoperfusion should be considered**

Drug	Serum Conc.[a] *mg/L*	Method of Choice
Phenobarbital	100	HP > HD
Glutethimide	30–40	HP
Methaqualone	40	HP
Salicylates	800	HD
Theophylline	40	HP > HD
Paraquat	0.1	HP > HD
Methanol	500	HD
Trichloroethanol	500	HP > HD
Meprobamate	100	HP

[a] Suggested concentrations only; clinical condition may warrant intervention
at lower concentrations (e.g., in mixed intoxications).
HD, hemodialysis; HP, hemoperfusion.

3. Hemoperfusion is a process whereby blood is passed through a cartridge packed with activated charcoal or carbon (Samtleben et al, 1996). Hemoperfusion is more effective than hemodialysis in clearing the blood of many protein-bound drugs because the charcoal in the cartridge will compete with plasma proteins for the drug, adsorb the drug, and remove it from the circulation. Similarly, hemoperfusion will remove many lipid soluble drugs from the blood much more efficiently than hemodialysis.

If a drug is removed from the blood by hemoperfusion and hemodialysis to the same extent, then hemodialysis is preferred as problems of cartridge saturation are avoided and any coexisting acid–base disturbance can be treated concomitantly.

4. Continuous hemodiafiltration and hemoperfusion may be particularly useful in hemodynamically unstable patients who cannot tolerate conventional treatment. Compared with conventional treatment, the rate of drug removal is lower; hence, plasma levels may decrease more slowly and longer treatment times are required. Prolonged continuous treatment is potentially useful in drugs with moderate volumes of distribution (V_D) and slow intercompartmental transfer time to prevent posttherapy rebound of plasma drug levels. Clear advantages of continuous treatment over repeated conventional treatment for drug rebound remains to be demonstrated. Continuous hemoperfusion has been used successfully in meprobamate, theophylline, and phenobarbital toxicity; continuous hemodiafiltration has been used successfully in ethylene glycol and lithium toxicity (Leblanc et al, 1996), and unsuccessfully in paraquat poisoning.

C. Importance of volume of distribution. The volume of distribution is the theoretical volume into which a drug is distributed. For example, heparin, a drug that is confined to the blood compartment, has a V_D of approximately 0.06 L per kg. Drugs distributed primarily in the extracellular water (e.g., cephalothin) will have a V_D of approximately 0.2 L per kg. Some drugs will have V_D exceeding the volume of total-body water (0.6 L per kg) because they are extensively bound to, or stored in, tissue.

With drugs that have a high V_D (e.g., digoxin, glutethimide, tricyclics), the amount of drug present in the blood represents only a small fraction of the total-body load. Thus, even if a hemodialysis or hemoperfusion treatment extracts most of the drug present in blood flowing through the extracorporeal circuit, the amount of drug removed during a single treatment session represents only a small percentage of the total-body drug burden. Subsequently, additional drug can enter the blood from tissue stores, causing a recurrence of toxic manifestations. On the other hand, even transiently lowering the plasma concentration of many drugs may mitigate certain important toxic effects of these agents. Hence, hemodialysis or hemoperfusion can sometimes effectively reduce drug toxicity even when the V_D is large.

D. Technical points

1. Vascular access for hemodialysis or hemoperfusion in poisoning. In patients without permanent vascular access in place, percutaneous cannulation of the large central veins with dialysis catheters is required. Techniques for obtaining vascular access are discussed in Chapter 4.

2. Choice of hemodialyzer. A high-efficiency dialyzer with a high urea clearance should generally be used. Biocompatible membranes may have theoretical advantages in unstable patients. A high-flux dialyzer should be used when the substance to be removed has a molecular weight greater than several hundred daltons.

3. Choice of a hemoperfusion cartridge. Some of the cartridges are listed in Table 12-3. Typical sorbents are activated carbons (charcoals), ion-exchange resins, or nonionic exchange macroporous resins. Sorbent particles have been rendered biocompatible by coating of the surface with a polymer membrane. The cartridges contain various amounts of sorbent, the smaller ones being designed for pediatric use. No controlled comparative evaluation of in vivo performance of the various brands of cartridges has been published.

4. The hemoperfusion circuit. The hemoperfusion circuit is similar to the blood side of a hemodialysis circuit and includes an air detector and a venous air trap. Standard hemodialysis blood pumps and machines (without use of dialysis solution) are often used to drive the blood through the tubing and cartridge.

5. Priming the hemoperfusion circuit. Setup and priming procedures differ depending on the brand of cartridge used, and the manufacturer's literature should be consulted in all instances. The hemoperfusion cartridge must be primed in a vertical position with the arterial side facing down. One manufacturer (Gambro) recommends that its cartridges be rinsed initially with 500 mL of 5% dextrose in water to load the charcoal with glucose. This maneuver is alleged to result in a smaller drop in the serum glucose level during the hemoperfusion treatment. Other manufacturers do not recommend a glucose rinse.

Table 12-3. Some available hemoperfusion devices

Manufacturer	Device	Sorbent Type	Amount of Sorbent	Polymer Coating
Asahi	Hemosorba	Charcoal	170 g	Poly-HEMA
Clark	Biocompatible system	Charcoal	50, 100, 250 mL	Heparinized polymer
Gambro	Adsorba	Charcoal	100 or 300 g	Cellulose acetate
Organon-Teknika	Hemopur 260	Charcoal	260 g	Cellulose acetate
Smith and Nephew	Hemocol or Haemocol	Charcoal	100 or 300 g	Acrylic, hydrogel
Braun	Haemoresin	XAD-4	350 g	None

N.B. Smaller devices are available for use in children.

After the glucose rinse (if one is used), the cartridge is rinsed with 2 L of heparinized (2,500 units per L) 0.9% sodium chloride solution at a flow rate of 50–150 mL per minute. In rinsing Clark cartridges, the manufacturer recommends that the final liter of rinsing fluid be infused at a relatively rapid rate (i.e., about 150% of the anticipated blood flow rate through the device, such as 300 mL per minute if the blood flow rate will be 200 mL per minute).

6. Heparinization during hemoperfusion. Once the cartridge has been primed, a bolus dose of heparin (usually 2,000–3,000 units) is administered into the arterial line, the cartridge is kept inlet side down, and blood flow through the cartridge is begun. As a rule, because of adsorption on the sorbent, more heparin is required for a hemoperfusion treatment (e.g., approximately 6,000 units per session for a charcoal cartridge, or 10,000 units per session for a resin cartridge) than for hemodialysis. Heparin should be given in amounts sufficient to maintain the patient's Lee–White clotting time (see Chapter 9 for description of the various clotting tests) at about 30 minutes, or the activated clotting time or whole-blood partial thromboplastin time at about twice the normal value.

7. Duration of hemoperfusion. Prolonged hemoperfusion (beyond 3 hours) is usually unnecessary. A single 3-hour treatment will substantially lower the blood levels of most poisons for which hemoperfusion is effective. More prolonged use of a hemoperfusion cartridge is inefficient because the charcoal tends to become saturated (especially when cartridges containing less than 150 g charcoal are used). Replacement of saturated devices with fresh devices is not usually required, and any rebound in plasma drug concentrations consequent to tissue release can be treated with a second hemoperfusion session. On the other hand, continuous treatments may be continued for several days until clinical improvement or non-toxic plasma level is achieved. During continuous treatment hemoperfusion devices may need to be changed every 4 hours.

E. Complications
  1. Hemodialysis
   a. Hypophosphatemia. In contrast with uremic patients, patients being dialyzed for poisoning will not usually have an elevated serum phosphate value. Because phosphate is not present in standard dialysis solutions, intensive dialysis can severely lower the serum phosphate level, resulting in respiratory insufficiency and other complications. Hypophosphatemia during dialysis can be avoided by supplementing the dialysis solution with phosphate (Chow et al, 1998; see Chapter 5).
   b. Alkalemia. Standard hemodialysis solutions contain unphysiologically high concentrations of bicarbonate and/or bicarbonate-generating base and are designed to correct metabolic acidosis. Using a standard hemodialysis solution to perform dialysis for poisoning in a patient with metabolic or respiratory alkalosis can provoke or worsen alkalemia unless a low-bicarbonate dialysis solution is used (see Chapter 5).
   c. Disequilibrium syndrome in acutely uremic patients. In patients with both acute uremia and poisoning,

it may be dangerous to carry out a prolonged high-efficiency dialysis session initially. The disequilibrium syndrome is discussed in Chapter 7.

2. Hemoperfusion. Mild transient thrombocytopenia and leukopenia can occur, but levels usually return to normal within 24–48 hours following a single hemoperfusion. Adsorption or activation of coagulation factors has also been observed rarely and may be clinically significant in patients with liver failure.

3. Continuous therapy. Fluid and electrolyte imbalance may be potential problems and require frequent monitoring. Prolonged anticoagulation may predispose to bleeding.

II.   Management of poisoning with selected agents

A.   Acetaminophen. Activated charcoal should be given to those presenting within 4 hours after poison ingestion. Serum levels should be measured and plotted against the Rumack–Matthew nomogram to establish the risk for hepatotoxicity and requirement for N-acetylcysteine (NAC) therapy. The risk of hepatic necrosis can be quite high when acetaminophen ingestion has been combined with ethanol abuse, even at relatively low acetaminophen serum levels. If serum acetaminophen levels are above 150 µg per mL at 4 hours, the likelihood of toxicity is high and NAC (PO or IV) should be given. NAC prevents the accumulation of the toxic byproducts by increasing reduced glutathione stores. Its efficacy in the prevention of liver failure declines if started more than 10 hours after ingestion, though it may still be worth giving even after 24 hours. Despite the fact that acetaminophen is moderately water-soluble, minimally protein-bound, and thus removed by dialysis or hemoperfusion, NAC remains the treatment of choice.

B.   Aspirin. In adults, severe aspirin poisoning is usually accompanied by metabolic acidosis with respiratory alkalosis, whereas in children isolated metabolic acidosis is often encountered. The appearance of central nervous system symptoms is a sign of severe poisoning. The Done nomogram (Done and Temple, 1971), relating serum levels and time of ingestion to outcome, gives some idea of the seriousness of salicylate poisoning in an individual patient. MDAC should be given and alkaline diuresis carried out if substantial urine output is achievable, particularly when symptoms are present and serum salicylate levels are greater than 50 mg per dL. Aspirin has a V_D of only 0.15 L per kg. Despite the fact that the drug is about 50% protein-bound, it is well removed by hemodialysis. Hemodialysis should be considered when the serum level exceeds 80 mg per dL or the condition of the patient warrants aggressive management.

C.   Barbiturates. Toxic serum levels of phenobarbital are greater than 3 mg per dL, and coma begins to appear at levels of 6 mg per dL. MDAC should be considered as first-line therapy and alkalinization of the urine may also be useful in the case of long-acting barbiturates. Phenobarbital is 50% protein-bound, but its V_D is only 0.5 L per kg, and phenobarbital is well removed by either hemodialysis or hemoperfusion. Hemodialysis should be contemplated when coma is prolonged, especially when complications of coma, such as pneumonia, threaten. There is, however, no evidence that hemodialysis will improve overall survival.

D.   Digoxin. The probabilities of digoxin-induced arrhythmias are 50% and 90% at serum levels of 2.5 and 3.3 ng per mL, respectively. Treatment includes correction of hypokalemia, hypomagnesemia, and alkalosis and administration of oral activated charcoal.

The V_D of digoxin is large (8 L per kg in normal patients, 4.2 L per kg in dialysis patients), and the drug is 25% protein-bound. For these reasons, only 5% of the body load will be removed by a 4-hour hemodialysis treatment. Although hemoperfusion is more effective and has been shown to improve symptoms, it is not routinely recommended in the treatment of digoxin toxicity as the V_D of the drug is so large that total-body clearance is limited. Digoxin-specific antibody fragments (Fab fragments) are indicated for massive ingestions, profound intoxication, or hyperkalemia in the presence of life-threatening arrhythmia (Martiny et al, 1988). Although Fab has been used successfully in patients with coexisting renal failure, digoxin may be released from the Fab–digoxin complex, leading to a rebound in toxicity (Ujhelyi et al, 1993). Plasmapheresis done soon after Fab fragment administration promotes removal of the Fab-digoxin complexes (Zdunek et al, 2000). In dialysis patients, a judgment to employ hemoperfusion (made easier by the presence of an arteriovenous access) or digoxin antibody is required.

E.   Toxic alcohols. Poisonings with toxic alcohols should be suspected in patients with unexplained metabolic acidosis accompanied by increases in anion and osmolal gaps. However, a normal osmolal gap does not eliminate the possibility of toxic alcohol ingestion (Jacobsen et al, 1997). Methanol and ethylene glycol are metabolized via alcohol dehydrogenase to produce toxic metabolites (formic acid and glycolic acid, respectively). Ethanol and fomepizole (4-methylpyrazole) have several-fold greater affinities for alcohol dehydrogenase and can be used as antidotes to delay the conversion to toxic metabolites and allow excretion of the parent drug. Hemodialysis may be required as it is effective in removing both toxic alcohols and their metabolites and in correcting metabolic abnormalities.

Early symptoms of toxicity due to ethylene glycol, which is contained in antifreeze, include confusion, convulsions, and coma, followed by signs of myositis and myocarditis. A severe acidosis commonly occurs. Renal failure often supervenes as a result of oxalate precipitation in the kidney, delaying the excretion of the poison. Gastric lavage should be instituted if the patient is seen within 1 hour, and early aggressive management of acidosis with sodium bicarbonate is essential. Indications for the administration of an antidote (ethanol or fomepizole) are shown in Table 12-4. Currently, there are insufficient data to define relative roles of fomepizole and ethanol in the treatment of ethylene glycol poisoning (Barceloux et al, 1999). Fomepizole has advantages over ethanol in terms of validated efficacy, predictable pharmacokinetics, ease of administration, and lack of adverse effects, whereas ethanol has advantages over fomepizole in terms of clinical experience and lower drug costs. Indications for hemodialysis are shown in Table 12-5. Traditionally, an ethylene glycol level above 50 mg per dL is an indication for dialysis. In the absence of both renal dysfunction

Table 12-4. Indications for treatment of ethylene glycol poisoning with an antidote

1. Documented plasma ethylene glycol concentrations > 20 mg/dL

or

2. Documented recent (hours) history of ingesting toxic amounts of ethylene glycol and osmolal gap > 10 mOsm/kg

or

3. History or strong clinical suspicion of ethylene glycol poisoning and at least two of the following criteria:
   A. Arterial pH < 7.3
   B. Serum bicarbonate < 20 mEq/L
   C. Osmolal gap > 10 mOsm/kg[a]
   D. Urinary oxalate crystals present

[a] Laboratory analysis by freezing point depression only.
Reproduced with permission from Barceloux DG, et al. *J Toxicol Clin Toxicol* 1999;37:537.

and metabolic acidosis, the use of fomepizole may obviate the need for dialysis, even in patients with serum ethylene glycol levels greater than 50 mg per dL. However, if patients with plasma levels of ethylene glycol levels greater than 50 mg per dL are not treated with hemodialysis, their acid–base balance should be monitored very closely and hemodialysis initiated promptly if acidosis develops. The dosing schedule for ethanol or fomepizole and the dose adjustments for hemodialysis are shown in Tables 12-6 and 12-7. Hemodialysis should be performed until acidosis has resolved and the ethylene glycol levels are lower than 20 mg per dL. If ethylene glycol levels are unavailable, dialysis should be performed for at least 8 hours. Redistribution of ethylene glycol may result in rebound elevation of ethylene glycol levels within 12 hours after cessation of dialysis, and repeat dialysis may be necessary. Thus, serum osmolality, electrolytes, and acid–base status should be monitored closely within 24 hours after dialysis. Pyridoxine (500 mg IM four times daily) and thiamine (100 mg IM four times daily) may be given to increase the metabolism of glyoxylate. In addition, judicious intravenous

Table 12-5. Indications for hemodialysis in patients with severe ethylene glycol poisoning

1. Severe metabolic acidosis (pH < 7.25–7.3) unresponsive to therapy
2. Renal failure
3. Ethylene glycol levels > 50 mg/dL unless fomepizole is being administered and patient is asymptomatic with a normal pH[a]

[a] Such patients should be monitored very closely and hemodialysis initiated if acidosis develops.
Reproduced with permission from Barceloux DG, et al. *J Toxicol Clin Toxicol* 1999;37:537–560.

Table 12-6.   Guidelines for use of ethanol in toxic alcohol poisonings

1. Loading dose 0.6 g/kg given intravenously (10% ethanol in D5W) or orally (20% ethanol in water).
2. Maintenance dose.
    A. In alcoholic patients 154 mg/kg/hr.
    B. In nonalcoholic patients 66 mg/kg/hr.
    C. During hemodialysis, either double the ethanol infusion rate from A. or B. or enrich dialysate with 100 mg/dL ethanol[a]
    D. Double the ethanol dose when ethanol is given orally with charcoal.
3. Adjust to maintain serum ethanol level of 100–200 mg/dL.

[a] Enrichment can be carried out by infusing 100% ethanol into dialysate or by adding 100% ethanol into either the "acid concentrate" or the "base concentrate" of a dual-concentrate, bicarbonate-based dialysate delivery system (Chow et al, 1997; Wadgymar and Wu, 1998; Noghnogh et al, 1999). Both ethanol (65%) and phosphorus can also be added to an acid concentrate to produce ethanol-enriched (125 mg/dL) and phosphorus-enriched (3 mg/dL) dialysates (Dorval et al, 1999).

fluids should be given to prevent calcium oxalate crystal deposition in the kidneys and acute renal failure. Hypocalcemia, which may be worsened by bicarbonate treatment, should be corrected if symptomatic or severe. It is uncertain if correction of hypocalcemia significantly increases calcium oxalate precipitation in tissues. Hypophosphatemia resulting from intensive dialysis may be corrected using a phosphate-enriched dialysis fluid (Chow et al, 1998).

Acidosis, altered mental status, and retinal involvement are the principal clinical manifestations of methanol toxicity. Initial management is similar to that for ethylene glycol toxicity, including correction of acidosis with sodium bicarbonate. Thereafter, ethanol should be administered as the antidote (Table 12-6). Although fomepizole has been used in a few patients with methanol toxicity, further studies are necessary before it can be recommended routinely for this purpose. Hemodialysis is indicated when (a) methanol levels are greater than 50 mg per dL; (b) visual, funduscopic, or mental status changes are present; (c) severe acidosis is present; (d) serum formic acid levels are

Table 12-7.   Guidelines for use of fomepizole in the treatment of ethylene glycol poisoning

1. Loading dose 15 mg/kg IV in 100 mL 0.9% saline over 30 min–1 hr
2. Maintenance dose: 10 mg/kg every 12 hr for 4 doses, then
3. 15 mg/kg every 12 hr until ethylene glycol concentration < 20 mg/dL and patient is asymptomatic with normal arterial pH
4. Dose adjustments during hemodialysis 15 mg/kg every 4 hr or 1–1.5 mg/kg/hr infusion during dialysis

Modified from Barceloux DG., et al. *J Toxicol Clin Toxicol* 1999;37:537.

elevated; or (e) the patient has consumed an equivalent of more than 30 mL of pure methanol. Hemodialysis should be continued until acidosis is corrected and serum methanol levels are lower than 20 mg per dL or for at least 8 hours if levels cannot be measured. Folic acid (50–70 mg IV every 4 hours for 24 hours) may promote metabolism of formate to carbon dioxide and water.

F.   Lithium carbonate. Most intoxications result from chronic accumulation, renal failure, diuretics and dehydration, interactions with angiotensin-converting enzyme inhibitors and nonsteroidal anti-inflammatory drugs. Mild (serum lithium 1.5–2.5 mEq per L) and moderate (serum lithium 2.5–3.5 mEq per L) lithium toxicity are characterized by neuromuscular irritability, nausea, and diarrhea. Severe toxicity (serum lithium greater than 3.5 mEq per L) can result in seizures, stupor, and permanent neurologic deficit. Initially, diuretics should be stopped and half normal saline should be used to rehydrate the patient. As lithium is 0% protein-bound, with a V_D of 0.8 L per kg, it is removed very well by dialysis. Hemodialysis should be considered when (a) serum lithium is greater than 3.5 mEq per L; (b) serum lithium is greater than 2.5 mEq per L in patients with appreciable symptoms, in patients with renal insufficiency, or in asymptomatic patients when levels are expected to rise (e.g., following recent massive ingestion) or when levels are not falling as rapidly as expected. As serum lithium may rebound following dialysis due to shift from the intracellular compartment, dialysis should be performed using a high-clearance dialyzer for 8–12 hours. Repeated dialysis may be necessary until the serum lithium level remains below 1.0 mEq per L 6–8 hours after dialysis. Prolonged continuous hemodiafiltration may reduce the rebound of lithium levels post treatment (Leblanc et al, 1995). Dialysate can be enriched with phosphorus if one anticipates the development of hypophosphatemia as a result of aggressive dialysis. However, further studies are needed to confirm the utility of this method.

G.   Mushroom poisoning. Ingestion of large numbers of poisonous mushrooms is associated initially with severe gastrointestinal symptoms followed by hepatic insufficiency and cardiovascular collapse. The toxins of these mushrooms (α-amanitin and phalloidin) are removed by hemodialysis and hemoperfusion in vitro, but the efficacy of hemodialysis or hemoperfusion in patients poisoned by mushrooms has been difficult to interpret because of lack of controls; some survival benefit has been alleged.

H.   Paraquat and diquat. Delayed toxicity with pulmonary fibrosis, renal and multiorgan failure can occur following ingestions of more than 10 mL of paraquat concentrate. Survival is dependent on amount ingested and plasma levels with respect to time of ingestion (Proudfoot et al, 1979). A plasma level above 3 mg per L regardless of time ingested is usually fatal. Initial management includes gastric lavage with administration of activated charcoal or Fuller's Earth with cathartic. Hemoperfusion is effective in drug removal and should be considered when the serum paraquat level is 0.1 mg per L or above. Repeated or continuous hemoperfusion may be needed for several days to maintain the serum level below 0.1 mg per L as paraquat has a large V_D and slow intercompartmental transfer rate. Although the evidence that hemoperfusion improves survival is controversial, hemoperfusion should be considered as occasional patients have recovered despite massive ingestions and pulmonary involvement.

I.   Phenothiazines and tricyclic antidepressants. These agents are highly protein-bound and have extremely large volumes of distribution (in the range of 14 to 21 L per kg). Hence, the total amount of these drugs removed by either hemodialysis or hemoperfusion is small. However, hemoperfusion can be useful in temporarily lowering the plasma drug level and reducing acute toxicity. Treatment of intoxication with these agents is largely supportive, including correction of acidosis with bicarbonate.

J.   Anticonvulsants

1.   Phenytoin. Nystagmus and ataxia occur at serum values greater than 20 and 30 mg per L, respectively. Phenytoin is 90% protein-bound (70% in uremic patients) and has a V_D of 0.64 L per kg. Phenytoin is removed poorly by hemodialysis but moderately well by hemoperfusion.

2.   Sodium valproate. Valproate sodium has a small V_D, is metabolized by the liver, and has significant protein-binding. In overdose, protein-binding becomes saturated and free valproate can be subjected to extracorporeal removal. High-flux hemodialysis with or without hemoperfusion should be considered when there is coma, severe liver dysfunction or other organ failure.

K.   Sedatives and hypnotics

1.   Chlordiazepoxide, diazepam, clonazepam, flurazepam. Treatment is largely supportive as the high degree of protein-binding and the high V_D of these drugs limits their removal by extracorporeal therapy. Flumazenil, a benzodiazepine antidote, can be used in severe benzodiazepine poisoning but might unmask seizures.

2.   Meprobamate and chloral hydrate. These sedatives are lipid-soluble, moderately protein-bound, and have V_D values of 0.7 and 1.6 L per kg, respectively. Hemoperfusion is indicated for patients who have been severely poisoned with these agents and who have not responded to standard intensive care.

3.   Glutethimide, methaqualone, methyprylon, ethchlorvynol. These sedatives are highly lipid-soluble and have a large V_D. They are poorly removed by hemodialysis and moderately well removed by hemoperfusion. After a hemoperfusion session, a rebound in plasma drug levels may occur, and this may be sufficient to put the patient back into coma, necessitating a second or even a third hemoperfusion session. Continuous hemoperfusion may be useful to prevent rebound, although more studies are needed.

L.   Theophylline. Toxic reactions occur when theophylline levels become greater than 25 mg per L (therapeutic dose is 10–20 mg per L). Chronic intoxication may have more pronounced symptoms. Seizures may occur with levels greater than 40 mg per L but may occur at levels as low as 25 mg per L. Cardiovascular collapse is rare until levels are greater than 50 mg per L. Theophylline has a V_D of 0.5 L per kg, poor intrinsic metabolism with 56% protein-binding, and is well adsorbed by charcoal, enabling its effective removal by MDAC and hemoperfusion. MDAC should be used in significant poisonings even if the overdosing is via the intravenous route. Propranolol (1–3 mg IV) may be used in tachyarrhythmia, and hypokalemia should be corrected. Hemoperfusion or high-efficiency hemodialysis is indicated if vomiting prevents the use of MDAC; either modality can be used in addition to MDAC in unstable patients with seizures, hypotension, or unstable arrhythmia. Hemoperfusion or hemodialysis should also be considered in patients with acute intoxication with levels above 100 mg per L (550 μmol per L), with chronic toxicity with levels above 60 mg per L (330 μmol per L) or above 40 mg per L (220 μmol per L) in the elderly or infants. Combining hemodialysis with hemoperfusion may further enhance clearance and prevent saturation of the hemoperfusion cartridge. Continuous hemoperfusion has also been used with success in severely toxic and hypotensive patients, but prolonged treatment is needed. Treatment should be continued until the plasma level is 25–40 mg per L.

M. Other drugs. Management of poisoning due to other agents is beyond the scope of this book. The reader is referred to Haddad et al (1998) and Tables 12-8 and 12-9.

Table 12-8. Drugs removed with hemodialysis

ANTIMICROBIALS/ ANTICANCER		
cefaclor	fosfomycin	(clarithromycin)
cefadroxil	gentamicin	metronidazole
cefamandole	kanamycin	nitrofurantoin
cefazolin	neomycin	ornidazole
cefixime	netilmicin	
cefmenoxime	sisomicin	sulfisoxazole
cefmetazole	streptomycin	sulfonamides
cefotiam	tobramycin	tetracycline
cefoxitin	bacitracin	(doxycycline)
cefpirome	colistin	(minocycline)
cefroxadine		
cefsulodin	amoxicillin	tinidazole
ceftazidime	ampicillin	trimethoprim
(ceftriaxone)[a]	azlocillin	aztreonam
cefuroxime	carbenicillin	cilastatin
cephacetrile	clavulinic acid	imipenem
cephalexin	(cloxacillin)	(chloramphenicol)
(cefonicid)	(dicloxacillin)	(amphotericin)
ceforanide	(floxacillin)	
(cefotaxime)	mecillinam	ciprofloxacin
cefotetan	(mezlocillin)	(enoxacin)
(cefoperazone)	(methicillin)	fleroxacin
cephalothin	(nafcillin)	(norfloxacin)
(cephapirin)	penicillin	ofloxacin
cephradine	piperacillin	
moxalactam	temocillin	isoniazid
	ticarcillin	(vancomycin)
amikacin		capreomycin
dibekacin	(clindamycin)	PAS
	(erythromycin)	pyrizinamide
	(azithromycin)	(rifampin)

Table 12-8. *Continued*

(cycloserine)
ethambutol

5-fluorocytosine
acyclovir
(amantadine)
didanosine
foscarnet
ganciclovir
(ribavirin)
vidarabine
zidovudine

(pentamidine)
(praziquantel)

(fluconazole)
(itraconazole)
(ketoconazole)
(miconazole)

(chloroquine)
(quinine)
(azathioprine)
bredinin
cyclophosphamide
5-fluorouracil
(methotrexate)

BARBITURATES
amobarbital
aprobarbital
barbital
butabarbital
cyclobarbital
pentobarbital
phenobarbital
quinalbital
(secobarbital)

**HYPNOTICS,
SEDATIVES,
TRANQUILIZERS,
ANTICONVUL-
SANTS**
carbamazepine
carbromal
chloral hydrate
(chlordiazepoxide)
(diazepam)
(diphenylhydantoin)
(diphenylhydramin)
ethiamate

ethchlorvynol
ethosuximide
gallamine
glutethimide
(heroin)
meprobamate
(methaqualone)
methsuximide
methyprylon
paraldehyde
primidone
valproic acid

**CARDIOVASCULAR
AGENTS**
acebutolol
(amiodarone)
atenolol
betaxolol
(bretylium)
(calcium channel
   blockers)
captopril
(diazoxide)
(digoxin)
enalapril
fosinopril
lisonopril
quinapril
ramipril
(encainide)
(flecainide)

(lidocaine)
metoprolol
methyldopa
(ouabain)
N-acetylprocainamide
nadolol
(pindolol)
practolol
procainamide
propranolol
(quinidine)
(timolol)
sotatol
tocainide

ALCOHOLS
ethanol
ethylene glycol
isopropanol
methanol

**ANALGESICS,
ANTIRHEUMATICS**
acetaminophen
acetophenetidin
acetylsalicylic acid
colchicine
methylsalicylate
(d-propoxyphene)
salicylic acid

ANTIDEPRESSANTS
(amitriptyline)
amphetamines
(imipramine)
isocarboxazid
MAO inhibitors
(pargylline)
(phenelzine)
tranylcypromine
(tricyclics)

SOLVENTS, GASES
acetone
camphor
carbon monoxide
(carbon tetrachloride)
(eucalyptus oil)
thiols
toluene
trichloroethyl

**PLANTS, ANIMALS,
HERBICIDES,
INSECTICIDES**
alkyl phosphate
amanitin
demeton sulfoxide
dimethoate
diquat
methylmercury
complex
(organophosphates)
paraquat
snake bite
sodium chlorate
potassium chlorate

MISCELLANEOUS
acipimox
allopurinol
aminophylline
aniline
borates

continued

Table 12-8. *Continued*

boric acid	folic acid	theophylline
(chlorpropamide)	mannitol	thiocyanate
chromic acid	methylprednisolone	ranitidine
(cimetidine)	potassium dichromate	
dinitro-*o*-cresol	sodium citrate	

PAS, para-amino salicylic acid.
a Drugs in parentheses are not well removed.
Reprinted with permission from Winchester JF. Active methods for detoxification. In: Haddad LM et al, eds. *Clinical management of poisoning and drug overdose*, 3rd ed. Philadelphia: WB Saunders, 1998.

Table 12-9.   Drugs and chemicals removed with hemoperfusion

Barbiturates
amobarbital
butabarbital
hexabarbital
pentobarbital
phenobarbital
quinalbital
secobarbital
thiopental
vinalbital

Nonbarbiturate hypnotics, sedative, and tranquilizers
carbromal
chloral hydrate
chlorpromazine
(diazepam)
diphenhydramine
ethchlorvynol
glutethimide
meprobamate
methaqualone
methsuximide
methyprylon
promazine
promethazine
(valproic acid)

Analgesics, antirheumatic
acetaminophen
acetylsalicylic acid
colchicine
d-propoxyphyene

methylsalicylate
phenylbutazone
salicylic acid

Antimicrobials/ anticancer
(adriamycin)
ampicillin
carmustine
chloramphenicol
chloroquine
clindamycin
dapsone
doxorubicin
gentamicin
isoniazid
(methotrexate)
thiabendazole
(5-fluorouracil)

Antidepressants
(amitryptiline)
(imipramine)
(tricyclics)

Plant and animal toxins, herbicides, insecticides
amanitin
chlordane
demeton sulfoxide
dimethoate
diquat
methylparathion

nitrostigmine
(organophosphates)
phalloidin
polychlorinated
biphenyls
paraquat
parathion

Cardiovascular
digoxin
diltiazem
(disopyramide)
flecainide
metoprolol
n-acetylprocainamide
procainamide
quinidine

Miscellaneous
aminophylline
cimetidine
(fluoroacetamide)
(phencyclidine)
phenols
(podophyllin)
theophylline

Solvents, gases
carbon tetrachloride
ethylene oxide
trichloroethane
xylene

Metals
(aluminum)[*]
(iron)[*]

() Not well removed; ()* removed by chelation.
Reprinted with permission from Winchester JF. Active methods for detoxification. In Haddad LM *Clinical management of poisoning and drug overdose*, 3rd ed. Philadelphia: WB Saunders, 1998.

SELECTED READINGS

Barceloux DG, et al. American Academy of Clinical Toxicology practice guidelines on the treatment of ethylene glycol poisoning. Ad Hoc Committee. *J Toxicol Clin Toxicol* 1999;37:537–560.

Chow MT, et al. Hemodialysis-induced hypophosphatemia in a normophosphatemic patient dialyzed for ethylene glycol poisoning: treatment with phosphorus-enriched hemodialysis. *Artif Organs* 1998;22:905–907.

Chow MT, et al. Treatment of acute methanol intoxication with hemodialysis using an ethanol-enriched, bicarbonate-based dialysate. *Am J Kidney Dis* 1997;30:568–570.

Chyka PA. Multiple-dose activated charcoal and enhancement of systemic drug clearance: summary of studies in animals and human volunteers. *J Toxicol Clin Toxicol* 1995;33:399–405.

Done AK, Temple AR. Treatment of salicylate poisoning. *Mod Treat* 1971;8:528–551.

Dorval M, et al. The use of an ethanol- and phosphate-enriched dialysate to maintain stable serum ethanol levels during haemodialysis for methanol intoxication. *Nephrol Dial Transplant* 1999;14: 1774–1775.

Gurland H, et al. Extracorporeal blood purification techniques: plasmapheresis and hemoperfusion. In: Jacobs C, et al, eds. *Replacement of renal function by dialysis*, 4th ed. Dordrecht: Kluwer Academic, 1996:472.

Haddad LM, et al, eds. *Clinical management of poisoning and drug overdose*, 3rd ed. Philadelphia: WB Saunders, 1998.

Jacobsen D, McMartin KE. Antidotes for methanol and ethylene glycol poisoning. *J Toxicol Clin Toxicol* 1997;35:127–143.

Ku Y, et al. Clinical pilot study on high-dose intraarterial chemotherapy with direct hemoperfusion under hepatic venous isolation in patients with advanced hepatocellular carcinoma. *Surgery* 1995;117:510–519.

Kulig K. Initial management of ingestions of toxic substances. *N Engl J Med* 1992;326:1677–1681.

Leblanc M, et al. Lithium poisoning treated by high-performance arteriovenous and venovenous hemodiafiltration. *Am J Kidney Dis* 1996;27:365–372.

Litovitz TL, et al. 1998 annual report of the American Association of Poison Control Centers toxic exposure surveillance system. *Am J Emerg Med* 1999;17:435–487.

Martiny SS, et al. Treatment of severe digitalis intoxication with digoxin-specific antibody fragments: a clinical review. *Crit Care Med* 1988;16:629–635.

Noghnogh AA, et al. Preparation of ethanol-enriched, bicarbonate-based hemodialysates. *Artif Organs* 1999;23:208–209.

Proudfoot AT, et al. Paraquat poisoning: significance of plasma paraquat concentrations. *Lancet* 1979;2:330–332.

Samtleben W, et al. Plasma therapy at Klinikum Grosshadern: a 15-year retrospective. *Artif Organs* 1996;20:408–413.

Ujhelyi MR, et al. Disposition of digoxin immune Fab in patients with kidney failure. *Clin Pharmacol Ther* 1993;54:388–394.

Wadgymar A, Wu GG. Treatment of acute methanol intoxication with hemodialysis. *Am J Kidney Dis* 1998;31:897.

Yip L, et al. Concepts and controversies in salicylate toxicity. *Emerg Med Clin North Am* 1994;12:351–364.

Zdunek M, et al. Plasma exchange for the removal of digoxin-specific antibody fragments in renal failure: timing is important for maximizing clearance. *Am J Kidney Dis* 2000;36:177–183.

III

Peritoneal Dialysis

Section Three

Physiology of Peritoneal Dialysis

Peter G. Blake and John T. Daugirdas

Peritoneal dialysis is the method of renal replacement therapy used by approximately 100,000 patients worldwide. In particular, since the introduction of continuous ambulatory peritoneal dialysis (CAPD) approximately two decades ago, its popularity has increased greatly, mainly because of its simplicity, convenience, and relatively low cost. Before describing the clinical application of peritoneal dialysis and its potential complications, it is important to have an understanding of the underlying anatomy and physiology on which peritoneal dialysis is based.

I.   What is peritoneal dialysis? In essence, peritoneal dialysis involves the transport of solutes and water across a "membrane" that separates two fluid-containing compartments. These two compartments are (a) the blood in the peritoneal capillaries, which in renal failure contains an excess of urea, creatinine, potassium, and so forth, and (b) the dialysis solution in the peritoneal cavity, which typically contains sodium, chloride, and lactate and is rendered hyperosmolar by the inclusion of a high concentration of glucose. The peritoneal membrane that acts as a "dialyzer" is actually a heteroporous, heterogeneous, semipermeable membrane with a relatively complex anatomy and physiology.

As is explained in detail in Chapter 14, chronic peritoneal dialysis is divided into CAPD and automated peritoneal dialysis (APD). CAPD typically involves four 2.0- to 2.5-L dwells daily, with each lasting 4–8 hours. In APD, anything from 3 to 10 dwells is delivered nightly using an automated cycler. In the daytime, the patient usually carries a dwell, which is drained each night before cycling recommences; this is called continuous cycling peritoneal dialysis (CCPD). Alternatively, the patient is left "dry" during the day, and this is termed nocturnal intermittent peritoneal dialysis (NIPD). Hybrid prescriptions between CAPD and APD, in which APD patients have daytime exchanges or CAPD patients have an extra automated exchange at night, are increasingly being used to augment clearance or fluid removal.

During the course of a peritoneal dialysis dwell, three transport processes occur simultaneously:

A.   Diffusion. Uremic solutes and potassium diffuse from the peritoneal capillary blood down the concentration gradient into the peritoneal dialysis solution, whereas glucose, lactate, and, to a lesser extent, calcium diffuse in the opposite direction.

B.   Ultrafiltration. Simultaneously, the relative hyperosmolarity of the peritoneal dialysis solution leads to ultrafiltration of water and associated solutes across the membrane.

C.   Absorption. Also simultaneously, there is constant absorption of water and solute from the peritoneal cavity both directly and indirectly into the lymphatic system.

In this chapter, the anatomy of the peritoneal membrane will be considered, as will the physiology of these three transport processes and the net fluid removal and clearances that result from their action.

II. Anatomy

A. Basic anatomy. The peritoneum is the serosal membrane that lines the peritoneal cavity (Fig. 13-1). It has a surface area that is thought to be approximately equal to body surface area and so typically ranges from 1 to 2 m^2 in an adult. It is divided into two portions:

1. The visceral peritoneum, which lines the gut and other viscera, and
2. The parietal peritoneum, which lines the walls of the abdominal cavity.

The visceral peritoneum accounts for about 80% of the total peritoneal surface area and receives its blood supply from the superior mesenteric artery, whereas its venous drainage is via the portal system. In contrast, the parietal peritoneum, which may be more important in peritoneal dialysis, receives blood

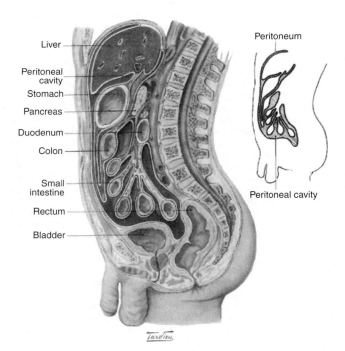

Liver

Peritoneal cavity

Stomach

Pancreas

Duodenum

Colon

Small intestine

Rectum

Bladder

Peritoneum

Peritoneal cavity

Tardieu

Figure 13-1. Simplified anatomy of the peritoneal cavity showing the visceral and parietal peritoneal membrane. (Adapted from Khanna R, et al, eds. *The essentials of peritoneal dialysis.* **Dordrecht: Kluwer, 1993.)**

from the lumbar, intercostal, and epigastric arteries and drains into the inferior vena cava. Total peritoneal blood flow cannot be directly measured but has been indirectly estimated at between 50 and 100 mL per minute. The main lymphatic drainage of the peritoneum and of the peritoneal cavity is via stomata in the diaphragmatic peritoneum, which ultimately drain via large collecting ducts into the right lymphatic duct. There is, however, additional drainage via lymphatics in both the visceral and parietal peritoneum.

The peritoneal membrane is lined by a monolayer of mesothelial cells that have microvillae and that produce a thin film of lubricating fluid. Under the mesothelium is the interstitium, which comprises a gel-like matrix containing collagenous and other fibers, and also the peritoneal capillaries and some lymphatics. The interstitium has been described as a two-phase system in which a colloid-rich, water-poor phase and a water-rich, colloid-poor phase are interspersed.

B.   The peritoneal membrane as a "dialyzer." The peritoneal membrane as a dialyzer can be thought of as comprising six resistances in series. These are:

1. The stagnant capillary fluid film overlying the endothelium of the peritoneal capillaries
2. The capillary endothelium itself
3. The endothelial basement membrane
4. The interstitium
5. The mesothelium
6. The stagnant fluid film that overlies the peritoneal membrane

Newer concepts, such as the three-pore model for peritoneal transport, have been developed in recent years and suggest that the major resistance to peritoneal transport is located in the peritoneal capillary endothelium and its basement membrane. There is also evidence that the interstitium, especially in its colloid-rich phase, offers significant resistance to solute transport. It is now thought that neither the mesothelium nor the stagnant fluid films offer significant resistance to transport.

C.   The three-pore model. This model, which has been well validated by clinical observations, suggests that the peritoneal capillary is the critical barrier to peritoneal transport and that solute and water transport across it is mediated by pores of three different sizes (Fig. 13-2). These are:

1. Large pores with a radius of 20–40 nm. Macromolecules, such as protein, are transported by convection through these pores, which likely are large clefts in the endothelium.
2. Small pores with a radius of 4.0–6.0 nm. There are large number of these which also likely correspond to interendothelial clefts; they are responsible for the transport of small solutes, such as urea, creatinine, sodium, and potassium.
3. Ultrapores with a radius of <0.8 nm. These are responsible for the transport of water only and are thought to correspond to aquaporins, which are known to be present in the peritoneal membrane; these ultrapores, or aquaporins, account for "sieving" by the peritoneal membrane (see below).

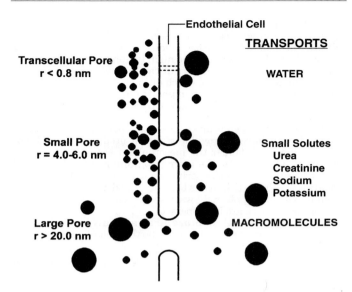

Figure 13-2.   Diagrammatic representation of the three-pore model of peritoneal transport. (Adapted from Flessner MF. *J Am Soc Nephrol* **1991;2:122.)**

D.   Effective peritoneal surface area. Given the central role of the peritoneal capillaries in peritoneal transport, it should not be surprising that transport is dependent on the surface area of the peritoneal capillaries rather than on the total peritoneal surface area. Furthermore, not all peritoneal capillaries are close enough to the mesothelium to be involved. The distance of each from the mesothelium determines its relative contribution and the cumulative contribution of all of the above capillaries determines the effective surface area and the resistance properties of the membrane. Thus, the concept of "effective peritoneal surface area" has arisen. This corresponds to the area of the peritoneal surface that is sufficiently close to peritoneal capillaries to play a role in transport. Therefore, two patients with the same peritoneal surface area may have markedly different peritoneal vascularity and so also have very different effective peritoneal surface areas. In a given patient, effective peritoneal surface area may vary in different circumstances, increasing, for example, in peritonitis when inflammation increases vascularity. The degree of vascularity of the peritoneum is thus more important than its surface area in determining the transport characteristics of an individual patient.

This concept of the importance of the distribution of capillaries in the peritoneal membrane and of the distance water and solutes have to travel from the capillaries across the interstitium to the mesothelium is termed the "distributed model" of peritoneal transport and represents a shift away from viewing the membrane as a discrete "dialyzer" of uniform thickness (Fig. 13-3).

III. Physiology of peritoneal transport. As mentioned above, peritoneal transport comprises three processes that take place simultaneously. These are (a) diffusion, (b) ultrafiltration, and (c) fluid absorption. For simplicity, these will be considered separately.

A. Diffusion. This process is critical for removal of uremic solutes in peritoneal dialysis. Diffusion typically occurs down the concentration gradient from peritoneal capillary blood to dialysis solution. Peritoneal diffusion depends on the following factors:

1. The concentration gradient. For a substance such as urea, this is maximal at the start of a peritoneal dialysis dwell, when the concentration in the dialysis solution is zero. It gradually decreases during the course of the dwell. This effect can be counteracted by the performance of more frequent exchanges, as is typically done in APD, or by increasing dwell volumes, which allows the gradient to remain greater for a longer time.

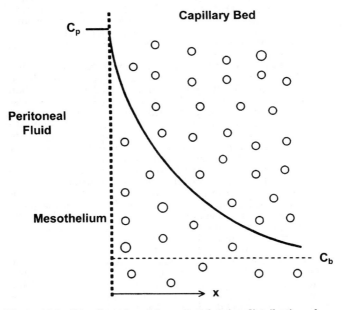

Figure 13-3. **Distributed model concept showing distribution of peritoneal capillaries in the interstitium and their distances from the mesothelium, represented by the dotted, vertical line. Cp, the solid, curved line, represents the efficiency of transport from a given capillary to the peritoneal space, increasing for capillaries located closest to the mesothelial boundary.** (Adapted from Flessner MF. *J Am Soc Nephrol* 1991;2:122.)

2.   Effective peritoneal surface area. As already stated, this depends not only on the total peritoneal surface area but also on the degree of vascularity, which may vary between patients and within a given patient under different conditions (e.g., peritonitis). It can also be increased by using larger fill volumes, which recruit more peritoneal membrane, but this effect is limited in most individuals once volumes reach 2.5–3 L.

3.   Intrinsic peritoneal membrane resistance. This parameter is not well characterized but may reflect differences in the number of pores per unit surface area of capillary available for peritoneal transport and the distance across the interstitium of these capillaries from the mesothelium.

4.   Molecular weight of the solute concerned. Substances with lower molecular weight, such as urea (MW 60), are more easily transported than those with higher molecular weights, such as creatinine (MW 113) or albumin (MW 69,000).

    a.   Mass transfer area coefficient. The combined effects of factors 2–4 are sometimes measured by an index called the mass transfer area coefficient (MTAC). For a given solute, the MTAC is equivalent to the diffusive clearance of that solute per unit time in a given patient if dialysate flow is infinitely high, so that the gradient is always maximal if ultrafiltration has not occurred. Typical MTAC values for urea and creatinine are 17 and 10 mL per minute, respectively. The MTAC is mainly a research tool and is generally not used in clinical practice.

    b.   Peritoneal blood flow. It is important to note that diffusion does not generally depend on peritoneal blood flow because 50–100 mL per minute is already more than adequate relative to MTAC values for even the smallest solutes. Thus, in contrast to the situation in hemodialysis, diffusion in peritoneal dialysis is dependent on dialysate rather than blood flow. The ability of vasoactive agents to influence peritoneal transport is not related to their ability to increase peritoneal blood flow per se but rather to the associated recruitment of larger numbers of peritoneal capillaries that increase effective peritoneal surface area. The same effect is seen in peritonitis where inflammation increases peritoneal vascularity, and there is a consequent increase in peritoneal diffusion. It should be noted that the proportion of peritoneal blood flow involved in peritoneal dialysis is unknown, and it is possible that in some areas of the peritoneum blood flow may limit diffusion.

B.   Ultrafiltration. This occurs as a consequence of the osmotic gradient between the relatively hypertonic dialysis solution and the relatively hypotonic peritoneal capillary blood. It is usually due to the presence of high concentrations of glucose in dialysate and depends on the following:

1.   Concentration gradient for the osmotic agent (i.e., glucose). Again, this is typically maximal at the beginning of a peritoneal dialysis dwell and decreases with time due to dilution of the glucose by ultrafiltrate and due to diffusion of the glucose itself from the dialysis solution into the blood (Fig. 13-4). The gradient is also less in the presence of marked hyperglycemia. The gradient can be maximized by

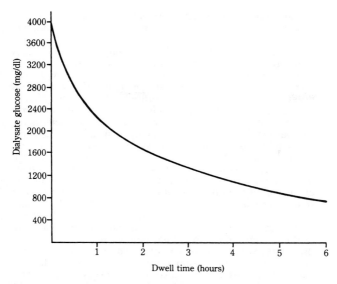

Figure 13-4.   Dialysate glucose level after instillation of a 4.25% dextrose (3.86% glucose) exchange into the peritoneal cavity. The initial level is close to 3,860 mg per dL.

using more hypertonic solutions of dextrose or by doing more frequent exchanges, as is done with APD.

   2.   Effective peritoneal surface area (as described above).

   3.   Hydraulic conductance of the peritoneal membrane. This differs from patient to patient and perhaps reflects the density of small pores and ultrapores in the peritoneal capillaries, as well as the distribution of distances of capillaries from the mesothelium.

   4.   Reflection coefficient for the osmotic agent (i.e., glucose). This measures how effectively the osmotic agent diffuses out of the dialysis solution into the peritoneal capillaries. It is between 0 and 1; the lower the value, the faster the osmotic gradient is lost and the less sustained ultrafiltration is. For glucose, this coefficient is typically low (approximately 0.03). Newer polyglucose preparations have values close to 1.

   5.   Hydrostatic pressure gradient. Normally, the capillary pressure (around 20 mm Hg) is higher than the intraperitoneal pressure (around 7 mm Hg), which should favor ultrafiltration. This effect is greater in an overhydrated and lower in a dehydrated patient. Rises in intraperitoneal pressure tend to oppose ultrafiltration, and this may occur when larger dwell volumes are used. This picture is complicated by the fact that interstitial pressure is less than both capillary and intraperitoneal pressures; therefore, hydrostatic pressure gradients alone do not explain ultrafiltration.

6. Oncotic pressure gradient. This tends to oppose ultrafiltration but operates to a lesser degree in a hypoalbuminemic patient.

a. Sieving. As is the case in hemodialysis, ultrafiltration in peritoneal dialysis involves not just water transport but also convective solute transport. However, during ultrafiltration, in contrast to the situation in hemodialysis, solute does not move across the membrane in direct proportion to its concentration in blood. This is because "sieving" of solute occurs at the peritoneal membrane. Sieving coefficients for the various solutes differ with molecular weight, charge, and so forth, as well as between patients. Values vary between 0 and 1, and the higher the sieving coefficient, the greater the convective transport for that solute. This sieving effect is accounted for by the ultrapores, which are responsible for about half of total ultrafiltration and which transport only solute-free water. Sieving makes ultrafiltration a less effective form of convective solute transport. However, without sieving, glucose-induced ultrafiltration itself could not occur as the membrane would not be "semipermeable."

b. Alternative osmotic agents. For many years, efforts have been made to develop alternative osmotic agents that may induce more effective ultrafiltration than glucose. The ideal osmotic agent would be safe, inexpensive, and would have a high reflection coefficient (i.e., would not diffuse out of the peritoneal cavity into the blood to dissipate the osmotic gradient). The recent development of a polyglucose molecule called "icodextrin" is of some promise in this regard. Icodextrin is a large molecule with a high reflection coefficient, and so ultrafiltration is sustained at a relatively steady level throughout even a long-duration dwell.

C. Fluid absorption. This occurs via the lymphatics at a relatively constant rate and with little or no sieving, so that its net effect is to counteract both solute and fluid removal. It has been increasingly recognized that only a small proportion of this absorption occurs directly into the lymphatics. The majority is absorbed across the parietal peritoneum into the tissues of the abdominal wall, from where it is subsequently taken up by the lymphatics and perhaps even by peritoneal capillaries. Typical values for peritoneal fluid absorption are 1.0–2.0 mL per minute, of which 0.2–0.4 mL per minute go directly into the lymphatics. The determinants of this process are:

1. Intraperitoneal hydrostatic pressure. The higher this is, the greater the amount of fluid that is absorbed; intraperitoneal hydrostatic pressure is raised by increasing intraperitoneal volume as a result of more effective ultrafiltration or the use of larger infusion volumes. It is also higher when patients are sitting than when they are standing, and it is lower when they are supine (Fig. 13-5).

2. Effectiveness of lymphatics. The effectiveness of lymphatics absorbing fluid from the peritoneal cavity may differ markedly from person to person, but this is not well understood.

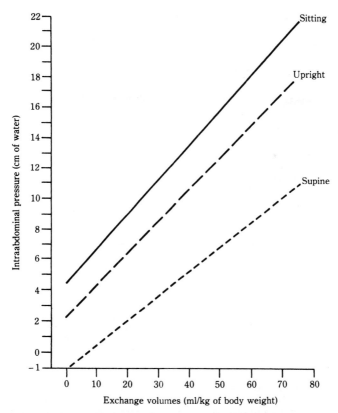

Figure 13-5. **Intra-abdominal pressure after infusing various volumes of dialysis solution. (Modified from Diaz-Buxo JA. Continuous cycling peritoneal dialysis. In Nolph KD, ed. *Peritoneal dialysis*. Hingham: Martinus Nijhoff, 1985.)**

IV. Clinical assessment and implications of peritoneal transport

A. **Peritoneal equilibration test (PET).** In clinical practice, indices such as the MTAC and hydraulic conductance of the peritoneal membrane are too complex for routine measurement and peritoneal transport is assessed using equilibration ratios between dialysate and plasma for urea (D/P urea), creatinine (D/P Cr), sodium (D/P Na), and so forth (Fig. 13-6). Equilibration ratios measure the combined effect of diffusion and ultrafiltration rather than either in isolation. However, they correlate well with MTAC values for the corresponding solutes, suggesting diffusion as their primary determinant. They thus are greatly influenced by the molecular weight of the solute

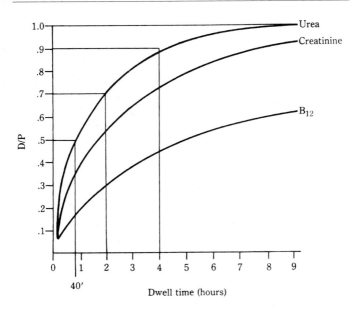

Figure 13-6. **Rate of entry of urea, creatinine, and vitamin B_{12} into peritoneal dialysis solution that has been left in the abdomen. Results are expressed as the ratio of the level in dialysate (D) to the level in plasma (P). Typical D/P ratios for urea at time points of 40 minutes, 2 hours, and 4 hours are indicated.**

concerned as well as by the membrane permeability and effective surface area. Interestingly, body size tends to have little relation to equilibration ratios despite its supposed equivalence to peritoneal surface area, presumably indicating that actual and effective peritoneal surface areas correlate poorly.

Conventionally, equilibration ratios are measured in a standardized PET that involves a 2-L 2.5% dextrose dwell with dialysate samples taken at 0, 2, and 4 hours and a plasma sample at 2 hours. A PET is also used to measure net fluid removal and the ratio of dialysate glucose at 4 hours to dialysate glucose at time zero (D/D_0 G). Patients are classified principally on the basis of their 4-hour D/P Cr into one of four categories: high, high-average, low-average, and low transporters (Fig. 13-7). The protocol for performing a PET and its use in the evaluation of ultrafiltration failure is further discussed in Chapter 18, whereas its role in peritoneal dialysis prescription is described in Chapter 17.

1. **High transporters** achieve the most rapid and complete equilibration for creatinine and urea, presumably because they have a relatively large effective peritoneal surface area or high intrinsic membrane permeability (i.e., low membrane resistance). However, high transporters rapidly lose their osmotic gradient for ultrafiltration because the dialysate glucose dif-

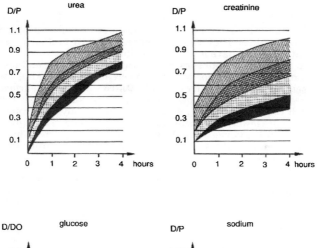

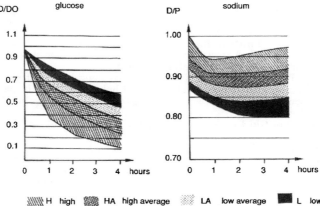

Figure 13-7. Standard peritoneal equilibration curves for urea, creatinine, and sodium, as well as glucose absorption showing ranges of values for high, high-average, low-average, and low transporters. (Modified from Twardowski et al. Peritoneal equilibration test. *Perit Dial Bull* 1987;7:138.)

fuses into the blood through the highly "permeable" membrane. Thus, high transporters have the highest D/P Cr, D/P Ur, and D/P Na values but have low net ultrafiltration and D/D_0 G values. They also have higher dialysate protein losses and so tend to have lower serum albumin values.

2.   Low transporters, in contrast, have slower and less complete equilibration for urea and creatinine, reflecting low membrane permeability or small effective peritoneal surface area. They thus have low D/P Ur, D/P Cr, and D/P Na and high D/D_0 G with good net ultrafiltration. Dialysate protein losses are lower, and serum albumin values tend to be higher.

3.   High-average and low-average transporters have intermediate values for these ratios and for ultrafiltration and protein losses.

In practice, high transporters tend to dialyze relatively well but to ultrafiltrate poorly, whereas low transporters ultrafiltrate well but dialyze poorly, although these issues are often masked while residual renal function is still substantial. Thus, high transporters tend to do best on peritoneal dialysis regimens that involve frequent short-duration dwells (e.g., APD), so that ultrafiltration is maximized. Low transporters, in contrast, tend to do best on regimens based on long-duration, high-volume dwells, so that diffusion is maximized. Average transporters can do well on any of a variety of peritoneal dialysis regimens.

Therefore, the PET is useful because it guides prescription of peritoneal dialysis and because it helps to predict the particular complications that a given patient will be prone to develop.

B.   Net fluid removal. As already stated, net fluid removal in peritoneal dialysis depends on the balance between peritoneal ultrafiltration and peritoneal absorption and thus on the determinants of these two processes. As lymphatic flow and the transport qualities of the membrane are not amenable to alteration, fluid removal in peritoneal dialysis can, in clinical practice, be enhanced by:

    1.   Maximizing the osmotic gradient

        a.   Higher tonicity dwells (e.g., 4.25% dextrose)

        b.   Shorter duration dwells (e.g., APD)

        c.   Higher dwell volumes

    2.   An osmotic agent with a higher reflection coefficient (e.g., polyglucose)

    3.   Increasing urine output (e.g., with diuretics)

As is shown in Fig. 13-8, the net fluid removal with a 1.5% 2-L dextrose dwell is maximal in the first hour and intraperitoneal volume is greatest after 90 minutes. After this time, the volume being ultrafiltered is less than that being resorbed, and by 6–10 hours, the intraperitoneal volume falls below 2 L, and the patient is achieving net fluid gain. If the more hypertonic 4.25% dextrose dialysis solution is used, initial fluid removal is greater and more sustained, and intraperitoneal volume is greatest after about 3 hours and will not fall below 2 L until after many hours.

The effect of larger dwell volumes on net fluid removal is complex. On the one hand, fluid removal increases because the

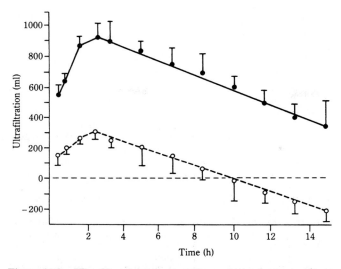

Figure 13-8.   Ultrafiltration volume (volume drained minus volume instilled) as a function of time after infusion of dialysis solution containing 1.5% dextrose (1.35% glucose, *open circles*) or 4.25% dextrose (3.86% glucose, *closed circles*). (Modified from Diaz-Buxo JA. Intermittent, continuous ambulatory and continuous cycling peritoneal dialysis. In: Nissenson AR, et al, eds. *Clinical dialysis*. Norwalk, CT: Appleton-Century-Crofts, 1984.)

osmotic gradient persists longer due to the greater quantity of glucose in the peritoneal cavity and because the effective surface area over which water is transported is likely increased. On the other hand, fluid removal decreases because intraperitoneal pressure rises (Fig. 13-5), thereby decreasing the hydrostatic gradient that favors ultrafiltration and promoting peritoneal fluid absorption into the tissues and lymphatics. The net effect of these forces varies and is difficult to predict.

   C.   Peritoneal clearance. Clearance for a given solute is defined as the volume of plasma cleared of that solute per unit time. It is thus equal to the quantity of solute removed in a given time divided by the plasma concentration of that solute during that time. It is typically measured in milliliters per minute or, in peritoneal dialysis, as liters per week. In peritoneal dialysis, clearance of a given solute is the net result of the effects of diffusion plus ultrafiltration minus fluid absorption.

   In hemodialysis, clearance for a small solute, such as urea, is relatively constant during the treatment; however, with peritoneal dialysis, it changes, being maximal at the start of a dwell, when both diffusion and ultrafiltration are greatest, and being less as the dwell proceeds and both ultrafiltration and diffusion decline due to loss of the urea concentration gradient and the glucose osmotic gradient, respectively. In practice, however, peritoneal clearance is measured per day or per week rather than per minute or per hour, and peritoneal dialysis is best described as a modality in which a low level of clearance is delivered continuously, as compared with hemodialysis where a high level of clearance is delivered intermittently.

Clearance in peritoneal dialysis is influenced by all of the factors that determine diffusion, ultrafiltration, and absorption. In clinical practice, peritoneal clearance can be increased by:

1. Maximizing time on peritoneal dialysis (i.e., no "dry time")
2. Maximizing concentration gradient (i.e., more frequent exchanges as in APD and larger dwell volumes)
3. Maximizing effective peritoneal surface area (i.e., larger dwell volumes)
4. Maximizing peritoneal fluid removal (as described above)

The mechanism by which increasing dwell volumes augment clearance is sometimes confusing. Larger dwell volumes enhance urea and creatinine diffusion from blood to dialysate because the greater volume makes the gradient stay higher for longer. However, the corollary of this is that D/P ratios tend to be a little lower with larger dwell volumes. Effective peritoneal surface area may also increase because of recruitment of more membrane by the greater fluid volume, and consequently MTAC values may rise. This effect tends to be modest or absent once volumes exceed 2.5 L in adults, presumably because all of the available membrane has been recruited. These two effects increase diffusive clearance even though D/P ratios may be lower. An additional effect is that, as already described, the larger dwell volume may in some patients diminish ultrafiltration slightly. Thus, a switch from 2.0- to 2.5-L dwells represents a 25% increase in infused volume but might, for example, be associated with a decrease in D/P ratios by 3% and of ultrafiltration by 5%, leading to a net increase of about 20% in clearance.

It should also be noted that changes in the peritoneal dialysis prescription alter urea and creatinine clearances to different degrees because the latter is more time-dependent than the former. Thus, a switch from CAPD to NIPD may lead to a much more marked decrease in creatinine than in urea clearance, whereas a switch from NIPD to CCPD will cause a disproportionately greater enhancement in creatinine clearance. These effects are especially marked in low transporters whose creatinine clearance is particularly time-dependent, as reflected by the flat shape of the creatinine equilibration curve.

    1. Measurement of clearance. Peritoneal clearance per day in peritoneal dialysis is easily measured and corresponds to the total daily dialysate drain volume multiplied by the solute concentration in that dialysate and divided by the simultaneous plasma concentration of the same solute. Stated more simply, clearance equals the drain volume multiplied by the D/P ratio for the solute concerned.

In CAPD, it is presumed (quite reasonably) that the plasma urea does not alter significantly during the day because dialysis is continuous. Thus, the plasma sample can be taken at any convenient time during the day concerned. In APD, there is significantly more intense dialysis at night than in the daytime; therefore, a constant plasma urea cannot be assumed. It is recommended that the plasma sample be taken in the middle of the noncycling period (usually midafternoon) when the urea is about halfway between its lowest level (in the morning after cycling) and its highest level (at night before cycling).

Clearance is measured per day but expressed per week. It is conventional to normalize urea clearance to total-body water (V), which is typically estimated using the Watson nomogram (see Table 17-4). Creatinine clearance is normalized to 1.73 m^2 surface area, which is estimated using the formula of DuBois (see Table 17-4).

2. Examples of peritoneal clearance calculations. See Table 17-4.

D. Sodium removal. In peritoneal dialysis, it is helpful to consider sodium removal separately from water removal. As already mentioned, ultrafiltration in peritoneal dialysis involves sodium sieving, so that water losses are proportionately greater than sodium losses. At the end of a 4-hour dwell, dialysate sodium levels will have fallen from the initial 132 mEq per L to about 120–125 mEq per L (Fig. 13-7). In the early part of a dwell, dialysate sodium falls rapidly because it is diluted by ultrafiltrate containing only about 80 mEq sodium per L. This effect is partly counteracted by diffusion, which becomes more significant as the concentration gradient for sodium widens. Thus, late in the dwell, when ultrafiltration is much lower, diffusion raises the dialysate sodium back up to about 125 mEq per L. Overall, net sodium removal with a 4-hour, 1.5% dextrose, 2-L exchange is minimal, although with a 4-hour, 4.25% dextrose, 2-L dwell, it is typically in excess of 70 mEq. Thus, in an anuric patient, sodium removal requires the use of more hypertonic solutions. Lowering the sodium concentration in the dialysis solution would increase diffusive sodium removal but would require greater concentrations of glucose to achieve the same osmotic effect. Such solutions can be made up but are not commercially available.

E. Protein losses. Obligatory dialysate protein losses are a feature of peritoneal dialysis and typically average 5–10 g daily of which half is accounted for by albumin. These losses are probably the major cause of the lower serum albumin levels seen in peritoneal dialysis, as compared with hemodialysis patients. Losses are greatest and serum albumin is lowest in high transporters. The losses or clearances of large molecular weight proteins such as albumin are relatively constant during the course of a dwell, but low molecular weight proteins such as lysozyme behave more like small solutes such as creatinine in that their clearance falls markedly as the dwell proceeds.

As already mentioned, protein losses are believed to occur via a relatively small number of large pores that correspond to interendothelial clefts. Peritoneal absorption of fluid is a form of "bulk flow" and so involves protein, as well as other solutes. It thus acts to decrease net peritoneal protein losses.

During peritonitis, protein losses increase markedly for a number of days, presumably due to an increase in effective peritoneal surface area consequent to increased vascularity. This effect is in part mediated by prostaglandins. Protein losses on intermittent peritoneal dialysis regimens appear to be no less per day than those on continuous regimens, presumably because the losses continue even during the "dry" interdialytic periods.

V.   Residual renal function. There is evidence that residual renal function persists longer and at a higher level in chronic peritoneal dialysis patients than those on hemodialysis and that this plays an important part in the success of peritoneal dialysis. Residual function contributes to salt and water removal and to clearance of both small and medium-size molecular weight solutes. Creatinine clearance is disproportionately high with residual renal function as tubular secretion contributes to the overall clearance to a greater extent. The opposite is the case with urea clearances where tubular resorption is significant. There is evidence that the mean of urea and creatinine clearance is a reasonable estimate of true glomerular filtration rate in the failing kidney; this estimate is used when calculating the renal contribution to total creatinine clearance in patients on peritoneal dialysis. Residual renal function has been shown to be predictive of patient outcome in peritoneal dialysis, perhaps because it is associated with better preserved renal endocrine and metabolic function and superior volume homeostasis, as well as greater small- and large-molecule clearance.

SELECTED READINGS

Flessner MF. Peritoneal transport physiology: insights from basic research. *J Am Soc Nephrol* 1991;2:122–135.

Flessner MF, et al. Blood flow does not limit peritoneal transport. *Perit Dial Int* 1999;19(Suppl 2):S208.

Heimburger O, et al. A quantitative description of solute and fluid transport during peritoneal dialysis. *Kidney Int* 1992;41:1320–1332.

Keshaviah P, et al. Relationship between body size, fill volume and mass transfer area coefficient in peritoneal dialysis. *J Am Soc Nephrol* 1994;4:1820–1826.

Krediet RT, et al. Icodextrin's effect on peritoneal transport. *Perit Dial Int* 1997;17:35–41.

Krediet RT. The peritoneal membrane in chronic peritoneal dialysis. *Kidney Int* 1999;55:341–356.

Mactier RA, et al. Influence of dwell time, osmolality, and volume of exchanges on solute mass transfer and ultrafiltration in peritoneal dialysis. *Semin Dial* 1988;1:40.

Rippe B, et al. Computer simulations of peritoneal transport in CAPD. *Kidney Int* 1991;40:315–325.

Rippe B, et al. A three-pore model of peritoneal transport. *Perit Dial Int* 1993;13(Suppl 2):S35–S38.

Rippe B, et al. Role of transcellular water channels in peritoneal dialysis. *Perit Dial Int* 1999;19(Suppl 2):S95–S101.

Ronco C. The "nearest capillary" hypothesis: a novel approach to peritoneal transport physiology. *Perit Dial Int* 1996;16:121–125.

Twardowski ZJ, et al. Peritoneal equilibration test. *Perit Dial Bull* 1987;7:138.

14

Apparatus for Peritoneal Dialysis

Michael I. Sorkin and Peter G. Blake

In this chapter, solutions and equipment for the various forms of peritoneal dialysis are described. Continuous ambulatory peritoneal dialysis (CAPD), automated peritoneal dialysis (APD), and hybrids of the two are discussed. Apparatus for acute peritoneal dialysis is reviewed in Chapter 16.

I. CAPD. In CAPD, dialysis solution is constantly present in the abdomen. The solution is typically changed four times daily, with a range of three to five times depending on individual patient requirements. Drainage of "spent" dialysate and inflow of fresh dialysis solution are performed manually, using gravity to move fluid into and out of the peritoneal cavity (Fig. 14-1). Technically, peritoneal dialysis solution flows into the peritoneal cavity, and dialysate drains out (i.e., the solution does not become dialysate until dialysis has occurred, although the term "dialysate" is commonly used for fresh as well as for used [or "spent"] solution). In this chapter, the term dialysate is used correctly to refer only to peritoneal dialysis solution after it has been instilled into the peritoneal space.

A. Dialysis solutions. CAPD solutions are packaged in clear, flexible plastic bags or, less commonly, in semirigid plastic containers.

1. Dialysis solution volumes. For adult patients, CAPD solutions are available in volumes of 1.5, 2.0, 2.25, 2.5, or 3.0 L, depending on the manufacturer. The commonly used bags are routinely overfilled by about 100 mL to allow for flushing, as will be described in a subsequent section. The standard volume prescribed has been 2.0 L, but 2.5 L is increasingly replacing it. Generally, larger volumes are desirable because they optimize solute clearance, but they may not always be tolerated by smaller patients.

2. Dialysis solution electrolyte concentrations. The electrolyte concentrations of CAPD solutions vary little by manufacturer. The three standard formulations are shown in Table 14-1.

All commonly marketed CAPD solutions contain lactate as the bicarbonate-generating base, and acetate is no longer used. There is interest in the use of bicarbonate-based peritoneal dialysis solutions; such preparations have recently become available in some European countries. A two-compartment bag system is used to keep the bicarbonate separate from the calcium and magnesium until just before use. The hope is that bicarbonate solutions will be more biocompatible, with consequent improvement in peritoneal host defenses and/or peritoneal membrane longevity.

With the widespread use of calcium carbonate or calcium acetate as a phosphate binder, CAPD solutions containing

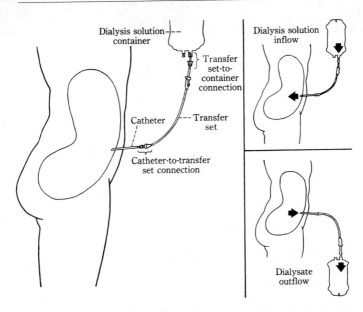

Figure 14-1.   Basic continuous ambulatory peritoneal dialysis (CAPD) system, with catheter, a "straight transfer set, and dialysis solution container. On the right, inflow and outflow are depicted. (Modified from Cogan MG, Garovoy MR, eds. *Introduction to dialysis.* New York: Churchill Livingstone, 1985.)

Table 14-1.   Three standard peritoneal dialysis solution formulations (mEq/L)[a]

Component	Solution		
	1	2	3 (low calcium)
Sodium	132.0	132.0	132.0
Potassium	0.0	0.0	0.0
Magnesium	1.5	0.5	0.5
Calcium	3.5	3.5	2.5
	(1.75 mmol/L)	(1.75 mmol/L)	(1.25 mmol/L)
Chloride	102.0	96.0	95.0
Lactate	35.0	40.0	40.0

[a] Values in mmol/L are identical except for calcium, where mmol/L values are shown in parentheses.

2.5 mEq per L (1.25 mmol per L) rather than 3.5 mEq per L (1.75 mmol per L) calcium are increasingly used with the goal of reducing the incidence of the hypercalcemia that is sometimes associated with oral calcium administration (see Chapter 21).

3. Dialysis solution dextrose concentrations. Dextrose is the osmotic agent commonly used in CAPD solutions, and preparations containing 1.5%, 2.5%, and 4.25% dextrose are routinely available and are labeled as such in North America. The true anhydrous dextrose or glucose concentrations in these solutions are 1.36%, 2.27%, and 3.86%, respectively, and this is how they are typically labeled in Europe. The approximate osmolarities of these solutions are 345, 395, and 484 mOsm per L, respectively.

Dextrose as an osmotic agent in peritoneal dialysis has the advantage of being familiar, relatively safe, and inexpensive and also is a source of calories. There is concern, however, that it predisposes patients to hyperglycemia, dyslipidemia, obesity, and possibly to long-term peritoneal membrane damage. In addition, it is not very effective in some patients, especially high transporters, and inadequate ultrafiltration may result. Alternative osmotic agents would be potentially helpful, and some have recently become available commercially. Amino acid based solutions are used for nutritional supplementation as they are largely absorbed by the end of a 4- to 6-hour dwell. Studies have shown them to be modestly effective in nutritionally compromised patients. They are reasonably effective osmotically but can be only used once or twice daily because they tend to cause some degree of acidosis, as well as a rise in the blood urea. These side effects may have to be addressed with oral alkali therapy and more dialysis, respectively.

Polyglucose preparations, such as icodextrin, are now available in some countries. Because they are not significantly absorbed, their osmotic effect is more sustained. Their main use is thus in the long nocturnal dwell in CAPD and in the long day dwell in APD, especially in patients with ultrafiltration failure (see Chapter 18). Their use is associated with unphysiologic blood levels of maltose, but no associated toxicity has been identified. One potential advantage for icodextrin is a reported reduction in glucose-induced lipid abnormalities.

4. Dialysis solution pH. In the manufacturing process, the pH of CAPD solutions is lowered to about 5.5 to prevent caramelization of glucose during heat sterilization. The acidic pH of peritoneal dialysis solution is normally well tolerated, and the pH of the dialysate rises rapidly as it accumulates bicarbonate from the patient. However, some patients complain of pain during inflow of dialysis solution. Sometimes this pain can be relieved by neutralizing the dialysis solution pH with alkali prior to instillation.

The low pH of peritoneal dialysis has an adverse effect on leukocytes. Even brief exposure to such low-pH solutions in vitro causes "stunning" of leukocytes, impairing their ability for phagocytosis, bacterial killing, and superoxide generation. As mentioned above, newer bicarbonate-based solutions with a physiologic pH are being studied and may soon be commercially available.

5.   Glucose degradation products. The heat sterilization process leads to generation of glucose degradation products which have toxic effects on the peritoneal membrane.
New strategies to deal with this include multicompartmental
solution bags where the glucose, having been heat-sterilized
at a pH that retards the formation of glucose degradation
products (e.g., in the neighborhood of pH 3.2), is kept separate
from the rest of the solution which can then be maintained at
a higher pH (e.g., pH 6.7). At the time of use, the glucose is
allowed to mix with the rest of the solution, bringing the pH
of the resultant mixture to close to 6.3–6.4. A higher pH and a
reduced amount of glucose degradation products are advantages of this particular solution.

6.   Sterility and trace metals. The preparation of peritoneal dialysis solutions is carefully regulated to ensure that
the final product is bacteriologically safe and has very low concentrations of trace metals.

7.   Dialysis solution temperature. CAPD solutions are
usually warmed to body temperature prior to inflow. They can
be instilled at room temperature, but uncomfortable lowering
of the body temperature and shivering can result. The best
warming method is to use a heating pad or special oven. Microwave ovens are frequently used, but this is not recommended
by most manufacturers because "hot spots" may be produced
during heating. When using a microwave oven, great care
must be taken to avoid overheating of the dialysis solution
as this can chemically alter the dextrose and may cause discomfort on instillation. Also, accidental boiling of the solution
in a confined space may cause an explosion. Heating methods
that involve immersing the peritoneal dialysis solution container completely in water are also not recommended because
contamination can result.

B.   Transfer sets. The CAPD solution bag is connected to the
patient's peritoneal catheter by a length of plastic tubing called
a "transfer set" (also sometimes called a "giving set"). There are
three major types of transfer sets, each requiring a different
method of performing the CAPD exchange. For the purpose of
discussion, we will refer to them as the straight transfer set, the
Y transfer set, and the double-bag system. Note that some transfer sets are connected to the peritoneal catheter via a short extension or adapter tubing (see below).

1.   Straight transfer set (Fig. 14-1). This system is now
rarely used because it is associated with high rates of peritonitis. However, a brief description is helpful in understanding
how more modern systems have evolved.

a.   Design. The straight transfer set is a simple plastic
tube. One end connects to the peritoneal catheter and the
other end to the dialysis solution bag. All exchanges are performed by making and subsequently breaking the connection between the transfer set and the bag. This connection
typically involves a spike or a Luer lock.

b.   Exchange procedure. Dialysis is performed as
follows:

(1)   Dialysis solution is instilled by gravity.
(2)   The empty bag and transfer set are rolled up and
stored in a pouch carried on the patient's body.
(3)   Dwell time is typically 4 to 8 hours.

(4)   The bag is unrolled and placed on the floor. The dialysate is drained into the bag. The bag is then disconnected from the transfer set and discarded.

(5)   A new bag is attached to the transfer set using a spike or Luer lock.

(6)   Fresh dialysis solution is instilled.

Once every several months, the transfer set is changed. Extended-life transfer set tubing allows patients to dialyze for 6 months between transfer set changes.

2.   **The Y Set** (Fig. 14-2)

   a.   Design. This is a Y-shaped piece of tubing that is attached by its stem to the patient's catheter or extension tubing at the time of each solution exchange. During the exchange, the afferent and efferent limbs of the Y are attached to a bag of fresh peritoneal dialysis solution and to a drain bag, respectively. In some cases, the drain bag is the empty solution bag that was used in the previous exchange. Most Y sets are not attached directly to the catheter but rather to a short (15 to 24 cm) adapter or extension tubing inserted between the catheter and the stem of the Y set. This extension tubing is sometimes confusingly called a transfer set, but in this chapter that term is reserved for the tubing that connects the solution bag and drain bag to the extension tubing and catheter. The extension tubing avoids the need for, and the risk of damage associated with, repeated clamping of the catheter.

   b.   Exchange procedure

   (1)   Spike/lock: The fresh bag of dialysis solution is attached to the afferent limb of the Y set via a spike or Luer lock.

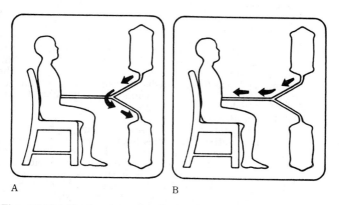

A   B

Figure 14-2.   **Y-set system using flush-before-fill. A: A small volume of fresh dialysis solution is drained directly into the drainage container (either before or just after drainage of the abdomen). This act washes away any bacteria that may have been introduced in the limb of the Y leading to the new bag at the time of connection. B: Fresh solution is introduced through the rinsed connector. Double-bag system differs only in that the fresh dialysis solution bag is incorporated into the Y tubing, and no connection to it is needed.**

(2)   Connect: The stem of the Y set is connected to the adapter tubing.

(3)   Drain: The stem and efferent limb of the Y are unclamped and the spent dialysate is drained from the peritoneal cavity into the drain bag.

(4)   Flush: With the stem of the Y set clamped, approximately 100 mL of fresh solution is flushed from the new bag through the afferent limb of the Y into the efferent limb and so into the drain bag.

(5)   Fill: The efferent limb is clamped and the stem unclamped, and the peritoneal cavity is filled from the new bag of dialysis solution.

(6)   Disconnect: The Y set is then disconnected from the adapter tubing.

The Y set was developed to free patients from the requirement to remain attached to the transfer set and empty bag between exchanges. Early studies revealed a more important benefit—a peritonitis rate significantly lower than that with the straight set. This is thought to be due to the flush-before-fill procedure used to prime the tubing. Bacteria that may be introduced during the connection procedure are washed out of the Y set into the empty drainage bag rather than into the patient, as happens with the straight set. Also, because the tubing and bags are disconnected from the patient between exchanges, less mechanical stress may be placed on the catheter exit site and tunnel. This may result in fewer episodes of minor trauma to the catheter exit site and tunnel and therefore to fewer exit site and tunnel infections. This, in turn, may reduce the peritonitis rate.

Because of this lower peritonitis rate and the convenience of allowing the patient to disconnect between exchanges, Y-set systems increasingly displaced the straight system as the transfer set of choice from the mid-1980s on. Nondisconnect Y sets, which are filled with sodium hypochlorite between exchanges, were initially popular but are now less so due to their complexity, lack of apparent additional benefit, and risk of painful accidental intraperitoneal hypochlorite infusion. Similarly, removable, reusable Y sets, called "O sets" in which the disconnected Y was filled with disinfectant between exchanges and stored with the two limbs connected to form an "O" are now of mainly historical interest.

3.   Double-bag systems

   a.   Design. These systems are a variant of the Y set in which the solution bag comes preattached to the afferent limb of the Y, so obviating the need for any spike or Luer lock connection. The drain bag is similarly preattached to the efferent limb, and the only connection the patient needs to make is thus between the transfer set and the extension tubing. A flush-before-fill step is still performed, but the purpose is only to flush out residual air and not to prevent peritoneal cavity contamination, as this is no longer relevant in the absence of a need to make a transfer set–to–solution container connection.

   These are now most popular systems because of their ease of use and because of evidence that they are associated with even lower rates of peritonitis than the standard Y sets.

Their only disadvantage is that their disposability results in increased cost as compared to older reusable systems.

b.   Exchange procedure

(1)   Connect: The patient connects the new transfer set to the extension tubing.

(2)   Drain: The stem and efferent limb are unclamped and spent dialysate is drained from the peritoneal cavity into the drain bag.

(3)   Flush: The stem is clamped, and the afferent limb of the Y is opened by breaking a "frangible" in the tubing. Then 100 mL of peritoneal dialysis solution is flushed through from the fill bag to the drain bag to remove residual air from the tubing.

(4)   Fill: The efferent limb is clamped, the stem is unclamped, and fresh peritoneal dialysis solution is run into the peritoneal cavity.

(5)   Disconnect: All limbs are clamped, and the transfer set is disconnected from the extension tubing.

C.   Various connectors for peritoneal dialysis. Over the years, a number of connectors and associated devices have been developed and marketed in an attempt to reduce the possibility of bacterial contamination while making either the catheter–to–transfer set or the transfer set–to–container connections.

1.   Catheter–to–transfer set (or extension tubing–to–transfer set) connection

a.   Catheter connector. Early in the history of CAPD, simple, plastic, plug-in connectors were used at the catheter–to–transfer set junction. Cracking of the plastic connector and accidental disconnection were frequent events that often led to peritonitis. A special Luer lock connector made of titanium was developed to prevent such problems. Titanium was chosen for its light weight and resistance to electrolyte-containing solutions. Designed for easier handling and a tighter connection, the new product functioned very well. Catheter–to–transfer set connectors constructed from more durable plastics are also available.

b.   Quick connect–disconnect systems. With the advent of the disconnect Y sets and double bags, the need for easy yet sterile connection at the catheter–to–transfer set joint (or adapter–to–transfer set joint) has arisen. A number of new connectors for this purpose are now available.

2.   Transfer set–to–container connection. With the advent of double-bag systems, technologies to facilitate the connection between the transfer set and the peritoneal dialysis solution container are less relevant. However, some of them are still used, and brief mention will be made of them.

a.   Spike-and-port design. The spike-and-port design is the oldest and simplest system used to connect the transfer set to the dialysis solution container. It is operated by pushing a spike located at the end of the transfer set into a port on the dialysis solution container.

b.   Easy-lock connectors. Spiking the container is difficult for many patients because it requires reasonably good vision, depth and sensory perception, and strength. Mistakes can result in contamination and subsequent peritonitis. The spike has thus been replaced in many transfer sets by a Luer lock or screw type system, resulting in easier insertion. A modified form contains a recessed fluid pathway to prevent accidental contamination, a reservoir that can be filled with an antiseptic solution (e.g., povidone–iodine), and a silicon O-ring to provide a tight seal.

   c.   Specialized connection devices can reduce the risk of peritonitis associated with CAPD. However, most of the devices are bulky and cumbersome, and some require use of an electric power outlet or a somewhat heavy portable battery. These include:

   (1)   Mechanical devices to assist in spike–port insertion. Available devices make use of levers or gears to assist blind or arthritic patients in inserting the transfer set spike into the port on the dialysis solution container.

   (2)   Ultraviolet (UV) light sterilization device. This device combines a mechanical system that assists in spiking the port with UV light irradiation of the spike and port just before the connection is made.

II.   Automated peritoneal dialysis. APD is now the fastest growing peritoneal dialysis modality, and in some programs, the majority of peritoneal dialysis patients are treated with it. It is traditionally divided into continuous cycling peritoneal dialysis (CCPD) and nocturnal intermittent peritoneal dialysis (NIPD). In CCPD, the patient carries peritoneal dialysis solution in the abdominal cavity throughout the day but performs no exchanges and is not attached to a transfer set. At bedtime, the patient hooks up to an automated cycler that will change the dialysis solution in his or her abdomen three or more times in the course of the night. In the morning, the patient, with the last dwell remaining in the abdomen, disconnects from the cycler and is free to go about daily activities. In NIPD, the patient drains out fully at the end of the cycling period, and so the abdomen is "dry" all day. Because of the absence of a long-duration day dwell, clearances are generally lower on NIPD than on CCPD, but patients may prefer it instead in case there is good residual renal function or because of mechanical contraindications to walking about with solution in the abdominal cavity (e.g., leaks, hernias, back pain).

   A.   Cyclers. These are machines that automatically cycle dialysis solution into and out of the abdominal cavity. For safety purposes, instillation and drainage have typically been performed using only the force of gravity. However, a pump is sometimes used to deliver the solution up to a raised container from which it will be allowed to enter the abdomen. Cyclers also warm the dialysis solution before inflow. With the aid of clamps and timers, they regulate the time of inflow, dwell, and outflow of dialysis solution.

   More recent cycler models are small and light enough to pack in a large suitcase and carry on trips. They use air pressure to pump fluid into and out of the patient and into and out of the warming device and so are not gravity-dependent. Advanced design and computer technology make them simple to set up and operate. The patient typically sets only the start time, volume of solution, dwell time, and length of dialysis or stop time desired. The cycler calculates the timing of the exchange, measures volume of ultrafiltrate, and optimizes drain and inflow time by measuring flow rates and changing from drain to fill when flow stops rather waiting for a preset time. It also tests to determine whether flow has stopped because of obstruction. More recent models incorporate 'smart cards' which can be used to program the cycler prescription and to record the actual prescription delivered to the patient.

An extremely useful feature is the ability to draw dialysis solution from a separate solution container for the last instillation in the morning, called the "last bag option," because this last inflow, which will be in place throughout the day, often requires a higher dextrose concentration than the other exchanges.

Typically, patients spend 8–10 hours a night cycling. Dwell volumes range from 1.5 to 3.0 L, and the number of cycles usually varies from 3 to 10 per night. The amount of fluid used is between 8 and 20 L but averages 10–14 L.

B.   Dialysis solution. Dialysis solution for APD is the same as that used for CAPD. Most cyclers are fed by a tube containing a multipronged manifold that can attach to as many as eight dialysis solution containers simultaneously to provide sufficient solution for the night. The total number of containers required, and thus the cost, can be reduced by using large containers holding 3 or 5 L of dialysis solution, although lifting these can be a problem for older and frailer patients. Because the cycler can be fed from two or more containers simultaneously, with appropriate selection of the dextrose concentrations of the containers being hung, a number of intermediate dextrose concentrations (e.g., between those commercially available) can easily be delivered.

C.   APD connections

  1.   Transfer sets. One set of plastic tubing serves to interconnect several dialysis solution containers to the cycler and to connect the cycler to the patient. Shorter, simpler, and less expensive solution delivery sets are constantly being developed.

  2.   Catheter–to–transfer set connection. The catheter–to–transfer set connection must be made every night and broken every morning. Previously, many patients had a standard Luer lock connector at the end of the peritoneal catheter. The procedure for connecting the catheter connector to the transfer set was tedious because it required sterile procedure and a lengthy antiseptic scrub. This older connector has largely been replaced by new, quick connect–disconnect systems that require no manual disinfection and therefore are much easier to use. Some of these systems also may fit CAPD transfer sets, allowing APD patients to use the CAPD method whenever desired (e.g., when traveling).

  3.   Transfer set–to–container connections. The standard spike-and-port or Luer lock connections are most often used to connect the multipronged transfer set to the dialysis solution containers. In order to minimize the risk of contamination, the newer cyclers allow for a flush option after this connection has been made. The same connection technologies used to assist CAPD patients with visual impairment, arthritis, or neuropathy (see above) can also assist APD patients in making the transfer set–to–container connections.

D.   Tidal peritoneal dialysis (TPD). This form of APD was designed to optimize solute clearance by leaving a large volume of dialysis solution in the peritoneal cavity throughout the dialysis session. Initially, the peritoneal cavity is filled with a volume of dialysis solution selected to be as large as possible without causing discomfort. The volume used depends on patient size and habitus but is typically up to 2–3 L. During the drain phase, only about half of the dialysate is drained, leaving the other half in the peritoneal cavity. If 3 L is being used, the next fill volume (the tidal volume) is 1.5 L, the next drain volume is about 1.5 L, and so on. Cycles are quite short, usually totaling less than 20 minutes with dwell times for the replacement aliquot being only 4–6 minutes. Usually, 26–30 L of dialysate is exchanged over an 8- to 10-hour dialysis session. The peritoneal cavity is drained completely only at the end of the dialysis session. At this stage, as in standard NIPD, the peritoneal catheter can be capped and the peritoneal cavity left empty until the next treatment. Alternatively, fluid can be left in the cavity as in CCPD.

The high dialysate flow rate provides increased diffusion gradients between blood and dialysate and minimizes the formation of unstirred layers of dialysate next to the peritoneal membrane. The presence of half the initial fill volume provides continuous contact between dialysate and peritoneal membrane. As a result, solute and water removal occur continuously, not just during the dwell period.

   1.   Technical problems. TPD has a number of technical problems, making it difficult to recommend for routine use.

      a.   Peritoneal catheter. The peritoneal catheter must have excellent inflow and drain characteristics because up to 30 L of dialysate is exchanged nightly. This usually means that dialysate flow must be 180–200 mL per minute during the drain phase.

      b.   Cost. In adults, the advantages of TPD in terms of clearance are only seen when 20–30 L of dialysis solution is used each day, and this is very expensive.

      c.   Ultrafiltration computations. The ultrafiltration volume must be calculated and added to the drain volume with each exchange; otherwise, the intra-abdominal volume will become progressively larger. TPD is best performed with newer cyclers that have been modified, so that the outflow volume can be set to trigger a change to dialysate inflow mode. When the preset outflow volume is reached (e.g., 1.5 L), the machine changes immediately to inflow to infuse a fresh 1.5 L of dialysis solution. This system is quite different from that in most early cyclers, in which inflow/outflow cycles are regulated only by preset timers, not by volume.

At present, TPD as described above is not widely used, and a recent multicenter study has shown that clearance is not really much improved using TPD compared with standard APD (Rodriguez et al, 1998).

In small children, the lower volumes required and the good clearances that can be achieved make TPD a more attractive option. In adults, low-volume TPD (i.e., 10–15 L per night) using a residual volume of only 200–500 mL can be useful to deal with the common APD complication of pain at the end of each drain cycle. By always keeping some solution in the abdominal cavity, these TPD-type regimens can minimize this pain.

III. Hybrid regimens. In an effort to improve the clearances and ultrafiltration associated with standard CAPD and APD without infringing unduly on patient lifestyle, a number of hybrid methodologies between CAPD and APD have evolved.

A. Night exchange device

1. This system was designed to provide a single extra exchange for CAPD patients. This is delivered automatically at a predetermined time, most often while the patient is asleep at night. In essence, it is a cycler that provides one exchange cycle. Its uses are to allow a fourth exchange for a patient who cannot manage four during regular waking hours, to provide a fifth exchange for a patient who needs additional exchanges but does not have time to do five during waking hours, or to provide more even spacing of five exchanges to enhance clearance. Splitting the long nocturnal CAPD dwell in two also enhances ultrafiltration, and so the device may be useful for patients, typically high transporters, who have net fluid resorption after long dwells.

2. The device simply holds and warms a single bag. It is typically set up before the patient goes to bed, just like a cycler, but it uses standard CAPD tubing rather than a special manifold. It allows the patient to drain at a predetermined time and then to fill automatically. The patient performs a routine exchange upon awakening and continues the CAPD routine manually during the day. The device does not supply any information about fluid removal. The same effect could be obtained using any one of the standard cyclers set for a single exchange, but this would be more complicated and time consuming as well as more costly (i.e., in terms of the expense of the additional multipronged manifold as well as of the cycler itself).

B. APD with daytime exchanges. Even CCPD does not provide adequate clearances for some patients once residual renal function is lost. Additional day exchanges may be required. These exchanges improve clearance as the typical 14- to 16-hour, single day dwell in CCPD is unduly long and does not provide significant additional dialysis after the first 4–6 hours. These additional day exchanges also improve ultrafiltration as the single day dwell is also too long for effective net fluid removal. Indeed, in many patients, especially higher transporters, a single day exchange can result in significant net fluid resorption to a degree that is medically unacceptable. Additional day exchanges can be done manually using standard CAPD transfer sets, but this is relatively expensive in terms of solution and tubing costs and may be inconvenient for patients.

An alternative strategy, originally described as "PD Plus," involves using the cycler tubing to deliver the additional exchange(s). Thus the patient returns to the cycler in the afternoon or evening, reattaches to the transfer set, drains the dialysate that has been in the peritoneal cavity since that morning, and then refills from the large-volume solution containers (3–5 L) that will be used to provide solution for cycling that night. The patient then detaches from the transfer set but is able to reattach to the same tubing later, either to do another exchange or to commence cycling that night. This is made possible by a modification of the transfer set that allows serial connections and disconnections to be performed or by simply using "caps" to protect the respective endings of the transfer set and adapter tubing while disconnected. This strategy, which is sometimes described as using the cycler as a "docking station," can be easily performed with the newer generation of cyclers and is less costly because no additional transfer set is required and because the solution can be drawn from more economical, large-volume solution bags. It has the additional advantage that it can be set up for the patient in advance by a relative or a helper. However, for the working patient, the requirement to return to the cycler during the noncycling period may be a disadvantage, and in such cases, a manual CAPD type exchange may be preferred.

In some patients, a second day dwell is not required but a single long day dwell leads to net fluid resorption. In these cases, the cycler tubing can be used to drain the day dwell early without any subsequent fill.

SELECTED READINGS

Bargman JM. Peritoneal dialysis catheter connection devices: what have we learned? *Perit Dial Int* 1992;12:9–11.

Chagnac A, et al. Calcium balance during pulse alfacalcidol therapy for secondary hyperparathyroidism in CAPD patients treated with 1.0 and 1.25 mmol/L dialysate calcium. *Am J Kidney Dis* 1999;32:82–86.

Chandra D, et al. A randomized multicenter clinical trial comparing isosmolar icodextrin with hyperosmolar glucose solutions in CAPD. *Kidney Int* 1994;46:496–503.

Coles G, et al. A randomized controlled trial of a bicarbonate- and a bicarbonate/lactate-containing dialysis solution in CAPD. *Perit Dial Int* 1997;17:48–51.

Gokal R, et al, and the MIDAS Study Group. Improvement of hyperlipidemia with icodextrin use in CAPD patients. *J Am Soc Nephrol* 1998;9:283A.

Jones M, et al. Treatment of malnutrition with 1.1% amino acid peritoneal dialysis solution: results of a multicenter outpatient study. *Am J Kidney Dis* 1998;32:761–767.

Kiernan L, et al. Comparison of continuous ambulatory peritoneal dialysis–related infections with different "Y-tubing" exchange systems. *J Am Soc Nephrol* 1995;5:1835–1838.

Kopple, et al. Treatment of malnourished CAPD patients with amino acid based dialysate. *Kidney Int* 1995;47:1148–1157.

Li PK, et al. Comparison of double-bag and Y-set disconnect systems in continuous ambulatory peritoneal dialysis: a randomized prospective multicenter study. *Am J Kidney Dis* 1999;33:535–540.

Misra N, Nolph KD, Khanna R. Will automated peritoneal dialysis be the answer? *Perit Dial Int* 1997;17:435–439.

Port FK, et al. Risk of peritonitis and technique failure by CAPD connection technique: a national study. *Kidney Int* 1992;42:967–974.

Rodriguez AM, et al. Automated peritoneal dialysis: a Spanish multicentre study. *Nephrol Dial Transplant* 1998;13:2335–2340.

Peritoneal Access Devices

Stephen R. Ash and John T. Daugirdas

A good peritoneal catheter should allow adequate rates of solution inflow and outflow and be of such design as to minimize infection at the skin exit site and to allow for successful resolution of peritonitis should it occur. Finally, it should be safely implantable without major surgery.

I. Types of catheters. Peritoneal catheters may be categorized as acute or chronic.

A. Acute catheters. All acute catheters have the same basic design: a length of straight or slightly curved, relatively rigid tubing with numerous side holes at the distal end. A metal stylet or flexible wire over which the catheter slides is used to guide insertion. Acute catheters are designed to be placed "medically" at the bedside because even the short delays associated with surgical consultation and implantation may not be acceptable for patients in acute renal failure. Because acute catheters do not have cuffs to protect against bacterial migration, the incidence of peritonitis increases prohibitively beyond 3 days of use. Also, risk of bowel perforation increases with duration of use. If extended dialysis is necessary, the acute catheter must be removed periodically and replaced by a new catheter in a different abdominal wall location.

B. Chronic catheters. Chronic peritoneal catheters are constructed from silicone rubber or polyurethane and have one or two Dacron cuffs. Like acute catheters, most chronic catheters have numerous side holes at the distal end. The silicone rubber or polyurethane surface promotes development of squamous epithelium in the subcutaneous "tunnel" next to the catheter, at the exit site, and within the abdominal wall. The presence of this epithelium increases the resistance to bacterial penetration of the tissue near the skin exit and peritoneal entry sites. The Dacron cuffs provoke a local inflammatory response that progresses to form fibrous and granulation tissue within 1 month. This fibrous tissue serves to fix the catheter cuff in position and to prevent bacterial migration from the skin surface or from the peritoneal cavity (in cases of peritonitis) past the cuff into the subcutaneous tunnel.

Chronic peritoneal catheters, protected against migration of bacteria and fixed in position, are not restricted to a 3-day period of use as are the uncuffed acute catheters. Peritonitis can usually be treated successfully without catheter removal. Chronic catheters function successfully for 2 or more years, on average, before complications precipitate their removal.

A chronic catheter is usually implanted by surgical dissection in the operating room. Effective and safe techniques for bedside placement, utilizing guide wire and dilators or peritoneoscopy, also exist. When it is anticipated that the need for peritoneal dialysis will be longer than a few days, a chronic catheter should be placed initially, obviating the necessity for periodic replacement of acute catheters.

   1.   Tenckhoff catheter. A typical two-cuff straight Tenckhoff catheter is shown in Fig. 15-1. For obese patients with pendulous abdomens, the distance between the two cuffs of a standard Tenckhoff catheter may be inappropriately short; extralong catheters with more widely spaced cuffs are available. Single-cuff catheters are also available and can function as well as double-cuff catheters when the single cuff is in the deep position, that is, when it is sewn into the abdominal musculature and the distance from the cuff to the skin exit site is relatively short (5 cm or less). Some advocate placing the single cuff in the superficial position, especially when using these catheters to perform acute peritoneal dialysis, in order to facilitate their subsequent removal.

   2.   Alternate chronic catheter designs
   a.   Modifications aimed at improving outflow. The standard Tenckhoff catheter almost always allows easy inflow of fluid. However, effective drainage of the abdomen may be variable and difficult. This is especially so in the later stages of the drain when resistance to fluid outflow increases as the omentum and bowel loops are brought close to the catheter tip and sides by Bernoulli (suction) forces near the catheter entry holes and by the diminished volume of fluid in the abdomen. To minimize outflow obstruction, a number of alternative catheters have been devised (Fig. 15-2). The curled Tenckhoff catheter provides an increased bulk of tubing to separate the parietal and visceral layers of the peritoneum. Flow into and out of the catheter tip is more protected, and there are more side holes for outflow. The Toronto Western catheter (TWH, left column in Fig. 15-2) makes use of two perpendicular silicone disks to hold omentum and bowel away from the exit holes. The T-fluted catheter (Fig. 15-2, bottom left) has grooves (flutes)

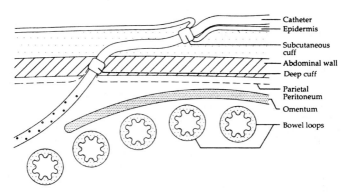

Figure 15-1.   Schematic drawing of a straight Tenckhoff peritoneal catheter showing its proper relationship to adjacent tissues.

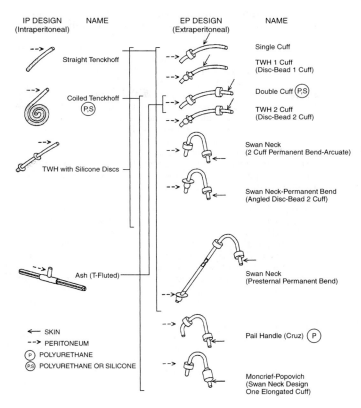

Figure 15-2. Currently available chronic peritoneal catheters showing their intraperitoneal (left) and extraperitoneal (right) portions.

on the surface of its two limbs to distribute flow widely. The "T" shape of the catheter places the limbs next to the parietal peritoneum so that external migration of the catheter is not possible. In spite of the various intraperitoneal (IP) shapes, all peritoneal dialysis catheters have roughly the same outflow characteristics, though some have more reproducible and consistent outflow.

b. Modifications of the deep cuff. In addition to its unique IP design, the Toronto Western catheter has a deep cuff in the form of a Dacron disk especially fashioned to minimize leakage and fix the catheter's position (TWH1 and TWH2, right column, in Fig. 15-2). A silicone bead next to the disk is designed to allow the peritoneum and sometimes the posterior fascia to be closed around the catheter between the bead and disk. This method of fixing the deep cuff is different from the technique of placing Tenckhoff catheters, in which the deep cuff rests entirely in the rectus muscle.

The bead-and-disk type of deep cuff is also available on the straight Tenckhoff catheter (the so-called Missouri catheter), with the disk affixed to the bead at a 45-degree angle (Fig. 15-3). As a result, when the disk is placed next to the posterior rectus fascia, the IP part of the catheter naturally tends to angle downward into the pelvis and should have less tendency to migrate into the upper abdomen.

c.   The swan-neck catheters. These have a V-shaped arc (150 degrees) between the deep and superficial cuffs (Fig. 15-2, right). The bend allows the catheter to exit the skin facing downward yet enter the peritoneum facing toward the pelvis, as Tenckhoff originally suggested (1974). In some studies, lower rates of cuff extrusion and exit site infection have been found for catheters with downward-facing exit sites compared with those that have laterally directed or upwardly directed exit sites. **Presternal** swan-neck catheters have an added subcutaneous extension (Fig. 15-2, right), allowing tunneling of the catheter under the skin to exit at the upper chest. Such catheters are especially useful for obese patients, where the shifting of the abdominal wall would otherwise create excessive movement at the exit site and predispose to infection. Presternal catheters also are useful for patients wishing to bathe in a tub, provided that patients do not immerse the presternal exit site in the bath water.

d.   Pail-handle (Cruz) catheter. This catheter (Fig. 15-2, right) has two right-angle bends: one to direct the IP portion parallel to the parietal peritoneum and one to direct the subcutaneous portion downward toward the skin exit site. It is available only in polyurethane. Its clinical

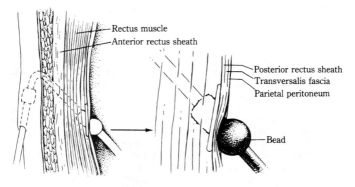

Figure 15-3.   Missouri catheter, featuring a swan-neck shape and a deep cuff composed of an angled disk and ball. (Modified from Twardowski ZJ, et al. The need for a "swan neck" permanently bent, arcuate peritoneal dialysis catheter. *Perit Dial Bull* 1985;5:219.)

benefits have not been well defined. Its larger internal diameter and position of the coil near the parietal peritoneum allows more rapid outflow than standard silicone catheters, and its shape facilitates placement in obese patients.

   e.   Moncrief–Popovich catheter. This catheter is very similar to the standard swan-neck Tenckhoff, except that the external cuff is much longer (Fig. 15-4). When the catheter is first implanted with 1,000 units of heparin instilled, the external segment is buried subcutaneously (initially there is no exit site) for a period of 2 to 8 weeks or longer to allow tissue ingrowth into the external cuff in a sterile environment. Subsequently, a small incision is made in the skin through which the external segment of the catheter is brought out.

   f.   Critical comparison of catheter designs. To what extent the new catheter designs are improvements over standard straight and curled Tenckhoff catheters has not been determined, despite a large number of retrospective studies and a few prospective trials. The standard curled and straight silicone Tenckhoff catheters still enjoy wide use and remain the standards against which the newer designs are judged. Prospective studies have demonstrated small but significant advantages to two-cuff and to coiled catheters.

   Catheters with deep cuffs or larger IP portions, such as the Toronto Western and Missouri models, require surgical dissection for placement, whereas standard Tenckhoff-type catheters and the T-fluted catheter can also be placed blindly or peritoneoscopically. The Toronto Western catheter does not diminish outflow failure, may have increased incidence of omental attachment, and is more difficult to remove. Fixation of the deep cuff by disk and bead methods does result in fewer exit site infections or pericatheter hernias. Only preliminary data are available on the new Moncrief–Popovich catheter and technique. These data suggest a reduced incidence of peritonitis but no decrease in exit site infection.

   Several catheters are now available in polyurethane as well as in silicone rubber. Polyurethane is a stronger and smoother material than silicone, and the hope was that it would reduce the formation of biofilm. However, polyurethane catheters have not been shown to have a lower incidence of recurrent peritonitis, outflow obstruction, or mechanical failure; indeed, they may be more susceptible to damage by chemicals, such as alcohol and polyethylene glycol, and to disruption of the bond between the catheter and its cuffs.

II.   Placement procedures

A.   Acute catheters. The acute peritoneal catheter is designed to be placed blindly into an abdomen that has been prefilled with fluid. Insertion is guided by either a sharpened stylet or flexible guide wire. Examples of acute catheters with stylets are the Stylocath (Abbott Laboratories, North Chicago, IL) and the Trocath (Baxter Healthcare, Deerfield, IL). An acute catheter designed to be inserted over a flexible guide wire is available from Cook Co. (Bloomington, IN).

   The potential complications of acute catheter placement (see below, II.A.2) should be understood. The incidence of complica-

IMPLANTATION

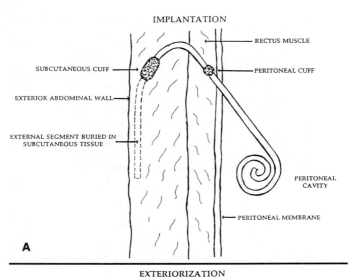

EXTERIORIZATION

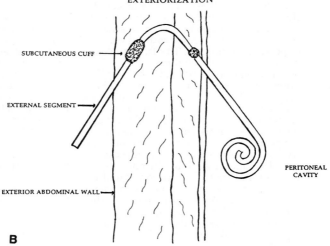

Figure 15-4.   Technique of peritoneal catheter implantation advocated by Moncrief et al. (1993). A: Initially, there is no exit site. B: Two to eight weeks later, the external end of the catheter is exteriorized.

tions is increased in patients with ileus or adhesions from previous abdominal surgery. Placement is also difficult in comatose or uncooperative patients who cannot tense the abdominal wall during insertion of the catheter or prefilling needle. Surgical or peritoneoscopic placement of a chronic peritoneal catheter should be considered for such patients.

1.   Procedure. Either a midline or a lateral abdominal entry site can be chosen (Fig. 15-5, solid black squares). The midline site is about 3 cm below the umbilicus. The lateral site is just lateral to the border of the rectus muscle, on a line between the umbilicus and the anterior superior iliac spine. On the right, the lateral site is thus approximately situated at McBurney's point. The left lateral site is considered preferable because it avoids the cecum. When choosing an insertion site, avoid areas of previous catheter insertion or scars by at least 2 to 3 cm. The bladder must be empty, as a full bladder can inadvertently be penetrated by the stylet during insertion. The abdomen should be carefully examined to exclude the presence of massive enlargement of the liver, spleen, bladder, or other organs and to exclude other remarkable pathology (e.g., abdominal carcinomatosis).

a.   Don mask, cap, gown, and sterile gloves. Wash, prepare, and drape the skin overlying the desired insertion site. Anesthetize the full depth of the abdominal wall liberally at the desired site, using approximately 10 mL of local anesthetic agent.

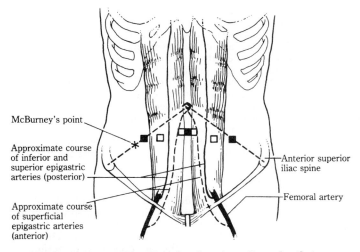

Figure 15-5.   Deep-cuff locations for chronic peritoneal catheters. The solid squares show deep-cuff locations for catheters placed by peritoneoscopic or blind techniques. These are also the usual placement sites for "acute" catheters. The hollow squares locate alternative placement sites for chronic catheters placed by surgical dissection, as described in the text.

b. Make a 1- to 2-cm skin incision over the desired entry site. (Some prefer to make a smaller, e.g., 3-mm, incision.) Dissect down to the level of the fascia using a blunt hemostat. While asking the patient to tense the abdominal wall, insert a small needle or plastic tube into the abdomen (e.g., a 16-gauge Angiocath or a 14-gauge Voorhees needle). The needle or tubing should be at least 6 to 8 cm long in order to reach the peritoneal space. If an Angiocath was used, remove the needle at this time, leaving the plastic tube in place. By gravity, infuse 1–2 L of 1.5% dextrose dialysis solution into the abdomen until the abdomen becomes moderately tense. Observe the patient carefully for signs of respiratory embarrassment while the abdomen is being filled.

c. The subsequent steps now depend on whether a stylet or wire will be used to guide catheter insertion:

(1) Stylet method (for Stylocath or Trocath catheters)

(a) Remove the plastic tubing or needle used for filling. Place fingers of one hand on the catheter in such a way as to limit the initial depth of penetration to a few centimeters beyond the estimated location of the parietal peritoneum (usually about 6–8 cm from the tip of the catheter). While the patient again tenses the abdominal wall, push the stylet–catheter through the abdominal wall, aiming 20 degrees off the perpendicular toward the patient's coccyx. Remove the stylet immediately while holding the catheter in place. Peritoneal fluid should now escape through the catheter.

(b) Replace the stylet partially, stopping 1 cm short of full insertion. Aim the stylet and catheter toward the left inguinal ligament, and angle the stylet to a plane as close as possible to that of the abdominal wall. Advance the catheter over the stylet down into the abdominal cavity without advancing the stylet itself until the catheter meets firm resistance, or until the "wings" or suture points descend to the skin surface.

(c) Remove the stylet, connect the catheter to the dialysis tubing, and immediately begin drainage of the peritoneal fluid. If no flow occurs, rotate or withdraw the catheter slightly.

(d) Adjust the position of the catheter support wings so that they lie against the skin, and suture the catheter in place.

(2) Guide wire method (for Cook peritoneal dialysis catheters)

(a) Insert the guide wire through the plastic tubing or needle that was used to fill the abdomen with fluid. Remove the plastic tubing or needle.

(b) Insert the catheter over the guide wire into the abdominal cavity in the same general direction as described for the stylet method. If it is necessary to reposition the catheter, reinsert the wire and readvance the catheter over the wire.

(c) Suture the catheter in place.

2. Complications of acute catheter insertion
a. Preperitoneal placement
(1) Of the filling tubing or needle. Inflow of the fluid used to fill the abdomen will be slow, local swelling may be noted, and pain during filling may occur. It is important to recognize preperitoneal placement at this point and not proceed with catheter insertion at this site. The plastic tubing or needle should be removed and reinserted at another site.

(2) Of the catheter itself. Dialysis solution outflow will be minimal and the return will quickly become blood-tinged. Remove the catheter and insert another. The second catheter can be inserted at the same site if filling of the abdomen went well, or at a second site if there was any question about whether the filling tubing or needle was also placed preperitoneally.

b. Blood-tinged dialysis solution return.
In addition to preperitoneal placement of the catheter, blood-tinged outflow through the catheter can occur due to injury of a vessel in the abdominal wall or mesentery. The return will usually clear with continued dialysis. Use of room temperature dialysate may slow or stop capillary bleeding.

c. More serious complications.
Grossly bloody effluent, a fall in the hematocrit, or shock signal that a larger intra-abdominal blood vessel has been punctured; this usually requires urgent performance of a laparotomy. Unexplained **polyuria** and **glycosuria** can reflect inadvertent puncture of the urinary bladder. Feces or gas in the effluent or watery diarrhea having a high glucose concentration indicates bowel perforation. In case of bowel perforation, it is sometimes possible merely to remove the catheter and observe the patient carefully while treating with intravenous antibiotics. Peritoneal dialysis should be delayed for several days unless the bowel has been surgically repaired.

B. Chronic catheters.
There are four options for placement of chronic peritoneal catheters: (a) surgical placement by dissection, (b) blind placement using the Tenckhoff trocar, (c) blind placement using a guide wire, and (d) minitrocar placement using peritoneoscopy. The larger catheters, such as the Toronto Western and Missouri models (Figs. 15-2 and 15-3), must be placed surgically. Straight and curled Tenckhoff catheters (Fig. 15-2), with or without a swan-neck section, may be placed by any technique.

1. Surgical implantation.
This is still the most popular method for placement of chronic peritoneal catheters. It begins with either extensive local anesthesia or light general anesthesia. There are two general approaches: the **lateral** and the **paramedian**. Either can be used with any of the catheters, although Toronto Western and Missouri catheters are usually placed using the paramedian technique.

a. Lateral approach.
The abdominal entry site is through the lateral border of the rectus sheath (Fig. 15-5).

(1) Procedure for insertion of straight and curved Tenckhoff catheters

(a) The skin, subcutaneous tissue, and rectus sheath over the desired entry site are dissected, resulting in creation of the primary incision. The peritoneum is identified, lifted, and opened using a 1- to 2-cm incision. The space between the anterior abdominal wall and the mass of bowel and omentum is identified.

(b) If the omentum is prominent, one can perform a local **omentectomy** by pulling out 7–10 cm of omentum and resecting it. Some advocate routine partial omentectomy at the time of catheter insertion as a means of improving long-term catheter survival (Nicholson et al, 1991).

(c) The catheter is prepared by wetting and squeezing all air bubbles out of the cuffs to promote better tissue ingrowth. It is washed with sterile normal saline, 20 mL of which is injected through it to remove particulates. It is then advanced through the incision into the peritoneal cavity by feel using an internal stylet or a large, curved, blunt clamp. The curled Tenckhoff model must be advanced over a stylet, uncoiling the catheter within the peritoneal space. With the standard Tenckhoff catheter, with the stylet held stationary, the proper location of the catheter tip should be just beneath the left inguinal ligament, between the anterior abdominal wall and the mass of omentum and bowel loops. In this location, there is less chance of functional outflow obstruction from bowel loops and omentum. Location of the catheter tip deep in the cul-de-sac of the pelvis, as originally emphasized by Tenckhoff (1974), is rarely feasible due to inadequate catheter length and if achieved will often result in pain during inflow.

(d) After proper positioning of the catheter tip, the peritoneum is closed tightly around the catheter below the level of the deep cuff using a running lock stitch. The incidence of subsequent leakage will depend largely on the care and skill used to fashion this suture line.

(e) The abdominal musculature and fascia are closed around the cuff with interrupted sutures.

(f) The skin exit site must be selected. The location can be estimated by laying the outer part of the catheter over the skin, accommodating for a V bend to direct the exit toward the patient's feet. If the catheter does not have a preformed V bend, create a gentle bend in the subcutaneous tract to direct the exit site laterally or downward. A sharply arcuate subcutaneous course of a straight catheter creates tension between the two cuffs and tends to displace the intra-abdominal portion from the pelvis. The skin exit site should be exactly 2 cm distant from the location of the superficial cuff. This distance is necessary to allow proper epithelialization of the tract down toward the superficial cuff.

(g) A tunneling tool is then passed subcutaneously from the primary incision to the skin exit site from below. The skin is nicked over the tool to create the exit site, and the catheter is pulled through the tunnel by attachment to the tunneling tool. The tunnel is widened through the primary incision with hemostats lightly attached to the catheter to facilitate passage of the superficial cuff through the tunnel to its proper position.

(2) Procedure for insertion of bead disk catheters. The same general technique is followed. The skin incision should be longer (about 4 cm) and the peritoneal incision larger (about 2 cm). The peritoneum, alone or with the posterior rectus sheath, is pulled between the bead and the disk as shown in Fig. 15-3. Placement is otherwise as already described.

b. Paramedian approach. The paramedian approach places the deep cuff at the medial border of the rectus muscle. Care must be taken to avoid transsecting the inferior epigastric or superficial epigastric artery in this approach (Fig. 15-5).

(1) Procedure. The general procedure is as described above.

2. Blind placement using the Tenckhoff trocar. This method is still used to place straight and curved Tenckhoff catheters though less frequently than other methods.

a. Procedure

(1) A 2- to 3-cm skin incision is made and blunt dissection carried out down to the fascia. A plastic tube or needle is inserted in the peritoneal cavity, which is then filled with dialysis solution as for acute catheter placement. The plastic tube is removed.

(2) The patient is asked to tense the abdomen, and the abdominal wall is penetrated in a perpendicular direction using the Tenckhoff trocar. This is a 6-mm-diameter trocar surrounded by two half-cylinders, which are, in turn, surrounded by an external housing. After insertion of the entire device, the trocar is removed, leaving the half-cylinders in place within the housing. Peritoneal fluid should now well up into the housing.

(3) An obturator is inserted into the cuffed peritoneal catheter to reinforce it, stopping 2–3 cm short of the tip, leaving the catheter with a soft, pliable, leading end. The housing is aimed caudad at the left lower quadrant, and the stiffened catheter is inserted through the housing into the abdomen until the cuff comes to rest against the narrowed "shoulder" of the half-cylinders. The cuff is now near the outer surface of the abdominal wall.

(4) The housing and half-cylinders are carefully removed from around the cuff and catheter, leaving the cuff in position next to the abdominal wall on the outer rectus sheath.

(5) Creation of the subcutaneous tunnel and exit site then proceeds as for surgical implantation.

3. Blind placement using a guide wire. This technique is a modification of that used for wire-guided placement of acute catheters and can be used to place straight or curled Tenckhoff catheters. The necessary equipment is available from the Cook Company (Bloomington, IN) or Quinton Instruments (Seattle, WA).

a.   Procedure

(1)   The abdomen is prefilled with dialysis solution as for acute catheter insertion.

(2)   The guide wire is inserted through the same needle or tubing that was used to fill the abdomen.

(3)   A dilator, jacketed in a longitudinally scored sheath, is inserted over the guide wire.

(4)   After the dilator–sheath is inserted, the dilator is removed, leaving the sheath in place.

(5)   The Tenckhoff catheter, stiffened by a partially inserted obturator, is directed down into the sheath. As the cuff advances, the sheath is split by pulling tabs on its opposing sides. Splitting the sheath allows the cuff to advance to a position next to the abdominal wall.

(6)   By further splitting and retraction, the sheath is removed from its position around the catheter.

(7)   The subcutaneous tunnel is then created, as in surgical placement.

4.   Use of the minitrocar and peritoneoscopy. This method can be used to place straight or curled Tenckhoff catheters, or, with some modifications, to place the T-fluted catheter. The necessary equipment (Y-TEC system) is available through Medigroup Inc. (Aurora, IL) (Fig. 15-6).

a.   Procedure (for Tenckhoff catheters). The steps are shown in Fig. 15-7.

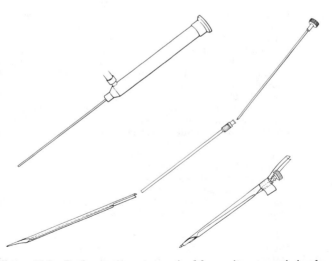

Figure 15-6.   Basic components required for peritoneoscopic implantation of a chronic peritoneal catheter, showing the stylet, the cannula, the catheter guide, and the 2-mm-diameter peritoneoscope. (Courtesy of Medigroup Inc., Aurora, IL.)

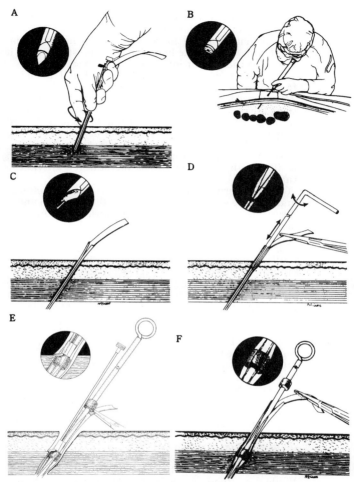

Figure 15-7. Implantation of a peritoneal catheter using the Y-TEC system and peritoneoscope. A: Initial insertion of the trocar cannula and plastic catheter guide with a rotating motion. B: After removal of the trocar, initial visual confirmation of peritoneal penetration and air insufflation (not shown). Visual examination of the abdomen locates an area relatively free from adhesions and omentum. C: The catheter guide is left in place after the peritoneoscope and cannula have been removed. D: First of the two-step dilation procedure of the catheter guide and the surrounding hole in the abdominal wall. E: Insertion of the Tenckhoff catheter through the dilated catheter guide with the cuff implanter advancing the cuff into the musculature. F: After proper placement of the deep cuff of the catheter in the musculature, the catheter guide is removed by a steady upward pull. Subsequently, the external end of the catheter is tunneled under the skin to place the superficial catheter cuff 2 cm from the exit site (Courtesy of Medigroup Inc., Aurora, IL.)

(1)   The abdomen is not prefilled with dialysis solution. The abdominal wall is first penetrated by a 2.2-mm mini-trocar (stylet) housed in a metal cannula (Fig. 15-7A). The cannula has a thin plastic guide, coiled around it in a spiral. The catheter guide has a longitudinal slit to allow it to expand radially during catheter insertion.

(2)   After penetration of the abdominal wall, the mini-trocar is removed from the cannula and replaced with the 2.2-mm peritoneoscope. When fully inserted, the sighted tip of the peritoneoscope is located just past the tip of the cannula. The IP location of the cannula tip is confirmed under direct vision by observing the motion of smooth, glistening surfaces and blood vessels during respiration.

(3)   The peritoneoscope is removed, and the abdomen is filled with 600–1,000 mL of microfiltered air via the cannula.

(4)   The peritoneoscope is reinserted into the cannula, and both are advanced together into the abdomen under direct vision (Fig. 15-7B). Bowel loops, omentum, and adhesions are identified and avoided. The clearest, longest open space is selected for catheter positioning, regardless of direction. The peritoneoscope and cannula are advanced until the cannula tip reaches the end of the selected space or until the hub of the cannula reaches the skin.

(5)   At this point, the peritoneoscope and cannula are both removed, leaving only the plastic catheter guide in place (Fig. 15-7C). Although the diameter of the longitudinally slit catheter guide is only 2.7 mm, dilation to 6 mm is performed using two dilators of graded diameter (Fig. 15-7D). The dilators are then removed, leaving the dilated catheter guide in place (Fig. 15-7E).

(6)   An obturator is inserted into the Tenckhoff catheter to stiffen it, stopping short of the catheter tip to leave the latter soft and flexible. The catheter and obturator are then inserted into the abdomen through the dilated catheter guide, until the cuff is firmly seated against the abdominal musculature (for the curled Tenckhoff, the catheter is advanced into the abdomen during intermittent retraction of the obturator).

(7)   With the obturator still in place, the cuff implanter is placed around the catheter adjacent to the deep cuff. While the catheter guide is held stationary, the cuff implanter is advanced 1 cm, bringing the deep cuff into the musculature.

(8)   The plastic catheter guide is carefully removed (Fig. 15-7F), leaving the cuff implanter, catheter cuff, and obturator in place. The obturator and, finally, the cuff implanter are then removed.

(9)   A small skin exit site incision is made with a no. 11 scalpel blade, and a tunneling tool is pushed into the skin exit site and through the primary incision. The end of the tool is attached to the outer end of the catheter, which is then pulled out through the skin exit site. Dilation of the subcutaneous tract and placement of the superficial cuff is performed as for surgical placement.

b. Procedure for placement of the T-fluted catheter.
The initial placement steps are the same as for Tenckhoff catheters, up to the step where the dilators are removed and the dilated plastic catheter guide is left in place (Fig. 15-7E). Then the T-fluted catheter, with the two limbs folded forward, is inserted into a special spiral-shaped guide that also incorporates a steel tube with wings (to aid in cuff implantation). The whole assembly is introduced through the dilated plastic catheter guide, both guides are removed, and in the process, the internal limbs open against the parietal peritoneum. For more details, see the Internet References.

5. Relative advantages and disadvantages of various methods of chronic catheter placement
a. Surgical placement. One **advantage** is that a sharp trocar or introducing needle is not used, greatly reducing the risk of bowel perforation or bleeding. Also, the catheter tip can enter the abdomen under direct vision, avoiding local adhesions. If the peritoneal incision is widened to 2 cm, the course of the catheter can sometimes be inspected. If the peritoneum and musculofascial layers are tightly closed against the catheter, the incidence of subsequent leakage can be lower than when a Tenckhoff trocar is used. The **disadvantages** of surgical placement include the requirement for more anesthesia (with subsequent risk of postoperative ileus), a larger incision relative to the other methods, higher overall cost, and difficulty scheduling an operating room.

b. Blind Tenckhoff trocar placement. The principal **advantage** is that the catheter can be placed by a nephrologist, thereby reducing delay. Also, the required equipment is relatively inexpensive. The **disadvantages** are a higher incidence of early leakage (the trocar creates a relatively large hole in the abdominal wall) and more frequent outflow obstruction due to misplacement of the catheter.

c. Blind guide wire placement. The principal **advantages** are that the catheter may be placed by a nephrologist, and early leakage is probably less than with either surgical placement or Tenckhoff trocar placement due to the relatively small hole made in the abdominal wall during insertion. One **disadvantage** is that the introducing needle may enter the abdomen in a less than optimal direction, leading the guide wire into position between bowel loops. Another is possible perforation of bowel or blood vessels by the sharp introducing needle.

d. Minitrocar peritoneoscopy (Y-TEC procedure).
The **advantages** are direct visualization of the site where the Tenckhoff catheter tip will reside and use of a small-diameter minitrocar and dilatable guide, which creates a tight fit of the abdominal wall around the Tenckhoff catheter and cuff, reducing the chance of leakage. Also, placement can be carried out by either a nephrologist or a surgeon, and it can be done in a procedure room. **Disadvantages** include the modest cost of the equipment and the need for the nephrologist or surgeon to be trained in peritoneoscopic procedures.

6.   Prophylactic antimicrobial drugs. Because the catheter is a foreign body, prophylactic antimicrobials are recommended for all methods of chronic catheter placement. A cephalosporin can be administered orally 1–2 hours before, or parenterally 30 minutes before, the procedure. After implantation, a cephalosporin may be added to the dialysis solution for the first one or two exchanges.

III.   Catheter break-in procedures. The break-in period for a peritoneal catheter is the time between catheter insertion and routine catheter use. During this period every effort is made to avoid leakage of fluid around the new catheter. Leaks not only delay ingrowth of fibrous tissue into the cuffs but also provide a medium for bacterial growth and movement, thus increasing the risk of peritonitis and exit site infection.

A.   Acute catheters. Acute catheters require no break-in, although some physicians use reduced volumes (500 mL, then 1,000 mL) for the initial four to eight exchanges before proceeding to the standard 2,000- or 2,500-mL exchange volumes. For further discussion, see Chapter 16.

B.   Chronic catheters

1.   Principles. A variety of break-in strategies for new chronic catheters have been proposed. These include:

a.   When practical, peritoneal dialysis exchanges are delayed for 2–4 weeks.

b.   At least once per week during the break-in period, heparinized saline is infused into the abdomen.

c.   When peritoneal dialysis has to be started within a week of catheter placement, the abdomen is drained and left dry for part of each day.

d.   Patient activity is initially restricted to minimize IP pressure, especially when fluid volumes are high.

e.   The patient is instructed to avoid straining and coughing during the break-in period.

The purpose of step b is to clear IP blood and fibrin from the catheter and to minimize the chances of omental adhesion. The purpose of steps a, c, d, and e is to reduce the incidence of leakage by minimizing the intra-abdominal pressure, which is highest during ambulation or straining or when the abdomen contains dialysis solution. Catheters placed and buried (the Moncrief–Popovich technique) require no break-in technique at all yet function well without omental obstruction after exteriorization.

2.   Practice. The type of break-in procedure used depends primarily on whether peritoneal dialysis is needed for treatment and support of the patient at the time of catheter insertion.

a.   For a patient requiring immediate, intensive dialysis. In this situation, a break-in period is not feasible unless temporary hemodialysis is used. However, because such a patient is usually on bed rest, the intra-abdominal pressure rise during filling is limited, and leakage is not usually a problem. Some nephrologists set the exchange volume at 500 mL for the first four exchanges, 1,000 mL for the next four, and then proceed to the desired exchange volume, if tolerated. Others proceed directly to 2,000-mL exchanges in patients who are supine and inactive. Heparin (500 units per L) is added to each solution bag for the first few exchanges. Once the need for acute dialysis has subsided, break-in can be instituted according to the most appropriate option described below.

b. For a patient requiring maintenance dialysis, already trained for continuous ambulatory peritoneal dialysis (CAPD)

(1) First 24 hours. Immediately after insertion, 2 L of 1.5% dextrose dialysis solution containing 500 units per L heparin is infused and immediately drained.

(2) Days 2–14 (or longer). Manual or automated nocturnal intermittent peritoneal dialysis (NIPD) is begun using a schedule such as the following: three exchanges per 24 hours, using 2-L volumes: First inflow at 6 p.m., exchange at 9 p.m., another exchange at 11 p.m., outflow in the morning. The abdomen is left dry during the day. Activity is forbidden while the abdomen contains dialysis solution.

3. For a patient requiring maintenance dialysis, not yet trained for CAPD

a. First 24 hours. Same as described in Section b(1) above.

b. Days 2–14 (or longer). There are three options:

(1) NIPD using a cycler. Heparin optional, exchange volume normally 2 L, three to five exchanges during the night. Drain in morning, and leave abdomen dry during the day.

(2) Intermittent peritoneal dialysis. Rapid exchanges in a dialysis unit using a cycler for 8–12 hours, 3 days per week.

(3) Hemodialysis. Performed as needed using a temporary vascular access. At least weekly, an in–out exchange is performed using 1 L of normal saline containing 500 units per L heparin.

c. For a patient not yet requiring maintenance dialysis

(1) First 24 hours. Same as b(1) above.

(2) Day 2 until the start of maintenance dialysis. At least once per week, perform an in–out exchange (zero dwell time) using 1 L of sterile saline solution containing 500 units per L heparin.

IV. Complications of peritoneal catheters. The three major catheter-related complications are pericatheter leak, outflow failure, and infection of the exit site or tunnel. With Tenckhoff double-cuff catheters, these complications occur with incidence rates of 7%, 17%, and 14% of insertions, respectively, during the first year. These complications are significant problems with other peritoneal catheters as well. Peritoneoscopically placed catheters have a lower incidence of these complications (Gadallah et al, 1999).

A. Pericatheter leak. These usually present in the first weeks after insertion but may not become apparent until after the patient begins CAPD. In addition to overt leakage at the skin exit site, leaks may manifest more subtly as asymmetrical subcutaneous swelling and edema, weight gain, and diminished outflow volume. The risk of leakage is increased if there is little or no break-in period. Management of leaks is discussed in Chapter 20.

B. Outflow failure. Outflow failure is usually detected when the drainage volume is substantially less than the inflow volume and there is no evidence of pericatheter leakage. It usually occurs soon after catheter placement, but it may also commence during or after an episode of peritonitis, or at any time during the life of the catheter. Outflow failure is often preceded by irregular drainage, increased fibrin in the dialysate, or constipation.

There are several approaches to treatment, which vary according to whether peritonitis is present. The management strategy includes the following:

1. Check for kinking. Kinking of the catheter in the subcutaneous tunnel sometimes occurs with double-cuff catheters when the cuffs have been implanted too close to each other. Obstruction due to kinking usually becomes apparent soon after catheter placement. Functional obstruction is present during both inflow and outflow. The degree of obstruction may be variable, depending on patient position. Pressing the subcutaneous tunnel may increase flow.

Management consists of catheter replacement or removal of the superficial cuff. The latter can be accomplished as described in Section IV.D.1, below.

2. Treatment of constipation. Constipation due to decreased bowel motility is a common cause of outflow obstruction. Thus, a logical early step in treatment of outflow obstruction is to administer a laxative (either a single 10-mg bisacodyl suppository or two 5-mg bisacodyl tablets). If necessary, these may be repeated or a saline enema can be given. Laxatives containing magnesium and enemas containing phosphate, such as the Fleet enema, should be avoided in renal failure patients. After a bowel movement is achieved, outflow is again attempted. Correction of constipation resolves approximately 50% of catheter outflow obstructions.

3. Heparin. Heparin should be added to peritoneal fluid (250–500 units per L) whenever plugs or strands of fibrin are visible in the outflow fluid. Heparin is more useful prophylactically than therapeutically; once outflow obstruction is established, irrigation of the catheter with heparin is often unsuccessful in relieving the obstruction.

4. Thrombolytic agents. If heparin is ineffective, the next step is to try a thrombolytic agent. Tissue plasminogen activator and streptokinase are both available. Urokinase is temporarily not available in the United States, but the imminent availability of recombinant urokinase is anticipated. Streptokinase is the least expensive but entails a slight risk of inducing an anaphylactic reaction. Protocols for using these agents are in Table 15-1.

5. Catheter reposition. If obstruction is not relieved by any of the above techniques, it is likely to be due to attachment of omentum or other tissues to the catheter tip. Catheters that have migrated and show poor outflow are usually tightly attached to omentum, and it is this rather than the actual migration that is the principal cause of the outflow obstruction.

Table 15–1.   Protocols for streptokinase, urokinase, or tissue plasminogen activator infusion for treatment of peritoneal catheter outflow obstruction

A. Streptokinase

1. *Testing for streptokinase allergy.* Because of the slight risk of an anaphylactic reaction, a scratch test, followed by an intradermal test, should be performed prior to IP infusion. A 100 IU/mL solution is prepared. After the skin has been scratched with a 25-gauge needle, a drop of solution is placed over the scratch. If no wheal and flare appear within 15 min, then 0.1 mL of the same solution is injected intradermally. If no wheal and flare appear, then IgE-mediated allergy to streptokinase is unlikely (Dykewicz et al, 1986).

2. *Infusion protocol.* Streptokinase is available as a lyophilized powder in both 250,000-and 750,000-IU vials. We reconstitute 750,000 IU (with sterile saline), dilute it to 30–100 mL in 0.9% saline, inject the total volume into the peritoneal catheter, clamp the catheter, wait 2 hrs and assess drainage. If drainage is still poor, repeat the protocol once.

B. Urokinase

Urokinase is available as a lyophilized powder in vials containing 250,000 IU (reconstitute using sterile water) and also in liquid form as vials of 5000 IU/mL. Both 75,000 IU diluted to 40 mL in 0.9% saline and 5,000 IU diluted to 40 mL in 0.9% saline, injected into the peritoneal catheter as described above for streptokinase, have been used successfully. As in the case of streptokinase, the treatment can be repeated if initially unsuccessful, using a larger dose of urokinase if desired.

C. Tissue plasminogen activator

Introduction into the catheter lumen of a concentration of 1 mg/mL for a period of 1 or more hours has been effective (Sahani et al, 2000).

The position of the Tenckhoff catheter tip can be determined by an abdominal radiograph and should vary less than 4 cm in 1 month. All recently manufactured catheters incorporate a radiopaque stripe. If the catheter does not have such a stripe, a very low x-ray dose will allow visualization of a plain silicone catheter.

Whether or not the catheter has migrated, the next step in the attempt to relieve obstruction is to move the catheter to a different location in the abdomen, in the process attempting to free it of its omental attachments. There are three methods of moving the catheter: (a) blind techniques (radiographic monitoring is desirable but not essential), (b) peritoneoscopic techniques, and (c) surgical "stripping."

   a.   Blind or fluoroscopic techniques. These are feasible with nonarcuate Tenckhoff catheters. The abdomen, if not already distended, is filled with dialysis solution. The patient is premedicated because IP manipulation of a catheter is often painful. A sterile, malleable metal rod, bent into a curve to facilitate passage through the catheter, is advanced to within 4 cm of the catheter tip. Using the skin site as a fulcrum, the catheter is rotated gently until the distal tip lies in another IP location. The function of the catheter in the new position can be tested by infusing and draining heparinized saline or dialysis solution.

Even though the catheter can be moved by this technique, breaking omental adhesions to the catheter is difficult, and catheter outflow is restored only about 30% of the time.

b.   Reposition using peritoneoscopy. Microfiltered air (about 600 mL) is insufflated into the abdomen through the obstructed Tenckhoff catheter, which is then clamped. Using the Y-TEC minitrocar and plastic catheter guide, the abdomen is punctured about 5 cm from the malfunctioning catheter. Ideally, the puncture site position is such that it would be appropriate for a new catheter so that, if repositioning of the existing catheter is unsuccessful, a new one can be placed through this puncture site. The minitrocar is removed and the IP position of the cannula is confirmed by insertion of the peritoneoscope. The catheter and attached omentum are inspected. A sterile, malleable, curved metal rod (such as a Foley catheter guide) is inserted into the catheter, which is then moved to a location free of adhesions, under observation through the peritoneoscope. If the catheter cannot be freed from the attached omentum, it should be manipulated under vision, by advancing the peritoneoscope underneath the catheter, between the adhesion and the peritoneal penetration point, and rotating it into the contralateral quadrant while avoiding contact of its tip with visceral or parietal peritoneum. This movement displaces the catheter and attached omentum. The catheter is then reinspected to determine its position and to ascertain if the omentum has been removed. In our experience, reposition using peritoneoscopy is successful in relieving outflow obstruction about 50% of the time, with the best results being reported for straight Tenckhoff catheters. If repositioning is unsuccessful, a new catheter can be placed through the catheter guide that was inserted along with the minitrocar, as already described, and the old dysfunctional catheter can then be removed.

c.   Surgical stripping of the catheter. It is possible surgically to remove omentum from a catheter while leaving the catheter in place. Under general anesthesia, a 3- to 5-cm incision is made in the midline or next to the site of the deep cuff. The catheter is identified and attached omentum is removed, using a specially designed stripping tool if desired. Performing a local omentectomy at the same time diminishes the chances of reocclusion.

6.   Catheter replacement. These strategies fail in more than 20% of cases of catheter outflow obstruction. The only remaining option is to surgically remove the obstructed catheter and replace it with a new one.

7.   Treating peritonitis. Outflow obstruction is sometimes a consequence of acute peritonitis. Peritonitis changes the management of outflow obstruction for several reasons. In such instances, obstruction is unlikely to be due to kinking or constipation. Manipulation of the catheter can be especially painful and should not be tried until the infection is under control. Finally, rapid correction of catheter obstruction is desirable because IP administration of antimicrobials is preferable when treating peritoneal dialysis–associated peritonitis, especially during the initial few days. The following management plan is proposed:

a. Infuse a loading dose of antimicrobials IP (see Chapter 19) mixed with dialysis solution. The volume of solution given should depend on the degree of abdominal distention. Also, add 1,000 units of heparin to the initial exchange and after any exchange in which fibrin is seen.

b. Infuse streptokinase, urokinase, or tissue plasminogen activator as described in Table 15-1.

c. If adequate outflow is not established within 24 hours (after two infusions of thrombolytic agent), place an acute peritoneal catheter, or a second chronic catheter, by peritoneoscopy (with or without an attempt at reposition). Treat peritonitis promptly with IP antimicrobials. Add heparin 500 units per L to all subsequent exchanges. The obstructed chronic catheter can be left in place if tunnel infection is not present.

d. After 2–3 days, when symptoms have subsided and fluid is clearing, if an acute catheter was inserted it should be removed. Repositioning of the chronic catheter can then be attempted using either fluoroscopy or peritoneoscopy to guide the manipulation, but a low success rate should be anticipated. If function of the original catheter can be restored, continue to treat peritonitis as usual. If repositioning fails and fluid is clear or nearly clear, catheter removal and placement of a new catheter can be performed in the same operative setting.

e. If peritonitis fails to clear in 2 or 3 days, or if fungal or pseudomonal organisms are cultured, remove the peritoneal dialysis catheter (see Chapter 19).

C. Catheter infection

1. Exit site infection. This presents as redness, swelling, and tenderness at the exit site, somtimes with a large amount of crusting or purulent exudate. Treatment is discussed in Chapter 19.

2. Tunnel infection. Tunnel infection can present as an extension of skin exit-site infection, with pain, swelling, nodularity, and redness over the subcutaneous portion of the catheter. Systemic signs, such as fever, may also be present. Alternatively, tunnel infection can result in "relapsing" peritonitis caused by the same organism. It may be visualized on high-frequency ultrasonography as a lucent space around the outer cuff or tunnel of the catheter. Management of tunnel infection is discussed in Chapter 19.

D. Other complications related to peritoneal catheters. Other catheter-related complications include cuff erosion, pain on dialysis solution inflow, and abdominal wall hernias.

1. Cuff erosion. The superficial cuff can erode through the skin because of exit site infection or because it initially was located too close to the skin exit site. Late erosion of the superficial cuff can also occur if the deep cuff separates from the abdominal musculature. The entire catheter can then be extruded outward, pushing the superficial cuff through the skin. Treatment consists of removal of the superficial cuff, which should be done as soon as inflammation appears around the cuff. This is done by anesthetizing the exit site, widening it with a scalpel, and separating the cuff from the subcutaneous tissues. The cuff is then trimmed with a cold-sterilized safety razor and a forceps is used to remove the fragments. A double-cuff catheter is thus converted to single-cuff. If subcutaneous tunnel infection subsequently becomes apparent, the catheter must be removed.

2. Pain during dialysis solution inflow. This common symptom may be related to the low dialysis solution pH, to abnormally high dialysis solution temperature, to omental attachment to the catheter, or to pressure created in a neighboring structure (rectum, vagina, spermatic cord) during inflow. The last two causes are the most common, and catheter reposition is often required to cure the condition.

a. Addition of alkali to the dialysis solution. Alteration of dialysis solution pH by addition of sodium hydroxide or sodium bicarbonate can sometimes reduce inflow pain. The titratable acidity in most dialysis solutions is between 1 and 2 mmol per L. Addition of an equivalent amount of sodium hydroxide will neutralize the dialysis solution pH to 7.0, but this is not commercially available in sterile, pyrogen-free form. Also, addition of excess sodium hydroxide can quickly raise the dialysis solution pH to very alkaline values, and the final pH should be verified before infusion.

b. Addition of sterile, pyrogen-free sodium bicarbonate to the dialysis solution (Henderson et al, 1986) is more convenient. The titratable acid in the dialysis solution reacts with some of the bicarbonate added to generate PCO_2, which acts to increase the acidity of the dialysis solution, so limiting the rise in pH. Thus, addition of the usual amount of bicarbonate (4–5 mEq per L) does not neutralize the pH of the dialysis solution completely, but overalkalinization is avoided. If bicarbonate is added to the dialysis solution, increased transfer of base to the patient should be anticipated. In the near future, bicarbonate-based solutions may become available commercially and facilitate the management of this problem.

3. Abdominal hernias. These are discussed in Chapter 20.

V. Care of peritoneal catheters. The exit site and related incisions should be cared for in the same manner as other fresh surgical wounds. For the first few days after placement, the exit site should be covered by gauze bandages and the bandages changed whenever they are noted to be discolored by exudate or blood. Occlusive, air-impermeable coverings should never be used, nor should ointments. The dressing should immobilize the catheter against the skin.

The patient should be instructed to avoid catheter movement at the exit site as much as possible because movement delays healing and can lead to infection. When necessary, the catheter can be anchored to the skin at a second site to minimize motion at the exit site. As the patient begins to care for the catheter, bandage changes may be made less frequently. After a few weeks, the catheter exit site may be left unprotected and open to the air, but it is generally preferable to cover it with a gauze dressing to minimize irritation. The optimal method of exit site care is controversial. By 1–2 months after insertion, we believe that the least exit site treatment is the best. However, one randomized study showed that thrice-weekly applications of a povidone–iodine solution followed by a dry gauze dressing reduced exit site infection compared with a daily wash with nonbacterial soap (Luzar et al, 1991). Training patients to observe their catheters regularly for signs of exit site and tunnel infection is important. The role of *Staphylococcus aureus* nasal carriage and exit site infection is discussed in Chapter 19.

CAPD patients may shower a few weeks after catheter placement if the catheter site is well sealed. The exit site should be dried thoroughly after a shower. Baths are also allowed if the catheter exit site is only briefly wetted. Patients typically are not permitted to swim. The risk of infection increases with the bacterial count of the water.

VI. Catheter removal and replacement

A. Acute catheters. As noted above, acute uncuffed catheters should be removed within 3, or at most 4, days of insertion. After the abdomen has been drained and the sutures removed, the catheter is gently pulled out. It is best to let the peritoneum rest for a day or so before inserting a new acute catheter, if possible. The replacement catheter should be inserted at least 2–3 cm from the original site, preferably alternating medial and lateral locations.

B. Chronic catheters. Chronic catheters that have been in place for more than 3 months should be removed by surgical dissection in either an outpatient surgical suite or an operating room. Removal of catheters with IP disks or with a bead disk at the deep cuff is more complicated, and the procedure is best done in a well-equipped surgical facility. The defect left in the abdominal wall after removal of the catheter should be repaired carefully to avoid subsequent hernia or leakage. A T-fluted catheter is removed by traction after first freeing the deep cuff from the musculature.

SELECTED READINGS

Ash SR. Chronic peritoneal dialysis catheters: effects of catheter design, material, and location. *Semin Dial* 1990;3:39.

Ash SR, et al. Clinical trials of the Ash Advantage peritoneal dialysis catheter. *Perit Dial Int* 2000;20:S46.

Ash SR. Peritoneal access devices for intraperitoneal chemotherapy. In: Sugarbaker PH, ed. *Peritoneal carcinomatosis: principles of management.* Boston: Kluwer Academic, 1996.

Ash SR. Peritoneal access devices and placement techniques. In: Nissenson AR, Fine RN, eds. *Dialysis therapy,* 2nd ed. St Louis: Mosby–Year Book, 1993.

Ash SR, et al. Peritoneoscopic placement of the Tenckhoff catheter: further clinical experience. *Perit Dial Bull* 1983;3:8.

Ash SR, Janle EM. T-fluted peritoneal dialysis catheter. *Adv Perit Dial* 1993;9:223–226.

Ash SR, Nichols WK. Placement, repair and removal of chronic peritoneal catheters. In: Gokal R, Nolph KD, eds. *Textbook of peritoneal dialysis.* Boston: Kluwer Academic, 1994.

Chadha V, et al. Tenckhoff catheters prove superior to cook catheters in pediatric acute peritoneal dialysis. *Am J Kidney Dis* 2000;35: 1111–1116.

Degesys GE, et al. Tenckhoff peritoneal dialysis catheters: the use of fluoroscopy in management. *Radiology* 1985;154:819–820.

Diaz-Buxo JA, et al. Single cuff versus double cuff Tenckhoff catheter. *Perit Dial Bull* 1984;4:S100.

Dykewicz MS, et al. Identification of patients at risk for anaphylaxis due to streptokinase. *Arch Intern Med* 1986;146:305–307.

Gadallah MF, et al. Peritoneoscopic versus surgical placement of peritoneal dialysis catheters: a prospective randomized study on outcome. *Am J Kidney Dis* 1999;33:118–122.

Gokal R, et al. Peritoneal catheters and exit-site practices: towards optimal peritoneal access. *Perit Dial Int* 1993;13:29–39.

Henderson IS, et al. Potentially irritant glucose metabolites in unused CAPD fluid. In: Maher JF, Winchester JF, eds. *Frontiers in peritoneal dialysis.* New York: Field, Rich & Associates, 1986.

Luzar MA, et al. Exit-site infection in continuous ambulatory peritoneal dialysis: a review. *Perit Dial Int* 1991;11:44.

Moncrief JW, et al. The Moncrief–Popovich catheter: a new peritoneal access technique for patients on peritoneal dialysis. *ASAIO J* 1993; 39:62–65.

Nicholson ML, et al. The role of omentectomy in continuous ambulatory peritoneal dialysis. *Perit Dial Int* 1991;11:330–332.

Park MS, et al. Effect of prolonged subcutaneous implantation of peritoneal catheter on peritonitis rate during CAPD: a prospective, randomized study. *Blood Purif* 1998;16:171–178.

Parsoo I, et al. Urokinase infusion for obstructed catheter in CAPD. *Perit Dial Bull* 1986;6:105.

Prischl FC, et al. Initial subcutaneous embedding of the peritoneal dialysis catheter: a critical appraisal of this new implantation technique. *Nephrol Dial Transplant* 1997;12:1661–1667.

Sahani MM, et al. Tissue plasminogen activator can effectively declot peritoneal dialysis catheters [Letter]. *Am J Kidney Dis* 2000;36:in press.

Song JH, et al. Clinical outcomes of immediate full-volume exchange one year after peritoneal catheter implantation for CAPD. *Perit Dial Int* 2000;20:194–199.

Tenckhoff H, et al. *Chronic peritoneal dialysis: a manual for patients, dialysis personnel and physicians.* Seattle: University of Washington School of Medicine Press, 1974.

Twardowski ZJ, et al. Long-term experience with swan neck Missouri catheters. *ASAIO Trans* 1990;36:M491–M494.

Twardowski ZJ, et al. Six-year experience with swan neck presternal peritoneal dialysis catheter. *Perit Dial Int* 1998;18:598–602.

Wiegmann TB, et al. Effective use of streptokinase for peritoneal catheter failure. *Am J Kidney Dis* 1985;6:119–123.

Zappacosta AR, et al. Seldinger technique for Tenckhoff catheter placement. *ASAIO Trans* 1991;37:13–15.

Internet Reference

Peritoneal catheter trials, insertion methods (http://www.hdcn.com/pd/cath)

Acute Peritoneal Dialysis Prescription

Stephen M. Korbet and Nouhad O. Kronfol

I. Introduction. Acute peritoneal dialysis provides the nephrologist with a nonvascular alternative for dialysis. Peritoneal dialysis, like other continuous renal replacement therapies used in the intensive care setting, is acutely less efficient than conventional hemodialysis; however, because of its continuous nature, its efficiency may ultimately be comparable or superior to that of hemodialysis (depending on the hemodialysis regimen being used) in the management of acute renal failure, as well as toxic/metabolic, electrolyte, or volume problems in critically ill patients.

A. Advantages. The performance of peritoneal dialysis is technically simpler than that of hemodialysis or other forms of continuous renal replacement therapy, as peritoneal dialysis does not require highly trained personnel or expensive, complex equipment. As a result, peritoneal dialysis can be instituted quickly. Acute peritoneal dialysis is usually performed manually but can be done with the assistance of a cycler (see below). It avoids the potential problems related to vascular access (hemorrhage, air embolism, thrombosis, infection) and does not require anticoagulation. The gradual but continuous nature of the procedure results in effective removal of fluid and solute with less hemodynamic instability. Lack of a blood–hemodialyzer interaction and the lower likelihood of hypotensive episodes may lessen ongoing insults to the already acutely damaged kidneys.

B. Disadvantages. Peritoneal dialysis is less efficient than hemodialysis in the treatment of acute problems (i.e., flash pulmonary edema, poisonings or drug overdose, and hyperkalemia) and may not be the dialytic therapy of choice for extremely catabolic patients when daily hemodialysis or continuous renal replacement therapy is feasible. Protein losses can be substantial in peritoneal dialysis and could complicate the care of already malnourished, critically ill patients. Serious morbidity (30%) and mortality (5%) attributed to the use of acute peritoneal dialysis and hemodialysis are similar.

C. Indications. Acute peritoneal dialysis is most often used in the setting of acute renal failure, but it is also beneficial in the control of volume overload states in patients with cardiovascular compromise, such as those with congestive heart failure, and in the treatment of hypothermia or hemorrhagic pancreatitis (where peritoneal lavage may be beneficial). It is most beneficial in the treatment of hemodynamically unstable patients or patients in whom vascular access is problematical.

D. Contraindications. There are few absolute contraindications to the use of peritoneal dialysis, but the most obvious are recent surgery requiring abdominal drains; known fecal or fungal peritonitis (the catheter acts as a foreign body, delaying therapeutic response); and a known pleuro-peritoneal fistula. Relative contraindications for peritoneal dialysis include abdominal wall cellulitis (may lead to peritonitis), adynamic ileus (results in technical problems that decrease the efficiency of peritoneal dialysis), and a new aortic prosthesis (may result in infection of the prosthesis). The presence of abdominal adhesions or fibrosis is often considered a relative contraindication as it decreases the efficiency of peritoneal dialysis. Peritoneal dialysis can complicate the care of patients with underlying respiratory failure as it may mechanically interfere with respiration and may increase the production of carbon dioxide resulting from the metabolism of absorbed glucose.

II. Peritoneal catheter. For many patients, such as those with multiorgan system failure, a prolonged period of renal failure can be anticipated, and initial insertion of a Tenckhoff catheter (rather than use of an uncuffed temporary catheter, which will have to be replaced after 3 days) is recommended. If a shorter course is expected or if peritoneal dialysis must be started before such a catheter can be placed, a temporary stylet catheter is a reasonable choice (see Chapter 15).

III. Use of automated cyclers. Acute peritoneal dialysis has traditionally been done using manual exchanges. Automated cyclers can be used instead, with considerable savings in nursing time, especially when a short (30–60 minutes) exchange time is required. However, temporary peritoneal catheters sometimes function erratically with cyclers, triggering the cycler alarm system and causing frequent interruptions of dialysis. Tenckhoff catheters are preferable in this setting.

IV. Prescribing acute peritoneal dialysis

A. Session length. In the setting of acute renal failure, continuous removal of fluids and solutes is required in a patient who often is catabolic, oliguric, and in need of ongoing nutritional and therapeutic support. This commonly results in the need for hourly exchanges on a continuous basis for days or weeks. As the dialysis requirements of a patient may change from day to day, it is prudent to write peritoneal dialysis orders for only 24 hours at a time, reassessing and altering the prescription as indicated. A standardized form with "Acute Peritoneal Dialysis Orders" is helpful in assuring that the specifications of the procedure are complete and clear for the nursing staff responsible for its delivery (Table 16-1).

B. Exchange volume. Choice of exchange volume is dictated primarily by the size of the peritoneal cavity. An average-sized adult can usually tolerate 2-L exchanges, but in smaller patients, those with pulmonary disease (in whom a large exchange volume might contribute to respiratory difficulty), and those with abdominal wall or inguinal hernias, the exchange volume should be reduced.

Initiating acute peritoneal dialysis with a 2-L exchange volume is standard. However, after the placement of a peritoneal dialysis catheter, some nephrologists prefer to start with smaller volumes (1–1.5 L) for the first few exchanges in the hope of minimizing the risk of leaks. Otherwise, one should not reduce the exchange volume without good reason as the larger the volume is, the greater the clearance and ultrafiltration rates that can

Table 16–1. Acute peritoneal dialysis orders

PERITONEAL DIALYSIS ORDERS
A. Nursing orders:
  1. Dialysis to run _____ hours
  2. Exchange volume: _____ L
  3. Warm dialysis fluid to 37°C.
  4. Exchange time: Inflow 10 minutes
              Dwell _____ minutes
              Outflow 20 minutes or as long as fluid
              drains freely
              DO NOT LEAVE FLUID IN ABDOMEN
  3. Strict intake and output to be kept on fluid intake–output record.
  4. Dialysate balance to be recorded on peritoneal dialysis record.
  5. Dialysis fluid running balance to be maintained at: _____ L.
  7. Dialysate solution: _____%
  8. Additives to dialysate:
     Medication   Dose   Frequency
     _____   _____ /2L   q exchange **or** x _____ exchanges
     _____   _____ /2L   q exchange **or** x _____ exchanges
  9. Heparin: 1,000 units/2 L q exchange: yes/no
  10. Turn and position patient p.r.n. for optimum outflow.
  11. Vital signs q _____ hours
  12. Catheter care and dressing change qod.
  13. Withdraw 15 mL dialysis fluid from catheter port q AM during dialysis and send for cell count with differential, and culture and sensitivity: yes/no
B. Blood draw orders:
  1. BUN, creatinine, HCO_3, Na, K, Cl, and glucose 8 AM and 6 PM each day during dialysis
C. Notify physician immediately for:
  1. Poor dialysate flow
  2. Severe abdominal pain or distention
  3. Bright red blood or cloudy dialysate drain
  4. Dialysate leak or purulent drainage around catheter exit site
  5. Blood pressure of less than _____ mm Hg systolic
  6. Respiration rate of greater than _____ /min, or severe shortness of breath
  7. Temperature of greater than _____ °C
  8. Two consecutive positive exchanges
  9. Single positive exchange balance (dialysate-IN *minus* dialysate-OUT) of ≥1,000 mL
  10. If negative balance exceeds _____ L over _____ hours

be achieved. In large or very catabolic patients, an exchange volume of 2.5–3 L may be required (if tolerated) to augment the efficiency of dialysis.

 C. Exchange time. This is the combined time required for inflow, dwell, and drain. To maximize dialysis efficiency in acute peritoneal dialysis, the exchange time most commonly used is 1 hour, although 2-hour exchange times also are commonly used in patients who are not overly catabolic.

  1. Inflow time. Inflow is by gravity and usually requires about 10 minutes (200 mL per minute). Inflow time is dictated by the volume to be infused and the height of the dialysis solution above the patient's abdomen. It may be prolonged due to kinking of the tubing or increased inflow resistance by intra-abdominal tissues in close proximity to the catheter tip. On initiation of acute peritoneal dialysis, some patients may experience pain or cramping with inflow of dialysis solution. This may result from the hypertonic and acidic nature of the peritoneal dialysis fluid or distention of tissues around the catheter by rapidly inflowing fluid. These problems often improve with time but when severe may be relieved by slowing the dialysate inflow rate for several exchanges. Otherwise, inflow time should be kept to a minimum to maximize dialysis efficiency. Cold dialysate solution also results in discomfort, and for this reason, the solution should be warmed to 37°C before infusion.

  2. Dwell time. The dwell period is the time during which the total exchange volume is present in the peritoneal cavity (i.e., the time from the end of inflow to the beginning of outflow).

   a. Standard dwell period. When initiating peritoneal dialysis in acutely ill and catabolic patients, the usual dwell time is 30 minutes to achieve an exchange time of 60 minutes. With a 2-L exchange volume, 48 L of fluid will thus be exchanged daily. Given a peritoneal membrane with average transport characteristics, the urea concentration in the drained dialysate will be approximately 50%–60% of that in the plasma (D/P ratio of 0.5–0.6 at 1 hour) (see Fig. 13–6). Thus, with an aggressive dialysis exchange rate of 2 L per hour, the plasma urea clearance could approximate 24–29 L per day (0.5–0.6 × 48 L per day), or 168–202 L per week. This is at the lower end of the clearances normally obtained with blood-based CRRT therapies (see Chapter 10).

   b. Dwell period for more stable patients. If the patient is not extremely catabolic, a longer dwell time (e.g., 1.5–5 hours) can often be used. With a 4-hour exchange time (dwell time 3.5 hours), the dialysate urea concentration is, on average, 90% of that in the plasma (D/P ratio of 0.9 at 4 hours). This leads to a plasma urea clearance of at least 11 L per day (0.9 × 12 L per day), or 77 L per week. In terms of weekly $(K \times t)$ / V, the weekly clearance of 77 L is the $(K \times t)$ term. For a 72 kg patient with a V of 38 L, weekly $(K \times t)$ / V would be 77/38 or 2.0.

  3. Outflow time. Outflow of spent dialysate is by gravity and usually requires 20–30 minutes. Outflow time depends on the total volume to be drained, the resistance to outflow, and the difference in height between the patient's abdomen and the drainage bag. In many patients, particularly those with large abdomens, the first exchange may not drain completely (often only 1–1.5 L is retrieved) due to initial filling of poorly draining areas of the abdomen. As long as marked abdominal distention is not present, a second exchange of 2 L can be cautiously instilled. Subsequent drainage usually proceeds normally. If outflow continues to be poor, then outflow obstruction should be managed according to the guidelines described in Chapter 15. Pain during outflow is unusual, but localized pain may occasionally be noted at the end of a drain due to a siphoning effect of the catheter on the peritoneum.

D. Choosing the dialysis solution dextrose concentration

1. Standard 1.5% dextrose (glucose monohydrate). This concentration of dextrose [approximately 1,360 mg glucose per dL (75 mmol per L)] will exert an osmotic force sufficient to remove 50–150 mL fluid per hour when using a 2-L exchange volume and a 60-minute exchange time (Table 16-2). That is, the volume drained exceeds the volume instilled by 50–150 mL. (The mechanism of osmotic ultrafiltration during peritoneal dialysis is discussed in Chapters 13 and 18.) This ultrafiltration rate translates into fluid removal of 1.2–3.6 L per day.

2. Higher concentrations of dextrose. Greater fluid removal can be achieved with higher dextrose concentrations (Table 16-2). A 4.25% dextrose solution can result in an ultrafiltration rate of 300–400 mL per hour. Acutely, this degree of fluid removal can be required for the treatment of congestive heart failure. However, continued use of the 4.25% solution could theoretically result in the removal of 7.2–9.6 L per day and cause marked hypernatremia. In practice, this degree of fluid removal is not often required. Available dextrose solutions used alone or in combination (i.e., either 1.5% or 2.5% exchanges used continuously or some combination of 1.5% and 4.25% exchanges) can be adjusted to provide the level of ultrafiltration desired. Once the patient is euvolemic, one can resume using 1.5% solution for all exchanges.

Table 16–2. Estimated ultrafiltrate volume during acute peritoneal dialysis

Dextrose[a]		Glucose			Osmolarity[b]	Ultrafiltrate Volume[c]	
g/dL	mg/dL	g/dL	mg/dL	mOsm/L	(mOsm/L)	mL/exchange	L/d
1.5	1,500	1.36	1,360	76	346	50–150	1.2–3.6
2.5	2,500	2.27	2,270	126	396	100–300	2.4–7.2
4.25	4,250	3.86	3,860	215	485	300–400	7.2–9.6

[a] Glucose monohydrate, weighing 10% more than anhydrous glucose.
[b] Solution osmolarity = electrolyte osmolarity (270 mOsm/L) + glucose osmolarity.
[c] 2-L exchange volume, 60 min exchange time.

3. When very rapid fluid removal is required. The osmotic effect of a high-dextrose dialysis solution diminishes rapidly as the glucose is absorbed and as the glucose concentration is further diluted by fluid movement into the peritoneal space. Thus, high-dextrose dialysis solution is most effective during the initial 15–30 minutes. Occasionally, a patient in severe pulmonary edema will require very rapid fluid removal. Such patients can be treated initially with two or three in–out (zero dwell time) 2-L exchanges of 4.25% solution. Each exchange will still remove approximately 300 mL of fluid, so that almost 1 L may be removed over a 1-hour period.

4. Effect of peritonitis. During peritonitis, inflammation of the peritoneum leads to enhanced absorption of glucose from the dialysate, rapidly reducing the osmotic gradient. In such patients, maintaining the efficiency of ultrafiltration may require that the exchange time be reduced and/or that more hypertonic exchanges (2.5% or 4.25%) be used.

E. Dialysis solution additives. When injecting any additive into dialysis solution containers, meticulous sterile technique must be followed in order to prevent bacterial contamination of the dialysis solution and peritonitis.

1. Potassium. Standard peritoneal dialysis solutions contain no potassium, but when the patient is hypokalemic, potassium chloride (3.5–4 mEq per L) can be added. Even in normokalemic patients, failure to add potassium chloride may result in hypokalemia (especially with 60-minute exchanges) if the patient's total-body potassium content is normal or low and the oral intake is poor. It must also be remembered that glucose absorption and correction of acidosis with peritoneal dialysis promotes a shift of extracellular potassium into cells, lowering the serum concentration. If moderate to severe metabolic acidosis is being corrected, addition of even 4 mEq per L of potassium to dialysis solutions may not prevent hypokalemia, and parenteral supplementation may be required.

2. Heparin. Sluggish dialysate flow from catheter obstruction by fibrin clots may occasionally be seen in acute peritoneal dialysis. This is usually a result of the slight bleeding that may accompany catheter insertion or irritation of the peritoneum by the catheter. Heparin (1,000 units per 2 L) added to the dialysis solution can be helpful in preventing or treating this problem. Because heparin is not absorbed through the peritoneum, there is no increased risk of bleeding.

3. Insulin. Because glucose is absorbed from the dialysis solution, supplemental insulin administration may be required for the diabetic patient undergoing acute peritoneal dialysis. Regular insulin may be added to the dialysis solution (Table 16-3) before infusion. The blood glucose level must be monitored closely, and the dose of insulin tailored to the needs of the patient. To minimize the risk of hypoglycemia after di-alysis has been stopped, insulin should not be added to the last exchange of a treatment session.

4. Antibiotics. Intraperitoneal administration of antibiotics is efficient and provides an alternative route for patients with poor vascular access and for those with peritonitis (see Chapter 19). Intraperitoneal administration or more

Table 16–3. Insulin addition to peritoneal dialysis solutions

Dialysate Dextrose Conc. (%)	Amount of Regular Insulin to Add (Units/2 L)
1.5	8–10
2.5	10–14
4.25	14–20

frequent IV or PO dosing may be required for antibiotics (e.g., aminoglycosides) whose clearances are enhanced by peritoneal dialysis (see Chapter 28).

V. Monitoring fluid balance. Monitoring fluid balance during acute peritoneal dialysis can be difficult. However, it is important to maintain an accurate flow sheet of all fluid intake and output (Table 16-4) to determine not only the adequacy of dialysate drainage during each exchange but the patient's overall fluid balance as well. Weighing the patient daily is helpful but should be done in the same phase of the fill–drain cycle (preferably at the end of drainage). Because neither the fluid balance nor the weight is completely reliable, the nephrologist must use both along with clinical assessment to monitor the patient for signs of fluid overload and dehydration.

VI. Monitoring clearance. It is important to ensure that acute peritoneal dialysis is delivering adequate clearance to the patient with acute renal failure. There are, however, no validated definitions of what adequate clearance is in this context. In general, the blood urea nitrogen level should be maintained below 80 mg per dL, (28 mmol per L). Formal clearance measurements are not practical, but clearance can be estimated by measuring the urea nitrogen concentration in representative samples of dialysate and plasma in order to calculate a D/P ratio for urea. This is multiplied by the total daily dialysate drain volume to give daily urea clearance. This should be at least 10 mL per minute (14 L per day) and may need to be 20–30 mL per minute (28–42 L per day) in larger, highly catabolic patients. Clearance can be raised by increasing dwell volumes to 2.5–3 L or by decreasing dialysis exchange time as described above.

VII. Complications. A number of problems may arise during the course of acute peritoneal dialysis. To minimize the potential for complications, clearly defined indications for immediate physician notification should be provided in the nursing orders (Table 16-1).

A. Abdominal distention. Incomplete drainage may lead to progressive intraperitoneal accumulation of dialysate, with attendant discomfort, distention, and even respiratory compromise. Thus, one should observe the drainage cycle and make sure that the patient is emptying completely during the allowed drainage period. A properly trained nurse will know this, but for extra security, the dialysis orders should require the nephrologist to be called immediately for any technical problems related to the dialysis procedure.

Table 16-4. Peritoneal dialysis record

	Intake (mL)									Output (mL)									Totals	
Date	Dialysis Solution									Dialysis solution										
				Time IN								Time OUT								
	Ex #	Sol, %	Medications	Start	End	PD vol.	Oral	IV	Other	Total IN	Start	End	PD vol.	Urine	Other	Total OUT	Exchange balance	Running balance	Weight (kg)

B.   Peritonitis. Peritonitis may complicate acute peritoneal dialysis in up to 12% of cases. This occurs most often within the first 48 hours and is more common with open- than closed-drainage systems. Although infections from gram-positive organisms dominate (more than 50%), there is a higher incidence of fungal-related peritonitis in acute peritoneal dialysis. This may be a reflection of the severity of illness in patients requiring acute peritoneal dialysis as well as predisposing factors, such as the prolonged use of multiple antibiotics.

C.   Hypotension. Rapid removal of large amounts of fluid can lead to hypovolemia with consequent hypotension, arrhythmia, and even death. In some patients (e.g., those with hypoproteinemia), large amounts of fluid can be removed even when using exclusively 1.5% dextrose solutions. Immediate administration of intravenous fluid (0.9% normal saline) to correct hypotension, along with decreasing the dextrose concentration of the dialysate and/or increasing the dwell time to limit ongoing excess fluid removal, is indicated in this setting. To avoid such catastrophes when using high-dextrose solutions, it is best to write orders for a period of only a few hours at a time, reassessing and adjusting the dialysis solution concentration depending on the patient's condition.

D.   Hyperglycemia. In the diabetic or prediabetic patient, the high-dextrose solutions used for peritoneal dialysis can result in hyperglycemia. Blood glucose levels should therefore be monitored closely in such patients and treated with insulin accordingly. Intraperitoneal instillation of regular insulin may enhance the ease of glucose management (Table 16-3; see Chapter 25).

E.   Hypernatremia. Due to the low sieving coefficient for sodium (ultrafiltrate concentration/plasma concentration = 0.5), the ultrafiltrate generated in peritoneal dialysis has a sodium concentration of approximately 70 mEq per L (0.5×140 mEq per L). Increased losses of water associated with frequent hypertonic exchanges can therefore lead to hypernatremia. Implementing intravenous replacement of losses with 0.45% normal saline or replacing half of the losses with 5% dextrose water prevents the development of hypernatremia.

F.   Hypoalbuminemia. With the frequent exchanges utilized in acute peritoneal dialysis, protein loss via the dialysate can be as high as 10–20 g per day and up to twice this amount if peritonitis supervenes. Thus, oral or parenteral hyperalimentation should be instituted early. Metabolism of carbohydrate absorbed from the dialysis solution combined with metabolism of carbohydrate supplied by hyperalimentation can lead to excessive generation of carbon dioxide, which can be problematic for patients with respiratory compromise or failure. Intensive peritoneal dialysis coupled with hyperalimentation can result in hypophosphatemia, hyperglycemia, hypokalemia, or hypomagnesemia.

SELECTED READINGS

Health and Public Policy Committee, American College of Physicians. Clinical competence in acute peritoneal dialysis. *Ann Intern Med* 1988;108:763–765.

Leblanc M, Tapolyai M, Paganini EP. What dialysis dose should be provided in acute renal failure? *Adv Ren Replace Ther* 1995;2:255–264.

Manji S, et al. Peritoneal dialysis for acute renal failure: overfeeding resulting from dextrose absorbed during dialysis. *Crit Care Med* 1990;18:29–31.

Nolph KD, Sorkin MI. Peritoneal dialysis in acute renal failure. In: Brenner BM, Lazarus JM, eds. *Acute renal failure,* 2nd ed. New York: Churchill Livingstone, 1988:809–838.

Valeri A, et al. The epidemiology of peritonitis in acute peritoneal dialysis: a comparison between open- and closed-drainage systems. *Am J Kidney Dis* 1993;21:300–309.

Adequacy of Peritoneal Dialysis and Chronic Peritoneal Dialysis Prescription

Peter G. Blake and Jose A. Diaz-Buxo

The prescription of chronic peritoneal dialysis involves a number of elements. Initially, there is the choice of peritoneal dialysis modality; then there is the selection of a prescription based on clearance and ultrafiltration requirements. Additional issues are the choice of the giving set (for continuous ambulatory peritoneal dialysis, or CAPD), the cycler (for automated peritoneal dialysis, or APD), and the composition of the dialysis solution with particular reference to calcium concentration, the osmotic agent, and the buffer used; however, these have already been dealt with in Chapter 14 and will not be further addressed here.

I. Choice of a treatment modality (Table 17-1). This should take into consideration both patient preferences and the need to provide a medically optimal peritoneal dialysis prescription. Patient preferences may be based on issues such as lifestyle, ability to perform self-dialysis, family and social support, and geographic factors. Medical requirements of the prescription typically include the provision of adequate clearances and fluid removal. A third issue to be remembered is the relative costs of different prescriptions, as many programs have to deal with financial constraints. Ultimately, the final modality selection should rest with the patient, to the extent possible.

A. Modalities of peritoneal dialysis therapy

1. CAPD. The simplicity of CAPD, its relatively low cost, and the associated freedom from dialysis machinery have combined to make it the most popular chronic peritoneal dialysis modality. It provides continuous therapy and a steady physiologic state. Control of body fluid volume can usually be achieved, and normalization of blood pressure is possible in most patients. Reasonable glycemic control in diabetic patients can be obtained in a relatively physiologic manner with the use of intraperitoneal insulin.

Disadvantages of CAPD includes a need for multiple procedural sessions (usually four per day), limitations on dwell volumes due to increased intraperitoneal pressure, and a limited range of solute clearance. Episodes of peritonitis occurring as often as once every 12 months were a significant disadvantage in the past; however, with improved transfer sets and connecting devices, such occurrences have been markedly reduced.

2. APD. This has become very popular in recent years and in many countries is being used in 20%–40% of all peritoneal dialysis patients. It has classically been divided into contin-

Table 17-1. Comparison of typical CAPD and APD prescriptions

	CAPD	CCPD	NIPD
PD solution used (L/wk)	56–72	70–120	84–120
Dialysis time (hr/wk)	168	168	70
Time on machine (hr/wk)	0	63–70	63–70
Number of procedures/wk	28	14	14
Kt/V urea/wk	1.5–2.4	1.5–2.6	1.2–2.0
CrCl (L/wk)	40–70	40–70	25–50

CAPD, continuous ambulatory peritoneal dialysis;
CCPD, continuous cycling peritoneal dialysis;
NIPD, nocturnal intermittent peritoneal dialysis.
CrCl, Creatinine clearance.

uous cycling peritoneal dialysis (CCPD) and nocturnal inter-mittent peritoneal dialysis (NIPD). These modalities have already been described in Chapter 14.

The main advantage of CCPD is the ability to provide con-tinuous therapy without the need for on—off procedures dur-ing the day. All connections and preparation of equipment usually take place at bedtime in the privacy of the home, so that psychological adjustment is facilitated, and patient fatigue and "burnout" may be reduced. CCPD is an attractive treatment option for active individuals who are being in-convenienced by the interruptions in daily routine that are re-quired with CAPD. It is also the therapy of choice for most pa-tients who require assistance in carrying out their dialysis (e.g., children, the dependent elderly, nursing home residents).

The main disadvantages of CCPD are the need for a cycler, the slightly greater complexity and cost, and the complications associated with a prolonged day dwell, which may result in excessive resorption of dialysate. Variants of CCPD in which the day dwell is only kept in place for part of the day are useful in high and high-average transporters or in those with mechan-ical symptoms or complications.

NIPD is similar to CCPD, except that there is no dialysis fluid in the abdomen during the daytime. Ideally, the number of cycled exchanges done at night is increased to compensate for the lack of a day dwell, and cycler dwell times are corre-spondingly shorter; however, in practice, the cycler prescrip-tions used are often no different from those in CCPD. NIPD is particularly suitable for patients with high peritoneal trans-port status who have problems with ultrafiltration due to rapid absorption of glucose (see Chapter 18). It is also useful in pa-tients with mechanical complications (e.g., hernias, leaks, back pain) that prevent them from having fluid in their abdomen while they are ambulatory. Other theoretical benefits of NIPD include a lower overall glucose absorption rate, due to the ab-sence of a day dwell, and better peritoneal immunologic de-fenses, due to the lack of peritoneal lavage during the day.

The main disadvantages of NIPD are its relatively high cost and its inability in most patients to provide adequate small solute clearance because of the absence of a day dwell.

An alternative form of APD is tidal peritoneal dialysis (TPD). This modality uses an initial fill volume followed by partial drainage at periodic intervals. The volume that is intermittently cycled is called the "tidal volume," and the volume that remains in the peritoneal cavity is the "reserve volume." The ratio of tidal to reserve volume can vary, but a 50% tidal is recommended for maximum clearances in most patients. As explained in Chapter 14, the principal purpose of TPD is to enhance clearance of small solutes by avoiding the normal loss of dialytic time that is associated with inflow and drainage of solution on standard APD. However, in terms of clearance, the advantage of TPD over standard APD is not seen unless very large quantities of dialysis solution are used. The main disadvantage of high-volume TPD is increased cost and complexity, and it is not widely used.

3. Hybrid forms of peritoneal dialysis. Hybrid forms between CAPD and APD have become popular in recent years, principally to achieve higher clearances and better ultrafiltration. These hybrid forms can be divided as follows:

a. CAPD with automated nocturnal exchanges. This is done with a night exchange device that can be set up at bedtime to do an exchange while the patient sleeps. It has the advantage of breaking up the long nocturnal dwell, thus increasing ultrafiltration as well as clearance. The disadvantage is that it increases both the cost and the complexity of CAPD and requires the patient to be attached to a device while sleeping.

b. APD with additional exchanges during the day. This is a strategy to break up the long diurnal dwell of APD with a view to improving both clearance and ultrafiltration. Typically, the first day dwell is left in by the cycler as a last exchange ("last-bag option"). The second diurnal exchange can either be a manual CAPD-type exchange or can be done with the cycler tubing, using the cycler as a sort of "docking station." The advantage of this strategy is that it maximizes the clearances that can be achieved on peritoneal dialysis. The disadvantages are that it requires more procedures than standard CCPD and is more costly. The use of the docking-station approach rather than manual exchanges can, however, decrease this extra cost.

II. Choice of a prescription

A. Clearance targets. A critical issue in selection of a peritoneal dialysis prescription is the clearance requirements of the patient. In general, optimal clearance can be defined as that clearance above which further increments do not lead to clinically significant improvements in patient outcome. Minimum targets are best defined as those that allow the patient to be maintained in reasonably good health without significant uremic symptoms and with patient outcomes at least as good as those associated with well-prescribed chronic hemodialysis. These target clearances have not yet been well characterized, and the existing literature is confounded by the major contribution of residual renal clearance, which may not be equivalent in significance to peritoneal clearance. A present consensus, expressed in the National Kidney Foundation Dialysis Outcomes Quality Initiative (DOQI) peritoneal dialysis adequacy guidelines, based on the available data and on a combination of mathematical theories and uncontrolled clinical outcome studies, are that minimum acceptable doses for CAPD are a fractional urea clearance *(Kt/V)* of 2.0 per week and a creatinine clearance, corrected for 1.73 m² body surface area (CrCl), of 60 L per week. On the basis that CCPD and NIPD are relatively intermittent therapies and are therefore less efficient, target clearances with these therapies have been set at higher levels (Table 17-2). More recent recommendations from the Canadian Society of Nephrology keep the targets the same for CAPD, CCPD, and NIPD on the basis that all are daily therapies but suggest that the CrCl target for low and low-average transporters should be set at 50 rather than 60 L per week. The rationale for the latter recommendation is that low transporters have difficulty achieving a CrCl of 60 L per week once residual renal function is lost but have been shown to have superior outcomes, thus justifying the lower but more realistic target.

   B.   Measurement of clearance (Table 17-3). Clearance in peritoneal dialysis is typically measured either by *Kt/V* or CrCl. Both comprise a peritoneal and a residual renal component. The latter is frequently very important in peritoneal dialysis as residual renal function lasts longer than in hemodialysis and accounts for a greater proportion of total clearance.

      1.   Measurement of *Kt/V*. *Kt/V* is a dimensionless index that measures fractional urea clearance. Peritoneal *Kt/V* is calculated by performance of a 24-hour collection of dialysate effluent and measurement of its urea content. This is then divided by the average plasma urea level for the same 24-hour period to give a clearance term, *Kt*. The timing of the plasma

Table 17-2.   Clearance targets for peritoneal dialysis

(1) DOQI

Factor	CAPD	CCPD	NIPD
Kt/V per wk	2.0	2.1	2.2
CrCl L per wk	60	63	66

(2) Canadian Society of Nephrology

Factor	High/high-average transporters (CAPD, CCPD, NIPD)	Low/low-average transporters (CAPD, CCPD, NIPD)
Kt/V per wk	2.0	2.0
CrCl L per wk	60	50

CAPD, continuous ambulatory peritoneal dialysis; CCPD, continuous cycling peritoneal dialysis; NIPD, nocturnal intermittent peritoneal dialysis; DOQI, Dialysis Outcomes Quality Initiative.

Table 17-3.   Formulas for calculating clearance indices in peritoneal dialysis

Kt/V:
Kt = Total ***Kt*** = peritoneal ***Kt*** + renal ***Kt***
Peritoneal ***Kt*** = 24-h dialysate urea nitrogen content/serum urea nitrogen
Renal ***Kt*** = 24-hr urine urea nitrogen content/serum urea nitrogen

V (by Watson formula):
$V = 2.447 - 0.09516\,A + 0.1074\,H + 0.3362\,W$ (in males)
$V = -2.097 + 0.1069\,H + 0.2466\,W$ (in females)
  where A = age (yr); H = height (cm), and W = weight (kg)

CrCl (creatinine clearance)
CrCl = total **CrCl** corrected for 1.73 m^2 body surface area (BSA)
Total **CrCl** = peritoneal **CrCl** + renal **CrCl**
Peritoneal **CrCl** = 24-hr dialysate creatinine content/serum creatinine
Renal **CrCl**[a] = 0.5 [24-hr urine creatinine content/serum creatinine
  + 24-hr urine urea nitrogen content/serum urea
  nitrogen]

Body Surface Area (BSA, duBois formula):
BSA (m^2) = $0.007184 \times W^{0.425} \times H^{0.725}$
  where BSA = body surface area (m^2), W = Weight (kg),
  and H = height (cm)

[a] For PD adequacy purposes, renal "CrCl" is the average of the urinary creatinine and urea creatinine clearances.

urea sample is not critical in CAPD because it is relatively constant at all times. In CCPD and, especially, NIPD, blood urea is not constant throughout the day; therefore, it is best to take a measurement in the middle of the noncycling daytime period, which is typically between 1:00 and 5:00 pm and is thought to represent approximately the average blood urea for the day for a patient.

Residual renal *Kt* is calculated in the same way using a 24-hour collection of urine. The two *Kt* terms are then combined to give total *Kt* and are normalized to *V*, which represents total-body water. It is recommended that *V* be estimated using one of the standard formulas for total-body water, such as those of Watson or of Hume-Weyers. These are based on the age, sex, height, and weight of the patient (Table 17-3). This normalization will give a daily *Kt/V*, which is then multiplied by 7 to give a weekly value because this is how clearance is conventionally expressed in peritoneal dialysis.

2.   **CrCl.** The measurement of CrCl is similar to that of *Kt/V* (Table 17-3). Again, the peritoneal component is calculated by measuring creatinine content of a 24-hour collection of dialysate effluent, and this is then divided by the serum creatinine. The residual renal CrCl is known to markedly overestimate true glomerular filtration rate in most patients; therefore, it is conventional to add the mean of the urinary urea and creatinine clearances to the peritoneal clearance to give the total creatinine clearance. This is then corrected for

1.73 m^2 body surface area, with the latter estimated using the formula of DuBois (Table 17-3 and Fig. 17-1).

The high glucose levels found in dialysate artifactually elevate the measurement of creatinine in some biochemical assays, and each laboratory should make a correction for this based on its own experience. This may be done by measuring the apparent creatinine content in unused bags of dialysis solution with various dextrose concentrations, so that a correction factor can be calculated.

3. Frequency of measurements. It is recommended by the DOQI peritoneal dialysis work group that in peritoneal dialysis patients both *Kt/V* and CrCl should be measured three times during the first 6 months on peritoneal dialysis and every 4 months subsequently, as well as after every significant change in the peritoneal dialysis prescription or in the patient's clinical status. Urinary clearance should be measured every 2 months until residual renal function is negligible. Some will find these requirements unduly onerous, and a compromise in more stable patients who have been achieving their targets would be to measure clearances every 6 months. If an incremental approach to peritoneal dialysis is being used (see Section E), it is particularly important that measurements of urinary clearance be done every 2 months.

4. Examples of clearance calculations. See Table 17-4.

5. Discordance between *Kt/V* and CrCl. A frequent finding when measuring clearances in patients on peritoneal

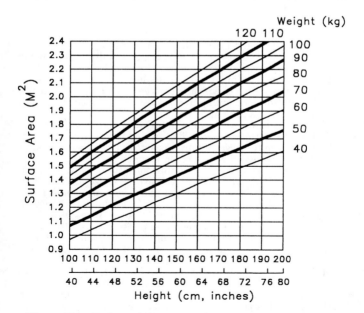

Figure 17-1. Body surface area as a function of body weight (kg) and height (inches and centimeters).

Table 17-4.   Examples of clearance calculations in continuous ambulatory peritoneal dialysis and automated peritoneal dialysis

(1) A 50-year-old man weighing 66 kg has no residual renal function. He is on CAPD with four 2.5-L exchanges daily, and his net UF is 1.5 L. His V by the Watson formula is 36 L, and his BSA by the DuBois formula is 1.66 m². Serum urea nitrogen is 70 mg/dL (25 mmol/L), and serum creatinine is 10 mg/dL (884 μmol/L). The urea nitrogen and creatinine (after correction for glucose) levels in the 24-hr dialysate collection are 63 mg/dL (22.5 mmol/L) and 6.5 mg/dL (575 μmol/L), respectively. Calculate his Kt/V and CrCl.

Kt urea/d = 24-hr drain volume x D/P urea = 11.5 Liters × 63/70 = 10.35 L/d. Daily Kt/V = 10.35 L/36 L = 0.288 L.

Weekly Kt/V = 0.288 × 7 = 2.02 L.

Creatinine clearance per day = 24-hr drain volume × D/P creatinine = 11.5 L × 6.5/10 = 7.48 L/d. Corrected for 1.73 m² BSA = 7.48 × 1.73/1.66 = 7.80 L/d. Weekly CrCl = 7.8 × 7 = 55 L/wk.

(2) A 48-year-old woman on APD weighs 63 kg and does five 2.4-L cycles nightly plus a 6-hr 2-L day dwell. Her V by Watson is 32 L, and her BSA by DuBois is 1.60 m². Her 24-hr dialysate drain volume is 15 L, indicating 1 L net UF. Her pooled dialysate collection has a urea nitrogen level of 48 mg/dL (17.1 mmol/L) and a creatinine level (after correction for glucose) of 4.5 mg/dL (398 μmol/L). Her mid-afternoon serum urea nitrogen is 65 mg/dL (23.2 μmol/L), and serum creatinine is 9 mg/dL (796 μmol/L). Her urinary urea and creatinine clearance are 2 and 4 mL/min, respectively.

Calculate her total weekly Kt/V and creatinine clearance.

Peritoneal Kt = daily drain volume × D/P urea = 15 Liters × 48/65 = 11.1 L

Peritoneal Kt/V = 11.1 L/32 L = 0.35 per d = 2.45 per wk.

Renal urea clearance = renal Kt urea = 2 mL/min = 20 L/wk.

Renal Kt/V = 20/32 = 0.63 per wk.

Total Kt/V = peritoneal plus renal Kt/V = 2.45 + 0.63 = 3.08 per wk

Peritoneal creatinine clearance = daily drain volume × D/P creatinine

= 15 L × 4.5/9 = 7.5 L. Corrected for 1.73 m² BSA = 7.5 × 1.73/1.60 = 8.1 L/d = 57 L/wk.

Renal creatinine clearance (for this purpose) = mean of renal urea and renal creatinine clearance = mean of 2 and 4 mL/min = 3 mL/min = 30 L/wk. Corrected for 1.73 m² BSA = 30 × 1.73/1.60 = 32.4 L/wk.

Total creatinine clearance = 57 + 32.4 = 89.4 L/wk.

CAPD, continuous ambulatory peritoneal dialysis; UF, ultrafiltration; BSA, body surface area; D/P, dialysate/plasma.

dialysis is that the Kt/V target is being achieved but not the CrCl one, or vice versa. The first scenario is most common and typically occurs in patients who have lost residual renal function, which contributes disproportionately to creatinine clearance as compared with urea clearance. The same discordance is frequently seen in patients on APD because the short dwells contribute disproportionately to urea clearance as compared with creatinine clearance. It may also be seen in low transporters where creatinine equilibration is disproportionately low in comparison with urea equilibration. The opposite situation, where CrCl, but not Kt/V, targets are achieved is most commonly seen in patients who have substantial residual renal function. The issue that arises in all of these cases is whether it is important to achieve both targets or whether one target suffices. In general, it would seem reasonable to continue a patient on peritoneal dialysis if one of the two clearance targets are being achieved and if the patient is doing well clinically. If possible, however, the prescription should be altered to allow achievement of both targets. If neither clearance target is being achieved despite maximal efforts, and if the patient is not clinically well, transfer to hemodialysis should be considered. If, however, the patient is doing well, a dilemma arises. A clinical judgment has to be made, in discussion with the patient, as to whether transfer to hemodialysis is indicated. In many such cases, it may be justifiable to continue with peritoneal dialysis, paying close attention to the development of uremic and nutritional complications. In making these decisions, factors other than clearances often have to be taken into account. These include fluid removal and the patient's general medical state and personal and social circumstances.

C. Determinants of clearance (Table 17-5). The total weekly Kt/V achieved on standard peritoneal dialysis prescriptions typically varies from as little as 1.2 to as much as 2.8 a week. Similarly, CrCl can vary from as little as 30 L per

Table 17-5. Factors determining clearance peritoneal dialysis patients

1. Nonprescription factors:
   Residual renal function
   Body size
   Peritoneal transport characteristics
2. Prescription factors:

(a) CAPD:	(b) APD:
Frequency of exchanges	Number of day dwells
Dwell volume	Volume of day dwells
Tonicity of dialysis solution	Tonicity of day dwells
	Time on cycler
	Cycle frequency
	Cycler dwell volumes
	Tonicity of cycler solution

CAPD, continuous ambulatory peritoneal dialysis; APD, automated peritoneal dialysis.

week to as much as 150 L per week. The major source of this variation is residual renal function. This and the other determinants of clearance are now reviewed:

1.   Residual renal function. This typically accounts for as much as 50% of total clearance at the initiation of peritoneal dialysis and tends to decline at a significantly slower rate than in hemodialysis. A large proportion of the differences between the clearances that patients achieve in peritoneal dialysis is accounted for by differences in residual renal function. As already mentioned, studies that have shown a correlation between clearances achieved and subsequent patient outcome have been somewhat confounded by this issue, and it appears that residual renal function is a much more potent predictor of outcome than peritoneal clearance per se. However, to date there have been no good studies in which differences in outcome associated with a wide range of peritoneal clearances have been examined.

2.   Peritoneal transport status. This is an important determinant of clearances that can be achieved, especially in APD where solute equilibration between plasma and dialysate is very time-dependent. Peritoneal transport is measured by the peritoneal equilibration test (PET), as discussed in Chapter 13. In general, low transporters do best with high-volume, long-duration dwells, whereas high transporters do best with high-frequency, short-duration dwells. What determines transport status is not well understood. Transport status is now recognized as a determinant of patient and technique survival on CAPD, with low transporters doing best despite clearances that tend to be lower than those their high-transport counterparts achieve. In all likelihood, this is at least partially due to the critical importance of ultrafiltration and its interaction with cardiovascular morbidity.

3.   Body size. Given that clearance indices are normalized to body surface area or total-body water, this is an important determinant.

4.   Prescription. See Section D below.

D.   Prescription strategies to achieve clearance targets in chronic peritoneal dialysis

1.   CAPD. In attempting to increase peritoneal Kt/V in CAPD patients, there are three options. One is to increase the frequency of daily exchanges, the second is to increase the individual dwell volumes, and the third is to increase the tonicity of the solutions, thereby augmenting ultrafiltration .

a.   Increasing exchange volumes. This usually results in only a small decrease in urea and creatinine equilibration so that the percentage increase in Kt/V and CrCl will be close to the percentage increase in the exchange volume, especially in larger patients. However, in smaller patients, and especially when 3-L dwell volumes are used, there may be some fall-off in equilibration. To achieve clearance targets it is typically necessary to use at least 2.5-L dwell volumes in patients who weigh more than 65 kg. Some programs prefer to initiate such patients on the larger dwell volumes, whereas others use 2-L volumes until residual renal function fades out and then make the switch.

The main disadvantage of increasing exchange volumes is that a minority of patients may complain of back pain, abdominal distention, even shortness of breath. This can be minimized if the increased volumes are introduced at the time of initiation of peritoneal dialysis, before the patient becomes accustomed to smaller volumes. Theoretically, there may be an increased risk of hernias and leaks due to the rise in intraperitoneal pressure. This may also theoretically impair ultrafiltration, but this effect is usually more than offset by the longer persistence of the glucose osmotic gradient when higher volumes are used.

b.   Increasing the frequency of daily exchanges. Most CAPD patients do four exchanges daily. Some smaller patients with significant residual renal function are commenced on three exchanges daily, but this has become less common. Increasing the number of exchanges from four to five per day generally does not have a major effect on urea equilibration, which remains at approximately 90% in patients with average transport characteristics. However, this will not be the case if patients do not ensure that the five daily exchanges are well spaced, with at least a 4-hour dwell time for each. For creatinine, however, there will be a noticeable drop in creatinine equilibration in the drained effluent because the equilibration curve for creatinine is typically still rising 4 hours after the dwell commences. Thus, increasing the frequency of exchanges is less effective than increasing dwell volumes, especially where CrCl is concerned.

An additional disadvantage of increasing the frequency of exchanges to five daily is that it may interfere unacceptably with a patient's lifestyle and lead to noncompliance or burnout. However, night exchange devices make a fifth exchange more practical. These devices can be set up before the patient goes to bed and will deliver the additional exchange halfway through the night. This strategy has the added advantage of increasing net ultrafiltration, as well as clearance.

c.   Increasing the tonicity of the dialysis solutions. This strategy increases both ultrafiltration and clearance. It is used in many centers, but there are concerns that it may lead to a higher incidence of hyperglycemia, hyperlipidemia, obesity, and, perhaps, long-term peritoneal membrane damage. The introduction of icodextrin based dialysis solution (see Chapter 14) for long dwells may be a simpler way to increase both ultrafiltration and clearance, although the effect on the latter is usually modest. The safety/adverse effect profile of icodextrin is still being developed. Blistering or exfoliative skin reactions have been reported (Goldsmith et al, 2000). Absorbed icodextrin metabolites can cause falsely high serum glucose measurements (Wens et al, 1997) and falsely low serum amylase determinations (Schonicke et al, 1999).

2.   APD. Peritoneal clearance in APD can be increased using a number of different strategies. In order of importance, these are:

a.   Introduction of a day dwell. In NIPD patients, the best way to increase clearance is to add a day dwell. This raises both Kt/V and CrCl, but the effect on CrCl is greater because creatinine equilibration is more dependent on longer dwell times. Typically, adding a day dwell in an NIPD patient will increase daily peritoneal Kt/V and CrCl by 25% to 50% and so is very cost-effective. The main disadvantage is that the long day dwell frequently results in net fluid resorption, particularly in high and high-average transporters. This can be dealt with by shortening the day dwell from 16 hours to 2–8 hours, depending on membrane characteristics, perhaps using the docking-station approach mentioned above. Thus, the day dwell can be done in the first part of the day (i.e., directly after coming off the cycler) or, alternatively, in the evening, before using the cycler. This allows both clearance and ultrafiltration to be maintained.

Further increases in clearance can be achieved by adding a second or even a third day dwell. Again, these can be done using the docking-station approach or, if it suits the patient better, using manual CAPD tubing in the conventional way. These strategies are relatively cost-effective in increasing clearance but do have the disadvantage of requiring patients to have fluid in their peritoneal cavity for at least part of the day. Day dwell volumes can be titrated to maximize clearance while minimizing mechanical symptoms.

b.   Increase dwell volumes on cycler. This increases clearance in APD, just as it does in CAPD. Because patients are supine during cycling, they can usually tolerate larger dwell volumes, and 2.5 L should be considered standard. Greater clearances will be achieved if the same total amount of dialysis solution is delivered in a smaller number of larger aliquots (i.e., 4×2.5 L per session is better than 5×2 L per session). In some patients, however, the rise in intraperitoneal pressure with increased dwell volume may impair ultrafiltration, but this is not usually clinically significant because its effect is offset by the longer lasting glucose osmotic gradient.

c.   Time on cycler. In general, the longer the time the patient spends on APD the better the clearance because individual dwell times are longer, allowing more complete equilibration.

d.   Increasing frequency of cycles. In general, doing more frequent cycles increases clearances on APD because it maximizes the concentration gradient between blood and dialysate. However, when the number of cycles in a given time period is increased, an increasing proportion of that period is spent draining and filling, and as a result some dialysis time is lost. Thus, there is a point beyond which increasing the number of cycles further is counter-productive in terms of cost and clearance achieved, and this is in the range of six to nine cycles per 9-hour cycling session. It tends to be higher in high transporters and lower in low transporters and is higher for urea than for creatinine. It may also be influenced by catheter function. To get around this problem, tidal peritoneal dialysis can be used, but it is only effective in raising clearance when very large volumes of dialysis solution are delivered (e.g., greater than 20–25 L per session) and therefore is not very cost-effective.

e. Increasing dialysis solution tonicity. As in CAPD, clearance can be augmented in APD by increasing ultrafiltration. Again, however, the same concerns about complications arise, and the use of icodextrin for the APD day dwell may be a better approach.

3. Recommended prescriptions by peritoneal transport type (Table 17-6).

a. Low transporters. In general, low transporters require long high-volume dwells to achieve clearance targets. Therefore, ideal prescriptions might include:

(1) CAPD with four 2.5- to 3-L exchange daily.

(2) CAPD with five 2.5- to 3-L exchanges daily, with the fifth delivered by a night exchange device.

(3) APD with a small number of large volume cycles at night and one or more day dwells (e.g., three 3-L dwells over 9 hours plus two 2.5-L day dwells done using the cycler tubing).

b. High transporters. High transporters generally do best with more frequent short-duration dwells, which achieve clearance targets without compromising ultrafiltration. Ideal prescriptions might include:

(1) APD with four to seven 2.5- to 3-L dwells over 9 hours plus or minus a short (3–4 hours) day dwell done using the cycler tubing.

(2) APD with icodextrin for the long day dwell.

Table 17-6. Recommended prescriptions by peritoneal transport type

a) *Low transporters.* In general, low transporters require long high-volume dwells to achieve clearance targets. Therefore, ideal prescriptions might include:

i) CAPD with four 2.5- to 3-L exchanges daily

ii) CAPD with five 2.5- to 3-L exchanges daily, with the fifth delivered by a night exchange device

iii) APD with a small number of large-volume cycles at night and one or more day dwells [e.g., three 3-L cycles over 9 hr plus two 2.5-L day dwells done using the cycler tubing]

b) *High transporters.* High transporters generally do best with more frequent short-duration dwells, which achieve clearance targets without compromising UF. Ideal prescriptions might include:

i) APD with four to seven 2.5- to 3-L dwells over 9 hr plus or minus a short 3- to 4 hr day dwell done using the cycler tubing.

ii) APD with icodextrin for the long day dwell.

c) *Average transporters.* Average transporters can generally be managed on the PD prescription that most suits their lifestyle. In some cases, they will have trouble with net resorption of the long day dwell on APD, and it may be helpful to shorten this or to use icodextrin.

CAPD, continuous ambulatory peritoneal dialysis; APD, automated peritoneal dialysis; UF, ultrafiltration.

    c. Average transporters. Average transporters can generally be managed on the peritoneal dialysis prescription that most suits their lifestyle. In some cases, they will have trouble with net resorption of the long day dwell on APD, and it may be helpful to shorten this or to use icodextrin.

E. Incremental versus maximal prescription. There are two distinct approaches to prescription of peritoneal dialysis when clearance targets are being considered. The incremental approach, which is particularly suitable when dialysis is being initiated early, suggests that peritoneal dialysis should be used to make up the difference between residual renal clearances and targeted clearances. Thus, patients may initially require only two or three CAPD exchanges daily or a low-volume, day-dry APD prescription. The alternative is the so-called maximal approach in which patients are at the outset given a sufficient prescription to meet their targets with peritoneal dialysis alone. This approach considers residual renal function as a temporary bonus that inevitably deteriorates with time.

    The advantages of the incremental approach are that it is initially less costly and less onerous for the patient. A disadvantage is that it requires regular monitoring of residual function to ensure that the total clearance achieved does not fall below target levels. The advantage of the maximal approach is that it delivers the largest amount of dialysis possible from the beginning, with potential benefits in patient well-being. It does, however, increase the cost and possibly the risk of patient burnout. In addition, the extra number of exchanges may increase the risk of peritonitis, obesity, hyperlipidemia, and so forth. There is no evidence as to which approach is superior, and in clinical practice, a compromise between the two is often preferred.

F. Empirical versus modeled approach. Another decision when prescribing peritoneal dialysis is whether to use commercially available software programs for modeling appropriate prescriptions or whether to proceed in an empirical manner. The modeled approach involves collecting patient anthropometric data, measuring peritoneal transport with a PET, and quantifying residual renal function. It also typically involves collection of 24-hour dialysate effluent to make particular calculations about peritoneal fluid removal and absorption. The computer program uses the data to predict, with reasonable accuracy, the clearances that will be achieved with various potential prescriptions. Alternatively, the program can suggest appropriate prescriptions to achieve the desired clearances. With this approach, the actual clearances still have to be measured as there is sometimes a discrepancy between the modeled and actual clearances achieved.

    The alternative approach is empirical, in which the physician uses knowledge of the patient's size, residual renal function, and peritoneal transport status to choose a reasonable prescription. This is then tested, clearances are assessed, and the prescription is adjusted if necessary. The modeled approach has the advantage that it may involve less trial-and-error and so result in earlier identification of an appropriate prescription for the patient, with consequent decreases in cost as well as inconvenience to the patient. However, even with the modelled approach, the initial prescription has to be selected empirically because peritoneal transport status will not yet have been determined. The empirical method has a theoretical advantage that it focuses the physician's attention on the patient rather than on purely numerical data. In practice, a combination of both approaches is frequently used, with the modeled approach being of particular use in complex cases and in patients on APD.

G.   Prescription pitfalls in peritoneal dialysis. There are a number of common pitfalls that physicians face in attempting to achieve adequate clearances and fluid removal on peritoneal dialysis.

1.   Loss of residual renal function. A common problem is that residual renal function is not monitored often enough and drops to a very low level without the physician being aware. Thus, the patient is left on an inadequate prescription for a significant period of time. This is best avoided by measuring residual clearance every 2–3 months or by adopting a maximal prescription approach that gives sufficient peritoneal clearance independent of residual function.

2.   Noncompliance. A chronic peritoneal dialysis patient may sometimes appear uremic despite measured clearances that exceed recommended targets. A strong possibility here is noncompliance. On the day that collections are performed, the patient is fully compliant with the prescription and appears to have excellent clearances. On other days, however, the patient is omitting exchanges or shortening time on the cycler. There is no single test that identifies this particular problem, and a high index of suspicion is required. Serial measurements of 24-hour dialysate plus urinary creatinine excretion may help identify the problem. Patients in whom the total creatinine excretion has increased in comparison with a baseline value should be suspected of noncompliance. The rationale here is that on the day of the collection, creatinine that has accumulated on previous noncompliant days is being dialyzed out, giving an artificially high value. The alternative explanation for an increase in total creatinine excretion is a gain in lean body mass, but this probably does not occur with any frequency in chronic-dialysis patients. There are a number of patterns of noncompliance in peritoneal dialysis patients that should be borne in mind. These include:

a.   Skipping CAPD exchanges

b.   Having inadequate spacing of CAPD exchanges

c.   Reducing the dwell volume of CAPD exchanges by flushing fresh dialysis solution directly into the drain bag

d.   Shortening of cycler time in APD

3.   Inappropriate switch from CAPD to APD. It is sometimes presumed that APD is a panacea for inadequate dialysis on CAPD, but the problem can actually become worse on APD if prescriptions are inappropriate. This is particularly likely in low transporters who are unlikely to achieve higher clearances on APD than CAPD, unless 2-day dwells are prescribed. It should be remembered that CrCl targets in particular may be difficult to achieve in APD. The point here is that creatinine equilibration is much more time-dependent than urea equilibration; therefore, the shorter duration dwells of APD typically lead to a fall in creatinine relative to urea clearance. Thus, a patient who has the same Kt/V urea after a switch from CAPD to APD will have a lower CrCl. This effect is most marked in low transporters and in NIPD.

H. Inadequate attention to fluid removal. Fluid removal is frequently neglected in prescriptions for peritoneal dialysis. Prescriptions that yield good clearances may not give sufficient ultrafiltration to keep the patient euvolemic and free from hypertension. This is particularly so in high and high-average transporters, especially if long dwells are used. Short day dwells in APD or a night exchange device in CAPD dwell are two strategies that may be useful. This is discussed in detail in Chapter 18.

I. Early initiation of peritoneal dialysis. Peritoneal dialysis may be particularly suitable when early initiation of dialysis is being practiced. This strategy, recommended by DOQI, suggests that dialysis be initiated when residual renal Kt/V is less than 2.0 per week, on the rationale that the clearance at which dialysis is commenced should not be lower than the level targeted when the patient is on dialysis. An exception can be made for patients who are asymptomatic and nutritionally stable. If peritoneal dialysis is used in this setting, an incremental approach may be useful, with an initial prescription of two exchanges per day or of NIPD being feasible options. Alternatively, a maximal approach can be used from the beginning as discussed in Section II.E, above. Early initiation is supported by evidence from retrospective analysis of data only, and more rigorous prospective studies are required. However, there is little doubt that, at present, many patients start dialysis much too late, and a move toward an earlier, healthier start is to be welcomed.

III. Nutritional issues in peritoneal dialysis. Nutritional measures in peritoneal dialysis patients have been repeatedly shown to predict patient survival and other outcomes. It is recommended that a number of these be routinely monitored to identify high-risk patients with a view to appropriate interventions.

Indices followed include normalized protein equivalent of nitrogen appearance (nPNA), serum albumin, subjective global assessment, and lean body mass as estimated from creatinine excretion.

A. Nutritional indices

1. nPNA. This is easily measured using the same 24-hour collections of dialysate and urine as are used to calculate Kt/V and CrCl. The rationale is that, in steady state, nitrogen excretion is proportional to protein intake. A variety of formulas have been derived to estimate nPNA from nitrogen and protein excretion, but there is evidence that the best of these may be those of Bergström (see Table 17-7) for formula and sample calculation). Previously, PNA estimates were normalized to actual body weight, but this can lead to misleadingly high nPNA values in wasted malnourished patients and to inappropriately low values in obese patients. Normalization to standard or ideal weight based on anthropometric tables is now preferred. Recommended target nPNA for peritoneal dialysis patients is 1.2 g per kg per day, but this may be unnecessarily and unrealistically high for many patients who achieve nitrogen balance at lower intakes. However, a falling nPNA or a level less than 0.8–0.9 g per kg per day should be a cause for concern.

Table 17-7.   Calculation of normal protein nitrogen appearance with example

Bergström formulas:

(1) PNA (g/d) = 20.1 + 7.5 UNA (g/d)

or

(2) PNA (g/d) = 15.1 + 6.95 UNA (g/d) + dialysate protein losses (g/d)

UNA (g/d) = urinary urea losses (g/d) + dialysate urea losses (g/d)

Use formula (1) if dialysate protein losses are unknown and formula (2) if they are known.

Normalization of PNA to body weight gives nPNA. Actual body weight, if used, can give a misleadingly high value in malnourished patients and a misleadingly low one in obese patients.

Normalization to standard body weight based on anthropometric tables is preferable.

Example:

A 60-kg man on CAPD 4 × 2.5 L daily has 24-hr dialysate effluent volume of 12 L which contains 58.3 mg/dL urea nitrogen so that total content = 12 × 58.3 × 10 = 7,000 mg = 7 g of urea nitrogen.

The 24-hr urine has a 500-mL volume and contains 560 mg/dL = 2,800 mg = 2.8 g of urea nitrogen

Total UNA = 7 + 2.8 = 9.8 g/d

Dialysate protein losses are measured at 8 g/d

Thus;

PNA = 15.1 + 6.95 (9.8) + 8 = 91.2 g/d

nPNA based on actual weight = 91.2/60 = 1.52 g/d

Patient has lost weight, however, and anthropometric tables suggest that his standard weight is 72 kg

nPNA based on this weight is 91.2/72 = 1.27 g/kg/d

PNA, protein nitrogen appearance; UNA, urinary nitrogen appearance; nPNA, normal protein nitrogen appearance; CAPD, continuous ambulatory peritoneal dialysis.

2.   Caloric intake. This is sometimes neglected in dialysis patients because it cannot be as easily measured as protein intake and there are no data correlating it to outcome. In peritoneal dialysis, caloric intake is a combination of dietary intake plus calories from the glucose absorbed from the dialysis solution.

The suggested target is 35 kcal per kg per day; typically, 10%–30% of this comes from the glucose, with the exact amount depending on the tonicity, dwell times, and volume of solutions used and on the patient's PET characteristics, which also influence the percentage of infused glucose absorbed. Measurement requires dietary assessment plus quantification of the glucose absorbed, reached by subtraction of the amount of glucose in the effluent from the amount delivered.

3.   Serum albumin. This is one of the most potent predictors of patient survival on peritoneal dialysis. It has become apparent that it is mainly influenced by PET status, which influences dialysate albumin losses, and by the presence of systemic illness or inflammation, as judged by the serum levels of acute-phase reactants, such as C-reactive protein. Compared with these factors, protein intake and delivered clearances have only a minor effect on serum albumin. Thus, it can be said that serum albumin in this population is much more than a nutritional marker.

4. Subjective global assessment. This simple clinical tool has become popular because it is easily done at the bedside, promotes history taking and physical examination, and has been shown to predict patient outcome. It is described in both the DOQI and Canadian Society of Nephrology references (see "Selected Readings").

5. Creatinine excretion. The total creatinine content measured in the same 24-hour urine and dialysate collections done to calculate clearance can be used to estimate lean body mass using the method of Keshaviah et al, 1995 (see "Selected Readings"). These estimates are predictive of patient outcome, and a low or falling value identifies a patient at risk.

B. Treatment of malnutrition. This is reviewed in Chapter 30.

SELECTED READINGS

Bergström J, et al. Calculation of the protein equivalent of total nitrogen appearance from urea appearance. Which formulas should be used? *Perit Dial Int* 1998;18: 467–473.

Bernardini J, et al. Pattern of noncompliance with dialysis exchanges in peritoneal dialysis patients. *Am J Kidney Dis* 2000;35:1104–1110.

Blake PG, et al. Recommended clinical practices for maximizing PD clearances. *Perit Dial Int* 1996;16:448–456.

Blake PG, et al. Clinical practice guidelines for adequacy and nutrition in peritoneal dialysis. *J Am Soc Nephrol* 1999;10(Suppl 13): S311–S321.

Churchill DN, et al. Adequacy of dialysis and nutrition in continuous peritoneal dialysis. *J Am Soc Nephrol* 1995;7:198–207.

Diaz-Buxo JA. Enhancement of peritoneal dialysis: the "PD Plus" concept. *Am J Kidney Dis* 1996;27:92–98.

Diaz Buxo JA, et al. PD adequacy: a model to assess feasibility with various modalities. *Kidney Int* 1999;55:2493–2501.

Goldsmith D, et al. Allergic reactions to the polymeric glucose-based peritoneal dialysis fluid icodextrin in patients with renal failure. *Lancet* 2000;355:897.

Harty JC, et al. The normalized protein catabolic rate is a flawed marker of nutrition in CAPD patients. *Kidney Int* 1994;45:103–109.

Keshaviah PR, et al. The peak concentration hypothesis: a urea kinetic approach to comparing the adequacy of continuous ambulatory peritoneal dialysis and hemodialysis. *Perit Dial Int* 1989;9:257–260.

Keshaviah PR, et al. Lean body mass estimation by creatinine kinetics. *J Am Soc Nephrol* 1995;4:1475–1485.

Keshaviah P. Timely initiation of dialysis: a urea kinetic approach. *Am J Kidney Dis* 1999;33:344–348.

National Kidney Foundation. DOQI Peritoneal Dialysis Adequacy Work Group. NKF DOQI clinical practice guidelines for adequacy of peritoneal dialysis. *Am J Kidney Dis* 1997;30(Suppl 2):S67–S136.

Sarkar S, et al. Tolerance of large exchange volumes by peritoneal dialysis patients. *Am J Kidney Dis* 1999;33:1136–1141.

Schonicke G, et al. Interference of icodextrin with serum amylase measurement. *J Am Soc Nephrol* 1999;10:229a (abstr).

Teehan BP, et al. A quantitative approach to the CAPD prescription. *Perit Dial Bull* 1985;5:152–156.

Wens R, et al. Overestimation of blood glucose measurements by auto-analyser method in CAPD patients treated with icodextrin. *J Am Soc Nephrol* 1997;8:275a (abstr).

Williams PF. Improved survival of high transporter peritoneal dialysis patients with individualized dialysis prescription. *J Am Soc Nephrol* 1999;10:231a (abstr).

Woodrow G, et al. Comparison of icodextrin and glucose solutions for daytime dwell in automated peritoneal dialysis. *Nephrol Dial Transplant* 1999;14:1530–1535.

Yeun JY, . Acute phase proteins and peritoneal dialysate albumin loss are the main determinants of serum albumin in peritoneal dialysis patients. *Am J Kidney Dis* 1997;30:923–927.

Internet References

Peritoneal dialysis adequacy links (http:// www.hdcn.com/pd/adequacy)

Peritoneal dialysis adequacy DOQI guidelines (http://www.kidney.org.)

Assessing Peritoneal Ultrafiltration, Solute Transport, and Volume Status

Dimitrios G. Oreopoulos and Panduranga S. Rao

An important purpose of peritoneal dialysis is to gain control of fluid balance. Fluid overload may play a role in the high cardio-vascular morbidity and mortality in dialysis patients in general, and may be involved in the relatively high mortality seen in continuous ambulatory peritoneal dialysis (CAPD) patients with high peritoneal transport characteristics on the peritoneal equilibration test (PET) (see Chapter 17).

Fluid overload is a clinical diagnosis based on the presence of edema and hypertension that would be expected to resolve with fluid removal. It is often, but not always, due to ultrafiltration (UF) failure. UF failure can be defined as fluid overload in association with net UF less than 400 mL after a 4-hour, 2-L, 4.25% dextrose dwell. The latter finding suggests that the fluid overload is at least partly related to a problem with UF rather than to dietary indiscretion or some other non–membrane-related cause.

Fluid overload and UF failure are important causes of peritoneal dialysis technique failure. One study, using as a definition of UF failure, an inability to achieve the target weight despite three or more hypertonic exchanges per day for more than a month, showed that 2.6% of peritoneal dialysis patients developed this complication in the first year on peritoneal dialysis and this number reached 31% by the sixth year (Heimburger et al, 1990). Other investigators report that 1.3%–6% of all patients on CAPD have this complication. Accordingly, in 1998, the International Society of Peritoneal Dialysis (ISPD) set up a committee to make recommendations on the management of fluid overload in peritoneal dialysis which were published in the year 2000.

Understanding the physiologic basis of UF and solute transport across the peritoneal membrane helps physicians to prescribe the appropriate type of peritoneal dialysis for an individual patient and to devise strategies to overcome poor UF when it occurs.

I. Physiology of UF. This is discussed in more detail in Chapter 13. UF in peritoneal dialysis is governed principally by the osmotic gradient for glucose between the blood in the peritoneal capillary and the hypertonic dialysate. This gradient, and hence UF, are maximum at the beginning of a dwell but decline with time due to (a) absorption of glucose from dialysate into blood and (b) dilution of dialysate due to movement of water from blood into dialysate (Figs. 13-4 and 13-8). UF can be maintained for longer by using more hypertonic solutions or by shortening the dwell time. The same effect can be achieved by using alternative osmotic agents with high molecular weight, such as glucose polymers (e.g., icodextrin), which are poorly absorbed and so exert a higher colloid osmotic pressure for a longer time. The transport characteristics of the peritoneal membrane are also important in determining UF when glucose is the osmotic agent. Low transporters absorb glucose slowly and so maintain the osmotic gradient with consequently greater UF. High transporters lose the gradient rapidly and have poor UF once the dwell time exceeds 2 to 4 hours. The final drain volume also depends on another variable: absorption of dialysate from the peritoneal cavity. This occurs via direct lymphatic flow and by tissue absorption of peritoneal fluid. This absorption, which averages about 120 mL per hour, significantly lowers the overall or net UF volume.

II. Measurement of peritoneal UF function. The function of the peritoneal membrane can be assessed by a number of standardized tests. The most commonly used tests involve infusion of a 2-L dwell of either 4.25% or 2.5% dextrose peritoneal dialysis solution. The solution is drained 4 hours later, and the solute concentration of the retrieved dialysate is analyzed. A low recovered volume can be an indication of a problem with UF, and reasons for this can be inferred by examining the concentrations of glucose, creatinine, and urea in the dialysate, and comparing them with plasma concentrations of the same solutes obtained during the 4-hour dwell. Traditionally, a 2.5% solution has been used to assess UF. However, a 4.25% test is now being advocated to screen for poor UF as it is more reliable. Thus, when the drainage volume fails to exceed the instilled volume by at least 400 mL 4 hours after instillation of a 4.25% 2-L test exchange, some problem with UF is likely. The 4.25% test also can be used to determine the cause of poor UF due to inadequate number or function of ultrapores in the peritoneal dialysis membrane by comparing the sodium concentration of dialysate with that of plasma (see below). A 2.5% test exchange exerts insufficient osmotic stress to provide this information.

A. Peritoneal equilibration test (PET). Notwithstanding the above recommendation to use 4.25% dextrose to assess UF and the likelihood that its use will increase in the future, the standard assessment of UF and peritoneal transport in North America and elsewhere is still most frequently fast PET based on 2.5% dextrose. The test is generally accurate (Twardowski, 1990), but it is important that one be familiar with the PET protocol and follow it closely to ensure accurate reproducible results.

B. Protocol

1. The patient's peritoneal cavity is drained for at least 20 minutes, ideally after an 8- to 12-hour overnight dwell using 2 L of 2.5% dextrose dialysis solution.

2. Weigh a 2-L bag of warmed 2.5% dextrose dialysis solution, including its attached port clamps.

3. The contents of the bag (the volume can be as high as 2,070 mL) are infused over 10 minutes. After each 400 mL of dialysis solution is infused, the patient should roll from side to side.

4. A blood sample is taken during the dwell period. Four hours after the end of the infusion, the dialysate is drained over a 20-minute period. After mixing, a drainage fluid sample is aspirated from the medication port of the drainage bag.

The blood and dialysate samples are analyzed for creatinine and glucose concentrations.

5. After drainage, the bag containing the drained effluent with its port clamp is again weighed. By subtracting the weight of the bag and its contents before infusion from this figure, one can calculate the weight and thus the volume of UF in the drainage bag.

C.   Interpretation of results (Table 18-1)

1.   UF volume. Drainage volume in a PET with 2.5% dextrose solution averages 2,370 mL. As 2-L bags of dialysate contain about 2,050 mL of dialysis solution, this equals 320 mL of UF. In patients who have difficulty with fluid removal during dialysis, the drainage volume may actually be less than that instilled.

2.   Drainage fluid glucose level. The mean 4-hour glucose level in the dialysate is 720 mg per dL (40 mmol per L). Values above 950 mg per dL (53 mmol per L) and below 500 mg per dL (28 mmol per L) are typically seen in low and high transporters, respectively.

3.   Dialysate/plasma creatinine (D/P Cr) (Fig. 18-1). The mean D/P Cr ratio at 4 hours is 0.65. High and low transporters typically have ratios above 0.82 and below 0.49, respectively. Usually the UF, glucose absorption, and D/P Cr ratios from the PET correlate and, according to Twardowski et al (1987), four groups of patients can thus be defined, as shown in Table 18-1. Patients with **very high** or **high-average** transport characteristics show a rapid drop in dialysate glucose, a high D/P Cr, and less UF due to rapid dissipation of the glucose gradient between blood and dialysate. Patients with **low-average** or **very low** transport characteristics show the opposite pattern, with a well-preserved glucose gradient and good UF. In some patients, however, UF does not follow this pattern, as there are other causes of UF failure. If 4.25 dextrose is used for the PET, the expected UF volumes will change, with less than 400 mL net UF being suggestive of UF failure. Equilibration ratios will be only slightly lower than those for 2.5% dextrose.

Table 18-1.   Classification of a patient's peritoneal transport using fast peritoneal equilibrium test

Transport Classification	D/P Creatinine	Dialysate Glucose (mg/dL)	Drainage Vol. (mL)	Net Ultra-filtration[a]
High	0.82–1.03	230–501	1,580–2,084	−470–35
High-average	0.66–0.81	502–722	2,085–2,367	35–320
Mean	**0.65**	**723**	**2,368**	**320**
Low-average	0.50–0.64	724–944	2,369–2,650	320–600
Low	0.34–0.49	945–1,214	2,651–3,326	600–1,276

[a] Assumes a fill volume of 2,050 mL. This may vary from 2,000 mL to 2,050 mL depending on manufacturer, fill volume of connecting tubing, and other factors. D/P, dialysate/plasma.

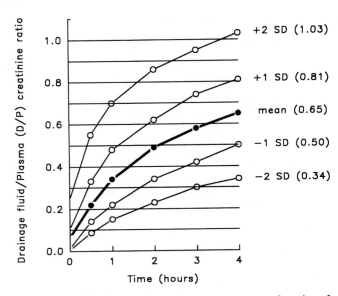

Figure 18-1. Dialysate/plasma creatinine (D/P Cr) as a function of time during the 4-hour peritoneal equilibration test (PET). The mean D/P ratio at 4 hours is about 0.65. (From Twardowsky ZJ, et al. Peritoneal equilibration test. *Perit Dial Bull* 1987;7:138.)

4. Pitfalls. Several factors can cause the PET test to yield misleading results. Table 18-2 lists the most common pitfalls of the PET:

a. Residual volume. Calculations of UF volume depend on the assumption that the residual volume (averaging 200 mL, but ranging from 50 to 700 mL or more) is similar before instillation and after drainage of the test exchange. Thus, the PET is less reliable in patients whose peritoneal catheters drain poorly. To standardize the residual volume in patients on intermittent or automated peritoneal dialysis (APD), who might otherwise start the test with a very low residual volume, it is best to prefill the abdomen with 2 L of 2.5% dextrose dialysis solution at least 2 hours before

Table 18-2. Factors that may affect the measurement of peritoneal ultrafiltration and solute diffusion

1. Residual volume
2. State of hydration
3. Plasma glucose levels
4. Incomplete intraperitoneal mixing
5. Handling of peritoneal effluent
6. Errors pertaining to glucose and creatinine estimation

starting the test. Indeed, prescription modeling computer programs that use PET results to predict clearances require a prolonged dwell (more than 8 hours) prior to the actual 4-hour PET, and this should be the recommended practice. This prefill is allowed to drain for at least 20 minutes before infusion of the 2.5% dextrose test exchange. Often the residual volume after drainage depends on patient position; the latter should be the same while draining the prefill exchange and the test exchange.

b. State of patient hydration. At the time of the test, the patient should be as close to euvolemia as possible. Dehydration may reduce UF, probably because UF will then be opposed by dehydration-induced increases in plasma and interstitial oncotic pressures, by decreases in capillary hydrostatic pressure, and, possibly, by increased reabsorption of peritoneal fluid. Paradoxically, overhydration also may reversibly reduce peritoneal UF by interfering in some unclear manner with water transport.

c. Plasma glucose levels in diabetics. During the PET, in nondiabetic patients, the plasma glucose level may reach 160 mg per dL (9 mmol per L). However, in diabetic patients with poorly controlled hyperglycemia, the concentration gradient for glucose may be much less, and so UF will decrease. Thus, one should perform the PET only after ensuring adequate control of plasma glucose.

d. Incomplete intraperitoneal mixing. During the PET, it is important that full mixing of the intraperitoneal dialysate occur, and to facilitate this, rolling of the patient from side to side during the infusion phase is important.

e. Storage of peritoneal effluent specimens

(1) Stability. The urea nitrogen and creatinine levels in the effluent may diminish on storage (due to bacterial breakdown) unless the sample is assayed promptly, and even refrigerated samples should ideally be analyzed within several days. If longer storage is anticipated, the samples should immediately be stored in a freezer.

(2) Assaying thawed samples. Before assaying thawed effluent specimens, the specimen should be mixed with a vortex; during thawing, concentration gradients commonly develop in the specimen, producing a nonhomogeneous solute distribution. This is an important potential source of error.

f. Laboratory errors

(1) Errors pertaining to glucose determination. Because ordinarily the glucose level in the effluent will be quite high (500–2,000 mg per dL, or 28–112 mmol per L), the sample for glucose is best diluted (e.g., 1 : 10) with saline before it is measured in the clinical laboratory.

(2) Errors pertaining to creatinine determination. With some methods of creatinine determination, the high dialysate glucose levels will interfere with the assay, resulting in falsely high creatinine readings (about 0.5 mg per dL for every 1,000 mg per dL glucose is typical). The exact correction factor for a given reference laboratory can vary greatly and is determined by measuring creatinine standards in different solutions containing 500, 1,000, 2,000, or 4,000 mg per dL glucose. Ideally, the newer creatinine assays that show very little interference by glucose should be used (Larpent and Verger, 1990).

D. Evaluation of fluid overload and UF failure. Once the diagnosis of fluid overload is made, the initial step is to search for reversible, non–membrane-related causes by taking a history from the patient, doing a physical examination, and checking the dialysis records to identify the time course and appropriateness of the patient's response to the problem. Often there are obvious non–membrane-related causes, which may include excess salt and water intake, severe hyperglycemia, noncompliance with exchanges, and failure to select appropriately hypertonic dialysis solutions. They may also include mechanical causes, such as leaks or catheter obstruction, entrapment, or malposition, which may be suspected after observing the patient do a quick fill and drain in the clinic.

If such problems are not immediately apparent, the next step is to evaluate UF more formally. This can be done by measuring the drain volume after a 2-L, 4-hour, 4.25% dextrose dwell, with a diagnosis of UF failure being made if the net UF is less than 400 mL. Alternatively, fast PET can be done with net UF less than 200 mL being consistent with UF failure. In either case, the equilibration ratios for urea, creatinine, and glucose should also be measured.

Causes of fluid overload and UF failure can be classified on the basis of the PET. The demonstration of a change in the PET may be more useful than a single PET reading taken in isolation. Therefore, all patients should have a "baseline" PET 3–6 weeks after starting peritoneal dialysis (Rocco et al, 1995). In patients with fluid overload, the assessment of UF and equilibration will typically fall into one of four categories.

1. Normal UF volume. A patient who has evidence of fluid overload but has a normal test result does not have truly diminished UF capacity. There are several reasons why such a patient can have clinical difficulty with fluid overload.

a. Excessive salt and water ingestion. With commonly used peritoneal dialysis regimens, patients with normal peritoneal membranes may produce up to 2.5 L of UF per day. In anuric patients, fluid ingestion above this level often leads to fluid overload.

b. Loss of residual renal function. This is an important and frequently overlooked cause of fluid overload in the face of normal UF. The patient is accustomed to a high fluid intake, and when urine output is lost, fluid overload will result if intake is not reduced or if the peritoneal dialysis prescription is not altered accordingly.

c. Noncompliance with the dialysis prescription. If the UF test is normal, one should suspect noncompliance with dialysis (e.g., two to three exchanges per day). Also, one may detect other clinical or laboratory signs consistent with inadequate dialysis.

d. Failure to use appropriately hypertonic dialysis solution. Some patients are concerned about using hypertonic bags because of fear of hyperglycemia, dehydration, or long-term side effects; pain on infusion, or because of lack of understanding. In the anuric patient, it is very difficult to achieve good salt and water balance without using hypertonic dialysis solution.

e.   Leakage. Occult leakage of dialysate through the abdominal wall into the subcutaneous issues may mimic fluid overload or suggest diminished UF. Often such patients will give a history of sudden diminution in their usual drain volume. When measuring UF with the PET, the volume drained may be normal or subnormal, depending on the size of the leak and whether it is active when the test is being performed. (For the diagnosis of leakage, see Chapter 20.)

f.   Excessive fluid absorption during the long-dwell exchange. In some patients, UF on the PET is normal but there is marked net fluid resorption during the long dwell exchange (i.e., the night exchange in CAPD patients and the daytime dwell in continuous cycling peritoneal dialysis patients). This is diagnosed by measuring the drainage volume after the long dwell exchange.

2.   Low UF volume, high solute transport

a.   Test results. Typically, the 4-hour drainage volume will be below 2,080 mL, the dialysate glucose level will be less than 500 mg per dL (28 mmol per L) and D/P Cr is 0.8 or higher. This constellation of findings has been called type I UF failure.

b.   Pathophysiology. The primary mechanism for type I UF failure is dissipation of the osmotic gradient due to absorption of glucose from the dialysate. The rapid reabsorption is likely due to increased vascular permeability and/or increased vascularity, which produces an increase in effective peritoneal surface area. The cause of type I UF failure is unknown, but the condition may be intrinsic (present from the initiation of peritoneal dialysis though often disguised by the presence of a significant urine output). Alternatively, it may be acquired as a result of membrane damage due to peritonitis, or perhaps due to chronic exposure to dialysate or to chronic release of exotoxin/endotoxin from the peritoneal catheter biofilm. It can also be transient, as is seen during and for a few weeks after episodes of peritonitis. Permeability to other solutes, such as urea and creatinine, also rises, so that solute removal is typically not a problem with this type of UF failure.

c.   Incidence. Type I UF failure is uncommon at the initiation of peritoneal dialysis (less than 3%) but increases in prevalence with time (up to 30% after 6 years).

3.   Low UF volume, reduced solute transport

a.   Test results. In these patients, the D/P Cr often is less than 0.5, and the dialysate glucose level is relatively high due to decreased absorption. This scenario would be expected to lead to a high UF volume due to a well-maintained osmotic gradient. However, these particular patients have low UF, and this relatively uncommon constellation of findings has been called type II UF failure.

   b.   Pathophysiology. In these patients, UF fails because of reduced peritoneal membrane water permeability or because of a decrease in the surface area of the membrane. It has been proposed that a number of irritants can stimulate peritoneal macrophages to secrete lymphokines, thus activating fibroblasts to cause peritoneal fibrosis. It may also result from severe or inadequately treated peritonitis, extensive adhesion formation after an abdominal operation, or intra-abdominal inflammation of any cause. Also, sclerosing encapsulating peritonitis is a rare and progressive complication of long-term peritoneal dialysis that can manifest as type II UF failure. The peritoneum in such patients is thickened and encapsulates the bowel loops like a cocoon. This usually fatal condition has characteristic computed tomography findings.
   c.   Incidence. Type II UF failure is much less common than type I.
4.   Low UF volume, normal solute transport
   a.   Excess lymphatic transport or dialysate resorption. Increased resorption of dialysate from the peritoneal cavity due to increased lymphatic flow or resorption into the abdominal wall is an important factor in some cases of UF failure and has been termed type III UF failure. The usual dialysate absorption rate may be around 60–100 mL per hour. Thus, over a 4-hour dwell, there would be about 250–400 mL of dialysate absorption. Given that the mean 4-hour drainage volume is about 320 mL, true UF may be 600–700 mL of UF over the 4-hour period. It is not clear why fluid resorption and/or lymphatic flow varies between patients. It is, however, recognized that higher intraperitoneal pressures, as may be seen in the supine position or with larger dwell volumes, may increase dialysate absorption (Durand et al, 1992).
   b.   Incidence. It is unclear what proportion of UF problems is due to type III UF failure. In one study, such failure accounted for two of nine cases.
   c.   Loss of aquaporins. A recently recognized cause of UF failure in patients whose solute transport may be normal, thus mimicking type III UF failure, is the loss or dysfunction of peritoneal membrane aquaporins. These water transport molecules are found in the peritoneal mesothelium and vascular endothelium, as well as elsewhere in the body, and correspond to the "ultrapores" in the three-pore model of peritoneal transport (see Chapter 13). These molecules transport water without any accompanying sodium (they have a very high sodium sieving coefficient) or other solute and are responsible for about half of true peritoneal UF. If they malfunction, water transport is diminished and dialysate sodium is relatively higher because sodium sieving is much less. To diagnose this, the dialysate and plasma sodium are measured after 60 minutes with a 1.5%, 2-L dextrose dwell and then after 60 minutes with a 4.25% dwell. Normally, the plasma-to-dialysate sodium gradient is at least 5 mEq per L greater with the 4.25% solution, due to marked sodium sieving through the aquaporins, but if these aquaporins are

decreased or dysfunctional, the gradient may be less than 5 mEq per L. In one recent study, 3 of 8 patients with UF failure had gradients less than 5 mEq per L, suggesting that aquaporin dysfunction was contributing to the problem.

    d. Mechanical problems. Leaks and catheter dysfunction are part of the differential diagnosis of low UF and normal membrane function. Again, clinical examination and imaging investigations, as described in Chapter 20, should allow this diagnosis to be made.

III. Management (Table 18-3)

  A. Normal test result. If noncompliance with fluid restriction or exchanges is diagnosed, patient education is required. If hyperglycemia is part of the problem, it should be corrected. If a catheter problem or leak is identified as the cause of fluid overload, this should be managed as discussed in Chapters 15 and 20, respectively. If the drainage volume of the long-dwell exchange is reduced despite good UF on the PET, the long-dwell exchange should be replaced by one or more exchanges of appropriately shorter duration. Strategies to do this are discussed below as part of the management of type I UF failure.

  B. Type I UF failure. Several management strategies can be tried:

    1. Reducing dwell time. Switching the patient from CAPD to APD eliminates several relatively long-dwell exchanges and usually increases total daily UF in patients with type I UF failure. On APD, it may help to increase the number of cycles to as many as one per hour so that the glucose gradient never has time to dissipate. However, this switching is expensive and may even decrease solute clearance because of the greater proportion of time being spent draining and filling.

    2. Eliminating long-dwell exchanges. Another option for the CAPD patient is to use a nighttime-exchange device to break up the long nocturnal dwell and so prevent excess fluid resorption. If the patient switches to or is already on APD, the long day dwell will be a problem. Going "day-dry"

Table 18-3. Treatment of net ultrafiltration failure

Type I UF failure:
Avoid long dwells
Glucose polymers
Type II and III UF failure
Avoid long dwells
Avoid very large dialysate volumes
Phosphatidylcholine?
Associated with impaired aquaporin function/transcellular water transport:
Avoid glucose?
Discontinue CAPD temporarily?
Glucose polymers

UF, ultrafiltration; CAPD, continuous ambulatory peritoneal dialysis.
Adapted from Krediet et al, 1996 with permission from Blackwell Scientific.

is one option, but in most patients, this will not provide adequate clearance. A better idea is to break up the long day dwell with one or more exchanges. These can be done by using manual CAPD tubing or by using the cycler tubing followed by a disconnection for 3 or 4 hours prior to cycling. If only one day dwell is required, this can be left in when coming off the cycler and drained with the APD tubing 3–4 hours later. Alternatively, the patient can go day-dry until 3–4 hours before cycling when the cycler tubing can be used to run in a dwell after which the patient disconnects. These short-duration dwells will not only prevent fluid resorption but will also give significant solute clearance in this high-transporter population.

3. "Resting" the membrane. For unknown reasons, stopping peritoneal dialysis for several weeks or months can sometimes reduce peritoneal hyperpermeability to glucose, with partial or complete restoration of UF capacity.

4. Alternative osmotic agents. An ideal solution to this problem would be to have a nonabsorbable osmotic agent, instead of glucose, in the dialysate. One such agent that is now being used in many countries is a polyglucose preparation known as icodextrin. This allows good UF to be maintained even over long dwells in high transporters. One theoretical concern is that some is absorbed and broken down to maltose, which cannot be further metabolized and so accumulates in the body. However, as no toxic effects have been identified even with long-term use, this appears to be a promising strategy. Typically, the polyglucose is used for long dwells only (the day dwell in APD or the nocturnal dwell in CAPD).

C. Type II and type III UF failure. With type II UF failure, switching to APD with consequent short dwell times may increase net UF. In mild cases, fluid restriction and use of a short cycle time may be sufficient to maintain euvolemia. In many of these patients, however, solute transport is also impaired, and transfer to hemodialysis becomes necessary. With type III UF failure, the short cycles of APD may also help, but, again, the long day dwell may have to be replaced by one or two shorter ones. Agents that decrease lymphatic flow would be ideal; phosphatidylcholine may do this, but there is limited evidence for its effectiveness in clinical practice.

D. Overhydration/edema. Of relevance to management of all causes of fluid overload is the observation that overhydration per se may reversibly impair the UF capability of the peritoneal membrane (Coli et al, 1986). In overhydrated patients, therefore, euvolemia should be restored, if possible, before performing the PET and diagnosing UF failure (Table 18-1). In the longer term, maintaining euvolemia in peritoneal dialysis patients may maximize UF. In addition to advising fluid restriction and appropriate choice of hypertonic dialysate, furosemide (e.g., 500 mg PO three times weekly or once daily) can increase the amount of urine output in patients with residual renal function.

E. Prevention of UF failure. While the etiology of UF failure is not clearly understood, a number of strategies can be used to prevent its occurrence. These involve protecting the peritoneal membrane or at least mitigating the effects of high-transport status. Membrane protection and preservation involves avoidance of peritonitis and, perhaps, limiting use of hypertonic dextrose dialysis solution, which is widely believed to damage the peritoneal membrane. Newer biocompatible solutions, based on bicarbonate buffer or different osmotic agents and now becoming available, may also better preserve the membrane, but this remains unproven.

Awareness of PET status and direction of high and high-average transporters to APD or icodextrin solution for long dwells may also help avoid fluid overload in this predisposed population. Given the poor outcomes described for these patients on standard CAPD, such an approach seems justified. Preservation of residual renal function and thus of urine output will also help. Preservation approaches include avoidance of nephrotoxins, such as aminoglycosides and nonsteroidal anti-inflammatory drugs, where possible. Again, the use of high-dose loop diuretics (e.g., furosemide 250–500 mg daily) should be considered in all peritoneal dialysis patients. Fluid and salt restriction should also be considered in patients at risk, such as high transporters and those who are anuric. Finally, glycemic control in diabetic patients may help maintain better UF.

IV. Hypertension and hypotension in CAPD

A. Hypertension. A substantial percentage of patients starting CAPD have hypertension, the pathogenesis of which is multifactorial. Proposed pathways for the genesis of hypertension include sodium and fluid overload, hyperstimulation of the renin–angiotensin system, and increased sympathetic activity. It would appear that the most important factor in CAPD influencing blood pressure is salt and fluid status. Indeed, in one report, improvement in blood pressure in the first 2 months of CAPD was related to the decrement in weight, suggesting that volume control was the critical factor (Saldanha et al, 1993).

Early reports suggested that peritoneal dialysis dramatically improved blood pressure control. However, this has not always been the experience in recent studies. It has been noted by some investigators that over a long duration of follow-up, CAPD patients require more classes of antihypertensive agents than patients on hemodialysis (Ritz et al, 1996). They were also less frequently off antihypertensive medications than hemodialysis patients. However, the same observations have not been made in other studies, some of which show better blood pressure control on peritoneal dialysis. It is likely that differences in patient case mix and in dialysis practices explain these contrasting findings.

Factors contributing to worsening of blood pressure control include loss of residual renal function and development of incipient UF failure with consequent salt and water overload, particularly in patients with high-transport status. Treatment with erythropoietin may be another important contributor to hypertension in peritoneal dialysis patients.

B. Hypotension. In contrast to the large number of peritoneal dialysis patients who are hypertensive, there is a proportion of patients who have chronic hypotension. In a retrospective analysis of 525 patients treated with CAPD, 65 were found to have hypotension (Shetty et al, 1996). The patients in this group tended to be sicker and had a higher mortality. Hypotension was attributed to hypovolemia in 25%, heart failure in 23%, and antihypertensive medications in 18%. There remained a category of patients (34%) in whom the cause was unclear. Correction of the underlying problem, where identifiable, could improve the hypotension. However, this is not always successful. Thus, in the above study, 88% of hypovolemic subjects responded readily to volume expansion, in contrast to the heart failure group in whom only 40% responded to therapeutic maneuvers. Overall, it appears that hypotension is not a good prognostic sign in CAPD patients.

SELECTED READINGS

Amann K, et al. Hypertension and left ventricular hypertrophy in the CAPD patient. *Kidney Int* 1996;50(Suppl 56):S37–S40.

Churchill DN, et al. Increased peritoneal membrane transport is associated with decreased patient and technique survival for continuous peritoneal dialysis patients. The Canada-USA (CANUSA) Peritoneal Dialysis Study Group. *J Am Soc Nephrol* 1998;9:1285–1292.

Coli U, et al. Role of peritoneal membrane hydration in UF capacity of patients on CAPD. In: Maher JF, Winchester JF, eds. *Frontiers in peritoneal dialysis.* New York: Field, Rich & Associates, 1986.

Durand PY, et al. Intraperitoneal pressure, peritoneal permeability and volume of ultrafiltration in CAPD. *Adv Perit Dial* 1992;8:22–25.

Heimburger O, et al. Peritoneal transport in CAPD patients with permanent loss of ultrafiltration capacity. *Kidney Int* 1990;38:495–506.

Ho-dac-Pannekeet MM, et al. Analysis of ultrafiltration failure by means of standard peritoneal permeability analysis. *Perit Dial Int* 1997;17:144–150.

International Society of Peritoneal Dialysis. Recommendations on management of fluid overload. *Perit Dial Int* 2000; in press.

Korbet SM. Evaluation of ultrafiltration failure. *Adv Ren Replace Ther* 1998;5:194–204.

Krediet RT, et al. Icodextrin's effect on peritoneal transport. *Perit Dial Int* 1997;17:35–41.

Krediet RT. The peritoneal membrane in chronic peritoneal dialysis. *Kidney Int* 1999;55:341–356.

Krediet RT, et al. Preservation of peritoneal membrane function. *Kidney Int* 1996;50(Suppl 56):S62–S68.

Larpent L, Verger C. The need for using an enzymatic colorimetric assay in creatinine determination of peritoneal dialysis solutions. *Perit Dial Int* 1990;10:89–92.

Lilaj T, et al. Influence of the preceding exchange on peritoneal equilibration test results: a prospective study. *Am J Kidney Dis* 1999;34:247–253.

Rippe B, et al. Role of transcellular water channels in peritoneal dialysis. *Perit Dial Int* 1999;19(Suppl 2):S95–S101.

Rocco MV, et al. Changes in peritoneal transport during the first month of peritoneal dialysis. *Perit Dial Int* 1995;15:12–17.

Saldanha L, et al. Effect of continuous ambulatory peritoneal dialysis on blood pressure control. *Am J Kidney Dis* 1993;21:184–188.

Shetty A, et al. Hypotension on continuous ambulatory peritoneal dialysis. *Clin Nephrol* 1996;45:390–397.

Twardowski ZJ. The fast peritoneal equilibration test. *Semin Dial* 1990;3:141.

Twardowski ZJ, et al. Peritoneal equilibration test. *Perit Dial Bull* 1997;7:138.

Peritonitis and Exit Site Infection

David J. Leehey, Vasant C. Gandhi, and John T. Daugirdas

I. Peritonitis

A. Incidence. Peritonitis remains the Achilles' heel of peritoneal dialysis. The overall incidence of peritonitis in continuous ambulatory peritoneal dialysis (CAPD) patients during the 1980s and early 1990s had averaged 1.1–1.3 episodes per year in the United States, but the introduction of Y-set and double-bag systems (see Chapter 14) has reduced this to approximately one episode every 24 months (Gahrmani et al, 1995; Monteon et al, 1998). The incidence rate in CAPD patients in the United States is now comparable to that seen in automated peritoneal dialysis (APD) patients. The same flush-before-fill methodology used in CAPD Y sets may also be used effectively in APD.

B. Pathogenesis

1. Potential routes of infection

a. Intraluminal. Peritonitis is thought to occur most often because of improper technique in making or breaking a transfer set–to–bag or catheter–to–transfer set connection. This allows bacteria to gain access to the peritoneal cavity via the catheter lumen.

b. Periluminal. Bacteria present on the skin surface can enter the peritoneal cavity via the peritoneal catheter tract. Infection of the peritoneum via this route may occur when:

(1) A permanent catheter is being used, and infection is present at the exit site or in the subcutaneous tunnel.

(2) A temporary catheter (which does not have a subcutaneous cuff) is employed for prolonged periods.

c. Transmural. Peritonitis may occur due to bacteria of intestinal origin that enter the peritoneal cavity by migrating through the bowel wall.

d. Hematogenous. Less commonly, peritonitis is due to bacteria that have seeded the peritoneum from a distant site by way of the bloodstream.

e. Transvaginal. Little is known about the possibility of ascending infection reaching the peritoneum from the vagina by way of the uterine tubes, but it may explain some instances of *Candida* peritonitis.

2. Bacteria-laden plaque. Within several months, the intraperitoneal (IP) portion of almost all permanent peritoneal catheters becomes covered with a bacteria-laden slime or plaque. It is unknown whether such plaque has an important role in the pathogenesis of peritonitis.

3. Role of host defenses. The peritoneal leukocytes are critical in combating bacteria that have entered the peritoneal space by any of the routes mentioned above. A number of factors are now known to alter their efficacy in phagocytosing and killing invading bacteria.

   a.   Dialysis solution pH and osmolality. Peritoneal dialysis solution has a pH close to 5.0 and an osmolality ranging from 1.3 to 1.8 times that of normal plasma, depending on the glucose concentration used. These unphysiologic conditions greatly inhibit the ability of peritoneal leukocytes to phagocytose and kill bacteria. High osmolality, low pH, and the presence of the lactate anion combine to cause inhibition of superoxide generation by neutrophils.

   b.   Peritoneal dialysis solution calcium levels. The antimicrobial actions of peritoneal macrophages are enhanced by both calcium and cholecalciferol. Use of a 2.5 mEq per L (1.25 mmol per L) calcium concentration in peritoneal dialysis solution has gained popularity (see Chapter 14). However, an increased risk of *Staphylococcus epidermidis* peritonitis has been associated with use of such low-calcium dialysis solutions, presumably because peritoneal macrophage function is impaired in the reduced-calcium environment (Piraino et al, 1992).

   c.   Peritoneal fluid immunoglobulin G (IgG) levels. The level of IgG in the peritoneal fluid correlates with the ability of peritoneal leukocytes to phagocytose bacteria. Patients with abnormally low levels may be prone to having more frequent episodes of peritonitis.

   d.   Human immunodeficiency virus (HIV) infection. The overall incidence of peritonitis does not appear to be higher in HIV-infected patients (Kimmel et al, 1993); however, infection with fungal species is probably more common.

C.   Etiology. Using appropriate culture techniques, an organism can be isolated from the peritoneal fluid in over 90% of cases in which symptoms and signs of peritonitis and an elevated peritoneal fluid neutrophil count are present. The responsible pathogen is almost always a bacterium, usually of the gram-positive variety (Table 19-1). The occurrence of fungal peritonitis (e.g., *Candida*) is uncommon but by no means rare. Infection with

Table 19-1.   Incidence of organisms isolated in patients with peritonitis

Organism	(%)
Bacteria	80–90
Staphylococcus epidermidis	30–45
Staphylococcus aureus	10–20
Streptococcus species	5–10
Coliforms	5–10
Klebsiella and *Enterobacter*	5
Pseudomonas	3–8
Others	<5
Mycobacterium tuberculosis	<1
Candida and other fungi	<1–10
Culture negative	5–20

Mycobacterium tuberculosis or other type of mycobacteria has been reported but is unusual.

  D. Diagnosis
  1. Diagnostic criteria for peritonitis. At least two of the following three conditions should be present: (a) symptoms and signs of peritoneal inflammation, (b) cloudy peritoneal fluid with an elevated peritoneal fluid cell count (more than 100 per μL) due predominantly (more than 50%) to neutrophils, and (c) demonstration of bacteria in the peritoneal effluent by Gram's stain or culture.

    a. Symptoms and signs. The most common symptom of peritonitis is abdominal pain. However, peritonitis should be suspected whenever a chronic peritoneal dialysis patient suffers from generalized malaise, particularly if nausea, vomiting, or diarrhea is also present. The usual manifestations of peritonitis are listed in Table 19-2.

    b. Peritoneal fluid
      (1) Cloudiness of the fluid. The peritoneal fluid generally becomes cloudy when the cell count exceeds 50–100 per μL (50–100 × 10^6 per L). In most patients, sudden onset of cloudy fluid with appropriate abdominal symptoms is sufficient evidence of peritonitis to warrant initiation of antimicrobial therapy. However, peritoneal fluid cloudiness may be due to the presence of fibrin (or, rarely, chyle) rather than to an increase in the cell count, and therefore a cell count should be obtained whenever feasible. Occasionally, fluid drained after a prolonged dwell period (such as after the daytime dwell in APD patients) appears cloudy in the absence of peritonitis. On the other hand, a relatively translucent peritoneal fluid does not completely exclude the possibility that peritonitis is present; occasionally, early in the course of peritonitis, the cell count may be only modestly elevated

Table 19-2. Incidence of symptoms and signs of peritonitis

Symptoms/Signs	%
Symptom	
Abdominal pain	95
Nausea and vomiting	30
Feverish sensation	30
Chills	20
Constipation or diarrhea	15
Sign	
Cloudy peritoneal fluid	99
Abdominal tenderness	80
Rebound tenderness	10–50[a]
Increased body temperature	33
Blood leukocytosis	25

[a] Highly variable, depending on the severity of infection and the amount of time elapsed between onset and medical evaluation.

(not enough to cause marked cloudiness of the fluid), but the percentage of peritoneal fluid neutrophils will be increased.

(2)   Importance of performing a differential count of peritoneal fluid cells. Peritonitis is usually associated with an increase in the absolute number and percentage of peritoneal fluid neutrophils. On some occasions, a high peritoneal fluid cell count (causing cloudy fluid) will be present due to an increase in the number of peritoneal fluid monocytes or eosinophils (see below). Most such cases are not associated with peritonitis and do not require antimicrobial treatment. For this reason, one should perform a differential cell count on the peritoneal fluid sample. Prior to counting, the fluid is spun in a special centrifuge (e.g., Cytospin, Shandon, Inc., Pittsburgh, PA) and the sediment colored with Wright's stain.

(3)   Obtaining the specimen

  (a)   CAPD patients. After disconnecting the drain bag full of peritoneal effluent, the bag is inverted several times to mix its contents. A sample (7 mL) is aspirated from the port of the drain bag and transferred to a tube containing ethylenediamine tetraacetic acid (EDTA).

  (b)   APD patients. In continuous cycling peritoneal dialysis (CCPD) patients, a representative cell count can be obtained easily from the daytime dwell by first draining the abdomen and taking the sample from the drainage bag. In nocturnal intermittent peritoneal dialysis (NIPD) patients who go "dry" during the day, there will often be some residual fluid present in the abdomen at the time the patient is seen. In these patients, the peritoneal fluid sample can be obtained directly via the peritoneal catheter. After careful cleaning of the catheter with povidone–iodine, a syringe is attached using meticulous sterile technique and the 2- to 3-mL of fluid in the catheter lumen is withdrawn and discarded. The peritoneal fluid sample (7 mL) is then withdrawn from the catheter using a second syringe. The sample is injected into a tube containing EDTA. If insufficient fluid is obtained in this manner, one can infuse 1 L of dialysis solution and drain the abdomen, obtaining a sample from the effluent. Although the absolute peritoneal fluid cell count will be lower in this diluted specimen, the differential will be similar to that in a sample obtained directly via the catheter.

  (c)   Storage time. Morphologic identification of the various cell types can become quite difficult in peritoneal effluent samples that have been stored for more than 3–5 hours prior to injection into the EDTA-containing sample tube.

(4)   Normal peritoneal fluid cell count values and criteria for peritonitis. The absolute peritoneal fluid cell count in CAPD patients is usually less than 50 cells per μL and is often lower than 10 cells per μL. In NIPD patients going "dry" during the day, the absolute cell count may be much higher, especially in specimens obtained directly via the catheter when the residual peritoneal fluid volume is small. Normally, the peritoneal fluid contains predominantly mononuclear cells (macrophages, monocytes, and, to a lesser extent, lymphocytes). Eosinophils and basophils are usually absent. The percentage of neutrophils does not normally exceed 15% of the total nonerythrocyte cell count and a value greater than 50% strongly suggests peritonitis, whereas one greater than 35% should raise suspicion. The percentage of neutrophils will be increased with both bacterial and fungal peritonitis, and even in many cases of tuberculous peritonitis.

The percentage of neutrophils in the peritoneal fluid is rarely elevated in the absence of peritonitis, but there are exceptions: in patients with infectious diarrhea or active colitis, in those with pelvic inflammatory disease, and in women who are menstruating or ovulating or who have recently had a pelvic examination. Pseudoperitonitis (elevated cell count, negative peritoneal fluid cultures, and benign course) has even been reported in CAPD patients who travel long distances over bumpy mountain roads (Katirtzoglou et al, 1985).

(5) Peritoneal fluid monocytosis. Tuberculous peritonitis is rare in peritoneal dialysis patients. Nevertheless, in the presence of persistent peritoneal fluid monocytosis, a diagnostic evaluation to exclude this diagnosis is warranted. Peritoneal fluid monocytosis may also occur in conjunction with peritoneal fluid eosinophilia.

(6) Peritoneal fluid eosinophilia. The peritoneal fluid eosinophil count may become elevated in peritoneal dialysis patients, causing cloudy fluid and leading to a suspicion of peritonitis (Humayun et al, 1981). Usually, the peritoneal fluid monocyte number is elevated also. Peritoneal fluid eosinophilia/monocytosis occurs most often soon after peritoneal catheter insertion. The irritant effect of peritoneal air (e.g., introduced at time of laparotomy) (Daugirdas et al, 1987) and possibly of plasticizers leached into the peritoneum from peritoneal dialysis solution containers and tubings is a suspected cause. In such cases, the eosinophilia most often resolves spontaneously within 2–6 weeks. Peritoneal fluid eosinophilia can also occur (uncommonly) during the treatment phase of peritonitis; in other patients it occurs episodically for unknown reasons. There have been several case reports of its occurring in association with fungal and parasitic infections of the peritoneum, including *Aspergillus niger*, *Paecilomyces variotii*, and *Strongyloides stercoralis*.

c. Culture of peritoneal fluid

(1) Technique. The incidence of positive peritoneal fluid cultures in patients suspected of having peritonitis depends on culture technique. One effective culture method recommended by the International Society for Peritoneal Dialysis (ISPD) Advisory Committee on Peritonitis Management (Keane et al, 2000) is outlined below:

(a) Storage. Peritoneal fluid should be cultured promptly; however, infected fluid kept at room temperature or refrigerated for a period often grows pathogenic organisms on subsequent culture.

(b)   Sample volume. The volume of peritoneal effluent sent for culture should be at least 50 mL because larger volumes increase the yield of positive culture results.

(c)   Sample preparation. The aliquot is centrifuged (e.g., at 3,000 g for 15 minutes) to concentrate the organisms. The supernatant is decanted off and the pellet resuspended in 3–5 mL of sterile saline and inoculated into standard blood culture media (aerobic and anaerobic). Radioactive culture techniques (e.g., BACTEC) may be utilized.

(2)   Yield of positive cultures. Seventy percent to ninety percent of dialysate samples obtained from patients with clinical peritonitis yield positive cultures for a specific microorganism within 24–48 hours. A more prolonged incubation period may be needed for more fastidious organisms.

(3)   Improving culture yield. The yield of positive cultures may be improved by hypotonic lysis. The centrifuged sediment is resuspended in 100 mL of sterile water to cause osmotic lysis of its cellular elements. This may induce release of intracellularly located bacteria from peritoneal leukocytes, thus increasing the recovery rate and allowing earlier microbiologic diagnosis. Washing the sediment with sterile saline and/or using an antibiotic-removing resin may result in positive cultures in patients receiving antibiotics.

(4)   Incidence of false-positive results. When such sensitive culture methods are used, approximately 7% of cultures may be positive (sometimes prolonged incubation is required), even in asymptomatic peritoneal dialysis patients. Whether such "false-positive" cultures represent contamination or subclinical peritonitis is not known.

(5)   Gram stain. Gram stain of the peritoneal fluid sediment is useful but positive in less than half of cases of culture-proven peritonitis. Gram stain is also useful for making the diagnosis of fungal peritonitis. Staining with fluorescent acridine orange dye has been reported to increase the visibility of bacterial organisms.

(a)   Necessity of performing blood cultures. Routine blood cultures are unnecessary; however, they should be performed if a patient appears septic, especially if an acute abdominal source (such as appendicitis, cholecystitis, perforated viscus, etc.) is suspected.

E.   Treatment. Much of the discussion that follows is an adaptation of the ISPD recommendations by Keane et al (2000).

1.   Initial management of peritonitis

a.   Choice of antimicrobial therapy. A first generation cephalosporin such as cefazolin or cephalothin is used in combination with ceftazidime. It is now recommended that aminoglycosides be avoided if possible in patients with residual renal function because of their nephrotoxicity (Shemin et al., 1999). Aminoglycosides may be used in patients without residual renal function. The management decision tree is shown in Fig. 19-1.

(1) Gram-positive. Because of the emergence of vancomycin-resistant organisms (e.g., enterococci), vancomycin is no longer recommended for initial therapy. First-generation cephalosporins (e.g., cefazolin) are now preferred. Intraperitoneal cefazolin can be conveniently administered in a single daily dose of 15 mg/kg, although a 25% increase in dose is recommended in patients with substantial residual renal function (Manley et al., 1999). Alternatives to cephalosporins include nafcillin and clindamycin. Vancomycin should be reserved for patients harboring β-lactam–resistant organisms, especially methicillin-resistant *S. aureus* (MRSA), or with penicillin/cephalosporin allergy. Ciprofloxacin alone is not recommended to treat gram-positive infections (Waite et al, 1993).

(2) Gram-negative, indeterminate, or not done. In many instances, it may be impractical or impossible to perform a prompt Gram stain of the peritoneal fluid effluent. Moreover, Gram stain is positive in only 9%–40% of peritonitis episodes and treatment usually is begun without the assistance of Gram stain results. Therefore, it is usual practice to use an additional antibiotic to cover gram-

Initial empiric management of peritonitis

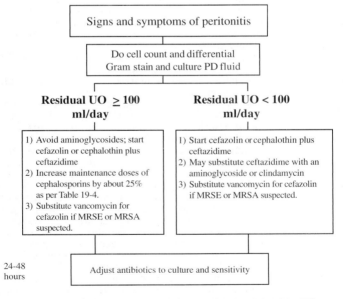

Figure 19-1. **Initial empiric management of adult peritonitis. UO, urine output. (Modified with permission from Keane W, et al. Adult peritoneal dialysis related peritonitis treatment recommendations. Update 2000.** *Perit Dial Int* 2000;20(4): in press.)

negative organisms (usually ceftazidime) until culture results are known. In Table 19-3 and Fig. 19-1 are listed sample prescriptions based on use of cefazolin in combination with ceftazidime.

(3) **Fungal organisms seen on Gram stain.** Strategies for treatment of fungal peritonitis are discussed later in this chapter.

b.   **Delivery methods and schedules for antimicrobial drugs.**

(1) **IP versus oral (PO) or intravenous (IV) antimicrobial therapy.** To treat peritonitis, antimicrobials have traditionally been administered IP rather than PO or IV, with the goal of maintaining constant and adequate drug levels in the dialysate. This remains the accepted approach, although some antimicrobials are more appropriately administered either IV (if the patient appears septic) or PO initially.

(2) **The loading dose.** A loading dose of antimicrobials is usually given IP when CAPD is the treatment modality (Table 19-4). If a patient appears toxic, we recommend giving a single loading dose IV [note that for aminoglycosides, we generally give 1.5 mg per kg (gentamicin, tobramycin) or 5 mg per kg (amikacin) IV]. Because many patients with peritonitis are in substantial pain, they may be unable to tolerate their usual exchange volume; for this reason, the IP loading dose is best administered in a bag containing only 1 L of dialysis solution. If the patient is to be treated for peritonitis while on APD, IP administration of the loading dose is less convenient. In such patients, we generally administer the loading dose IV.

(3) **Maintenance antimicrobial dose.** After the loading dose has been given, a CAPD or CCPD schedule is continued, with maintenance doses of antimicrobials added to each exchange (Table 19-4). One-liter exchange volumes may be used for several days to reduce patient discomfort. We prefer to use a CAPD regimen because of ease of antibiotic administration; however, this may result in fluid retention in rapid transporters.

(4) **Antimicrobial dosing guidelines.** Suggested loading and maintenance doses for a number of antimicrobial drugs are listed in Table 19-4. For maintenance doses added to the dialysis solution, there are two strategies. The first is to add the same dose to each dialysis solution bag. An alternative strategy is to add a larger dose to one bag only, every 12 or 24 hours (or, in the case of vancomycin, every 5–7 days). Single daily dose aminoglycosides have several advantages, including ease of administration (especially for outpatient therapy), increased efficacy (especially for organisms with relatively high mean inhibitory concentrations, i.e., greater than 2 μg per mL), and potentially less toxicity. Increased bacterial killing rates associated with prolonged postantibiotic effect are obtained using once-daily dosing. However, trough concentrations of antibiotic (i.e., 24 hours

Table 19-3. Sample prescriptions for initial treatment of adult peritonitis with unknown organism type

CAPD (continuous-dosing method)

1. Drain abdomen and obtain cell count and culture from drainage bag. Change the transfer set.
2. **Loading dose:** Infuse 2-L[a] of 1.5% dextrose dialysis solution containing:
   500 mg ceftazidime[b]
   1,000 mg cefazolin[b]
   1,000 units/L heparin

   Allow to dwell 3 hr. In patients who appear septic, administer loading doses IV (i.e., ceftazidime 1,000 mg, cefazolin 1,000 mg) rather than IP.
3. **Maintenance dose:** Continue regular CAPD schedule, using normal exchange volume if tolerated. Add 125 mg/L ceftazidime, 125 mg/L cefazolin[c], and 1,000 units/L heparin to each dialysis solution bag.

CAPD (intermittent-dosing method)

1. Drain abdomen and obtain cell count and culture from drainage bag. Change the transfer set.
2. **Loading dose:** Infuse 2-L[a] of 1.5% dextrose dialysis solution containing:
   1,000–1,500 mg ceftazidime[b]
   1,000 mg cefazolin[b,c]
   1,000 units/L heparin

   Allow to dwell 3 hr. In patients who appear septic, administer loading doses IV as per CAPD above.
3. **Maintenance dose:** Continue regular CAPD schedule, using normal exchange volume if tolerated. Administer 1,000–1,500 mg ceftazidime[b] and 1,000 mg cefazolin[b,c] to one exchange/day only (e.g., the long nocturnal exchange; the other exchanges contain no antibiotics!). If fibrin or blood is present in dialysate, add heparin to every exchange.

APD (continuous-dosing method)

Severe cases: Administer the loading doses of antimicrobials IV. Place on cycler for 24–48 hr continuously, using a 1- to 4-hr dwell time. Add maintenance doses of antimicrobials and heparin to each bag of dialysis solution as for CAPD.

Mild to moderate cases: Loading doses optional. Continue on usual CCPD or NIPD schedule; and maintenance doses of antimicrobials and heparin to each dialysis solution bag.

APD (intermittent-dosing method)

Severe cases: not recommended.

Mild to moderate cases: Treat with CCPD schedule; add 1,000–1,500 mg ceftazidime[b] and 1,000 mg cefazolin[b,c] to the long daytime dwell only (the other exchanges contain no antibiotics!)

---

[a] 2-L bags may initially cause discomfort. A 1-L bag can be used initially to administer the loading dose, but then the total amount of antibiotic in the loading exchange should be kept the same (e.g., the concentration in the bag will be doubled).

[b] Loading and intermittent IP doses listed are the amounts to be added to one exchange; i.e., to the whole bag of PD solution. Maintenance doses for the continuous dosing method are given as per L concentrations.

[c] Maintenance doses of cefazolin should be increased by about 25% in patients with substantial residual renal function as per Table 19-4.

This is the ceftazidime/cefazolin approach from Fig. 19-1. Aminoglycosides may be used initially in patients with residual urine output < 100 mL per day. Drug doses are approximate, based on a 70 kg patient.

CAPD, continuous ambulatory peritoneal dialysis; CCPD, continuous cycling peritoneal dialysis; NIPD, nocturnal intermittent peritoneal dialysis.

Table 19-4.   Antibiotic dosing recommendations for CAPD patients with and without residual renal function

Drug	CAPD Intermittent Dosing (once/d)		CAPD Continuous Dosing (mg/L unless stated)	
	Anuric	Non-anuric	Anuric	Non-anuric
Aminoglycosides				
Amikacin	2 mg/kg	Increase all doses by 25%	LD 25, MD 12	All LD same as anuric.
Gentamicin	0.6 mg/kg		LD 8, MD 4	Increase all MD by 25%
Netilmicin	0.6 mg/kg		LD 8, MD 4	
Tobramycin	0.6 mg/kg		LD 8, MD 4	
Cephalosporins				
Cefazolin	15 mg/kg	20 mg/kg	LD 500, MD 125	All LD same as anuric.
Cephalothin	15 mg/kg	ND	LD 500, MD 125	MD increase by 25%
Cephradine	15 mg/kg	ND	LD 500, MD 125	MD, ND
Cephalexin	500 mg PO qid	ND	As intermittent	MD, ND
Cefuroxime	400 mg PO/IV qd	ND	200, MD 100–200	MD, ND
Ceftazidime	1000–1500 mg	ND	LD 250, MD 125	MD, ND
Ceftizoxime	1000 mg	ND	LD 250, MD 125	MD, ND
Penicillins				
Piperacillin	4000 mg IV bid	ND	LD 4 g IV, MD 250	All LD same as anuric.
Ampicillin	250–500 mg PO bid	ND	MD 125; or 250–500 mg	MD, ND
Dicloxacillin	250–500 mg PO qid	ND	250–500 mg PO qid	MD, ND
Oxacillin	ND	ND	MD 125	MD, ND
Nafcillin	ND	No change	MD 125	MD, no change

Amoxicillin	ND	ND	LD 250-500, MD 50	MD, ND
Penicillin G	ND	ND	LD 50,000 units, MD 25,000 units	MD, ND
Quinolones				
Ciprofloxacin	500 mg PO bid	ND	LD 50, MD 25	ND
Ofloxacin	400 mg PO, then 200 mg PO qd	ND	As intermittent	ND
Others				
Vancomycin	15–30 mg/kg q5–7d	Increase doses by 25%	LD 1000, MD 25	All LD same as anuric. Increase MD by 25%
Teicoplanin	400 mg IP bid	ND	LD 400, MD 40[a]	ND
Aztreonam	ND	ND	LD 1000, MD 250	ND
Clindamycin	ND	ND	LD 300, MD 150	ND
Metronidazole	250 mg PO bid	ND	As intermittent	ND
Rifampin	300 mg PO bid	ND	As intermittent	ND
Antifungals				All LD same as anuric.
Amphotericin	NA	NA	1.5	NA
Flucytosine	2 g LD, then 1 g qd PO	ND	as intermittent	ND
Fluconazole	200 mg qd	ND	as intermittent	ND
Itraconazole	100 mg q 12 h	100 mg q 12 h	100 mg q 12 h	100 mg q 12 h
Anti-tuberculars	Isoniazid 300 mg PO qd + rifampin 600 mg PO qd + pyrazinamide 1.5 g PO qd plus Pyridoxine 100 mg/d	ND	As intermittent	ND

continued

Table 19-4.   *Continued*

Drug	CAPD Intermittent Dosing (once/d)		CAPD Continuous Dosing (mg/L unless stated)	
	Anuric	Non-anuric	Anuric	Non-anuric
Combinations				All LD same as anuric.
Ampicillin/ sulbactam	2 g q12h	ND	LD 1000, MD 100	ND
Trimeth/ sulphamethox	320/1600 mg q1-2d PO	ND	LD 320/1600, MD 80/400	ND

LD = loading dose; MD = maintenance dose; NA = not applicable; ND = no data; IV = intravenous; IP = intraperitoneally; PO = oral; qd = once a day; BID = twice a day; TID = three times a day; QID = four times a day.

The route of administration is intraperitoneal unless otherwise specified. The pharmacokinetic data and proposed dosage regimens presented here are based on published literature reviewed through January 2000, or established clinical practice. There is no evidence that mixing different antibiotics in dialysis fluid (except for aminoglycosides and penicillins) is deleterious for the drugs or patients. Do not use the same syringe to mix antibiotics.

Note: CAPD patients with residual renal function may require increased doses or more frequent dosing, especially when using intermittent regimens.

Anuric = < 100 mL urine/24 h. Non-anuric = > 100 mL/24 h.

For penicillins and cephalosporins: "no change" is for those predominantly hepatically metabolized, or hepatically metabolized and renally excreted; "ND" means no data, but these are predominantly renally excreted, therefore probably an increase in dose by 25% warranted; "NA" = not applicable, i.e. drug is extensively metabolized and therefore there should be no difference in dosing between anuric and non-anuric patients.

These data for CAPD only.

[a] This is in each bag × 7 d, then in 2 bags/d × 7 d and then in 1 bag/d × 7 d.

after a dose) will be low. The fact that the exact duration of the postantibiotic effect is unknown has led to some concern about the advisability of this type of regimen, especially in patients with residual renal function (Low et al, 1996).

There has been emerging interest in once-daily cefazolin dosing. Doses of 1.0–2.0 g IP daily have been utilized (Vas et al, 1997; Lai et al, 1997; Troidle et al, 1997). As there is no postantibiotic effect with cefazolin as there is with aminoglycosides, there is some concern that once-daily dosing may lead to more treatment failures than intermittent dosing. Therefore, convenience of administration must be balanced against the possibility of decreased efficacy.

c. Heparin. Peritonitis is often associated with formation of fibrinous clots in the peritoneal fluid, and the risk of catheter obstruction is high. For this reason, most add heparin (500–1,000 units per L) to the dialysis solution until signs and symptoms of peritonitis have resolved and until fibrinous clots are no longer visible in the peritoneal effluent.

d. Alterations in schedule for CAPD and APD. CAPD patients can generally continue their normal schedule of exchanges, unless, as discussed below, ultrafiltration becomes inadequate. Some physicians prefer to treat moderate to severe peritonitis in both CAPD and APD patients for the initial 24–48 hours with a series of 1- to 4-hour exchanges containing antimicrobials administered via a cycler. In CCPD patients with mild to moderate peritonitis, the usual CCPD schedule can be continued unchanged with antibiotics administered either continuously (added to all exchanges) or intermittently (added only to the daytime dwell). Alternatively, the patient can temporarily be converted to CAPD. In APD patients, it has been reported (Manley et al, 2000) that the initial intraperitoneal tobramycin dose should be 1.5 mg/kg, rather than 0.6 mg/kg as suggested by the ISPD Advisory Committee (Keane et al, 1996). Doses of selected antimicrobials in patients who remain on APD during treatment of peritonitis are given in Table 19–5. The decision to hospitalize a patient depends on many factors, including patient reliability, severity of peritonitis, and the type of treatment schedule chosen. In most centers, the majority of cases are now managed on an outpatient basis.

e. Consideration of secondary peritonitis. In a small but significant proportion of patients with peritonitis, a serious, underlying intra-abdominal disease process (e.g., perforated gastric or duodenal ulcer, pancreatitis, appendicitis, or diverticulitis) may be present. The presence of peritoneal fluid in the abdomen may mask the local tenderness commonly associated with some of these conditions. There is no easy method to detect these conditions at initial presentation. The presence of free IP air on upright chest radiograph is an unusual finding in CAPD patients, provided recent laparotomy or transfer set change has not been performed, and may suggest the presence of a

Table 19-5.   Dosing of antibiotics, by the intraperitoneal (IP) intermittent route, in automated peritoneal dialysis (APD)

Drug	
[a]Piperacillin	4000 mg IV bid
[a]Vancomycin	LD 35 mg/kg, MD 15 mg/kg IP qd
[b]Cefazolin	20 mg/kg qd, in first or second ambulatory dwell
[b]Tobramycin	LD 1.5 mg/kg d 1, MD 0.5 mg/kg qd, in first or second ambulatory dwell.
Fluconazole	200 mg IP q 24–48 h

Note: unless otherwise specified, IP doses to be added to the first ambulatory dwell after the automated exchanges. These data for APD only.
ID = insufficient data
[a] Unpublished data
[b] Manley HJ, et al, 2000.

perforated viscus. However, free IP air may occur more commonly in patients being treated with cyclers. A very high peritoneal fluid amylase level suggests pancreatitis or other serious intra-abdominal pathology. The interpretation of plasma amylase and lipase levels in dialysis patients with suspected pancreatitis is discussed in Chapter 24.

f.   Consequence of changes in peritoneal permeability. During peritonitis the permeability of the peritoneum to water, glucose, and proteins is increased. Rapid glucose absorption from the dialysis solution reduces the amount of ultrafiltration and can result in fluid overload. Higher dialysis solution glucose levels and shorter dwell times may be needed to maintain adequate ultrafiltration. Because glucose absorption is more rapid during peritonitis, hyperglycemia can result and may be severe in diabetics unless plasma glucose values are monitored with appropriate adjustments to the insulin dosage.

Protein losses during peritonitis are increased and should be dealt with by increasing dietary protein intake.

g.   Constipation. Constipation is a common associated complaint during peritonitis episodes. If present, phosphate binders (many of which can cause constipation) should be temporarily discontinued.

2.   Initial management of peritoneal contamination without peritonitis. After bacterial contamination of the peritoneal cavity, the incubation period for most organisms is about 12–48 hours. If a break in sterile technique has occurred, then it is advisable to institute antimicrobial therapy promptly in order to prevent peritonitis. The transfer set should be changed and the peritoneal cavity flushed with Ringer's lactate solution containing an antistaphylococcal antibiotic. A short (1- to 2-day) course of oral antimicrobial therapy may also be given. There is no documentation that these procedures are effective in preventing peritonitis.

3.   Change in management of peritonitis based on patient course and initial culture results. With effective treatment, the patient should begin to improve clinically within 12−48 hours, and the total cell count and percentage of neutrophils in the peritoneal fluid should begin to decrease.

Isolation of causative bacteria and determination of their antimicrobial sensitivity can generally be performed within 2−3 days. Longer growth periods may be needed for certain fastidious organisms (e.g., gentamicin- and methicillin-resistant *Staphylococcus aureus*). A single organism is isolated in 70%−90% of cases (Table 19-1).

a. Gram-positive organism cultured (Fig. 19-2). If *S. aureus*, *S. epidermidis*, or a *Streptococcus* species is identified, then continued therapy with a single antimicrobial agent is recommended. If an aminoglycoside was given initially, it can now be stopped. Many *S. epidermidis*-like organisms reported to be resistant to first-generation cephalo-

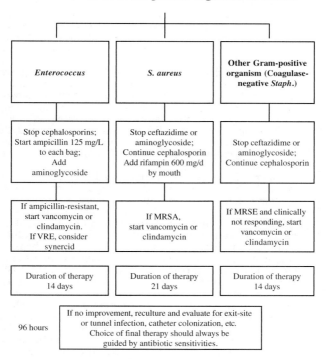

Figure 19-2. Management strategy of Gram-positive peritonitis. MRSA, methicillin resistant *Staph. aureus;* MRSE, methicillin resistant *Staph. epidermidis*. Modified with permission from Keane W, et al. Adult peritoneal dialysis related peritonitis treatment recommendations. Update 2000. *Perit Dial Int* 2000;20(4): in press.

sporins are sensitive to the levels achieved in the peritoneal cavity. Thus if the patient is clinically responding to treatment, there is usually no need to change the antibiotic regimen. If an *Enterococcus* species is cultured, ampicillin plus an aminoglycoside are generally employed.

(1) **Duration of therapy.** If patient improvement is prompt, antimicrobial therapy should be continued for a total of 14 days. If a cephalosporin is being used, then some physicians will switch to PO therapy after the first 5 days. Severe *S. aureus* infections require antimicrobials for 3 weeks, and treatment with one IP antistaphylococcal drug plus PO rifampin is recommended.

(2) **Nasal carriage and *S. aureus* infection.** Patients in whom *S. aureus* peritonitis develops not uncommonly are found to carry this organism in the nose. Eradication of nasal carriage may help prevent further peritoneal infections by this bacterium. This can be accomplished with intranasal mupirocin (bid for 5 days every 4 weeks) or oral rifampin (300 mg bid for 5 days every 3 months).

b.   Gram-negative organism cultured. Recovery of a gram-negative organism, even in a patient who is improving clinically, has several important implications: (a) gram-negative infections (especially *Pseudomonas* species) are hard to eradicate and may require treatment with several antimicrobial drugs for a prolonged duration, (b) gram-negative peritonitis may be a sign of unsuspected intra-abdominal pathology, and (c) prolonged treatment with aminoglycosides engenders the risk of otovestibular toxicity.

One decision tree for management is presented in Fig. 19-3. If a single, non-*Pseudomonas* species is recovered, the peritonitis can usually be treated by continuation of the IP aminoglycoside alone or by another single appropriate antibiotic.

If a *Pseudomonas* species is recovered, then the IP aminoglycoside should be continued with the addition of a semi-synthetic penicillin with anti-*Pseudomonas* activity (e.g., piperacillin) administered IV. Semisynthetic penicillins can inactivate aminoglycosides in vitro and thus should not be coadministered IP. Other alternatives are ceftazidime, ciprofloxacin, aztreonam, imipenem, and trimethoprim–sulfamethoxazole. *Pseudomonas* peritonitis requires catheter removal in up to two-thirds of cases (Bunke et al, 1995). However, the combination of ceftazidime and ciprofloxacin has been reported to be beneficial in a small series of patients (Shemin et al, 1996). Fluoroquinolones (such as ciprofloxacin and ofloxacin) have the advantage that effective dialysate levels can usually be achieved after PO dosing; however, concurrent administration with phosphate-binding antacids should be avoided to ensure adequate absorption from the gastrointestinal tract.

(1) **Duration of therapy.** In uncomplicated cases, duration of therapy for gram-negative peritonitis should be 21 days.

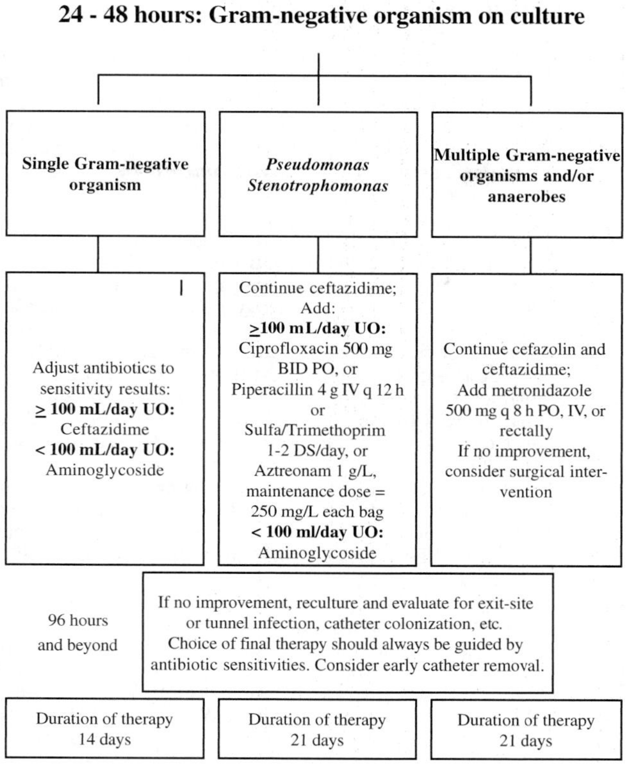

24 - 48 hours: Gram-negative organism on culture

Figure 19-3. Management strategy of Gram-negative peritonitis. UO, urine output. Modified with permission from Keane W, et al. Adult peritoneal dialysis related peritonitis treatment recommendations. Update 2000. *Perit Dial Int* **2000;20(4): in press.**

(2) IP aminoglycoside toxicity. To treat gram-negative peritonitis, a prolonged course (2 weeks) of aminoglycosides may be required. In the usual dosing strategy (after the loading dose), 4–6 mg per L of gentamicin, tobramycin, or netilmicin is added to the peritoneal dialysis solution. This results in constant serum drug levels, which may cause otovestibular toxicity. Adding a higher dose to a single bag only every 24 hours avoids constant serum levels above 2 mg per L and might reduce the toxicity of IP aminoglycosides.

(3) Alternative agents. Many gram-negative organisms are sensitive to aztreonam, newer cephalosporins, quinolones, imipenem, or the semisynthetic penicillins. Use of these alternative agents should be considered both initially and when prolonged therapy of gram-negative peritonitis is required.

(4)   Infection with *Pseudomonas cepacia*. A report of peritonitis with this agent traced the cause to contaminated povidone–iodine solutions (Panlilio et al, 1992). If this organism is cultured and if povidone–iodine was being used, contamination of the solution should be suspected.

(5)   Infection with *Xanthomonas* species. The major risk factor for infection with *Xanthomonas maltophilia* is the previous use of broad-spectrum antibiotics. These are usually very resistant organisms. Medical therapy must be extended to a minimum of 3–4 weeks, and catheter removal is usually required (Szeto et al, 1997).

(6)   Infection with *Campylobacter* species. *Campylobacter* is an unusual cause of peritonitis. There is a strong association with acute enterocolitis, which may precede the onset of cloudy dialysate by many days. The method of spread of these organisms from the gastrointestinal tract to the peritoneal cavity is unknown. Treatment can include an IP aminoglycoside in combination with PO erythromycin (Wood et al, 1992).

(7)   Infection with *Pasteurella multocida*. This is a gram-negative bacterium that resides in the upper respiratory tracts of animal hosts, especially dogs and cats. Peritonitis has been described after cat bites of the dialysis tubing.

c.   Polymicrobial peritonitis. Occasionally, more than one organism is recovered on culture. More than one gram-positive organism is not unusual and is suggestive of catheter involvement. About 60% of these infections can be resolved without catheter removal (Holley et al, 1992).

(1)   Secondary peritonitis. When one of the organisms recovered is gram-negative or an anaerobe such as *Clostridium* or *Bacteroides*, this is a poor prognostic sign, suggestive of the presence of an intra-abdominal abscess or a perforated abdominal viscus. Perforated diverticulum, tubo-ovarian abscess, cholecystitis, appendicitis, perforated ulcer, and pancreatitis must all be included in the differential diagnosis.

Management of secondary peritonitis must be individualized. Initial management can be accomplished by triple-antibiotic therapy aimed at gram-positive, gram-negative, and anaerobic organisms. Use of an IP aminoglycoside, IP vancomycin, and PO metronidazole as shown in Fig. 19-3 is one possible strategy. Although such conservative management may eventually be curative, a substantial percentage of patients receiving this treatment will need early laparotomy.

d.   Culture-negative peritonitis. If the culture results are negative at 24 hours, then the most likely explanation is that a bacterial infection was present but that the responsible organisms failed to grow in the culture sample. Sometimes growth appears only after 5–7 days, and cultures should be incubated for this length of time. Management depends on whether the patient is improving clinically and is shown in Fig. 19-4. Although the approach

24 - 48 hours: Culture negative

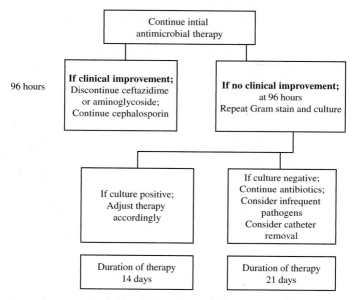

Figure 19-4. **Management strategy of culture-negative peritonitis. Modified with permission from Keane W, et al. Adult peritoneal dialysis related peritonitis treatment recommendations. Update 2000.** *Perit Dial Int* **2000;20(4): in press.**

presented in the figure is to continue both the initial aminoglycoside and cephalosporin for a full 14 days, some physicians either taper the aminoglycoside to a lower dose (e.g., 4 mg per L) or discontinue it entirely after 3 days if the patient is improving in order to limit the side effects.

Infection with *M. tuberculosis* or with nontuberculous mycobacteria sometimes presents as culture-negative peritonitis. Catheter removal is usually required but is not mandatory provided prompt therapy is carried out. This consists of a triple-drug regimen (usually isoniazid, rifampin, and pyrazinamide).

e. Fungal peritonitis. Factors predisposing to fungal peritonitis include prior antibiotic use, immunosuppression (e.g., immunosuppressive therapy, HIV infection), and malnutrition, especially a low serum albumin level. A variety of fungi are sometimes cultured, but *Candida* is the most prevalent species. Previous antibiotic therapy and diabetes mellitus are predisposing factors. There are two management strategies:

(1) Remove catheter; maintain patient on hemodialysis. Because the catheter is usually contaminated with fungi and because obstruction is common, the catheter is removed immediately. The patient is maintained on hemodialysis and usually improves, even when antifungal drugs are not administered. A new catheter can be inserted 4–6 weeks later, at least 1 week after all clinical evidence of peritonitis has subsided. Most clinicians believe this to be the optimal approach. In two recent studies (Goldie et al, 1996; Chan et al, 1994), catheter removal was necessary in 86% and 85% of patients, respectively.

One problem with simple removal of the catheter is that severe peritoneal adhesions can develop in patients with fungal peritonitis, precluding further peritoneal dialysis. In an attempt to limit adhesion formation, some physicians recommend, in addition to catheter removal, the PO or IV administration of antifungal drugs, such as amphotericin B, flucytosine, miconazole, fluconazole, or ketoconazole. The recommended dosages of these agents are the same as for patients with normal renal function, with the exception of flucytosine, for which the dosage must be reduced (see Chapter 28). However, penetration of many antifungal drugs (e.g., amphotericin B, ketoconazole) into the peritoneum after other than IP administration is poor. Penetration of flucytosine is relatively good, and a reduced incidence of peritoneal adhesion formation has been claimed after its use in fungal peritonitis.

(2) Continue peritoneal dialysis through the same catheter. Some have advocated administering IP and/or PO or IV antifungal drugs and leaving the original catheter in place if unobstructed. If there is no improvement after 4–7 days, the catheter should be removed.

4. Refractory peritonitis and indications for catheter removal. If by 48–96 hours there is no evidence of clinical improvement, then the peritoneal fluid Gram stain, cell count, and culture should be repeated. Antimicrobial removal devices should be used when culturing the peritoneal effluent to maximize the culture yield. Initially, one should attempt to readjust the antimicrobial therapy based on the culture results. If the refractory infection is due to staphylococcal species, rifampin 600 mg per day should be added if not already part of the regimen, especially if there is coexistent exit site infection. The presence of tunnel infection, intra-abdominal abscess, or gynecologic pathology should be suspected. Ultrasonography, computed tomography, or gallium scan are often helpful in diagnosis. Enterococcal peritonitis should be treated with ampicillin plus an aminoglycoside. *Pseudomonas* peritonitis is best managed by IV piperacillin plus an aminoglycoside. If anaerobic bacteria with or without multiple gram-negative organisms are cultured, surgical exploration should be considered.

With all of the above infections, if a 3- to 5-day course of the new, intensified antimicrobial regimen does not result in improvement, the peritoneal catheter should be removed and antimicrobial therapy continued for an additional 5–7 days.

After catheter removal, the safe time interval before a new catheter can be reinserted is a matter of controversy; it probably depends on the severity of the underlying peritonitis and whether fungal peritonitis or tunnel infection was present. A conservative approach is to wait several weeks, although in the absence of fungal infection it may be possible to insert a new catheter simultaneously with removal of the old catheter, obviating the need for hemodialysis (Posthuma et al, 1998). The new catheter should be inserted as far as possible from the old skin exit site.

5. Relapsing peritonitis. Relapsing peritonitis is defined as peritonitis with the same organism recurring within 4 weeks of stopping antimicrobial therapy. *S. epidermidis* or a gram-negative organism is usually involved, but "relapsing" culture-negative peritonitis is also common. The management strategy is similar to that for treating refractory peritonitis described above. That is, a trial of intensified antimicrobial therapy is given, but in the case of relapsing peritonitis, the total duration of treatment should be 2–4 weeks. In the case of relapsing gram-negative peritonitis, catheter removal with or without surgical exploration should be strongly considered, especially in patients with *Pseudomonas* infection. If it is elected to treat the patient medically, because of the dangers of prolonged aminoglycoside therapy, either the IP maintenance aminoglycoside dose should be administered intermittently or an alternative agent should be employed. As for refractory peritonitis, if antimicrobial therapy does not result in prompt clinical improvement (within 3–5 days), the peritoneal catheter should be removed and therapy continued for an additional 5–7 days.

a. Treatment with fibrinolytic enzymes. Streptokinase and urokinase have been used by some investigators in the treatment of relapsing peritonitis. These agents are utilized in an attempt to release bacteria entrapped in fibrin within the peritoneum or along the catheter, thus making it possible to eradicate the infection. Controlled studies on the use of enzymes in the treatment of relapsing peritonitis are warranted.

6. Peritonitis with catheter obstruction. Catheter obstruction frequently accompanies peritonitis. Management is discussed in Chapter 15.

7. Prophylactic antibiotic use. Prophylactic antibiotic use does not prevent peritonitis; this is probably true even for patients with exit site infections. However, short-term prophylactic antibiotics may be beneficial in the following settings: (a) before catheter placement; (b) after a technique break; (c) to prevent bacteremia during invasive procedures, such as colonoscopic polypectomy; and (d) to prevent exit site infection in the presence of *S. aureus* nasal carriage.

II. Exit site infection. Approximately one-fifth of peritonitis episodes are temporally associated with exit site and tunnel infections (Piraino et al, 1987).

A. Incidence. The incidence of exit site infections is approximately one episode every 24–48 patient-months. Patients with previous infections tend to have a higher frequency of occurrence.

B. Etiology and pathogenesis. Exit site infections are predominantly due to *S. aureus* or gram-negative organisms. In contrast to peritonitis, *S. epidermidis* is the causative organism in less than 20% of patients. *S. aureus* infections appear to have a distinct pathogenesis as they are associated with nasal and or skin carriage of the organism (Luzar et al, 1990a,b). Therefore, eradication of the carrier state is very helpful to effective management. Exit site infections due to gram-negative bacilli (enteric and pseudomonal organisms are most common) are also a source of considerable morbidity.

   C.   Therapy. Treatment is dependent on whether there is erythema alone or erythema in conjunction with purulent drainage (Fig. 19-5). In the former case, topical treatment with hypertonic saline compresses, hydrogen peroxide, or mupirocin 2% ointment

Diagnosis and Management of Exit-Site Infections

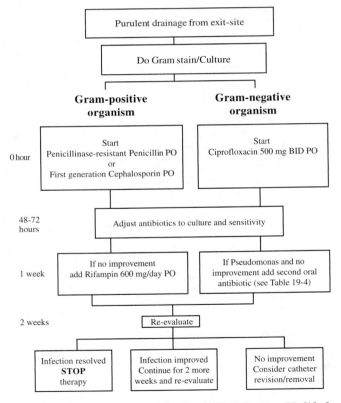

Figure 19-5.   Management strategy of exit site infections. Modified with permission from Keane W, et al. Adult peritoneal dialysis related peritonitis treatment recommendations. Update 2000. *Perit Dial Int* **2000;20(4): in press.**

is usually sufficient. Mupirocin ointment should not be used with polyurethane catheters (e.g., many catheters made by Vas-Cath or the Cruz catheter from Corpak) because the polyethylene glycol in mupirocin ointment will degrade the polyurethane and destroy the catheter. Ciprofloxacin otologic solution can be used with polyurethane catheters, but efficacy in treating exit-site infection is unknown (Montenegro et al, 2000). Treatment is more problematical and more prone to failure when there is purulent drainage. Moreover, some exit site infections extend into the subcutaneous tunnel, which may be evident only on ultrasonographic examination of the tunnel tract (Vychytil et al, 1999).

Therapy for purulent exit site infection should be based on results of Gram stain and culture. If gram-positive organisms are found, a cephalosporin or an antistaphylococcal penicillin PO is first-line treatment; IP vancomycin should be avoided unless necessary. If no improvement occurs after 1 week despite appropriate treatment based on culture and sensitivity, rifampin 600 mg per day PO may be added. If the infection has not resolved in 2 weeks, a surgical approach (deroofing, outer-cuff shaving, or catheter removal) is necessary. In the presence of tunnel infection, early cuff excision in combination with antibiotic administration results in a substantial rate of catheter salvage (Suh et al, 1997), although catheter removal is sometimes required, especially when there is coexisting peritonitis.

If gram-negative organisms are present, treatment should be based on sensitivity results. With more serious pseudomonal infections, IP ceftazidime or aminoglycoside may be necessary. Therapy should be continued until the exit site appears normal. If the exit site infection has not improved substantially within 4 weeks, catheter removal is generally required. *Pseudomonas* exit site infections often require catheter removal, although in one study, treatment with PO ciprofloxacin 500 mg bid and local care resolved the infection in the majority of patients (Kamzi et al, 1992). Magnesium–aluminum antacids as well as calcium salts, PO iron, and PO zinc may reduce the absorption of ciprofloxacin and should not be taken within 2 hours of antibiotic dosing.

D. Prevention. The major risk factor for exit site infection is staphylococcal nasal carriage. Persistently positive nasal cultures are associated with a threefold to fourfold increased risk of staphylococcal exit site infection. Therefore, it is logical to attempt to eradicate nasal carriage to prevent these infections. Protocols used include rifampin (600 mg PO for 5 days), mupirocin (2% ointment twice daily for 5 days every 4 weeks), and trimethoprim–sulfamethoxazole (one single-strength tablet three times weekly). In a randomized controlled trial, rifampin 600 mg PO for 5 days given every 3 months was effective in decreasing catheter infections (Zimmerman et al, 1991). In a recently published multicenter randomized trial (Mupirocin Study Group, 1996), use of nasal mupirocin in the regimen stated above in *S. aureus* nasal carriers resulted in a significant decline in exit site infections from this organism; however, the overall incidence of exit site infections was not decreased due to an increase in gram-negative infections, and rates of tunnel infection and peritonitis were not affected. In other trials, mupirocin ointment applied daily to the exit site decreased the rate of both exit site infections and peritonitis in comparison with a historical control group (Bernardini et al, 1996; Thodis et al, 1998).

There does not appear to be a difference in the incidence of exit site infections between double-cuff and single-cuff catheters, although the method of catheter placement may be important. Some advise leaving the catheter subcutaneously for several weeks after placement and then exteriorizing it prior to use. Use of chlorhexidine versus povidone–iodine solution is associated with a significant decrease in exit site infections in children (Jones et al, 1995). In an interesting study from Belgium, the use of protective dressing with a disinfectant was associated with a significantly decreased incidence of exit site infection compared with cleaning with regular soap and water (Luzar et al, 1990a). This difference did not apply to *S. aureus* infections—further evidence that measures in addition to local care are necessary to prevent exit site infections attributable to this organism.

SELECTED READINGS

Bernardini J, et al. A randomized trial of *Staphylococcus aureus* prophylaxis in peritoneal dialysis patients; mupirocin calcium ointment 2% applied to the exit site versus cyclic oral rifampin. *Am J Kidney Dis* 1996;27:695–700.

Bunke M, et al. *Pseudomonas* peritonitis in peritoneal dialysis patients: the Network 9 Peritonitis Study. *Am J Kidney Dis* 1995;25: 769–774.

Burkart JM. Significance, epidemiology, and prevention of peritoneal dialysis catheter infections. *Perit Dial Int* 1996;16:S340–S346.

Chan TM, et al. Treatment of fungal peritonitis complicating continuous ambulatory peritoneal dialysis with oral fluconazole: a series of 21 patients. *Nephrol Dial Transplant* 1994;9:539–542.

Daugirdas JT, et al. Induction of peritoneal fluid eosinophilia and/or monocytosis by intraperitoneal air injection. *Am J Nephrol* 1987; 7:116–120.

Gahrmani N, et al. Infection rates in end-stage renal disease patients treated with CCPD and CAPD using the UltraBag system. *Adv Perit Dial* 1995;11:164–167.

Goldie SJ, et al. Fungal peritonitis in a large chronic peritoneal dialysis population: a report of 55 episodes. *Am J Kidney Dis* 1996;28:86–91.

Holley JL, et al. Polymicrobial peritonitis in patients on continuous peritoneal dialysis. *Am J Kidney Dis* 1992;19:162–166.

Humayun HM, et al. Peritoneal fluid eosinophilia in patients undergoing maintenance peritoneal dialysis. *Arch Intern Med* 1981;141: 1172–1173.

Jones LL, et al. The impact of exit-site care and catheter design on the incidence of catheter-related infections. *Adv Perit Dial* 1995;11: 302–305.

Kamzi HR, et al. Pseudomonal exit site infections in continuous ambulatory peritoneal dialysis patients. *J Am Soc Nephrol* 1992;2:1498.

Katirtzoglou A, et al. "Pseudoperitonitis" in CAPD patients during travel. *Perit Dial Bull* 1985;5:140.

Keane W, et al, for the Advisory Committee on Peritonitis Management of the International Society of Peritoneal Dialysis. Adult peritoneal dialysis related peritonitis treatment recommendations. Updated 2000; *Perit Dial Int* 2000;20(4): in press.

Keane WF, et al. Peritoneal dialysis–related peritonitis treatment recommendations: 1996 update. *Perit Dial Int* 1996;16:557–573.

Kimmel PL, et al. Continuous ambulatory peritoneal dialysis and survival of HIV infected patients with end-stage renal disease. *Kidney Int* 1993;44:373–378.

Lai MN, et al. Intraperitoneal once-daily dosing of cefazolin and gentamicin for treating CAPD peritonitis. *Perit Dial Int* 1997;17:87–89.

Lampainen E, et al. Is air under the diaphragm a significant finding in CAPD patients? *ASAIO Trans* 1986;332:581–582.

Low CL, et al. Pharmacokinetics on once-daily IP gentamicin in CAPD patients. *Perit Dial Int* 1996;16:379–384.

Luzar MA, et al. Exit-site care and exit-site infection in continuous ambulatory peritoneal dialysis (CAPD): results of a randomized multicenter trial. *Perit Dial Int* 1990a;10:25–29.

Luzar MA, et al. *Staphylococcus aureus* nasal carriage and infection in patients on continuous ambulatory peritoneal dialysis. *N Engl J Med* 1990b;322:505–509.

Manley HJ, et al. Pharmacokinetics of intermittent intraperitoneal cefazolin in continuous ambulatory peritoneal dialysis patients. *Perit Dial Int* 1999;19:67–70.

Manley HJ, et al. Pharmacokinetics of intermittent intravenous cefazolin and tobramycin in patients treated with automated peritoneal dialysis. *J Am Soc Nephrol* 2000;11:1310–1316.

Millikin SP, Matzke GR, Keane WF. Antimicrobial treatment of peritonitis associated with continuous ambulatory peritoneal dialysis. *Perit Dial Int* 1991;11:252–260.

Monsen T, et al. Clonal spread of staphylococci among patients with peritonitis associated with continuous ambulatory peritoneal dialysis. *Kidney Int* 2000;57:613–618.

Montenegro et al. Exit-site care with ciprofloxacin otologic solution prevents polyurethane catheter infection in peritoneal dialysis patients. *Perit Dial Int* 2000;20:209–214.

Monteon F, et al. Prevention of peritonitis with disconnect systems in CAPD: a randomized controlled trial. The Mexican Nephrology Collaborative Study Group. *Kidney Int* 1998; 54:2123–2138.

Morduchowicz G, et al. Bacteremia complicating peritonitis in peritoneal dialysis patients. *Am J Nephrol* 1993;13:278–280.

Mupirocin Study Group. Nasal mupirocin prevents *Staphylococcus aureus* exit-site infection during peritoneal dialysis. *J Am Soc Nephrol* 1996;7:2403–2408.

Oxton LL, et al. Risk factors for peritoneal-dialysis related infections. *Perit Dial Int* 1994;14:137–144.

Panlilio AL, et al. Infections and pseudoinfections due to povidone–iodine solution contaminated with *Pseudomonas cepacia. Clin Infect Dis* 1992;14:1078–1083.

Piraino B. A review of *Staphylococcus aureus* exit-site and tunnel infections in peritoneal dialysis patients. *Am J Kidney Dis* 1990;16:89–95.

Piraino B, et al. A five-year study of the microbiologic results of exit site infections and peritonitis in continuous ambulatory peritoneal dialysis. *Am J Kidney Dis* 1987;4:281–286.

Piraino B, et al. Increased risk of *Staphylococcus epidermidis* peritonitis in patients on dialysate containing 1.25 mmol/L calcium. *Am J Kidney Dis* 1992;19:371–374.

Posthuma N, et al. Simultaneous peritoneal dialysis catheter insertion and removal in catheter-related infections without interruption of peritoneal dialysis. *Nephrol Dial Transplant* 1998;13:700–703.

Shemin D, et al. Effect of aminoglycoside use on residual renal function in peritoneal dialysis patients. *Am J Kidney Dis* 1999;34:14–20.

Shemin D, Maaz D. Gram-negative peritonitis in peritoneal dialysis: improved outcome with intraperitoneal ceftazidime. *Perit Dial Int* 1996;16:638–641.

Suh H, et al. Persistent exit-site/tunnel infection and subcutaneous cuff removal in PD patients. *Adv Perit Dial* 1997;13:233–236.

Szeto CC, et al. Xanthomonas maltophilia peritonitis in uremic patients receiving continuous ambulatory peritoneal dialysis. *Am J Kidney Dis* 1997;29:91–96.

Thodis E, et al. Decrease in *Staphylococcus aureus* exit-site infections and peritonitis in CAPD patients by local application of mupirocin ointment at the catheter exit site. *Perit Dial Int* 1998;18:261–270.

Troidle L, et al. Two gram intraperitoneal cefazolin for the treatment of peritonitis. *Perit Dial Int* 1997;17(Suppl 1):S40.

Vas S, et al. Treatment in PD patients of peritonitis caused by gram-positive organisms with single daily dose of antibiotics. *Perit Dial Int* 1997;17:91–94.

Vychytil A, et al. Ultrasonography of the catheter tunnel in peritoneal dialysis patients: what are the indications? *Am J Kidney Dis* 1999; 33:722–727.

Waite NM, et al. Poor response to oral ciprofloxacin in the treatment of peritonitis in patients on intermittent peritoneal dialysis. *Perit Dial Int* 1993;13:50–54.

Wood CJ, et al. *Campylobacter* peritonitis in continuous ambulatory peritoneal dialysis: report of eight cases and a review of the literature. *Am J Kidney Dis* 1992;19:257–263.

Yu AW, et al. Neutrophilic intracellular acidosis induced by conventional lactate-containing peritoneal dialysis solutions. *Int J Artif Organs* 1992;15:661–665.

Zimmerman SW, et al. Randomized controlled trial of prophylactic rifampin for peritoneal dialysis–related infections. *Am J Kidney Dis* 1991;18:225–231.

Internet Reference

Peritonitis and exit-site management protocols and links (http://www.hdcn.com/pd/peritonitis)

Mechanical Complications of Peritoneal Dialysis

Joanne M. Bargman

The instillation of dialysis fluid into the peritoneal cavity is accompanied by an increase in intra-abdominal pressure (IAP). The two principal determinants of the magnitude of the increased IAP are dialysate volume and the position of the patient during the dwell. The supine position is associated with the lowest IAP for a given dialysate volume; sitting entails the highest. Furthermore, actions such as coughing, bending, or straining at stool transiently cause very high levels of IAP. The increased IAP in peritoneal dialysis can lead to a variety of mechanical complications.

I. Hernia formation

A. Incidence and etiologic factors. The incidence and prevalence of hernias is difficult to assess. Hernias can be asymptomatic and difficult to diagnose on cursory examination. It has been suggested that as many as 10%–20% of patients may develop a hernia at some time on peritoneal dialysis.

Potential risk factors are listed in Table 20-1 and include large dialysate volumes and activities that involve isometric straining or the Valsalva maneuver. Furthermore, deconditioning of the musculature of the abdominal wall increases wall tension and predisposes to hernia formation.

B. Types of hernia. Many different types of hernia have been described in the peritoneal dialysis patient. These are listed in Table 20-2.

Indirect inguinal hernias are the result of bowel and/or dialysate tracking through the processus vaginalis, which has remained patent rather than obliterating normally. It is much more common in males. In boys, it is very likely that if one processus vaginalis is patent (causing inguinal hernia), then the other side is patent also, and repair (see below) should be done bilaterally.

C. Diagnosis. As mentioned above, hernias can be clinically occult. It is often better to have the patient stand and "bear down" as this increases IAP and makes a hernia even more obvious.

Pericatheter hernias need to be differentiated from masses caused by a hematoma, seroma, or abscess. Ultrasonography can distinguish the solid-appearing hernia from the fluid collections characterizing these other conditions. The scrotal fullness of an indirect inguinal hernia has in its differential diagnosis hydrocele (fluid/dialysate alone seeping through a patent processus vaginalis) and intrinsic scrotal or testicular pathology.

Delineation of a hernia can be aided by computed tomography (CT) scanning. One hundred milliliters of Omnipaque 300 is added to a 2-L bag of dialysate and then infused into the patient. **It is important that the patient then be as active and ambulatory as possible for the next 2 hours to facili-**

Table 20-1.   Potential risk factors for hernia formation

Large dialysate volumes
Sitting position
Isometric exercise
Valsalva maneuver (e.g., coughing, chopping wood)
Recent abdominal surgery
Pericatheter leak or hematoma
Obesity
Deconditioning
Multiparity
Congenital anatomical defects

tate the entry of dye into hernia sacs. CT scanning is then performed. In the case of inguinal hernias, it is important that the genitalia be scanned. The CT scan can indicate whether scrotal edema is the result of fluid tracking along a patent processus vaginalis or along the anterior abdominal wall (see below). This procedure can also help delineate anterior abdominal wall hernia from isolated leaks. In other types of hernia, such as umbilical hernia, CT scanning is not necessary because the diagnosis is usually obvious.

D.   Treatment. Small hernias pose the greatest risk of incarceration or strangulation of bowel. These should be repaired surgically. The patient should be warned that if a hernia stops being reducible, and especially if it becomes tender, medical consultation should be sought immediately. **Any patient presenting with peritonitis should be examined for the presence of small strangulated hernias, as these can lead to transmural leakage of bacteria and peritonitis.** Large hernias can also be repaired surgically, as can cystocele and enterocele. Uterine prolapse (not really a hernia) can sometimes be managed with a pessary, but ultimately hysterectomy may be necessary.

After surgical repair of a hernia, IAP must be kept as low as possible to facilitate healing. If the patient has significant residual renal function (e.g., 10 mL per minute or more), it may be pos-

Table 20-2.   Types of hernias reported in peritoneal dialysis patients

Ventral
Epigastric
Pericatheter
Umbilical
Inguinal (direct and indirect)
Femoral
Spigelian
Richter's
Foramen of Morgagni
Cystocele
Enterocele

sible to stop dialysis altogether for a week and then recommence with small volumes (e.g., 1 L) for another week. The patient must be watched for the development of uremic symptoms or hyperkalemia. If continuous cycling peritoneal dialysis (CCPD) is available, then the patient can dialyze supine and hence with lower IAP. If there is little or no renal function, low-volume peritoneal dialysis should be started postoperatively. An alternative is to hemodialyze the patient until wound healing is more complete (2–3 weeks).

Options for the patient with recurrent hernias includes a reduction in physical activities (e.g., stop chopping wood), more frequent dialysis exchanges with lower volumes (e.g., 5×1.5 L), CCPD with a small (e.g., 1 L) or short-duration day dwell or transfer to hemodialysis.

If the patient is too ill or refuses surgery, mechanical support of the hernia can be effected with a corset or truss. The patient should be warned about symptoms of incarceration and strangulation.

II.   Abdominal wall and pericatheter leak. The incidence of these complications is also unknown, but they are less common than hernias. Risk factors are similar to those outlined in Table 20-2, and surgical technique may play a role in the development of pericatheter leak.

   A.   Diagnosis. Abdominal wall leak may be difficult to diagnose clinically. It may be mistaken for ultrafiltration failure when dialysate returns are less than the instilled volume (Chapter 18). Weight gain is common as the dialysate accumulates in the tissues of the abdominal wall. The diagnosis should be considered with decreased effluent volumes, weight gain, protuberant abdomen, and absence of generalized edema. The patient should stand during the examination as this may reveal asymmetry of the abdomen. The abdominal wall itself may have a "baggy" look, with deep impressions made by waist bands, dialysate tubing, etc.

   Pericatheter leak is usually diagnosed by wetness (dialysate) on the exit site dressing. Diagnosis can be proven using contrast CT scanning as described under "Hernia formation" (Section I.C). Again, it is important to make sure that the patient is ambulatory for at least 2 hours after instillation of the dye to facilitate its movement into the abdominal wall.

   B.   Treatment. Pericatheter leak usually occurs as a postoperative complication of catheter implantation. It is not helpful to place purse-string sutures in response to the leak because the dialysate will then be diverted into the intervening tissue rather than exit around the catheter site. The patient should be drained and peritoneal dialysis stopped for at least 24–48 hours. The longer the patient can be left dialysate-free, the greater the chance that the leak will seal. If necessary, the patient should receive hemodialysis, and peritoneal dialysis can be recommenced several days later. In most cases, the leak seals spontaneously. If it persists, the catheter should be removed and reinserted at another site.

   In contrast to pericatheter leaks, abdominal wall leaks can occur early or late. CCPD in the supine position usually allows the dialysate accumulation to resolve. If the leak is the result of disruption of abdominal wall integrity, the patient should be converted to an NIPD regimen or to hemodialysis. Sometimes the abdominal wall defect heals after a transient course of NIPD, and CAPD can then be resumed. Sometimes surgical repair is feasible. Antibiotic prophylaxis is not usually necessary for peri-catheter leak unless there are obvious signs of infection.

Vaginal leaks can also occur. Some may result from tracking of dialysate through the fallopian tubes and may resolve with tubal ligation. Other incidents are due to dissection of dialysate through fascial defects and require patients to convert to NIPD or hemodialysis.

III.   Genital edema

A.   Pathogenesis. Dialysate can reach the genitalia by two routes: One is by traveling through a patent processus vaginalis to the tunica vaginalis, resulting in hydrocele. In this first route, the dialysate can also dissect through the tunica vaginalis, causing edema of the scrotal wall itself. The second route is through a defect in the abdominal wall, often associated with the catheter. In this instance, the dialysate tracks inferiorly along the abdominal wall and leads to edema of the foreskin and scrotum.

B.   Diagnosis. This complication is often painful and distressing to the patient who is quick to bring it to medical attention. CT peritoneography should be performed to distinguish which route has led to the genital swelling (i.e., anterior abdominal wall or processus vaginalis). Alternatively, 3–5 mCi of technetium-labeled albumin colloid can be injected into the dialysate and infused into the patient, and the route of leakage traced by scintigraphy.

C.   Treatment. Peritoneal dialysis should be temporarily stopped. Bed rest and scrotal elevation are helpful. Depending on the need, temporary CCPD with low volumes and with the patient supine can often be used without causing reaccumulation of genital edema. Hemodialysis can be used temporarily.

A leak via a patent processus vaginalis can be repaired surgically. If the leak is through the anterior abdominal wall, replacement of the catheter can be helpful. Allow time for healing of the previous defect with hemodialysis support. CCPD in the supine position allows lower IAP and decreases the chances of recurrent leakage.

IV.   Respiratory complications

A.   Hydrothorax. Under the influence of raised IAP, dialysate can travel from the peritoneal to the pleural cavity, leading to a pleural effusion composed of dialysis effluent. This complication is termed hydrothorax.

1.   Incidence and etiologic factors. The incidence of hydrothorax is unknown because the pleural effusion may be small and asymptomatic. It is less common than hernia.

There are defects in the hemidiaphragm that allow passage of dialysate. These defects may be congenital, in which case hydrothorax can occur with the first dialysis exchange, or acquired, whereby hydrothorax can be a late complication. They occur almost exclusively on the right side, probably because the left hemidiaphragm is mostly covered by heart and pericardium.

2.   Diagnosis. Symptoms of hydrothorax range from asymptomatic pleural effusion to severe shortness of breath.

Such symptoms may worsen with administration of hypertonic dialysate, which raises IAP.

Thoracentesis can be done for diagnosis or to relieve symptoms. The most diagnostic feature of the pleural fluid is the very high glucose level. It is otherwise typically transudative, with variable numbers of leukocytes.

Radionuclide scanning with technetium is also helpful. Technetium-labeled albumin colloid (5 mCi) is added to a dialysate bag, which is then infused into the patient. Posterior views are taken at 0, 10, 20, and 30 minutes and an anterior view at 30 minutes. It is important that the patient be ambulatory while the instilled tracer is dwelling to increase IAP and flux into the pleural cavity. Late (2–3 hours) views may be necessary if the movement of tracer into pleural cavity is not detected by gamma camera in earlier shots.

   3.   Treatment. If there are respiratory symptoms, peritoneal dialysis should be stopped immediately. Thoracentesis may be necessary; in which case, the diagnosis can be made by measuring glucose in the pleural fluid.

Definitive treatment entails repair of defects in hemidiaphragm or obliteration of the pleural space (pleurodesis). Rarely, the dialysate itself acts as an irritant in the pleural cavity and causes pleurodesis, so that peritoneal dialysis can be resumed 1–2 weeks later. Peritoneal dialysis with low IAP (small volumes, supine position) can sometimes be carried out without recurrence. Surgical options for treatment of hydrothorax are listed in Table 20-3.

B.   Altered mechanics of breathing. Pulmonary function is unchanged with peritoneal dialysis, except for a mildly decreased functional residual capacity. Arterial oxygenation has been observed to decrease slightly and transiently with start of CAPD.

Peritoneal dialysis does not worsen respiratory symptoms in patients with obstructive airways disease. The tonic stretch placed on the diaphragm by the raised IAP may actually facilitate the mechanics of breathing in these patients.

V.   Back pain

A.   Pathogenesis. The presence of dialysate in the peritoneal cavity both raises IAP and swings the center of gravity forward, producing lordotic stress on the lumbar vertebrae and paraspinal muscles. In predisposed individuals, the altered spinal mechanics can lead to exacerbation of sciatica or posterior facet symptoms. Lax anterior abdominal musculature will exacerbate this effect.

Table 20-3.   Surgical options for treatment of hydrothorax

Pleurodesis
   Talc
   Oxytetracycline
   Autologous blood
   Aprotonin–fibrin glue
Repair of hemidiaphragm
   Oversewing defects
   Reinforcement with patches

B. Treatment. Bed rest and analgesia are important when symptoms are acute. Some patients benefit by the performance of more frequent exchanges with smaller dialysate volumes. If possible, CCPD with a small day dwell is advisable for these patients in order to dialyze supine and so remove the lordotic stress on the lumbar spine. Ideally, the patient should undertake abdomen and back strengthening exercises, but this is not always feasible.

SELECTED READINGS

Cochran ST, et al. Complications of peritoneal dialysis: evaluation with CT peritoneography. *Radiographics* 1997;17:869–878.

Garcia Ramon R, Carrasco AM. Hydrothorax in peritoneal dialysis. *Perit Dial Int* 1998;18:5–10.

Hughes GC, et al. Thoracic complications of peritoneal dialysis. *Ann Thorac Surg* 1999;67:1518–1522.

Juergensen PH, et al. Value of scintigraphy in chronic peritoneal dialysis patients. *Kidney Int* 1999;55:1111–1119.

Khoury AE, et al. Hernias associated with CAPD in children. In: Khanna R, et al, eds. *Advances in peritoneal dialysis.* Toronto: University of Toronto Press, 1991:279–282.

Lieberman FL, et al. Pathogenesis and treatment of hydrothorax complicating cirrhosis and ascites. *Ann Intern Med* 1966;64:341–351.

Litherland J, et al. Computed tomographic peritoneography: CT manifestations in the investigation of leaks and abnormal collections in patients on CAPD. *Nephrol Dial Transplant* 1994;9:1449–1452.

Morris-Stiff GJ, et al. Management of inguinal herniae in patients on continuous ambulatory peritoneal dialysis: an audit of current UK practice. *Postgrad Med J* 1998;74:669–670.

Nomoto Y, et al. Acute hydrothorax in continuous ambulatory peritoneal dialysis: a collaborative study of 161 centers. *Am J Nephrol* 1989;9:363–367.

Okada H, et al. Thoracoscopic surgery and pleurodesis for pleuroperitoneal communication in patients on continuous ambulatory peritoneal dialysis. *Am J Kidney Dis* 1999;34:170–172.

Wanke T, et al. Diaphragmatic function in patients on continuous ambulatory peritoneal dialysis. *Lung* 1994;172:231–240.

21

Metabolic Complications of Peritoneal Dialysis

Sarah S. Prichard

Peritoneal dialysis is generally well tolerated and serves as an effective form of renal replacement therapy for most patients. However, peritoneal dialysis can be associated with a number of metabolic abnormalities that warrant attention and appropriate intervention.

   I.   Glucose absorption. Glucose remains the standard agent added to peritoneal dialysis fluid as an osmotic agent, although amino acids and polyglucose solutions have become available as alternatives. Glucose has the advantage of being cheap, stable, and relatively nontoxic to the peritoneum. However, it is easily absorbed across the peritoneal membrane. There is variability from patient to patient, depending on peritoneal transport characteristics, but as much as 60%–80% of the dialysate glucose is typically absorbed with each continuous ambulatory peritoneal dialysis (CAPD) exchange. This amounts to 100–150 g per day (500–800 kcal per day), which constitutes a significant portion of the recommended total energy intake of about 2,500 kcal per day (35 kcal per kg per day) in a 70-kg patient. In some patients, this provides a welcome source of calories and is likely responsible for the 5%–10% weight gain frequently seen during a patient's first year on peritoneal dialysis.

There are, however, disadvantages to dialysate glucose absorption. It results in increased insulin secretion, which together with insulin resistance (a common feature of chronic renal failure) results in plasma insulin levels that are persistently high. Hyperinsulinemia may be an independent risk factor for the development of atherosclerosis. In certain patients, the glucose loading can result in hyperglycemia severe enough to require the initiation of oral hypoglycemics or insulin therapy. Patients who were previously well controlled on oral hypoglycemics frequently require insulin therapy after the initiation of CAPD, and these patients should be advised of this possibility prior to starting peritoneal dialysis (see Chapter 25 regarding management of diabetes in peritoneal dialysis patients). The hypertriglyceridemia found in peritoneal dialysis patients is at least in part related to glucose absorption. To minimize glucose absorption, patients should be advised on appropriate salt and water management, which will diminish the need for hypertonic solutions. A more definitive solution may be the use of alternative osmotic agents, such as polyglucose or amino acids.

   II.   Lipid abnormalities. Patients on peritoneal dialysis have a variety of lipid abnormalities. Typically, they have high total and low-density lipoprotein (LDL) cholesterol, low high-density lipoprotein (HDL) cholesterol, high apolipoprotein B (apoB), low apoA-I, high triglycerides, and high lipoprotein(a) [Lp(a)] levels. Compared with hemodialysis patients, the most striking differences are the high apoB protein and LDL cholesterol levels, which are usually normal in hemodialysis patients. Levels of oxidized LDL and antibodies to oxidized LDL are elevated in end-stage renal disease (ESRD). These abnormalities are summarized in Table 21-1.

The lipoprotein profile of peritoneal dialysis is markedly atherogenic. The LDL particles are small and dense, indicated by the high apoB protein levels with modest elevations of LDL cholesterol. These small, dense LDL particles are particularly atherogenic in that they cross the endothelium with greater ease and are oxidized more readily than larger LDL particles. The pathogenesis of the overproduction of LDL particles in peritoneal dialysis remains obscure. Hypoalbuminemia secondary to peritoneal protein loss may at least partly contribute to the abnormality.

The hypertriglyceridemia seen in peritoneal dialysis results largely from the overproduction of the very low-density lipoproteins and a deficiency in lipoprotein lipase. There may also be a partial deficiency of hepatic lipase. The pathogenesis of these abnormalities is not understood, but the use of glucose-based peritoneal dialysis solutions and a variety of drugs, such as β-blockers, aggravate the problem. The usual level of triglycerides seen in peritoneal dialysis patients is 220–400 mg per dL (2.5–4.5 mmol per L), but levels greater than 530 mg per dL (6 mmol per L) are not unusual.

A. Treatment

1. Elevated LDL cholesterol/apoB protein. In the nonuremic population, there is compelling evidence that treatment that reduces elevated LDL cholesterol levels is associated with a significant reduction in the progression of coronary artery disease and a decrease in cardiac clinical events and deaths. Even patients with "normal" cholesterol and preexisting coronary artery disease benefit from treatment that reduces LDL cholesterol. Specifically, the hydroxymethylglutaryl coenzyme A (HMG-CoA) reductase group of drugs have been shown to be very efficacious. No equivalent studies have been done in dialysis patients. However, HMG-CoA reductase inhibitors have been demonstrated to be safe and effective in reducing LDL cholesterol and apoB protein

Table 21-1.   Lipid abnormalities in end-stage renal disease

Factor	PD	HD
Total cholesterol	↑	normal
LDL cholesterol	↑	normal
HDL cholesterol	↓	↓
Triglycerides	↑↑	↑
Apo A1 protein	↓	↓
Apo B protein	↑↑	normal
Lp(a)	↑↑	↑↑
LDL oxidation	↑	↑

PD, peritoneal dialysis; HD, hemodialysis; LDL, low-density lipoprotein; HDL, high-density lipoprotein; Lp(a), lipoprotein(a).

in this population. Therefore, it is reasonable to treat (a) peritoneal dialysis patients with known atherosclerotic heart disease and elevated LDL cholesterol and (b) peritoneal dialysis patients with elevated LDL cholesterol and other risk factors for coronary artery disease. The treatment of peritoneal dialysis patients with elevated LDL cholesterol/apoB without pre-existing coronary artery disease and/or other risk factors can be determined on a case-by-case basis. The HMG-CoA reductase drugs can cause a myopathy; consequently, muscles enzymes should be followed.

    2. Elevated triglycerides. Triglyceride elevation alone is a very weak independent risk factor for the development of coronary artery disease. Extreme elevations in peritoneal dialysis patients may predispose to pancreatitis. Carbohydrate loading from the dialysate cannot be avoided altogether in the peritoneal dialysis patients, although the use of polyglucose– and amino acid–based solutions may help. Sodium and water management to minimize the use of hypertonic solutions is advisable in the face of severe hypertriglyceridemia. As in the nonuremic population, ingestion of alcohol should be avoided because it can markedly increase triglycerides. Drugs known to exacerbate hypertriglyceridemia should also be avoided.

    There is no evidence in dialysis patients that treatment of hypertriglyceridemia is associated with improved clinical outcomes, although many physicians feel that treatment of levels greater than 350 mg per dL (4 mmol per L) is advisable. HMG-CoA reductase inhibitors also reduce triglyceride levels, although higher doses are often required. However, these are generally well tolerated. The fibrate drugs (benzofibrate, fenofibrate, gemfibrozil) also effectively reduce triglyceride levels. These drugs have a renal route of excretion, and the dosage therefore must be reduced by at least 25%. The major side effect is muscle toxicity, and therefore, muscle enzymes should be followed. Use of fibrates with HMG-CoA reductase inhibitors should be undertaken with caution.

    3. Low HDL cholesterol. The fibrate class of drugs raises HDL cholesterol levels. However, the value of raising HDL in reducing cardiac morbidity and mortality in ESRD has not been established.

    4. Antioxidants. In nonuremic patients, vitamin E, which is an effective antioxidant, may reduce cardiac events and mortality, although the usefulness of vitamin E for this purpose remains controversial. There are no equivalent studies for ESRD patients.

    5. Lp(a). There is no known treatment for the elevated Lp(a) seen in peritoneal dialysis patients.

III. Protein loss. Peritoneal dialysis is associated with significant loss of protein across the peritoneum. This loss is about 0.5 g per L of dialysate drainage, but may be higher and account for as much as 10–20 g per day. The major component of the protein losses is albumin, but immunoglobulin G (IgG) accounts for up to 15%. These losses are the major reason why peritoneal dialysis patients tend to have lower serum albumin levels than their hemodialysis counterparts, with typical values being 3.3–3.6 g per dL. Protein losses are greatest in high and high-average transporters and may contribute to the less successful outcomes seen with these patients on CAPD. Amino acid losses of approximately 2–3 g per day also occur. Acute inflammation, as seen in peritonitis, is associated with substantially greater protein losses, and a rapid reduction in serum albumin is common during episodes of peritonitis. Unresolving peritonitis is associated with protracted and exaggerated protein losses causing protein malnutrition. The protein loss itself may become an indication to terminate peritoneal dialysis temporarily or, on occasion, permanently. In addition, inasmuch as peritoneal dialysis may preserve residual renal function, in patients with nephrotic syndrome, this preserved renal function may be obtained at the cost of ongoing protein losses. Therefore, measurements of both peritoneal and urinary protein losses need to be evaluated in peritoneal dialysis patients, and appropriate dietary adjustments should be made.

IV. Hypo-/hypernatremia. Peritoneal dialysis solution typically contains 132 mmol per L of sodium. Most patients maintain a normal serum sodium on peritoneal dialysis. Those who are excessive water drinkers can get a dilutional hyponatremia. Conversely, with rapid ultrafiltration, hypernatremia may occur due to the sieving effect of the peritoneal membrane on sodium. In patients with marked hyperglycemia, hyponatremia may be seen as a result of water shifting into the extracellular fluid. Typically, the serum sodium falls about 1.3 mEq per L for each 100 mg per dL (5.6 mmol per L) rise in blood glucose.

V. Hypo-/hyperkalemia. Standard peritoneal dialysis solution contains no potassium. Potassium is removed during peritoneal dialysis by diffusion and convection; after a 4- to 6-hour exchange, the dialysate potassium level is usually close to that of plasma. In renal failure, gastrointestinal secretion of potassium is enhanced. Usually, only patients who are noncompliant in performing their dialysis exchanges have ongoing problems with hyperkalemia. However, hypokalemia has been reported in 10%–30% of CAPD patients. These cases are usually associated with poor nutritional intake, and most can be managed by liberalizing the diet, but persistent levels lower than 3 mmol per L should be managed with potassium supplementation.

VI. Hypo-/hypercalcemia. As discussed in Chapter 14, peritoneal dialysis solutions are available with 2.5 mEq/L (1.25 mmol per L) or 3.5 mEq/L (1.75 mmol per L) calcium concentrations.

Hypocalcemia, which is common in patients initiating dialysis treatment, is usually easily managed with calcium and vitamin D supplements together with the 1.75 mmol per L calcium dialysate. This high-calcium dialysate brings about a net transfer of calcium to the patient except in patients with a continuous high ultrafiltration. There are a few case reports of hypocalcemia post parathyroidectomy that was managed by the addition of calcium to the peritoneal dialysate.

Hypercalcemia is common in peritoneal dialysis patients on large doses of calcium supplements used as phosphate binders. The 1.25 mmol per L dialysate is indicated in such patients. Vitamin D supplementation may also have to be stopped to avoid elevated serum calcium levels. Peritoneal dialysis has been used in the treatment of severe hypercalcemia.

VII. Hypo-/hyperphosphatemia. See Chapter 30.

VIII. Elevated serum lactate. The usual base in peritoneal dialysis solutions is lactate. The lactate is metabolized by the liver to bicarbonate. Under most circumstances, the liver's ability to metabolize lactate easily exceeds the daily delivery of lactate. However, patients on oral hypoglycemic agents (metformin and related compounds) with advanced liver disease and thiamine deficiency may not have sufficient reserve to handle the lactate load of peritoneal dialysis, and a lactic acidosis may ensue. In patients with ongoing lactic acidosis, as with patients with acute hepatic failure or other conditions seen in the intensive care setting, the addition of lactate-containing peritoneal dialysis solutions may exacerbate the problem. In such cases, specially prepared bicarbonate-based solutions can be used. Soon commercially manufactured bicarbonate solutions will be widely available.

SELECTED READINGS

Appel G. Lipid abnormalities in renal disease. *Kidney Int* 1991;39: 169–183.

Attman PO, et al. Apolipoprotein B–containing lipoproteins in renal failure: the relation to mode of dialysis. *Kidney Int* 1999;55: 1536–1542.

Heyburn PJ, et al. Peritoneal dialysis in the management of severe hypercalcemia. *Br Med J* 1980;280:525–526.

Hutchison AJ, et al. Low-calcium dialysis fluid and oral calcium carbonate in CAPD. A method of controlling hyperphosphatemia whilst minimizing aluminium exposure and hypercalcaemia. *Nephrol Dial Transplant* 1992;7:1219–1225.

Joven J, et al. Lipoprotein heterogeneity in end-stage renal disease. *Kidney Int* 1993;43:410–418.

Lee MS, et al. Effects of gemfibrozil on lipid and hemostatic factors in CAPD patients. *Perit Dial Int* 1999;19:280–283.

Levine GN, Keaney JF, Vita JA. Cholesterol reduction in cardiovascular disease. Clinical benefits and possible mechanisms. *N Engl J Med* 1995;332:512–521.

Little J, et al. Longitudinal lipid profiles on CAPD: their relationship to weight gain, comorbidity, and dialysis factors. *J Am Soc Nephrol* 1998;9:1931–1939.

Maggi E, et al. Enhanced LDL oxidation in uremic patients: an additional mechanism for accelerated atherosclerosis? *Kidney Int* 1994; 45:876–888.

Murphy BG, et al. Increased serum apolipoprotein (a) in patients with chronic renal failure treated with continuous ambulatory peritoneal dialysis. *Atherosclerosis* 1992;93:53–57.

Prichard S, et al. Cardiovascular disease in peritoneal dialysis. *Perit Dial Int* 1996;16(Suppl 1):S19–S22.

Rajman I, et al. Low-density lipoprotein subfraction profiles in chronic renal failure. *Nephrol Dial Transplant* 1998;13:2281–2287.

Rostand S. Profound hypokalemia in continuous ambulatory peritoneal dialysis. *Arch Intern Med* 1983;143:377–378.

Scandinavian Simvastatin Survival Study Group. Randomised trial of cholesterol lowering in 4444 patients with coronary heart disease: the Scandinavian Simvastatin Survival Study (4S). *Lancet* 1994;344:1383–1389.

Sniderman AD, et al. Hyperapobetalipoproteinemia: the major dyslipoproteinemia in patients with chronic renal failure treated with chronic ambulatory peritoneal dialysis. *Atherosclerosis* 1987;65: 257–264.

Spital A, Sterns R. Potassium supplementation via the dialysate in continuous ambulatory peritoneal dialysis. *Am J Kidney Dis* 1985;6: 173–176.

Walker RJ, et al. Effect of treatment with simvastatin on serum cholesteryl ester transfer in patients on dialysis. PERFECT Study Collaborative Group. *Nephrol Dial Transplant* 1997;12:87–92.

Webb AT, et al. Lipoprotein (a) in patients on maintenance hemodialysis and continuous ambulatory peritoneal dialysis. *Nephrol Dial Transplant* 1993;8:609–613.

Wheeler DC. Abnormalities of lipoprotein metabolism in CAPD patients. *Kidney Int* 1996;50(Suppl 56):S41–S46.

IV

Special Problems
in the Dialysis Patient

Psychology and Rehabilitation

Paul L. Kimmel and Norman B. Levy

Dialysis patients lead a highly abnormal life. Those undergoing hemodialysis, continuous cycling peritoneal dialysis (CCPD), or nocturnal intermittent peritoneal dialysis (NIPD) are tethered to a machine to an extent unprecedented in the history of medical technology. Those treated by continuous ambulatory peritoneal dialysis (CAPD) are bound to a repetitive daytime ritual of solution changes. All dialysis patients find themselves abjectly dependent on a procedure, medical facility, or group of medical personnel and are exposed to other stresses as well (Table 22-1). Overall, the psychological response of a given patient to illness will depend on his or her premorbid personality, the extent of support by family and friends, and the course of the underlying disease.

I. Common psychological problems. Approximately 10% of medically hospitalized patients with end-stage renal disease (ESRD) have a psychiatric disorder. This probably underestimates the extent of mental illness prevalent in the entire population. The most important psychological problems encountered in dialysis patients are depression, dementia, drug- and alcohol-related disorders, and anxiety and personality disorders. Occasionally, patients with ESRD may have coexisting psychotic disorders. Uncooperative behavior can be a problem for patients and caregivers. Sexual dysfunction related to diabetes mellitus, atherosclerotic vascular disease, psychological problems, medications, or uremia can be a concern for patients that is not apparent to caregivers. Difficulties pertaining to occupation and rehabilitation are an ongoing concern for patients and staff alike and are expected to be a problem in an elderly, medically ill population. Depression is probably the most important psychological problem because it can progress to suicide or termination of dialysis if unrecognized or untreated.

A. Depression. Depression, the most common psychological complication in dialysis patients, is usually a response to real, threatened, or imagined loss. Manifestations include a persistent depressive mood, a poor self-image, and feelings of hopelessness. Physical complaints are not unusual and include sleep disorder, change in appetite and weight, dryness of the mouth and constipation, and diminution in sexual interest and ability (psychological causation of a physical complaint should not be assumed until the sign or symptom has received appropriate medical evaluation). Cognitive symptoms of depression, such as hopelessness and feelings of guilt or suicidal ideation, are important in helping the clinician distinguish between symptoms of uremia and a depressive disorder.

1. Suicide. Approximately 1 of every 500 dialysis patients commits suicide. A larger number attempt suicide on one or more occasions. An indeterminate number of deaths in dialysis patients brought on by dietary indiscretion or poor compliance

Table 22-1.   Psychological stresses of dialysis

Regimentation of dietary, fluid, and medication intake
Dialysis procedure
The illness
Multiple losses: job, freedom, life expectancy
Associated sexual dysfunction

with the dialysis prescription (shortening or skipping treatments) may also be related to suicidal intent, conscious or otherwise. The increased risk of suicide in this population should always be kept in mind.

B.   Dementia and delirious states. Dementia and delirious states may be related to an underlying or intercurrent medical disorder (such as hypothyroidism, hyperparathyroidism, septicemia, or hypoglycemia); to neurologic diseases (such as cerebrovascular disease, neurosyphilis, or subdural hematoma); to the use of prescribed or recreational medications; to alcohol use or its withdrawal; or to underdialysis. It is important for the physician caring for such a patient to ensure maximum effective dialysis (by reviewing the dialysis prescription, parameter of delivered dose of dialysis, and extent of recirculation) and nutrition, and to rule out the existence of progressive neurologic disorders, such as Alzheimer's disease. For patients with chronic, progressive, irreversible, untreatable dementia, the nephrologist should initiate discussions with family members regarding discontinuation of dialysis. In such patients, advanced directives are most helpful if completed before the onset of debilitating disease.

C.   Uncooperative behavior. Anger is common among patients suffering from chronic illness, and it is not surprising that a substantial minority of dialysis patients engages in behavior that vexes the dialysis staff. It is best not to be provoked by such behavior but to listen to the patient and attempt to understand him or her. Often the reasons for anger and uncooperative behavior are not known to the patient and must be carefully searched out in the context of the patient's home and work situations. However, under no circumstances should one tolerate behavior that may be dangerous to the patient or to other patients or staff in the dialysis unit. Patients with underlying psychosis may exhibit such behavior. In these cases, the assistance of a consultation–liaison psychiatrist is usually worthwhile.

D.   Sexual dysfunction. Dialysis patients of both genders frequently have sexual difficulties. Impotence eventually develops in approximately 70% of men treated with dialysis, and women on dialysis report diminution in the frequency of orgasm during intercourse. Patients of both genders engage in sexual intercourse much less frequently than they did prior to becoming uremic. The cause of sexual dysfunction is poorly understood. Psychological factors often play a role. In men, depression, reversal of family role due to loss of job, and the impact of cessation of urination (as the organ of urination is also the organ of sexuality) can all contribute to sexual dysfunction. In women, cessation of menses, diminution in fertility, and alteration in appearance may contribute to sexual dysfunction. The cause of impotence in male dialysis patients is often primarily organic, related to hormonal changes associated with uremia, to diabetes, to vascular insufficiency, or to the use of antihypertensive medications. The organic causes of impotence in dialysis patients and their management are detailed in Chapters 29 and 35.

E. Rehabilitation. About two-thirds of patients on dialysis do not return to the employment in which they had engaged prior to the onset of renal failure. The ability of individuals to return to work depends to a large degree on their socioeconomic status and the severity of illness at the time of initiation of ESRD therapy. It is much easier for a college professor or business executive on dialysis to work than for a patient qualified only for blue-collar employment because of greater flexibility of work schedule and because less physical exertion is usually required in white-collar jobs. In general, women have more options than men, especially married women for whom return to household work may be feasible. However, physical limitations may prevent patients from performing even light household duties. Loss of job is of extreme psychological import to all, but especially to men whose sense of masculinity is often directly tied to the work they perform.

The use of erythropoietin has been associated with improvement in physical capacity and may enhance the potential for rehabilitation of patients with ESRD. It is necessary to set realistic goals for rehabilitation. The gratification or lack thereof that the individual derived from work prior to illness is important. Individuals who never enjoyed their job will tend to curtail their work activities after initiation of dialysis therapy. It must not be forgotten that exercise is an important aspect of rehabilitation. Exercise programs can be designed for patients with even high degrees of physical limitation.

F. Quality of life (QOL). The proper means of measuring QOL in dialysis patients has not been established. Different scales (Sickness Impact Profile, Illness Effects Questionnaire, SF-36, Karnofsky Scale, Satisfaction with Life Scale, and the Kidney Disease Quality-of-Life Scale (KD-QOL) comprise subjective and objective measures and emphasize quantification of well-being, functional status, and patient satisfaction. Consensus is building that subjective measures are most important as QOL scales. The use of QOL scales to predict outcome is an area of active research investigation. The use of erythropoietin has been associated with improvement in ESRD patients' perception of QOL. Interestingly, most studies suggest ESRD patients have perceptions of QOL consistent with those of the general population. Exceptions noted are patients with successful renal transplants, who in aggregate tend to perceive higher QOL than the general population, and those with failed transplants, who tend to perceive a lower QOL compared with other ESRD patients. Interestingly, as in the general population, older (and sicker) hemodialysis patients may perceive an enhanced QOL. Such notions must be taken into consideration when discussing discontinuation of dialysis with patients and their families.

II. Treatment

A. Prevention. Much can be done to prevent the psychological problems that commonly arise. A modality of dialysis should be selected that best suits the personality and life situation of the patient. Patients who are very independent should be placed on forms of self-care dialysis or considered for early transplantation. Individuals who are at a high risk for psychological difficulties by past history should be identified early and monitored very closely. The use of glucocorticoids in patients with a history of psychosis when transplantation is considered may be problematical. Psychiatric consultations should be sought in such circumstances. All men starting dialysis should be informed of the possibility of eventual impotence. Should impotence occur, forewarned patients may be less upset and may more readily identify and discuss the problem with the physician. The informed patient will be more inclined to view impotence as a complication of his disease rather than as a reflection of deficient masculinity.

B. Psychotherapy. Several forms of psychological treatment are useful in this population. Some methods are best applied by the nonpsychiatric professional, whereas others are best left to a liaison psychiatrist.

  1. Individual psychotherapy is best used in a supportive sense and to treat specific psychological symptoms. Dialysis patients tend to be resistant to individual psychiatric treatment; they often feel overly doctored and frequently use denial as a mechanism of coping with their psychological difficulties. Talking therapies are often useful. For hemodialysis patients, such therapy is best scheduled during the dialysis treatment.

  2. Group therapy may also be beneficial. The most successful groups are those that are used for education, as well as for the uncovering of psychological problems.

  3. Sexual behavior therapy techniques first described by Masters and Johnson hold great promise for the treatment of sexual dysfunction in dialysis patients. It encourages patients to reenter sexuality by engaging in activity with their partners that does not necessarily include sexual intercourse or orgasm. A change in direction from avoidance to encounter is the therapeutic goal.

  4. Exercise that does not overtax the individual and is performed on a regular basis has been shown to diminish depression and anxiety in patients with ESRD.

C. Drug therapy. Drugs should be widely used to treat psychological problems in dialysis patients. Prime considerations in the choice of medications and dosage adjustment in patients with ESRD are whether the drug is metabolized by renal and hepatic routes (or both) and whether the drug is cleared by peritoneal dialysis or hemodialysis. Little information is available regarding clearance of many psychoactive drugs by newer, highly permeable membranes used in high-efficiency and high-flux hemodialysis and hemodiafiltration. If the clinician is concerned about the effects of nonadherence or clearance with highly efficient techniques, assessment of drug levels, where available, may be useful.

With the exception of lithium, virtually all of the psychiatrically active medications are fat-soluble, pass the blood–brain barrier, are detoxified by the liver, are eliminated in the bile in the feces, and are large molecules that are not dialyzable. Virtually all, again with the exception of lithium, have a great affinity for protein binding and require special consideration for patients with renal failure whose protein binding tends to be compromised. Chiefly for this reason, the rule of thumb is that one should not use on an individual with kidney failure more than two-thirds of the maximum dose that one would use on a patient with normal kidney function.

1. Anxiolytic agents. Anxiety states and repetitive panic attacks should initially be managed by psychotherapy and desensitization. Nevertheless, administration of short-acting benzodiazepines, such as lorazepam (Ativan) or alprazolam (Xanax), may be of benefit. Benzodiazepines that have pharmacologically active metabolites, such as chlordiazepoxide (Librium) and diazepam (Valium), should be avoided in dialysis patients. If given chronically, extremely high blood levels of active drug metabolites can occur, resulting in lethargy. Barbiturates should not be prescribed because they are less efficacious than the benzodiazepines; furthermore, the extent to which barbiturates are cleared by dialysis complicates proper dosage adjustment.

2. Antidepressants. Antidepressants can play a potentially large role in the treatment of depressive symptoms in dialysis patients. In general, dialysis patients tend to be undermedicated for their psychiatric problems. This is especially true for depression, which tends to be denied despite the fact that it is a very treatable illness. Because these patients have a high incidence of suicide usually secondary to depression, this is most regrettable. In general, greater attention should be paid to this illness and its treatment.

The emergence of the selective serotonin reuptake inhibitors and other newer antidepressants widens the medical armamentarium against depression. These medications, which include fluoxetine (Prozac), sertraline (Zoloft), paroxetine (Paxil), nefazodone (Serzone), and venlafaxine (Effexor), have attractive properties. They tend to have little or no anticholinergic effect, tend not to be sedative (with the possible exception of nefazodone), have a low incidence of side effects, and can be tolerated in extremely high doses, making them unsuitable as agents of suicide. They therefore contrast strongly with the original tricyclics (amitriptyline, desipramine, sinequan, and nortriptyline, to mention a few) and the monoamine oxidase inhibitors [phenelzine (Nardil) and tranylcypromine (Parnate)], which may be associated with a high incidence of side effects and are lethal in large doses. Of the newer antidepressants, the one with the longest track record (i.e., the highest number of dialysis patients treated with it and most widely studied in renal failure patients) is fluoxetine. There seems to no significant difference in the pharmacokinetics and levels of serum fluoxetine and norfluoxetine, its major metabolite, in depressed patients with normal kidney function and in depressed dialysis patients. A daily dose of 20 mg of fluoxetine is well tolerated, with few side effects and good efficacy. A significant shortcoming in the use of all antidepressants is the fact that they take 3 to 6 weeks to show efficacy. If a particular drug is not effective, another medication of the same or different family may be helpful, again after a 3- to 6-week trial period.

3. Lithium. Lithium is an exception to virtually all other psychotropic medications in terms of its being entirely eliminated by the kidney, non–protein-binding, and entirely dialyzable because it is a small molecule. As it is eliminated by the kidney only, in the face of total kidney failure, a single dose of medication produces a constant blood level pending the next hemodialysis treatment. That treatment should remove all of the lithium, enabling the use of a single dose, usually about 600 mg after the end of a hemodialysis run.

4. Major tranquilizers. Administration of a major tranquilizer is sometimes required for the control of symptoms of psychosis. This may be required for the treatment of patients in whom psychosis may be due to preexisting (functional) psychotic illness or psychosis precipitated by dementia or delirium-caused sepsis, uremia secondary to inadequate dialytic treatment, vascular disease, and endocrinopathies, just to mention a few major causes. As in the case of other psychotropic medications, these medicines, which include haloperidol, chlorpromazine, thioridazine, risperidone, and olanzapine, to mention a few, may be readily used in these patients. One should keep in mind that the maximum dose given should not exceed two-thirds of the maximum dose that would be prescribed to a patient with normal kidney function.

SELECTED READINGS

Fitts SS, Guthrie MR, Blagg CR. Exercise coaching and rehabilitation counseling improve quality of life for predialysis and dialysis patients. *Nephron* 1999;82:115–121.

Kennedy SH, et al. Major depression in renal dialysis patients: an open trial of antidepressant therapy. *J Clin Psychiatry* 1989;50:60–63.

Kimmel PL. Aspects of quality of life in hemodialysis patients. *J Am Soc Nephrol* 1995;6:1418–1426.

Kimmel PL, et al. Psychosocial factors, behavioral compliance and survival in urban hemodialysis patients. *Kidney Int* 1998;54:245–254.

Kimmel PL, et al. Psychiatric illness in patients with end-stage renal disease. *Am J Med* 1998;105:214–221.

Kutner NG, et al. Functional impairment, depression, and life satisfaction among older hemodialysis patients and age-matched controls: a prospective study. *Arch Phys Med Rehabil* 2000;81:453–459.

Levenson JL, Glocheski S. Psychological factors affecting end-stage renal disease. *Psychosomatics* 1991;32:382–389.

Levy NB, et al. Fluoxetine in depressed patients with renal failure and in depressed patients with normal kidney function. *Gen Hosp Psychiatry* 1996;18:8–13.

Levy NB. Psychiatric considerations. In: Massry SG, Glassock RJ, eds. *Massry and Glassock's textbook of nephrology*, 3rd ed. Baltimore: Williams & Wilkins, 1994.

Levy NB, et al. Psychopharmacology in patients with renal failure. *Int J Psychiatry Med* 1990;20:325–334.

Lo CY, et al. Benefits of exercise training in patients on continuous ambulatory peritoneal dialysis. *Am J Kidney Dis* 1998;32:1011–1018.

McClellan WM, et al. Functional status and quality of life: predictors of early mortality among patients entering treatment for end stage renal disease. *J Clin Epidemiol* 1991;44:83–89.

Milo E. Occupational therapy in the dialysis unit. *EDTNA ERCA J* 1996;22:41–42.

Oberly ET, et al. Renal rehabilitation: obstacles, progress, and prospects for the future. *Am J Kidney Dis* 2000;(4 suppl 1): S141–S147.

O'Brien ME. Compliance and long-term maintenance dialysis. *Am J Kidney Dis* 1990;15:209–214.

Painter P, et al. Physical functioning and health-related quality-of-life changes with exercise training in hemodialysis patients. *Am J Kidney Dis* 2000;35:482–492.

Rocco MV, et al. Prevalence of missed treatments and early sign-offs in hemodialysis patients. *J Am Soc Nephrol* 1993;4:1178–1183.

Sherman RA, et al. Deficiencies in delivered hemodialysis therapy due to missed and shortened treatments. *Am J Kidney Dis* 1994;24: 921–923.

Shidler NR, Peterson RA, Kimmel PL. Quality of life and psychosocial relationships in patients with chronic renal insufficiency. *Am J Kidney Dis* 1998;32:557–566.

Welch JL, Austin JK. Factors associated with treatment-related stressors in hemodialysis patients. *ANNA J* 1999;26:318–325.

White Y, Grenyer BF. The biopsychosocial impact of end-stage renal disease: the experience of dialysis patients and their partners. *J Adv Nurs* 1999;30:1312–1320.

Wolcott DL, et al. Relationship of dialysis modality and other factors to cognitive function in chronic dialysis patients. *Am J Kidney Dis* 1988;12:275–284.

Internet Reference

Dialysis rehabilitation links (http://www.hdcn.com/crf/rehab)

Nutrition

Michael V. Rocco and Michael J. Blumenkrantz

I. Causes of malnutrition in chronic dialysis patients. Malnutrition is a relatively common problem in chronic dialysis patients, affecting approximately one-third of both hemodialysis and peritoneal dialysis patients. Malnutrition can be secondary to poor nutritional intake, to increased losses, and/or to an increase in protein catabolism (Table 23-1). The sequelae of malnutrition are numerous and include increased mortality and hospitalization rates, impaired wound healing, increased susceptibility to infection, malaise, fatigue, and poor rehabilitation.

II. Nutritional assessment

A. Patient interview. Symptoms of nausea, vomiting, and anorexia, as well as recent changes in body weight, should be carefully evaluated with a view to ascertaining their cause. Nutritional status can also be affected by chronic medical conditions, such as severe congestive heart failure, diabetes, a variety of gastrointestinal diseases, and depression.

B. Assessment of food intake. Patient recall of food intake, determined on both dialysis and nondialysis days, can provide information on the intake of protein, fats, and carbohydrates. Food intake on dialysis days typically is about 20% lower than on nondialysis days. This is due to interruption of the patient's routine and perhaps to treatment-related side effects.

C. Medication intake. Dyspepsia due to ingestion of aluminum-containing antacids or oral iron supplements may limit food intake. Protein catabolism can be increased by the administration of medications such as prednisone and other catabolic steroids and tetracylines.

D. Physical examination, including anthropometry. General estimates of nutritional status may be obtained by comparing ideal to actual body weight and by evaluating the condition of mucous membranes, hair, and skin. Anthropometry can provide a reasonably accurate method for assessing body fat and protein stores. Skinfold thickness measured at the biceps or triceps provides an estimate of body fat, whereas midarm circumference can be used to estimate muscle mass. These measures can be compared to reference ranges established in well-nourished dialysis patients (Fig. 23-1; Nelson et al, 1990). Patients with values below the 25th percentile for either middle upper arm circumference or triceps skinfold thickness are at risk for malnutrition.

E. Bioimpedance. Bioimpedance analysis is based on the measurement of resistance and reactance when a constant alternating electrical current is applied to a patient. Empirical equations are used to predict total-body water from resistance and total-body mass from the ratio resistance/reactance or its geometrical derivative, the phase angle. Phase angle is strongly

Table 23-1. Causes of malnutrition

Decreased nutritional intake
    Overzealous dietary restrictions
    Delayed gastric emptying and diarrhea
    Other medical comorbidities
    Intercurrent illnesses and hospitalizations
    Decrease in food intake on hemodialysis days
    Medications causing dyspepsia (phosphate binders, iron
        preparations)
    Suppression of oral intake by peritoneal dialysate glucose load
    Inadequate dialysis
    Monetary restrictions
    Depression
    Altered sense of taste
Increased losses
    Gastrointestinal blood loss (100 mL blood = 14–17 g protein)
    Intradialytic nitrogen losses (HD 6–8 g amino acid/procedure;
        PD 8–10 g protein/d)
Increase in protein catabolism
    Intercurrent illnesses and hospitalizations
    Other medical comorbidities
    Metabolic acidosis (promotes protein catabolism)
    Catabolism associated with hemodialysis (controversial)
    Dysfunction of the growth hormone/insulin growth factor
        endocrine axis
    Catabolic effects of other hormones (PTH, cortisol, glucagon)

HD, hemodialysis; PD, peritoneal dialysis; PTH, parathyroid hormone.

correlated with other predictors of nutritional status, such as anthropometric measurements and serum albumin levels. In one study, there was a significant increase in mortality in hemodialysis patients with a phase angle below the 25th percentile (4.5 rad in men, 4.2 rad in women), compared with patients with higher phase angle values, even after correcting for other predictors of nutritional status, such as serum albumin levels (Maggiore et al, 1996).
  F.   Laboratory tests
    1.   Serum albumin. Low serum albumin levels are a strong predictor of mortality and hospitalization rates in chronic hemodialysis and peritoneal dialysis patients. The risk of mortality rises dramatically as serum albumin levels decline to less than 4.0 g per dL (Owen et al, 1993; Held et al, 1994; Churchill et al, 1996). Note that the method by which the serum albumin method is measured can result in levels that differ by up to 20%. The most commonly used method is that of bromocresol green (BCG); other methods include bromocresol purple (BCP) and nephelometry. In cross-sectional studies, serum albumin levels correlate poorly with actual caloric index or with nutritional indices, especially in continuous ambulatory peritoneal dialysis (CAPD) patients. Serum albumin levels are influenced by many factors, including hepatic synthesis, excretion, catab-

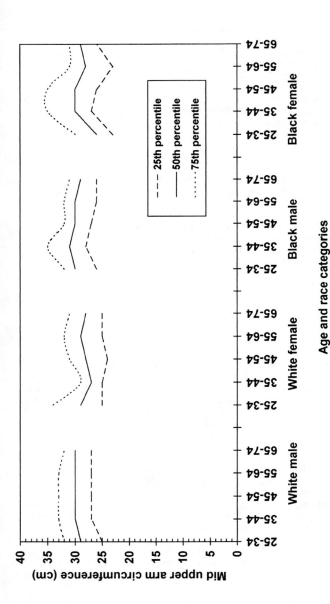

Figure 23-1. Middle upper arm circumference and triceps skinfold thickness, by percentiles, stratified by age, race, and gender, in nondiabetic hemodialysis patients. (Adapted from Nelson EE, et al. Anthropometric norms for the dialysis population. *Am J Kidney Dis* 1990;16:32.)

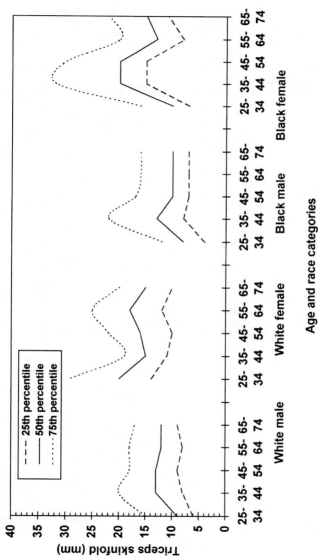

Age and race categories

Figure 23-1. Continued

olism, changes in plasma volume, and changes in the distribution of albumin between the extracellular and intracellular spaces. The serum level of acute phase proteins, such as C-reactive protein and serum amyloid A, have a greater impact on serum albumin levels than the protein catabolic rate (Kaysen et al, 1997). Despite these observations, serum albumin levels (or, according to some investigators, prealbumin levels) provide a consistent assessment of visceral protein stores. Furthermore, serum albumin levels decline in patients who manifest other signs of malnutrition, and increase as nutritional repletion occurs.

2.   Predialysis serum urea nitrogen (SUN). The predialysis SUN level reflects the balance between urea generation and removal. A low serum urea nitrogen (SUN) is often an important clue suggesting inadequate protein intake. Unless the patient has substantial residual renal function (greater than 2–3 mL per minute) or is receiving an unusually generous amount of hemodialysis, a predialysis SUN level of less than 50 mg per dL is often due to inadequate protein intake. Note, however, that the predialysis SUN level can rise into the "acceptable" range (e.g., 50–80 mg per dL) in a patient who has poor protein intake but who also is being inadequately dialyzed.

3.   Urea nitrogen appearance (UNA). The urea nitrogen output (or appearance), a readily measured parameter, should be equal to the urea nitrogen intake if the patient is in nitrogen balance. When a patient is not in nitrogen balance, caused by either catabolism or anabolism, then this relationship is not valid. The UNA is synonymous with the older term "protein catabolic rate." As discussed in Chapter 2, the UNA can be computed from blood-sided SUN measurements in either of two ways: (a) by using the predialysis SUN level and the Kt/V factored by the dialysis schedule and residual renal function (see Chapter 2) or (b) by computing the rise in SUN during all or part of an interdialytic interval. For the latter method, the UNA is calculated by the following equation:

UNA (g/d) = urinary urea nitrogen (g/d)
          + change in body urea nitrogen (g/d)

   where

Change in body urea nitrogen = $(SUN_f - SUN_i$ [g/L/d]$) \times BW_i$(kg)
          $\times$ (0.60 L/kg) + $(BW_f - BW_i$
          [kg/d]$) \times SUN_f$ (g/L) $\times$ (1.0 L/kg)

where i and f are the initial and final SUN values for the period of measurement, BW is body weight, 0.60 L/kg is an estimate of the fraction of body weight that is water and 1.0 is the volume of distribution of urea in the weight that is gained or lost. Another method used in computing the UNA for both hemodialysis and peritoneal dialysis patients is to collect aliquots of the spent dialysate and estimate weekly dialytic removal of nitrogen.

4.   Protein equivalent of total nitrogen appearance (PNA). Several formulas are available for the calculation of PNA from UNA. These are described in Table 17-7.

The PNA is normalized to body weight to obtain the nPNA, which is expressed as grams per kilogram body weight per 24 hours. There is, however, no generalized method of standardization for body weight. When actual patient weight is used for normalization, it does not account for the observation that obese subjects require fewer kilocalories per kilogram of body weight compared with lean subjects. Other methods include normalization to a standard body weight based on gender, age, and height or normalization to the hypothetical body weight of $V/0.58$, with V calculated from the Watson nomogram. Thus, whenever nPNA is reported, the method of normalization should be noted.

5. Other laboratory findings. Serum transferrin is low in almost all dialysis patients and may not be a good indicator of nutritional status in this population. Transferrin levels can be influenced by changes in iron stores, presence of inflammation, and changes in volume status. The serum prealbumin levels may be elevated due to interaction of prealbumin with retinol-binding protein.

III. Dietary needs of the chronic dialysis patient. The recommended average levels of nutritional intake are depicted in Table 23-2 and are similar to those recommended in the National Renal Diet (American Diabetic Association, 1993).

A. Need for individualization of the dietary prescription. Adherence to the renal diet is difficult and stressful, due to the numerous restrictions of this type of diet. The diet for each patient should be individualized to help accommodate each patient's unique circumstances in terms of palatability, cost, comorbid medical conditions, and cultural eating habits. Overly restrictive nutritional recommendations should be avoided as they may lead to poor intake!

The nutritional recommendations that are provided by the dietitian need to be reinforced by other members of the health care team. Compliance with the diet should be assessed on a regular basis, often monthly at the initiation of dialysis or for those patients who have a history of noncompliance with the renal diet. Patients with specific comorbid medical conditions may require additional dietary modifications. The special nutritional problems of the diabetic dialysis patient are discussed in Chapter 25.

B. Average rather than actual body weight. One problem with dietary intake recommendations for dialysis patients, who often are malnourished, is the choice of weight to use in the denominator. For example, if a patient has lost body mass such that his or her weight is now 50 kg instead of the usual 90 kg, ingestion of an "adequate" amount of protein and calories based on grams per kilogram or kilocalories per kilogram of the patient's actual weight may maintain the present weight, but this amount of food will not correct malnutrition. Kinetically modeled protein intakes (nPNA) for dialysis, as presented in Chapters 2 and 17, will yield protein intake normalized to actual weight. Protein and caloric recommendations should be based on the average body weight for healthy subjects of the same sex, height, age, and body frame size as the patient (Tables 23-3 and 23-4).

Example. A severely malnourished 35-year-old male hemodialysis patient who is 183 cm (72 in.) tall weighs 60 kg (132 lb).

Table 23-2.   Daily dietary recommendations for dialysis patients versus nonuremics[a]

Factor	Nonuremic	HD	PD
Protein (g/kg)	0.8	1.2	1.2–1.5
Calories (sedentary) (kcal/kg)	30	30[b]	30–40[b,c]
Protein (%)	15–20	15	15
Carbohydrate (%)	55–60	55–60[d]	55–60[c,d]
Fat (%)	20–30	Balance	Balance
Cholesterol (mg)	300–400	300–400	300–400
Polyunsaturated/ saturated fat ratio	2.0:1.0	2.0:1.0	2.0:1.0
Crude fiber (g)	25	25	25
Sodium (1 g = 43 mEq)	2–6 g	2 g + 1 g/LUO	2–4 g + 1 g/LUO
Fluids (L/LUO)	Ad lib	1 L + 1 L/LUO	1.0–2.5 L + 1 L/LUO
Potassium (1 g = 25 mEq)	2–6 g	2 g + 1 g/LUO	4 g + 1 g/LUO
Calcium (g)	0.8–1.2	Diet + 1.2	Diet + 1.2]
Phosphorus (g)	1.0–1.8	0.6–1.2	0.6–1.2
Magnesium (g)	0.35	0.2–0.3	0.2–0.3
Iron (mg)	10–18	See Chap. 27	See Chap. 27
Vitamin A	None	None	None
Beta carotene	None	None	None
Retinol	None	None	None
Thiamine (mg)	1.5	1.5	1.5
Riboflavin (mg)	1.8	1.7	1.7
Vitamin B_6 (mg)	10	10	10
Vitamin B_{12} (mg)	0.03	0.006	0.006
Niacin (mg)	20	20	20
Folic acid (mg)	1.0	>1.0	>1.0
Pantothenic acid (mg)	N/A	10	10
Biotin (mg)	N/A	0.3	0.3
Vitamin C (mg)	100	60–100	60–100
Vitamin E (mg)	N/A	None	None
Vitamin D		See Chap. 30	See Chap. 30
Vitamin K		See text	See text

[a] All intakes calculated on the basis of normalized body weight (i.e., the average body weight of normal persons of the same age, height, and sex as the patient).
[b] These levels of caloric intake are *rarely* attained in practice.
[c] Includes glucose absorbed from dialysis solutions.
[d] Carbohydrate intake should be decreased in patients with hypertriglyceridemia.
LUO, liters of urine output per day; HD, hemodialysis; PD, peritoneal dialysis.

Table 23-3. **Frame size as determined from elbow breadth**

Age (yr)	Frame Size		
	Small	Medium	Large
Men			
18–24	≤6.6	>6.6 and <7.7	≥7.7
25–34	≤6.7	>6.7 and <7.9	≥7.9
35–44	≤6.7	>6.7 and <8.0	≥8.0
45–74	≤6.7	>6.7 and <8.1	≥8.1
Women			
18–24	≤5.6	>5.6 and <6.5	≥6.5
25–34	≤5.7	>5.7 and <6.8	≥6.8
35–44	≤5.7	>5.7 and <7.1	≥7.1
45–54	≤5.7	>5.7 and <7.2	≥7.2
55–74	≤5.8	>5.8 and <7.2	≥7.2

Frame size by elbow breadth (cm) of U.S. male and female adults derived from the combined NHANES I and II datasets.
Data from Frisancho AR. New standards of weight and body composition by frame size and height for assessment of nutritional status of adults and the elderly. *Am J Clin Nutr* 1984;40:808.

From Tables 23-3 and 23-4, we find that the average weight for this medium-frame patient (were he healthy) would be about 84 kg (185 lb). From a urea kinetic modeling program, the patient's protein nitrogen appearance rate (which reflects protein intake in the absence of a catabolic state) is found to be 1.2 g per kg per day. Is this patient ingesting an adequate amount of protein?

The urea kinetic modeling–derived protein intake is based on the actual total-body water. With weight loss, total-body water does not decrease exactly in direct proportion to body weight, but let us assume that it does. If so, this patient's protein intake of 1.2 g per kg of actual body weight per day is equivalent to $1.2 \times 132/185 = 0.86$ g per kg per day based on the average healthy body weight of similar subjects: 84 kg (185 lb). The patient's dietary protein intake is inadequate and should be increased.

C. **Adequacy of dialysis.** The delivery of a dialysis dose that is less than adequate, as defined by National Kidney Foundation Dialysis Outcomes Quality Initiatives (DOQI) guidelines (Chapter 6 for hemodialysis and Chapter 17 for peritoneal dialysis), results in the patient having a difficult time achieving the recommended levels of protein and energy intake. It is suspected that the provision of adequate dialysis corrects subtle uremia and thus enables patients to have less anorexia.

D. **Protein**

1. **General considerations.** Recommended levels of protein intake are designed to balance the protein anabolism and amino acid losses during dialysis with phosphorus restrictions that inherently limit protein intake.

Table 23-4. Median weights for men and women in the United States by age, height, and frame size

Height		20–29			30–39			40–49			50–59			60–69			70–79		
									Frame size[a]										
in.	cm	S	M	L	S	M	L	S	M	L	S	M	L	S	M	L	S	M	L
													Weight (kg)						
Men																			
62	157	63	67	82	64	68	82	64	68	82	65	73	84	61	69	78	58	65	73
63	160	60	70	83	61	71	83	61	71	83	66	75	87	62	71	81	59	67	76
64	163	65	70	84	66	71	84	66	71	84	67	76	84	63	72	78	60	68	73
65	165	65	73	79	66	74	79	66	74	79	74	77	86	70	73	80	67	69	75
66	168	66	74	84	67	75	84	67	75	84	72	79	87	68	75	81	65	71	76
67	170	70	76	84	71	77	84	71	77	84	73	83	92	69	79	86	66	75	81
68	173	70	77	86	71	78	86	71	78	86	74	83	90	70	79	84	67	75	79
69	175	73	77	89	74	78	89	74	78	89	79	82	91	75	78	85	72	74	80
70	178	74	80	87	75	81	87	75	81	87	80	85	94	76	81	88	73	77	83
71	180	75	80	91	76	81	91	76	81	91	73	89	91	69	85	85	66	81	80
72	183	73	83	91	74	84	91	74	84	91	80	86	97	76	82	91	73	78	86
73	185	78	84	93	79	85	93	79	85	93	82	93	95	78	78	89	75	85	84
74	188	79	87	92	80	88	92	80	88	92	81	100	96	77	96	90	74	92	85

Women

58	147	50	60	83	52	63	85	53	65	88	54	59	98	54	57	93	54	55	88
59	150	51	63	75	53	66	77	54	68	80	55	64	84	55	62	79	55	60	74
60	152	51	57	84	53	60	86	54	62	89	54	67	84	54	65	79	54	63	74
61	155	52	58	78	54	61	80	55	63	83	56	66	85	56	64	80	56	62	75
62	157	53	58	78	55	61	80	56	63	83	58	66	88	58	64	83	58	62	78
63	160	53	59	80	55	62	82	56	64	85	58	67	86	58	65	81	58	63	76
64	163	55	59	76	57	62	78	58	64	81	60	68	83	60	66	78	60	64	73
65	165	58	60	78	60	63	80	61	65	83	60	69	86	60	67	81	60	65	76
66	168	56	60	72	58	63	74	59	65	77	68	68	88	68	66	83	68	64	78
67	170	57	62	77	59	65	79	60	67	82	61	74	86	61	72	81	61	70	76
68	173	60	64	73	62	67	75	63	69	78	61	72	85	61	70	80	61	68	75
69	175	61	65	76	63	68	78	64	70	81	62	74	91	62	72	86	62	70	81
70	178	62	67	73	64	70	75	65	72	78	63	75	91	63	73	86	63	71	81

a Frame size as defined in Table 23-3.

Data derived from the combined NHANES I and II datasets. *Data source:* Frisancho AR. New standards of weight and body composition by frame size and height for assessment of nutritional status of adults and the elderly. *Am J Clin Nutr* 1984;40:808–819.

2.   Hemodialysis patients. DOQI guidelines recommend that hemodialysis patients should ingest 1.2 g of protein per kilogram of average body weight per day. At least 50% of the protein ingested should be of high biologic value. This level of protein intake is often difficult to achieve in practice, however, with 30% to 50% of hemodialysis patients having a reported intake of less than 1.0 g of protein per kilogram of average body weight per day (Dwyer et al, 1998). Protein intake based on actual body weight can be predicted from predialysis SUN levels using urea kinetic modeling (see Chapter 2).

3.   Peritoneal dialysis patients. DOQI guidelines recommend that peritoneal dialysis patients should ingest 1.2 g of protein per kilogram of average body weight per day. Some physicians recommend that protein intake be as high as 1.5 g of protein per kilogram of average body weight per day for patients who are protein-depleted.

At least 50% of the protein ingested should be of high biologic value. The higher level of protein recommended for peritoneal dialysis patients is designed to account for protein losses in the dialysate. Protein intake can be estimated from urea levels in 24-hour dialysate and urine collections (see Chapter 17).

E.   Energy

1.   General considerations. Higher levels of caloric intake may be required for patients who perform strenuous labor, for patients who are well below their desired weight, and for patients who are hospitalized, have peritonitis, or have other causes of catabolic stress. DOQI guidelines recommend that all dialysis patients younger than 61 years ingest 35 kcal per kg per day. For patients older than 60 years, the recommended intake is 30–35 kcal per kg per day.

2.   Hemodialysis patients. Based on several small studies done in metabolic wards, a daily caloric intake of at least 35 kcal per kg average body weight has been proposed to maintain neutral nitrogen balance and prevent protein breakdown. However, this level of caloric intake is often difficult to achieve in practice because hemodialysis patients ingest on average less than 30 kcal per kg average body weight per day (Bergström et al, 1993). Also, there is no firm evidence in longitudinal studies that patients ingesting less than 30 kcal per kg subsequently lose dry weight or experience a decrease in serum albumin levels. In practice, caloric intake in several large hemodialysis populations has been found to average 23–27 kcal/kg when intake is based on dietary recall.

Carbohydrates should make up approximately 35% of nonprotein calories with fats providing the remainder of the nonprotein calorie intake. A modest amount of calories is absorbed during a typical hemodialysis session, usually in the range of 400 kcal per treatment when the dialysate glucose concentration is 200 mg per dL.

3.   Peritoneal dialysis patients. Total nonprotein calories (including calories from the dialysate glucose) should be approximately 30–40 kcal per kg average body weight per day. Up to 30% of a peritoneal dialysis patient's total caloric intake may be derived from glucose absorption from peritoneal dialysis fluid. Factors that influence the degree of glucose absorption include the percent dextrose used for each dwell, the length of each exchange, the volume of each dwell, the number of exchanges, and peritoneal membrane transport properties. In general, the higher the dialysate–to–plasma creatinine ratio (D/P Cr), the dwell volume, or the percent dextrose concentration, the higher the amount of glucose absorbed per exchange. Typical amounts of calories absorbed with various regimens are listed in Table 23-5. The values listed are derived from a computer simulation program.

    a.   CAPD and continuous cycling peritoneal dialysis (CCPD) regimens. With most CAPD and CCPD regimens that are made up primarily of 1.5% dextrose exchanges and include only one or two 4.25% exchanges per day, an amount of glucose providing about 500–600 kcal per day will be absorbed. Up to 700 kcal per day can be absorbed when the regimen consists almost exclusively of high-dextrose exchanges.

    b.   NIPD regimens. Assuming that 15 L of dialysis solution is used nightly, 390–860 kcal of glucose will be absorbed per night as the mean dextrose concentration ranges from 1.5% to 2.5% (Table 23-5).

    Note that these data provide only an estimate of calories from glucose absorption and that these estimates will vary depending on patient membrane characteristics and by variations in how the prescribed prescription is carried out by the patient.

F.   Lipids. Dialysis patients should follow the American Heart Association step I diet, which suggests that no more than 30% of total calories should be derived from fat and that less than 10% of calories should be derived from saturated fat. The ratio of polyunsaturated to saturated fats should be approximately 2 : 1 to help minimize elevations in triglyceride and cholesterol concentrations. Treatments for hypercholesterolemia and hypertriglyceridemia are discussed in Chapters 21 and 33.

G.   Carbohydrates. Patients with hypertriglyceridemia or impaired glucose tolerance may benefit from a diet that emphasizes complex carbohydrates over purified carbohydrates.

H.   Sodium and water. Sodium and water restrictions are individualized, depending on fluid status, the impact of sodium restriction on control of hypertension, and the extent of residual renal function.

    1.   Patients with substantial residual renal function. If urinary output is greater than 1 L per day, then mild fluid restriction (2 L per day) and sodium restriction (3–4 g per day, 120–160 mEq per day) is recommended. High-dose diuretic therapy (200–400 mg furosemide per day or equivalent) may assist in promoting diuresis.

    2.   Patients with anuria

        a.   Hemodialysis patients. Fluid intake should be restricted to about 1 L per day and sodium intake should be restricted to about 2 g per day (80 mEq per day). Interdialytic weight gain should be less than 5% of the patient's dry weight; however, minimal interdialytic weight gain has been associated with poorer nutritional status as assessed by lower PCRs and serum albumin levels (Sherman et al, 1995).

Table 23-5.   Estimated caloric value of absorbed glucose with various peritoneal dialysis regimens[a]

CAPD

Dextrose Daytime Exchanges			kcal Glucose Absorbed During the Daytime	Dextrose Nighttime Exchange	Night kcal Absorbed	Total kcal Absorbed
1st	2nd	3rd				
1.5%	1.5%	1.5%	250	4.25%	260	510
1.5%	2.5%	1.5%	310	4.25%	260	570
2.5%	2.5%	2.5%	420	4.25%	260	680
1.5%	4.25%	1.5%	400	4.25%	260	660
2.5%	4.25%	2.5%	510	4.25%	260	770

CCPD

Mean Dextrose Night Exchanges	Night kcal Absorbed	Dextrose Day Exchange	Day kcal Absorbed	Total kcal Absorbed
1.5%	250	4.25%	280	530
2.0%	340	4.25%	280	620
2.5%	410	4.25%	280	690

	Mean Dextrose Night Exchanges	kcal Absorbed Per Night
NIPD	1.5%	390
	2.0%	620
	2.5%	860

Acute Peritoneal Dialysis (60-min Cycle Time)

Exchange Schedule	kcal Absorbed/24 hr
All 1.5% dextrose exchanges	830
2.5% every 3rd exchange	990
4.25% every 3rd exchange	1,230
2.5% every exchange	1,320

[a] All calculations are based on a 2-L exchange volume. CAPD: four exchanges every 24 hr; CCPD: four nocturnal exchanges over 10 hr and one daytime exchange; NIPD: seven 2.14-L exchanges over 10 hr; acute peritoneal dialysis: 24 exchanges over 24 hr.
CAPD, continuous ambulatory peritoneal dialysis; CCPD, continuous cycling peritoneal dialysis; NIPD, nocturnal intermittent peritoneal dialysis.
Source: Values are derived from a computer simulation model developed by Baxter Healthcare, Inc. (Deerfield, IL) using glucose absorption constants in the literature. A 70-kg patient is assumed, with a 10-min fill and 20-min drain. Approximately 100 additional calories is absorbed in the form of lactate with each of these forms of dialysis.

   b.   Peritoneal dialysis patients. Dietary restrictions
   are usually less severe than those for hemodialysis patients
   due to the continuous nature of most peritoneal dialysis prescriptions as well as the ability to remove up to 2.5 L of ultrafiltrate per day. If ultrafiltration is easily removed, then fluid
   restriction should be about 2 L per day and sodium restriction should be about 3–4 g per day (120–160 mEq per day).
   Note, however, that the use of high dextrose concentrations
   in peritoneal dialysis dialysate should be minimized to help
   prevent the development of obesity and hypertriglyceridemia
   from the absorbed glucose.
I.   Potassium. Mild potassium restriction (4 g per day, or
100 mEq per day) is usually all that is needed in patients with
a moderate degree of residual renal function. Hyperkalemia
may be a problem in these patients only in the presence of
acidemia, hypoaldosteronism, or the administration of non-
steroidals, potassium-sparing diuretics, angiotensin-converting
enzyme inhibitors, or β-receptor blockers.
   The administration of angiotensin-converting enzyme inhibitors results in a decrease in the excretion of potassium into the
stool, a major source of potassium removal in patients on chronic
dialysis. Hyperkalemia in anuric peritoneal dialysis patients is
unusual because the dialysate contains no potassium and almost
all of these patients require only a modest potassium (4 g per day)
restriction. In hemodialysis patients, however, a more restricted
intake of potassium (2 g per day, or 50 mEq per day) is usually
required to prevent hyperkalemia.
J.   Calcium. The recommended intake for healthy nonuremic
persons is 1 g per day. Dialysis patients have an increased dietary
calcium requirement because of deficiency of vitamin D and resistance to the action of vitamin D. The renal diet tends to be low
in calcium because dairy intake is usually restricted to limit
the intake of phosphorus. To achieve calcium balance, dialysis
patients typically require supplementation with both calcium
and vitamin D. However, use of calcium and vitamin D in dialysis patients can result in severe hypercalcemia and must be
approached with caution. For details, see Chapter 30.
K.   Phosphorus. The usual dietary phosphorus intake in
nonuremic persons is 1.0–1.8 g per day. In dialysis patients, phosphorus intake needs to be restricted to maintain serum phosphorus levels in the 4.5- to 5.5-mg per dL range. Ideally, phosphorus
intake should be restricted to 0.6–1.2 g per day; however, as there
is a high correlation between the protein and phosphorus content,
adequate phosphorus restriction is often quite difficult to accomplish without unduly restricting the intake of protein. Consequently, virtually all chronic dialysis patients who are consuming an adequate amount of protein require the use of phosphate
binders to prevent hyperphosphatemia (see Chapter 30).
   Hyperphosphatemia is usually found in patients who are eating more than the prescribed amount of protein and/or dairy
products (some patients evidence a milk addiction!), are not taking a sufficient amount of phosphate-binding compound, and are
not timing ingestion of phosphate-binding compounds to coincide
with their meals. Inadequate dialysis can also be a factor. Dialysis patients should not ordinarily be given phosphate-containing
laxatives or enemas (e.g., the popular Fleet product line).

1. **Treatment.** Treatment is to reinforce compliance with the dietary phosphorus restriction and to ensure that the prescribed amount of phosphate-binding drug is being ingested at the proper times. Use of a large surface area dialyzer and provision of a longer dialysis session will increase the amount of phosphate removal during dialysis.

L. **Vitamins**

1. **Supplementation.** Dialysis patients may develop deficiencies of water-soluble vitamins unless daily supplements are given. Vitamin deficiencies are caused by poor intake, interference with absorption by drugs or uremia, altered metabolism, and losses to the dialysate. All dialysis patients should receive supplementary folic acid and B vitamins in the doses listed in Table 23-2 (Rocco et al, 1997). Vitamin replacement may have to be more intensive in patients undergoing high-flux dialysis due to increased losses (Kasama et al, 1996). In addition, the administration of higher doses of folate (10–15 mg per day) has been shown to decrease serum homocysteine levels, a risk factor for cardiovascular and peripheral vascular disease (Makoff et al, 1996). However, the long-term effects of high-dose folate supplementation are not known.

2. **Dangers associated with excess vitamin ingestion**

   a. **Vitamin C.** Ascorbic acid supplementation should be limited to 60–100 mg per day. Higher doses can result in the accumulation of a metabolite of ascorbic acid, namely, oxalate. Hyperoxalemia can result in the development of kidney stones, composed of calcium oxalate, and in the occurrence of calcium oxalate deposits in viscera, soft tissues, joints, and blood vessels. Intravenous ascorbic acid may be of value in treating erythropoieten-resistant anemia by increasing iron availability (see Chapter 27).

   b. **Vitamin A.** Serum vitamin A concentrations are almost always elevated in dialysis patients due to increased serum levels of retinol-binding protein, decreased renal catabolism, and the fact that dialysis cannot remove vitamin A. In addition to the multiple, serious adverse effects that hypervitaminosis A can induce in nonuremic persons, hypervitaminosis A in dialysis patients can also cause anemia and abnormalities of lipid and calcium metabolism.

   c. **Vitamin D.** Supplemental vitamin D is a valuable adjuvant in the treatment of secondary hyperparathyroidism. The dosage of vitamin D prescribed is based on the balance of decreasing parathyroid hormone levels while avoiding hypercalcemia or an elevated calcium–phosphorus product. Management of secondary hyperparathyroidism is discussed in more detail in Chapter 30.

   d. **Vitamin E.** Although several short-term studies have demonstrated that supplemental vitamin E can result in increased red cell survival, the long-term effects of vitamin E compounds in dialysis patients are not known.

   e. **Vitamin K.** Vitamin K deficiency can occur in patients receiving antibiotics that suppress the production of vitamin K by intestinal bacteria. Under these circumstances, supplementation with 7.5 mg of vitamin K per week may be beneficial.

3.   Commercial multivitamin preparations. All preparations containing vitamin A should be avoided. Also, preparations containing megadose quantities of any vitamin should not be used. One should especially avoid preparations containing high doses of vitamin C. Vitamin supplements formulated for the needs of dialysis patients are commercially available and should be used exclusively in this population.

M.   Trace minerals

1.   Iron. The treatment of iron deficiency is discussed in Chapter 27.

2.   Other trace elements. Little is known about the uptake and metabolism of other trace minerals in dialysis patients. In some instances, low serum values are accompanied by higher than normal levels in tissues; the clinical importance of this finding is not well understood. Therefore, it is difficult to make firm recommendations regarding the benefits and risks of supplementation of trace minerals in chronic dialysis patients.

IV.   Nutritional consequences of exercise. Endurance exercise training can improve several of the metabolic abnormalities that occur in dialysis patients. Exercise has been associated with an improvement in the rate of glucose disappearance and a reduction in fasting plasma insulin levels; in addition, plasma triglyceride values decrease and HDL cholesterol concentrations increase. Other benefits of exercise include an increase in muscle size and strength and improvement in endurance. Reductions in anxiety, hostility, and depression also have been reported.

V.   General considerations in the treatment of the malnourished dialysis patient

A.   Chronic renal failure patients. Reversible causes of malnutrition should be diligently pursued and corrected. The provision of adequate dialysis is a crucial first step in improving nutritional status. Other medical conditions should also be identified and treated if possible. Social considerations include access and preparation of food and consideration of ethnic and personal food preferences. Nutritional intervention in the form of oral or parenteral supplements should be considered after reversible causes of malnutrition have been identified and corrected.

B.   Acute renal failure patients. The degree of metabolic derangements and the amount of protein catabolism can vary greatly in individual patients with acute renal failure. Net protein degradation can be negligible or can be greater than 150 g per day; the latter is seen most often in patients with sepsis, shock, or rhabdomyolysis (Feinstein et al, 1983). The guidelines presented below are general principles that should be modified based on the individual patient's clinical condition.

C.   Energy requirements in hospitalized dialysis patients. Acute renal failure patients or hospitalized chronic dialysis patients often have high energy and nitrogen needs. Total nonprotein energy needs can be estimated by modifying the recommended energy intake for stable dialysis patients (30 kcal per kg) by an adjustment factor based on the patient's clinical condition. In the absence of sepsis (adjustment factor = 1.2–1.3) or severe burn (1.5–1.7), this adjustment factor usually is small, in the range of 1.1–1.2 (Table 23-6). Little information is

Table 23-6. Adjustment factors for determination of energy requirements

Clinical Condition	Adjustment Factor
Mechanical ventilation	
Without sepsis	1.10–1.20
With sepsis	1.25–1.35
Peritonitis	1.15
Infections	
Mild	1.00–1.10
Moderate	1.10–1.20
Sepsis	1.20–1.30
Soft-tissue trauma	1.10
Bone fractures	1.15
Burns (% of body surface area)	
0–20%	1.15
20–40%	1.50
40–100%	1.70

Recommendations adapted from Blackburn et al. *J Parenter Enteral Nutr* 1977; 1:11–22; Bouffard et al. *Intens Care Med* 1987; 13:401–404; Schneeweiss et al. *Am J Clin Nutr* 1990;52:596–601; Soop et al. *Clin Nephrol* 1989; 31:139–145.

available regarding the magnitude of these adjustment factors in patients receiving dialysis therapy, however. In general, energy expenditure in acutely ill patients with acute renal failure is 10%–15% less than in acutely ill patients without acute renal failure. In addition, hypermetabolism is about one-third less in patients with multiple organ failure including acute renal failure versus patients with multiple organ failure who have normal renal function (Soop et al, 1989).

Example. A 65-year-old man develops acute renal failure due to acute tubular necrosis and severe sepsis. He does not require mechanical ventilation; he weighs 70 kg and is 170 cm tall. What are his daily energy needs?

Using the adjustment factor:

Energy needs = basal energy needs × adjustment factor for sepsis

= 30 kcal/kg × 1.30 = 39 kcal/kg

In general, most patients with acute renal failure requiring dialysis have energy needs between 30 and 40 kcal per kg.

Higher levels of nutritional intake have not been shown to be beneficial from a nutritional standpoint and can cause hypercapnia, especially if patients have impaired pulmonary function. Little is known about the significance of the energy source used for supplementation in acute renal failure patients. Most authors recommend that both fat and glucose be given. The daily amount of glucose administered should not exceed 5 g per kg body weight as supplementation above this level results in incomplete oxidation of glucose and conversion of glucose to fat. The balance of energy requirements is provided by lipids (see Section E below). Some patients may need more frequent or intense dialysis once nutritional support is initiated to prevent a marked increase in BUN levels.

D.   Protein requirements. Amino acids are infused to help prevent protein breakdown, not to provide an additional source of calories; hence, they are not counted as part of the daily energy intake. The amino acid intake for patients with acute or chronic renal failure undergoing either chronic dialysis or one of the continuous renal replacement therapies should be in the range of 1.1–2.0 g per kg per day. There appears to be no benefit in using higher levels of protein supplementation, even in the face of very high nitrogen losses. When higher levels are given, there does not appear to be any additional improvement in nitrogen balance (Feinstein et al, 1983), and there is enhanced formation of urea and other nitrogenous waste products. The precise amount of protein given is derived from the amount of catabolic stress present; the guidelines are similar to that for catabolic patients without renal failure. Protein balance can be estimated from urea nitrogen appearance, as described in Section II.F.3.

E.   Lipid requirements. Energy requirements cannot usually be achieved by the administration of glucose infusions alone. Lipids have a high specific energy content as well as a low osmolality. The provision of 1.0 g or less of lipids per kg body weight usually prevents the development of a deficiency of essential fatty acids while decreasing the risk of the development of hypertriglyceridemia.

VI.   Specific agents for the treatment of the malnourished dialysis patient

A.   Oral supplements. The utilization of the gastrointestinal tract for nutritional support is preferred whenever possible because it is the most cost-effective method and provides the most physiologic means of providing nutrients. A number of different enteral formulas specifically formulated for chronic dialysis patients are available; some of the more common products are summarized in Table 23-7. Selection of an oral supplement in an individual patient should be based on the patient's specific nutritional needs as well as cost, palatability, lactose tolerance, and serum and supplement concentrations of sodium, potassium, and phosphorus.

B.   Intradialytic total parenteral nutrition (IDPN) in hemodialysis patients

1.   Indications and benefits. IDPN is indicated in the adequately dialyzed hemodialysis patient who has malnutrition and is unable to ingest or absorb sufficient food via the gastrointestinal tract. The largest study to date of patients receiving IDPN demonstrated that this procedure can decrease mortality in patients with an initial serum albumin level of less than 3.4 g per dL (Chertow et al, 1994).

2.   Composition, infusion, and complications. IDPN is performed by infusing an amino acid and protein solution during the hemodialysis procedure. The IDPN solution, which is usually composed of a 8.5% amino acid solution mixed with 250 mL of 50% dextrose, is infused in the venous drip chamber for the entire duration of the hemodialysis procedure. Additional energy can be provided by adding a lipid infusion to the IDPN solution; patients receiving lipids should be mon-

Table 23-7. Composition of enteral products commonly prescribed as an oral supplement for poorly nourished dialysis patients

Product	Source	Concentration (kcal/mL)	Protein (g/1,000 kcal)	CHO (g/1,000 kcal)	Fat (g/1,000 kcal)	Osmolality (mosm/kg H$_2$O)	Sodium [(mg)/1,000 kcal]	Potassium [(mg)/1,000 kcal]	Phosphorus [(mg)/1,000 kcal]
Amin-Aid	R&D Laboratories	2.0	9.7	182.8	23.1	700	<173	N/A	N/A
Comply	Mead Johnson	1.5	40	120	40.7	460	800	1,233	800
Deliver 2.0	Mead Johnson	2.0	37.5	100	51	640	400	850	500
Ensure Plus	Ross Products Division, Abbott Laboratories	1.5	36.6	133.3	35.5	690	700	1,293	470
Ensure Plus HN	Ross Products Division, Abbott Laboratories	1.5	41.7	133.3	33.3	650	787	1,213	704
Nepro	Ross Products Division, Abbott Laboratories	2.0	34.6	106.5	47.3	N/A	410	523	340
NuBasics Plus Drink	Nestle Clinical Nutrition	1.5	34.9	117.6	43.2	620–650	779	1,254	499
NuBasics 2.0 Drink	Nestle Clinical Nutrition	2.0	40	98	53	750	650	960	670
Nutren 2.0 diet	Nestle Clinical Nutrition	2.0	40	98	53	720	650	960	670
Nutren 1.5 diet	Nestle Clinical Nutrition	1.5	40	112.8	45.1	430–530	780	1,248	667

continued

Table 23-7. _Continued_

Product	Source	Concentration (kcal/mL)	Protein (g/1,000 kcal)	CHO (g/1,000 kcal)	Fat (g/1,000 kcal)	Osmolality (mosm/kg H₂O)	Sodium [(mg)/1,000 kcal]	Potassium [(mg)/1,000 kcal]	Phosphorus [(mg)/1,000 kcal]
Osmolite	Ross Products Divison, Abbott Laboratories	1.06	35	142.5	32.7	300	604	962	500
Renalcal Diet	Nestle Clinical Nutrition	2.0	17.2	145.2	41.2	600	N/A	N/A	N/A
ReNeph									
High Protein High Calorie	Nutra/Balance	2.12	32	128	40	N/A	360	40	96
High Protein High Calorie Sugar-Free	Nutra/Balance	2.12	10	160	40	N/A	100	4	24
Low Protein High Calorie	Nutra/Balance	2.03	33.3	125	41.7	N/A	312.5	104	150
Resource Plus	Sandoz Nutrition	1.5	36.7	133.3	35.3	600	867	1,400	473
Resource Standard	Sandoz	1.06	34.9	132.1	34.9	430	840	1,509	500
Sustacal Plus	Mead Johnson	1.52	40.1	125	37.5	630–670	559	974	559
TwoCal HN	Ross Products Division, Abbott Laboratories	2.0	41.9	108.7	45.5	690	728	1,228	526

CHO, carbohydrate.

itored closely for hypertriglyceridemia, changes in liver function tests, or compromise of the reticuloendothelial system. A typical composition of IDPN is outlined in Table 23-8.

Patients receiving high-flux hemodialysis of short duration may need to have their dialysis prescription modified to prevent painful arm cramps, which can occur when a high osmolality solution is rapidly infused, and to prevent hypoglycemia, which can occur when a rapid infusion of glucose is rapidly discontinued. In addition, patients should consume some carbohydrate within the last 30 minutes of the IDPN infusion to prevent hypoglycemia. Likewise, if patients dialyze against a glucose-free dialysate, the IDPN should not be discontinued until the conclusion of the hemodialysis procedure.

3. Effect of IDPN on *Kt/V*. When amino acids are given as part of IDPN, there typically will be about a 0.2 decline in the treatment *Kt/V* (McCann et al, 1999). This decline in *Kt/V* is due to the sudden increase in urea generation associated with amino acid infusion, which elevates the postdialysis BUN level.

C. Intraperitoneal infusion of amino acids in peritoneal dialysis patients

1. Indications and benefits. The utilization of amino acid dialysate in place of glucose-based dialysate has been proposed as a means to replace proteins lost in the dialysate and to help minimize complications associated with use of glucose-based dialysate solutions, including weight gain, hyperlipidemia, and glucose intolerance. In CAPD patients, the replacement of one or two of the four daily glucose dialysate exchanges with glucose-free, amino acid dialysate results in an improvement in nitrogen balance, greater net protein anabolism, and a significant increase in serum transferrin and total protein levels (Kopple et al, 1995).

Table 23–8. Composition of a "typical" solution for intradialytic parenteral nutrition

Component	Amount
50% Dextrose (D-glucose)	125 g (250 mL)
8.5% Crystalline amino acids (essential and nonessential)	42.5 g (500 mL)
20% Lipids	50 g (250 mL)
Electrolytes	Sodium phosphate, potassium chloride, and magnesium sulfate with amount per IDPN bag adjusted for serum electrolyte levels
Vitamins	See text and Table 23–2
Insulin, regular	Adjusted per blood glucose levels
Caloric content	
50% dextrose	425 kcal/treatment
20% lipid emulsion	500 kcal/treatment
Total	925 kcal/treatment

IDPN, intradialytic parenteral nutrition.

2. Composition, infusion, and complications. Usually, the amino acid dialysate solution consists of both essential and nonessential amino acids. It is given as the overnight exchange in CAPD patients or as the long daytime dwell in CCPD patients in order to maximize protein absorption. The osmotic effect of a 1.0% amino acid dialysate solution is similar to that of a 2.0% dextrose solution. Complications of utilizing amino acid dialysate solutions include anorexia, nausea, vomiting and an increase in BUN levels and are more common when patients receive two amino acid dialysate solutions per day versus one per day.

D. Parenteral supplements given by peripheral vein. In dialysis patients who are hospitalized and cannot ingest adequate calories by the enteral route, approximately 1,500 additional calories per day can be administered by peripheral vein using the solutions described in Table 23-9. Administration of calories by the peripheral route, supplemented by additional carbohydrate calories orally and from peritoneal dialysis or hemodialysis, often can obviate the need for insertion of a central line as long as the patient is not markedly catabolic. To prevent phlebitis, the osmolality of the solution should be less than 600 mOsm per kg. The serum triglyceride levels should be checked periodically to monitor for the development of marked hypertriglyceridemia.

E. Continuous total parenteral nutrition (TPN). TPN is used in patients with severe nutritional deficits who cannot re-

Table 23-9. Composition of a "typical" solution for parenteral supplements given by peripheral vein

Component	Amount
5% Dextrose (D-glucose)	12.5 g (250 mL)
8.5% Crystalline amino acids (essential and nonessential)	42.5 g (500 mL)
10% Lipids	25 g (250 mL)
Electrolytes	Sodium phosphate, potassium chloride, and magnesium sulfate with amount per IDPN bag adjusted for serum electrolyte levels
Vitamins	See text and Table 23-2
Insulin, regular	Adjusted per blood glucose levels
Heparin	1,000 units/L

Caloric content and osmolality
Administer solution at 40 mL/hr or 960 mL/d

	Caloric Content	Osmolality
5% dextrose	163 kcal/d	278 mOsm/kg H_2O
10% lipid emulsion	1,054 kcal/d	280 mOsm/kg H_2O
Total	1,217 kcal/d	558 mOsm/kg H_2O

IDPN, intradialytic parental nutrition.

ceive adequate nutritional intake from oral supplements, intraperitoneal amino acids, or IDPN. General guidelines for the formulation of a typical TPN solution are outlined in Table 23-10.

   1.   Carbohydrates. Approximately 50%–70% of nonprotein calories in TPN are provided from glucose. Glucose is
usually provided as 70% D-glucose to minimize the amount of
fluid administered. The precise amount of D-glucose given is
dependent on the calculated energy intake indicated for an
individual patient. Each milliliter of 70% dextrose provides
2.38 kcal.

   2.   Amino acids. There is much controversy regarding the
optimal mix of essential and nonessential amino acids used in
TPN solutions. Some authors report that essential amino acids

**Table 23–10.   Composition of "typical" total perenteral
nutrition solutions for hospitalized renal failure patients**

Component	Amount
70% Dextrose (D-glucose)	350 g (500 mL)
8.5% Crystalline amino acids (essential and nonessential)	42.5 g (500 mL)
20% lipids	50 g (500 mL)
or	
10% lipids	25 g (500 mL)
Electrolytes (general guidelines)[a]	
Sodium	40–80 mmol/L
Chloride	25–35 mmol/L
Potassium	<35 mmol/d
Acetate	35–40 mmol/d
Calcium	5 mmol/d
Phosphorus	5–10 mmol/d
Magnesium	2–4 mmol/d
Iron	2 g/d
Vitamins	See text and Table 23–2

Caloric content

Solution Administration Rate:	40 mL/h or 960 mL/d	60 mL/h or 1440 mL/day
70% dextrose	794 kcal/d	1,077 kcal/d
20% lipid emulsion	667 kcal/d	960 kcal/d
Total	1,461 kcal/d	2,037 kcal/d
70% dextrose	794 kcal/d	1,077 kcal/d
10% lipid emulsion	357 kcal/d	528 kcal/d
Total	1,141 kcal/d	1,605 kcal/d

[a] The specific amount of electrolytes given should be modified based on the
patient's clinical condition and serum concentration of electrolytes. The guidelines listed include electrolytes contributed by the infusion of amino acids. Use
of a TPN sodium level of about 130–135 mmol per L will prevent hyponatremia
but requires either daily dialysis or CCRT for adequate volume control.

can be used more efficiently than larger quantities of essential and nonessential amino acids, whereas others report the development of nausea, vomiting, and metabolic acidosis when only essential amino acids are administered. Most commercial crystalline amino acid solutions provide a mix of essential and nonessential amino acids.

3.   Lipids. Lipids can provide up to 50% of the non-protein calories in TPN solutions. Lipid emulsions are usually available in 10% and 20% solutions; the latter provides 2.0 kcal per mL. Lipids should be given over a 12- to 24-hour period to decrease the risk of decreased functioning of the reticuloendothelial system. Some authors recommend decreasing the amount of lipids given by 50% if the patient is septic or is at a high risk for sepsis. There is some controversy regarding the ratio of polyunsaturated to saturated fatty acids that is preferable in acutely ill dialysis patients, with most authors recommending a ratio between 1.0 and 2.0. If patients develop marked hypertriglyceridemia, lipid infusions can be provided either once or twice weekly instead of daily.

4.   Electrolytes. The amount of most electrolytes in TPN solutions should initially be moderately restricted, unless serum levels indicate a deficiency. Patients who are markedly catabolic can develop acidemia, hyperkalemia, hyperphosphatemia, or markedly elevated SUN levels very rapidly. On the other hand, the high glucose load plus the anabolism induced by TPN solutions can result in hypokalemia, hypophosphatemia, and hypomagnesemia. Therefore, blood levels of these electrolytes should be monitored frequently and adjustments in the electrolyte concentration made accordingly.

5.   Vitamins. Little research has been performed on vitamin requirements in patients with acute renal failure. In general, vitamin supplementation during TPN should be similar to that provided to chronic dialysis patients (Table 23-2).

6.   Minerals and trace elements. Iron should be supplemented to help provide for effective erythropoiesis. Zinc is sometimes given based on some evidence that it accelerates wound healing. Other trace elements probably need not be supplemented unless the patient receives TPN for more than 3 weeks.

SELECTED READINGS

American Diabetic Association. A healthy food guide: diabetes and hemodialysis. *Natl Ren Diet* 1993.

Bergström J, Heimbürger O, Lindholm B. Calculation of the protein equivalent of total nitrogen appearance from urea appearance: which formulas should be used. *Perit Dial Int* 1998;18:467–473.

Chertow GM, et al. The association of intradialytic parenteral nutrition administration with survival in hemodialysis patients. *Am J Kidney Dis* 1994;24:912–920.

Churchill DN, Taylor DW, Keshaviah PR for the Canada–USA (CANUSA) Peritoneal Dialysis Study Group. Adequacy of dialysis and nutrition in continuous peritoneal dialysis: association with clinical outcomes. *J Am Soc Nephrol* 1996;7:198–207.

Dwyer JT, et al. The hemodialysis pilot study: nutrition program and participant characteristics at baseline: the HEMO study group. *J Ren Nutr* 1998:8:11–20.

Eustace JA, et al. Randomized double-blind trial of oral essential amino acids for dialysis-associated hypoalbuminemia. *Kidney Int* 2000;57:2527–2538.

Feinstein EI, et al. Total parenteral nutrition with high and low nitrogen intakes in patients with acute renal failure. *Kidney Int* 1983; 24(Suppl 16):S319–S323.

Held PJ, et al. Continuous ambulatory peritoneal dialysis and hemodialysis: comparison of patient mortality with adjustment for comorbid conditions. *Kidney Int* 1994;45:1163–1169.

Johansen KL, et al. Anabolic effects of nandrolone decanoate in patients receiving hemodialysis. *J Am Med Assoc* 1999;281:1275–1281.

Johansen KL, et al. Physical activity levels in patients on hemodialysis and healthy sedentary controls. *Kidney Int* 2000;57:2564–2570.

Kasama R, et al. Vitamin B_6 and hemodialysis: the impact of high flux/high-efficiency dialysis and review of the literature. *Am J Kidney Dis* 1996;5:680–686.

Kaysen GA, Stevenson FT, Depner TA. Determinants of albumin concentration in hemodialysis patients. *Am J Kidney Dis* 1997;29: 658–668.

Kopple JD, et al. Treatment of malnourished CAPD patients with an amino acid based dialysate. *Kidney Int* 1995;47:1148–1157.

Maggiore Q, et al. Nutritional and prognostic correlates of bioimpedance indexes in hemodialysis patients. *Kidney Int* 1996;50: 2103–2108.

Makoff R, Dwyer J, Rocco M. Folic acid, pyridoxine, cobalamin and homocysteine and their relationship to cardiovascular disease in ESRD. *J Ren Nutr* 1996;6:2–11.

McCann L, et al. Effect of intradialytic parenteral nutrition on delivered Kt/V. *Am J Kidney Dis* 1999;33:1131–1135.

Nelson EE, et al. Anthropometric norms for the dialysis population. *Am J Kidney Dis* 1990;16:32–37.

Owen W, et al. The urea reduction ratio and serum albumin concentration as predictors of mortality in patients undergoing hemodialysis. *N Engl J Med* 1993;329:1001–1006.

Pierratos A, et al. Total body nitrogen increases on nocturnal hemodialysis. *J Am Soc Nephrol* 1999;10:299A (abstr).

Rocco MV, Makoff R. Appropriate vitamin therapy for renal dialysis patients. *Semin Dial* 1997;10:272–277.

Rocco M, et al, and the HEMO study group, NIDDK. Factors associated with dietary protein and energy intake and serum albumin levels in hemodialysis patients: An interim report from the HEMO study. *J Am Soc Nephrol* 1998;9:224A.

Sherman RA, et al. Interdialytic weight gain and nutritional parameters in chronic hemodialysis patients. *Am J Kidney Dis* 1995; 25:579–583.

Soop M, et al. Energy expenditure in postoperative multiple organ failure with acute renal failure. *Clin Nephrol* 1989;31:139–145.

Suda T, et al. The contribution of residual renal function to overall nutritional status in chronic hemodialysis patients. *Nephrol Dial Transplant* 2000;15:396–401.

Sunder-Plassman G, et al. Effect of high dose folic acid therapy on hyperhomocysteinemia in hemodialysis patients. *J Am Soc Nephrol* 2000;11:1106–1126.

Internet Reference

Nutritional guidelines, tables and links. (http://www.hdcn.com/crf/nutrition)

Serum Enzyme Levels

N. D. Vaziri and Cyril H. Barton

The concentrations of a number of serum enzymes commonly measured for diagnostic purposes can be abnormal in patients with end-stage renal disease (Table 24-1).

I. Acute myocardial infarction (MI). In dialysis patients undergoing acute MI, the time course of elevations in serum levels of creatine kinase (CK), aspartate aminotransferase (AST), and lactate dehydrogenase (LDH) is presumably similar to that in nonuremic patients, although no data to this effect have been published.

A. Creatine kinase

1. Elevated baseline serum total CK level. Baseline serum total CK values are elevated persistently in 10%–50% of dialysis patients. When elevation is present, it is usually mild (e.g., to values less than three times the upper limit of normal). Occasionally, CK levels of 5–10 times the upper limit of normal are encountered. Increases have been reported to be greatest in patients receiving injections of anabolic steroids.

The reason for the persistent elevation of total serum CK levels in some dialysis patients is unknown. CK levels are more often found to be elevated in hemodialysis patients than in those treated with continuous ambulatory peritoneal dialysis (CAPD). CK levels are higher in males than in females and higher in blacks than in whites; they correlate with arm circumference. Postulated causes for high levels include intramuscular injection of androgens or other drugs. No definite link has been established between elevated CK levels and any sort of dialysis-associated myopathy. After renal transplantation, elevated serum CK levels promptly return to the normal range.

2. Elevated percentage of CK-MB. In nonuremic patients, up to 5% of total serum CK is the MB isoenzyme. In the appropriate clinical circumstances, when serum total CK levels are elevated, a concomitant rise in the percentage of the MB isoenzyme is a highly specific indicator of myocardial damage. However, quantitation of the MB isoenzyme is fraught with potential pitfalls. The available assay methods rely on ion-exchange chromatography, electrophoresis, radioimmunoassay, or adsorption onto glass beads. With the chromatographic technique, false-positive elevations of the CK-MB value can occur due to the presence of nonmyocardial CK variants; the electrophoretic method can also give factitiously elevated CK-MB values in uremia. The remaining two methods appear to give relatively few false-positive results.

From 3%–30% of dialysis patients without evidence of myocardial ischemia have been reported to have an elevated percentage of CK-MB in their sera. Some of the higher numbers

**Table 24–1. Alterations of baseline
serum enzyme levels in dialysis patients**

Enzyme	Serum Level
CK	Increased in 10–50%
CK-MM	Increased in up to 40%
CK-MB	Increased in 3–30%
Cardiac troponin:	
Troponin T	Increased in up to 71%
Troponin I	Increased in up to 9%
LDH	Increased in about 35%
LDH isoenzymes (1–5)	Isomorphic pattern
Aspartate aminotransferase	Decreased in 10–90%
Alkaline phosphatase:	
Total	Increased in about 50%
Intestinal isoenzyme	Increased in about 50%
Bone isoenzyme	Increased in about 50%
Glutamyl transpeptidase	Increased in 10–15%
Amylase	Increased in about 50%
Lipase	Increased in about 50%
Trypsin(ogen)	Increased in up to 100%
Elastase	Increased in up to 43%
Phospholipase A_2	Increased in up to 100%

CK, creatine kinase; LDH, lactic dehydrogenase.

reported may have been due to methodologic problems discussed above; the more recent studies report an increase in the CK-MB percentage in 5% or less of dialysis patients. When the CK-MB percentage is increased in dialysis patients without MI, the elevation is slight (e.g., usually to less than 8% of the total CK value).

3. Elevated percentage of CK-BB in acute renal failure. Serum levels of the CK-BB isoenzyme have been reported to be increased in patients with acute renal failure, possibly due to release of the isoenzyme from damaged renal tubular tissue. In some assays, the CK-BB and CK-MB isoenzymes are not well separated. In stable hemodialysis patients, the serum CK-BB concentration is usually in the normal range.

B. Aspartate aminotransferase. See Section II.A.

C. Lactic dehydrogenase

1. Increased baseline serum LDH level. Serum levels of LDH may be elevated (to three times the upper limit of normal) in as many as 35% of patients with renal insufficiency, due either to a reduced elimination rate or to increased release from damaged renal tissue in patients with acute renal failure. The elevation is characterized by an "isomorphic" pattern; the LDH-1/LDH-5 ratio is less than 1, and there is a nearly proportional increase in the activities of the various LDH isoenzymes (Vaziri et al, 1990). Serum LDH levels also may increase acutely in the course of hemodialysis, consistent with a hemoconcentration effect, as well as release from leukocytes. For this reason, predialysis samples should always be used for evaluation of serum LDH (and other enzyme) levels.

2. Human cardiac myosin light chain 1. Enzyme immunoassay of cardiac myosin light chains has been proposed as a new, sensitive test for MI. Unfortunately, in dialysis patients, serum levels of this compound are elevated 40-fold over control values (Nakai et al, 1992); this test is not useful in the end-stage renal disease population.

D. Cardiac troponins

1. Cardiac troponin T is a regulatory contractile protein that is normally absent in blood, and its detection in blood serves as a specific and sensitive indicator of myocardial cell damage (Hamm et al, 1992). However, blood troponin T is elevated in a high percentage of patients with chronic renal failure with no clinical evidence of acute myocardial injury (Bhayana et al, 1995; Li et al, 1996; Frankel et al, 1996). The mechanism of elevated troponin T level in this population is unclear. However, the values are directly correlated to serum creatinine levels, suggesting but not proving impaired renal clearance as a possible cause. Blood troponin T levels are not altered by hemodialysis.

2. Cardiac troponin I is another cardiac specific regulatory contractile protein, elevated blood levels of which are a specific indicator of cardiac injury. However, elevated troponin I levels occur in up to 9% of patients with advanced renal failure in the absence of clinical evidence of myocardial injury (Li, et al, 1996). Nonetheless, troponin I appears to be a reasonably accurate predictor of myocardial injury in renal failure patients (Martin et al, 1998) and to be more specific than troponin T in this population. Hemodialysis does not significantly change the serum levels of troponin I.

II. Enzymes associated with hepatic disease

A. Alanine and aspartate aminotransferases (ALT and AST)

1. Low baseline serum ALT and AST levels. Serum aminotransferase values are sometimes depressed (e.g., by 20%–50%) in 10%–90% of dialysis patients. The reason is unknown. Many explanations have been advanced, including inhibition of transaminase activity in the serum by uremic toxins. When ALT and AST levels are measured by an ultraviolet method using the SMA 12/60 autoanalyzer, some degree of factitious underestimation may result due to the presence of materials in uremic serum that absorb ultraviolet light. Serum AST values have been shown to increase after dialysis; the increase is presumed to be due to (a) removal of a dialyzable inhibitor, (b) increased release of the enzyme from erythrocytes in the extracorporeal circuit, and/or (c) ultrafiltration-induced hemoconcentration.

Because of the low baseline serum aminotransferase levels in dialysis patients, the finding of a value slightly above the upper limits of normal or of a substantial rise within the normal range should alert the clinician to a possible underlying disease process.

2. Causes of mildly elevated serum aminotransferase levels. A common clinical problem is to evaluate the importance of mildly elevated aminotransferase levels (ALT, AST, or both) in a dialysis patient. The frequency with which acute viral hepatitis B or C becomes chronic is increased in dialysis patients, and an elevated serum ALT level must be considered to reflect possible hepatitis (especially hepatitis C) infection until proven otherwise. Herpes simplex hepatitis and cytomegalovirus hepatitis also present with elevated aminotransferases (AST > ALT). Other causes of elevated serum aminotransferase levels in dialysis patients include the effects of hepatotoxic drugs and iron overload (hemosiderosis).

B. Alkaline phosphatase

1. Sites of alkaline phosphatase production. Alkaline phosphatase is normally produced by cells lining the biliary tree. In obstructive jaundice, the serum level of alkaline phosphatase is increased. However, alkaline phosphatases are produced by many other tissues as well, including bone, intestine, lung, kidney, certain tumors of hepatic and extrahepatic origin, white blood cells, and placenta.

2. Elevated serum levels of bone- or intestine-derived alkaline phosphatase. Both bone and liver disease are common in dialysis patients; hence, an elevated unfractionated serum alkaline phosphatase level is often difficult to interpret. In dialysis patients, "intestine-derived" alkaline phosphatase often is elevated, and the source of this enzyme may be the kidney. An elevation of the intestinal isoenzyme rather than the presence of early metabolic bone disease or hepatic disease should be considered in renal failure patients with mildly elevated (up to 50% over normal) total serum alkaline phosphatase values (Alpers et al, 1988; Tibi et al, 1991).

The cause of alkaline phosphatase elevation in a given patient can usually be at least partially resolved by determination of the heat stability of the enzyme present in the serum specimen (the bone-derived enzyme will lose its activity after exposure to heat). In addition, concomitant elevation of other hepatobiliary enzymes (see below) increases the likelihood that an elevated serum alkaline phosphatase value is of hepatic origin.

C. Other hepatobiliary enzymes. Serum levels of 5′-nucleotidase, leucine aminopeptidase (LAP), and γ-glutamyl transpeptidase (GGT) are also increased in the presence of active hepatobiliary disease. Elevated serum values of these enzymes reflect hepatobiliary dysfunction somewhat specifically. One exception is pregnancy, in which serum concentrations of 5′-nucleotidase and LAP may be increased. Elevation of the serum GGT level can be caused by ingestion of certain drugs that induce hepatic microsomal enzymes (e.g., phenytoin and phenobarbital).

1. Levels of other hepatobiliary enzymes in dialysis patients. There are no good data available concerning baseline serum levels of 5′-nucleotidase and LAP in dialysis patients. For reasons that are not entirely clear, serum GGT levels may be significantly elevated (two to three times the upper limit of normal) in about 10%–15% of end-stage renal disease patients who do not abuse alcohol, who exhibit no clinical evidence of liver disease, and who are not known to be using drugs that affect hepatic microsomal enzymes.

III.   Enzymes associated with pancreatitis
A.   Amylase
1.   Elevated baseline levels of serum amylase. In most dialysis patients, due to the loss of urinary excretion, serum total amylase activity is elevated up to three times the upper limit of normal, even in the absence of clinical evidence of pancreatitis. The magnitude of elevation is higher in patients with acute renal failure than in chronic dialysis patients. Serum amylase levels may be spuriously low in peritoneal dialysis patients using icodextrin-containing dialysis solutions (Schonicke et al, 1999). Serum concentrations of the pancreas-specific P_3 isoenzyme have been variably reported to be increased or normal in asymptomatic dialysis patients. In fact, P_3 values exceeding three times the upper limit of normal are seen in up to 18% of asymptomatic dialysis patients. In contrast, in the nonuremic population, the P_3 amylase fraction is consistently absent and appears only with acute pancreatitis.

2.   Question of occult pancreatitis in dialysis patients. Autopsy studies of largely asymptomatic dialysis patients have revealed a high incidence of pancreatic abnormalities, including chronic pancreatitis. The extent to which persistent elevations of the serum amylase levels are due to decreased catabolism of the enzyme versus pancreatitis is not known.

3.   Serum and peritoneal fluid amylase levels during pancreatitis in dialysis patients. In a dialysis patient suspected of having pancreatitis, the finding of a serum total amylase value in excess of three times the upper limit of normal suggests that pancreatitis is present. Unfortunately, very severe pancreatitis can be present in dialysis patients with only slight, and therefore nondiagnostic, elevations in the serum total amylase level. We have found elevation of the plasma P_3 isoenzyme level to be a reliable indicator of pancreatitis in dialysis patients (Vaziri et al, 1988).

The peritoneal fluid amylase concentration, easily obtainable in patients receiving peritoneal dialysis, is not a sensitive indicator of pancreatitis because the peritoneal fluid amylase levels can be only slightly elevated in the presence of severe pancreatitis. Nevertheless, an effluent amylase level greater than 100 units per dL is suggestive of pancreatitis or some other intra-abdominal catastrophe (Caruana et al, 1987; Gupta et al, 1992).

B.   Lipase
1.   Elevated baseline serum lipase levels in dialysis patients. Serum lipase activity is elevated (as high as twice the upper limit of normal) in about 50% of dialysis patients. Serum lipase activity rises following hemodialysis due to (a) heparin-induced increase in lipolytic activity and (b) presumably, ultrafiltration-induced hemoconcentration. Therefore, predialysis samples should be used for this test.

C.   Serum pancreatic secretory trypsin inhibitor (PSTI). The plasma concentration of this inhibitory peptide (MW 6,000) is increased in acute pancreatitis. Unfortunately, PSTI is also markedly elevated in dialysis patients in the absence of dis-

cernible pancreatic pathology. Reduced renal degradation, possibly with increased pancreatic or extrapancreatic production, is involved.

D. Serum trypsin(ogen) rises in pancreatitis in concert with other pancreatic enzymes. However, trypsinogen level may be elevated in up to 100% of dialysis patients (Seno et al, 1995; Kimmel et al, 1995). The magnitude of elevation is greater in hemodialysis than in peritoneal dialysis patients.

E. Elastase I and phospholipase A_2 are two other pancreatic enzymes whose serum concentrations rise in acute pancreatitis. However, a large percentage of dialysis patients show marked elevations of these enzymes in the absence of clinical evidence of pancreatitis (Seno et al, 1995).

SELECTED READINGS

Alpers DH, et al. Intestinal alkaline phosphatase in patients with chronic renal failure. *Gastroenterology* 1988;94:62–67.

Bastani B, et al. Serum total amylase, pancreatic isoamylase and lipase activity in chronic renal failure patients on peritoneal dialysis, hemodialysis, or no dialysis. In: Khanna R, et al, eds. *Advances in continuous ambulatory peritoneal dialysis 1986*. Toronto: Peritoneal Dialysis Bulletin, Inc., 1987.

Bhayana V, et al. Discordance between results for serum troponin T and troponin I in renal disease. *Clin Chem* 1995;41:312–317.

Caruana RJ, et al. Serum and peritoneal fluid amylase levels in CAPD: normal values and clinical usefulness. *Am J Nephrol* 1987;7:169–172.

Chang BS, Barnes RV, Port EK. Transaminase levels in azotemia [letter]. *Ann Intern Med* 1976;85:255–257.

Cohen GA, et al. Observations on decreased serum glutamic oxalacetic transaminase (SGOT) activity in azotemic patients. *Ann Intern Med* 1976;84:275–280.

Fine A, McIntosh WB. Elevation of serum gamma-glutamyl transpeptidase in end-stage chronic renal failure. *Scott Med J* 1975l;20:113–115.

Frankel WL, et al. Cardiac troponin T is elevated in asymptomatic patients with chronic renal failure. *Am J Clin Pathol* 1996;106:118–123.

Gupta A, et al. CAPD and pancreatitis: no connection. *Perit Dial Int* 1992;12:309–316.

Hamm CW, et al. The prognostic value of serum troponin T in unstable angina. *N Engl J Med* 1992;327:146–150.

Horl WH, et al. Plasma levels of pancreatic secretory trypsin inhibitor in relation to amylase and lipase in patients with acute and chronic renal failure. *Nephron* 1988;49:33–38.

Kimmel PL, et al. Trypsinogen and other pancreatic enzymes in patients with renal disease: a comparison of high efficiency hemodialysis and continuous ambulatory peritoneal dialysis. *Pancreas* 1995;10:325–330.

Lal SM, et al. Total creatine kinase and isoenzyme fractions in chronic dialysis patients. *Int J Artif Organs* 1987;10:72–76.

Li D, et al. Greater frequency of increased cardiac troponin T than increased cardiac troponin I in patients with chronic renal failure [letter]. *Clin Chem* 1996;42:114–115.

Löwbeer C, et al. Increased cardiac troponin T and endothelin-1 concentrations in dialysis patients may indicate heart disease. *Nephrol Dial Transplant* 1999;14:1948–1955.

Martin GS, et al. Cardiac troponin-I accurately predicts myocardial injury in renal failure. *Nephrol Dial Transplant* 1998;13:1709–1712.

Mondelli MU, et al. Abnormal alanine aminotransferase activity reflects exposure to hepatitis C virus in haemodialysis patients. *Nephrol Dial Transplant* 1991;6:480–483.

Nakai K, et al. Increased serum levels of human cardiac myosin light chain 1 in patients with renal failure. *Rinsho Byori* 1992;40:529–534.

Roppolo LP, et al. A comparison of tropinin T and troponin I as predictors of cardiac events in patients undergoing chronic dialysis at a veteran's hospital: a pilot study. *J Am Coll Cardiol* 1999;34: 448–454.

Rutsky EA, et al. Acute pancresatitis in patients with end-stage renal disease without transplantation. *Arch Intern Med* 1986;146: 1741–1745.

Schonicke et al. Interference of icodextrin with serum amylase measurement. *J Am Soc Nephrol* 1999;10:229a(abstr).

Seno T, et al. Serum levels of six pancreatic enzymes as related to the degree of renal dysfunction. *Am J Gastroenterol* 1995;90:2002–2005.

Singhal PC, et al. Determinants of serum creatine kinase activity in dialysis patients. *Am J Nephrol* 1988;8:220–224.

Stanbaugh GH, Gillit DM, Holmes AW. Dialysis hemosiderosis mimicking non-A, non-B hepatitis. *Trans Am Soc Artif Intern Organs* 1984;30:217–221.

Tibi L, et al. Multiple forms of alkaline phosphatase in plasma of hemodialysis patients. *Clin Chem* 1991;37:815–820.

Vaziri ND, et al. Pancreatic enzymes in patients with end-stage renal diseases maintained on hemodialysis. *Am J Gastroenterol* 1988;83: 410–412.

Vaziri ND, et al. Serum LDH and LDH isoenzymes in chronic renal failure. Effect of hemodialysis. *Int J Artif Organs* 1990;13:223–227.

Diabetes

Antonios H. Tzamaloukas and Eli A. Friedman

More than 35% of all new patients starting dialysis are diabetic. Provision of maintenance dialysis for this group can be a challenging task. Morbidity and mortality are substantially higher in diabetic patients maintained on dialysis than in their nondiabetic counterparts, with cardiovascular disease and infection being the leading causes of death.

I.   When to initiate dialysis. Current guidelines emphasize initiation of dialysis prior to the appearance of frank uremic manifestations (at creatinine clearance equal to 9–14 mL per minute for a 70-kg patient) to prevent insidious malnutrition. In diabetic patients, dialysis should be initiated at a higher creatinine clearance, usually more than 15 mL per minute. There are several reasons for early dialysis of diabetic patients. Renal function deteriorates rapidly in this group. Hypertension, which is associated with rapid acceleration of diabetic retinopathy, is often difficult to control when the creatinine clearance falls below 15 mL per minute. Anecdotally, uremic symptoms may manifest at a less advanced degree of renal insufficiency in diabetic patients than in nondiabetic patients.

II.   Hemodialysis versus peritoneal dialysis. The problems with each form of dialysis are listed in Table 25-1. Long-term peritoneal dialysis in diabetic patients may complicate control of blood sugar because deranged glucose homeostasis is stressed further by the large amount of glucose administered via the dialysis solution. In addition, glucose absorption from the abdominal cavity decreases appetite. Many peritoneal dialysis patients have great difficulty ingesting the recommend amount of protein (1.2 g per kg daily). On the other hand, the incidence and severity of hypoglycemic episodes is reduced in continuous ambulatory peritoneal dialysis (CAPD) compared to that in hemodialysis patients due to the constant presence of glucose in the abdomen. Rates of infection (peritonitis, exit site and tunnel infections) and rates of catheter replacement are similar between diabetics and nondiabetics on peritoneal dialysis. With hemodialysis, coexisting blood vessel disease often hinders creation of an adequate, long-lasting vascular access. In diabetics, the survival rates of both arteriovenous (AV) fistulas and grafts are substantially reduced. Because of autonomic nervous system dysfunction or cardiac diastolic dysfunction, diabetics may be at increased risk for hypotension during dialysis. The poor vascular access and risk of hypotension combine to cause diabetics to receive a lesser amount of dialysis [in terms of fractional urea clearance (Kt/V)] than their nondiabetic counterparts. On the other hand, at least one group (Collins et al, 1991) has found excellent survival in diabetics who were given a generous amount $(Kt/V = 1.4)$ of hemodialysis.

No difference in the rate of progression of retinopathy between patients treated with hemodialysis and those treated

Table 25-1.   Dialysis modalities for diabetics

Modality	Advantages	Disadvantages
Hemodialysis	Very efficient Frequent medical follow-up (in center) No protein loss to dialysate Less need for leg amputation (?)	Risky for patients with advanced cardiac disease Multiple arteriovenous access surgeries often required; risk of severe hand ischemia High incidence of hypotension during dialysis session Predialysis hyperkalemia Prone to hypoglycemia
CAPD	Good cardiovascular tolerance No need for arteriovenous access Good control of serum potassium Good glucose control, particularly with use of intra-peritoneal insulin; less severe hypoglycemia	Peritonitis, exit site, and tunnel infection risks similar to those in nondiabetic dialysis patients Protein loss to dialysate Increased intra-abdominal pressure effects (hernias, fluid leaks, etc.) Schedule not convenient for helper if one is required (e.g., some blind patients)
CCPD	Good cardiovascular tolerance No need for arteriovenous access Good control of serum potassium Good glucose control with use of intraperitoneal insulin Good for blind diabetics	Protein loss to dialysate Peritonitis risk slightly less than for CAPD

CAPD, continuous ambulatory peritoneal dialysis; CCPD, continuous cycling peritoneal dialysis.

with peritoneal dialysis has been demonstrated. Although visual impairment impedes training for CAPD and makes it difficult for the patient to perform the exchange procedure properly, blind diabetics can be trained to perform CAPD without a helper. When properly instructed, their risk of developing peritonitis is only slightly greater than the risk in sighted diabetics. A number of devices are available to help visually impaired patients connect the dialysis solution container to the peritoneal transfer set (see Chapter 14). Continuous cycling peritoneal dialysis (CCPD) is a good therapeutic choice for blind diabetic patients because it requires the performance of only one "on" and one "off" procedure daily.

Reports from the U.S. Renal Data System (USRDS) suggested that mortality is higher in diabetic subjects, and especially diabetic women, on peritoneal dialysis than in those on hemodialysis. Results from the Canadian Organ Replacement Registry did not support this finding. Patient selection biases may have affected these observations. Whether peritoneal dialysis is associated with higher mortality than hemodialysis in diabetics has not been clarified.

For either modality of dialysis, improvement in nutrition and small solute clearances and, particularly, meticulous management and prevention of cardiovascular and infectious morbidity may lead to substantial improvement in patient survival.

III. Diet. Whatever the mode of dialysis therapy, diabetic patients generally show evidence of wasting and malnutrition. Many factors contribute, including inadequate food intake, diabetic gastroparesis and enteropathy, and the catabolic stress associated with frequent intercurrent illness. In the event of serious illness, diabetic dialysis patients often require early and intensive nutritional support.

A. Routine dietary prescription. The diets advocated for nondiabetic hemodialysis and CAPD patients in Chapter 23 also apply to diabetics. In an anuric diabetic patient being treated with hemodialysis, the stringent sodium, potassium, and fluid restrictions listed in Table 23-2 should be applied. Special effort should be made to limit intake of simple sugars and saturated fats. Hypolipidemic drugs should be used if lipid control is not adequate based on diet and insulin schedule alone. In malnourished patients, nutrition can improve with the use of intradialytic parenteral nutrition in hemodialysis or one exchange per day with amino acid–containing dialysate in peritoneal dialysis.

B. Diabetic gastroparesis and enteropathy. Diabetic gastroparesis can be associated with poor food intake and unpredictable nutrient absorption; the result can be hypoglycemia alternating with hyperglycemia. In such patients, small, frequent (up to six times per day) feedings may improve symptoms. The pharmacologic treatment of gastroparesis in diabetics on dialysis is unsatisfactory. Cisapride should not be used in this population. It is associated with potentially fatal dysrhythmias, such as torsade de pointes, especially in subjects with prolonged QT interval or those taking medications inhibiting the cytochrome P450-3A4 enzymes, such as macrolide antibiotics, fluconazole and related antifungals, and idinavir and related antiretroviral agents.

Metoclopramide in a small starting dose (5 mg twice a day), with small increments until results are seen, is still used. This drug is associated with a high incidence of extrapyramidal complications in dialysis patients, particularly at higher doses. Its effects are often temporary. Other "prokinetic" gastrointestinal motility drugs, such as domperidone or the newer motilin antagonists, may be proven useful in the future. Diabetic enteropathy with resulting diarrhea can also complicate alimentation, causing debilitation, poor food intake, and hypoglycemia. Severe cases of diabetic enteropathy can be treated with a trial of a broad-spectrum antimicrobial (e.g., doxycycline in a dose of 50 or 100 mg daily) to combat bacterial overgrowth in the intestine. Loperamide hydrochloride (up to 10 mg daily) to decrease bowel motility is also useful.

IV.   Control of blood sugar

A.   Alteration in insulin metabolism. In uremic patients (both diabetic and nondiabetic), insulin secretion by the β cells of the pancreas is reduced and the responsiveness of peripheral tissues (e.g., muscle) to insulin is depressed. On the other hand, the rate of insulin catabolism (renal and extrarenal) is decreased, and therefore, the half-life of any insulin present in the circulation is prolonged. All of these abnormalities are only partially corrected after institution of maintenance dialysis therapy.

1.   Abnormal glucose tolerance tests in all dialysis patients. The glucose tolerance test cannot be used to diagnose diabetes in dialysis patients because the rise in serum glucose concentration will be greater and more prolonged than normal in all dialysis patients as a result of uremia-induced insulin resistance. However, fasting serum glucose concentrations are normal in nondiabetic hemodialysis patients; a high level suggests the presence of diabetes. In CAPD patients, a true fasting state is never achieved due to constant absorption of glucose from the dialysis solution. In this group, unless peritonitis is present, the "fasting" serum glucose value rarely exceeds 160 mg per dL, even when using 4.25% dextrose dialysis solution; higher levels suggest that the patient has diabetes. In CAPD patients using icodextrin, serum glucose values may be spuriously overestimated by auto-analyzers that use glucose dehydrogenase method of sample analysis (Wens et al, 1997).

2.   Increased sensitivity to insulin. In diabetic dialysis patients being treated with exogenous insulin, the importance of reduced insulin catabolism overrides the impact of insulin resistance; when exogenous insulin is administered, its effect may be intensified and prolonged. Thus, smaller than usual doses should be given. Bolus administration of moderately large intravenous doses (e.g., 15 units of regular insulin), even when ketosis is present, can result in severe hypoglycemia. Hypoglycemia can also occur after administration of the longer acting insulins, such as insulin zinc suspension (Lente) and isophane insulin (NPH).

3.   Hyperglycemia. The clinical presentation of hyperglycemia is modified when renal function is absent. The absence of the "safety valve" effect of glucosuria may result in the development of severe hyperglycemia (serum glucose level > 1,000 mg per dL). Severe hyperosmolality with accompanying alteration of mental status is unusual because of the absence of water loss induced by osmotic diuresis. Indeed, even extreme hyperglycemia is often asymptomatic in dialysis patients. However, manifestations can include thirst, weight gain, and, on occasion, pulmonary edema (see Kaldany et al, 1982). Also, diabetic ketoacidosis, frequently accompanied by severe hyperkalemia and coma, can develop in insulin-dependent dialysis patients. Management of hyperglycemia with or without ketoacidosis differs from that in patients without renal failure in that administration of large amounts of fluid is unnecessary and generally contraindicated. All of the clinical and laboratory abnormalities of hyperglycemia are corrected by insulin administration, which is often the only treatment needed. To manage severe hyperglycemia, one can administer a continuous infusion of low-dose insulin (starting at 2 units per hour) with close clinical monitoring and measurement of serum glucose and potassium concentrations at 2- to 3-hour intervals. If severe hyperkalemia is present, electrocardiography should also be done.

   4.   Hypoglycemia. Hypoglycemia can develop in diabetic patients treated with either hemodialysis or peritoneal dialysis; it is usually due to reduced insulin catabolism and to reduced intake and absorption of food. The risk of hypoglycemia is increased in malnourished diabetic patients with diminished glycogen stores and in diabetics receiving β-blocking drugs (which impair glycogenolysis). In diabetic patients, hemodialysis solution should always contain about 200 mg per dL glucose; if glucose is not added, then severe hypoglycemia during or soon after the hemodialysis session can result.

B.   Insulin therapy. Tight control of the serum glucose concentration is difficult to achieve in dialysis patients, primarily because of variations in dietary intake and food absorption and the confounding effect of dialysis therapy. Nevertheless, good glucose control is worthwhile. Prolonged hyperglycemia leads to the development and progression of all diabetic complications, which become irreversible only in their later stages. Irreversibly and slowly formed compounds that are the result of nonenzymatic glycosylation of proteins, the so-called advanced glycosylation end products (AGEs), alter the structure and function of vascular basement membranes, stimulate the production of growth factors, and alter the function of intracellular proteins (Brownlee, 1997). In peritoneal dialysis patients, AGE deposition in the peritoneal membrane is associated with an increase in peritoneal permeability and excessive protein losses in the dialysate. Many of the changes associated with AGE (e.g., vascular changes) may have reached an irreversible stage by the time patients start dialysis. However, it is conceivable that good glycemic control will prevent some of these changes because the morbidity and mortality of diabetics with good glycemic control are lower than those of subjects with poor control. A fasting serum glucose level of less than 140 mg per dL, a postprandial value of less than 200 mg per dL, and a glycosylated hemoglobin level in the range of 100%–120% of the normal range are reasonable therapeutic goals.

Hypoglycemia must be avoided. Regular verification of glycemic control is important. Usually, patients are taught to prick their fingers and impregnate a piece of test paper with their blood. An automated device can then estimate the serum glucose concentration. The serum glucose level is checked in this manner at least once daily, usually two or three times a day.

Glycosylated hemoglobin values can be used to follow the degree of glycemia; however, in uremia there is increased formation of carbamylated hemoglobin, which cannot be distinguished from glycosylated hemoglobin by assays utilizing ion exchange chromatography. Affinity chromatography, which is commercially available, and colorimetric or enzyme-linked immunoassay are more suitable for tracking glycosylated hemoglobin levels in diabetic dialysis patients.

1. Regimens for hemodialysis patients. The amount of insulin per day required for patients receiving maintenance hemodialysis is usually small; optimum control of glycemia is achieved by administration of long-acting insulin at two separate times during the day (split dosing) and by supplementing with regular insulin for meals as needed. The proportions of long-acting and regular insulin, as well as the total insulin doses vary widely among different patients.

2. Regimens for peritoneal dialysis patients. Despite the fact that variable amounts of insulin are adsorbed to the dialysis solution container and infusion lines, excellent control of the serum glucose level can be obtained with addition of regular insulin to peritoneal dialysis solutions. Relatively long (3.8-cm, or 1.5-in.) needles should be used to ensure that the full dose of insulin is injected into the dialysis solution container rather than being trapped in the infusion port. After injection, the dialysis solution container should be inverted several times to ensure proper mixing.

a. CAPD patients

(1) Intraperitoneal regimen. The total dose of intraperitoneal insulin added daily to all dialysis solution containers will often be two to three times the previous daily subcutaneous dose. A number of regimens have been proposed, one of which, the Toronto Western Hospital Protocol, is reproduced in Table 25-2. Other approaches have been described by Beardsworth et al (1988), Flynn (1981), and Legrain and Rottembourg (1981).

(2) Subcutaneous regimen. Some reports suggest that use of intraperitoneal insulin is associated with an increased incidence of peritonitis or with reduced efficacy (Selgas et al, 1988). This point of view is controversial, and we believe that intraperitoneal insulin should be tried first under ordinary circumstances. If intraperitoneal insulin fails, subcutaneous injection, in a schedule similar to that described for hemodialysis, can provide a satisfactory alternative.

b. CCPD or nocturnal intermittent peritoneal dialysis (NIPD) regimen

(1) Intraperitoneal regimen. The intraperitoneal insulin dose is added as regular insulin to any one of the nocturnal dialysis solution containers attached to the

**Table 25-2.   Toronto Western Hospital Protocol for
Intraperitoneal Insulin Administration in CAPD patients**

Goals of therapy: Fasting blood glucose < 140 mg/dL
1-h postprandial: < 200 mg/dL
  1. Hospitalize patient.
  2. The protocol is based on use of four 2-L exchanges/d (adapt if necessary).
  3. First three exchanges are performed 20 min before each of the major meals, the fourth exchange at approximately 11 pm. A snack, consisting of a sandwich and small glucose-containing soft drink, is given at that time.
  4. Target total caloric intake (diet + dialysate) is 35 kcal/kg/d. Target oral caloric intake is 25–30 kcal/kg/d, depending on the expected amount of glucose absorption from dialysis solution.
  5. Measure blood glucose four times a day: fasting in the morning, 1 h after breakfast, 1 h after lunch, 1 h after supper.

Day 1: To each 2-L dialysis solution container, add the following amounts of regular insulin:
  a. One-fourth of the total number of insulin units (all types of insulin) ordinarily given SC daily prior to starting peritoneal dialysis. (However, all units added to the bag are regular insulin.) This amount of insulin is designed to help metabolize the dietary carbohydrate intake.
  b. To each bag, in addition to the insulin dose in a, add an insulin supplement to help metabolize the glucose present in the dialysis solution. This supplemental regular insulin dose is as follows:
  To each 2-L 1.5% dextrose bag: 2 units
  To each 2-L 2.5% dextrose bag: 4 units
  To each 2-L 4.25% dextrose bag: 6 units

EXAMPLE
Patient previously receiving 20 units of NPH insulin plus 10 units of regular insulin in the morning and 10 units of NPH insulin in the evening:
  Total daily SC insulin dose is 40 units
If CAPD schedule is to use three 2-L 1.5% exchanges during the day and one 2-L 4.25% exchange at night, then:
  To each 2-L 1.5% container add 10 + 2 = 12 units regular insulin
  To the 2-L 4.25% container add 10 + 6 = 16 units regular insulin

Day 2: Adjust amount of insulin added to the dialysis solution containers according to serum glucose levels obtained the previous day. The fasting blood sugar will reflect the insulin dose added to the solution infused at 11 pm. The postprandial serum glucose concentrations will reflect the insulin added to the solutions administered 20 min prior to the respective meals. The adjustment is made according to the table below, using columns 1 versus 3 to adjust the nocturnal exchange and columns 2 versus 3 to adjust each of the daytime exchanges.

continued

Table 25-2.   *Continued*

EXAMPLE
On day 1, the serum glucose values were:

1 h after breakfast	220 mg/dL
1 h after lunch	350 mg/dL
1 h after supper	300 mg/dL
Fasting (day 2)	160 mg/dL

One could now add an extra 2 units to the first daytime exchange, an extra 4 units to each of the second and third daytime exchanges, and leave the insulin dose for the nocturnal exchange the same.

Fasting serum glucose level (mg/dL)	1-h postprandial serum glucose level (mg/dL)	Amount of insulin change (units/2-L bag)
< 40	< 40	−6
< 40	40–80	−4
40–80	80–120	−2
80–180	120–180	No change
180–240	180–240	+2[a]
240–400	240–300	+4[a]
> 400	> 300	Variable

[a] In type 1 diabetics, substantially less additional insulin may be required.
CAPD, continuous ambulatory peritoneal dialysis; SC, subcutaneous.
Modified from Amair P, et al. Continuous ambulatory peritoneal dialysis in diabetics with end-stage renal disease. *N Engl J Med* 1982;306:625.

cycler. Initially, the amount added will usually be equal to the total amount of insulin (regular plus long-acting) previously given subcutaneously. In cyclers that infuse the "final" long-dwell daytime exchange from a separate container, regular insulin should be added to the latter as well. The amount of insulin added to the nocturnal dialysis solution container subsequently can be adjusted as guided by the fasting morning serum glucose level. A supplemental subcutaneous insulin dose may be required during the day to help metabolize carbohydrate absorbed with meals.

   (2)   Subcutaneous regimen. An alternative strategy is to give subcutaneous insulin in the evening to help metabolize the nocturnal glucose load.

C.   Oral hypoglycemic agents. A common problem for all oral hypoglycemic agents is that there are no appropriate studies of their use in dialysis patients.

Nevertheless, these agents are useful adjuncts in the treatment of diabetics and are used by many nephrologists. The safety of sulfonylureas depends on their mode of metabolism and their half-life. Use of short-acting agents primarily metabolized by the liver is, in general, safer in dialysis patients. Acetohexamide, chlorpropamide, and tolazamide are excreted to a large extent in the urine. These drugs should not be used in dialysis patients because their half-lives will be greatly prolonged in the absence of renal function, possibly resulting in severe and prolonged hypoglycemia. The excretion of glyburide is 50% hepatic, and prolonged hypoglycemia has been reported using this drug in dialysis patients (Krepinsky et al, 1999). Metabolism of glipizide, tolbutamide, and glidazide is almost completely hepatic. Consequently, the last three drugs should be considered if an oral hypoglycemic agent is desired. Many drugs frequently used in dialysis patients either antagonize (phenytoin, nicotinic acid, diuretics) or enhance (sulfonamides, salicylates, warfarin, ethanol) the hypoglycemic action of sulfonylureas.

Metformin, a biguanide, is associated with increased incidence of lactic acidosis in dialysis patients and should not used. Acarbose inhibits α-glycosidase in the enteric mucosa and moderates post-prandial hyperglycemia. Its side effects are primarily gastrointestinal. It may prove to be a useful adjunct to other diabetic medications in dialysis patients. High-fiber diets have similar effects on postprandial hyperglycemia but may cause decreased absorption of vitamins and other nutrients.

Troglitazone and other thiazolidinediones sensitize the target tissues to insulin and may be of help in obese, type 2 diabetics with insulin resistance. However, the use of this class of drugs is associated with the risk of severe hepatotoxicity. Studies of the efficacy and safety of the oral hypoglycemic agents, inhibitors of AGE formation (aminoguanidines), and the new genetically engineered insulin analogs (e.g., Lyspro insulin) in diabetics on dialysis will clarify the uses and limitations of these agents in this population.

V. Hyperkalemia. Hyperkalemia occurs commonly in diabetic patients, especially those who are anuric and are being treated by maintenance hemodialysis. The etiologic factors include insulin deficiency and resistance, aldosterone deficiency, and intracellular-to-extracellular fluid shifts attendant to hyperglycemia.

VI. Hypertension and peripheral vascular disease

A. Control of hypertension. The incidence of hypertension is high in diabetic dialysis patients. Control of high blood pressure is very important for the prevention of cardiovascular sequelae and deterioration of vision. Most diabetics have volume-sensitive hypertension that can be controlled by appropriate sodium and fluid restriction and by removal of excess extracellular fluid by dialysis. If medications are needed, then several drugs can be used. Angiotensin-converting enzyme inhibitors or angiotensin receptor antagonists have the advantage of conferring cardioprotective effects but may lead to dangerous hyperkalemia. A vasodilator or calcium channel blocker can be used as an alternative first-choice agent. Many nephrologists prefer clonidine or labetalol. β-Blockers are usually avoided in diabetics because they interfere with the recognition of hypoglycemia by the patient (they block the epinephrine effect) and can aggravate hyperkalemia by inhibiting adrenergically mediated muscle uptake of potassium. If antihypertensive drugs are used, the smallest dose that can lead to the desired effect should be sought. It should also be kept in mind that dialysis hypotension may be aggravated by the use of antihypertensives; consequently, removal of excess fluid may become problematic.

B. Peripheral vascular disease. Diabetic patients on dialysis have a very high rate of amputation (Eggers, 1999). Frequent examination of the feet by a podiatrist is important in diabetic dialysis patients; with regular care focused on prevention of ulcer development, the risk of amputation can be minimized.

VII. Cerebrovascular disease. The incidence of stroke is higher in diabetic dialysis patients than in their nondiabetic counterparts. Although the use of aspirin has been shown to reduce the risk of stroke in nonuremic patients, the benefit of such therapy in diabetic dialysis patients is unknown, and the use of aspirin theoretically increases the risk of intraocular hemorrhage. The danger of intraocular bleeding also deters use of the coumarin anticoagulants in this population.

VIII. Eye problems in diabetics on dialysis. Diabetic patients on dialysis are subject to eye complications common to all patients on dialysis. Conjunctivitis and keratitis are treated with ophthalmic preparations of antibiotic, antifungal, or antiviral agents in the usual doses. The dose of antibiotics given systematically should be adjusted for dialysis. Certain pathogens grow well in glucose-containing media and create a risk of severe eye infection in diabetics on dialysis.

Another condition seen in diabetic as well as nondiabetic dialysis patients is band keratopathy (corneal–conjunctival calcification), seen more frequently in patients with elevated calcium–phosphorus product (greater than 70, when both calcium and phosphorus concentrations are expressed in milligrams per deciliter). Irritation of the conjunctiva ("red-eye syndrome") by calcium phosphate deposits may complicate band keratopathy. Renal transplantation is the best way to treat band keratopathy. Superficial keratectomy or chelation of the calcium deposits with local application of ethylenediamine tetraacetic acid (EDTA) can be used to treat refractory cases.

Glaucoma is treated in dialysis patients in the same ways as in the general population. However, timolol may be contraindicated in patients with severe obstructive pulmonary disease or severe congestive heart failure. Among carbonic anhydrase inhibitors, acetazolamide should not be used because its primary pathway of elimination is through renal excretion, whereas methazolamide, in the lowest recommended dose (25 mg bid), may be safer. One interesting observation is that intraocular pressure increases slightly during the course of a hemodialysis session and may decrease after prolonged ultrafiltration. Cataracts are treated in the same way in diabetic and nondiabetic patients on dialysis.

Diabetic patients on dialysis often have advanced retinal changes due to hypertension and diabetic retinopathy. Vascular events secondary to hypertensive retinopathy (branch retinal vein occlusion from obstruction at the site of an AV crossing) can cause sudden decreases in vision. Control of hypertension may prevent this complication, as well as the more rare central retinal vein and artery occlusion.

A. Diabetic retinopathy. Retinopathy is present in essentially every diabetic patient starting dialysis. One-third of these patients are legally blind. Retinopathy is the most common cause of blindness in diabetics on dialysis; less common causes of blindness include macular edema, glaucoma, cataracts, and corneal disease. The early stage of background retinopathy, with leakage and occlusion of small retinal blood vessels, can cause visual loss if the macular area is involved. Slowing the progression of this stage requires careful control of blood pressure and blood glucose, and, in pre-end-stage renal disease (ESRD) patients without protein malnutrition, restriction of daily dietary protein intake to about 0.6 g per kg.

Retinopathy progresses to a proliferative stage believed to be secondary to local hypoxia and characterized by intense proliferation of new blood vessels in the retina. These vessels, which are located in the surface layer of the retina, cause loss of vision through vitreous bleeding, macular distortion, or detachment. Discovery of proliferative retinopathy is an indication for laser treatment, which decreases the risk of detachment and the need for oxygen (by destroying nonessential parts of the retina). Vitreous hemorrhages from proliferative retinopathy obstruct the path of light and may lead to retinal detachment and blindness. Vitrectomy and other microsurgical techniques (removal of retinal membranes, reattachment of retina) can improve vision in one-third to one-half of patients.

Progression of retinopathy is associated with long duration of diabetes, poor blood pressure control, and female gender, but not with the use of heparin in hemodialysis. Good blood pressure control during the dialysis period is imperative. Systematic ophthalmologic examinations at frequent intervals combined with aggressive but judicious use of surgical techniques may restore vision in selected patients.

Despite the use of heparin in hemodialysis, there is no evidence that the progression of retinopathy in diabetics on hemodialysis differs from that in diabetics on peritoneal dialysis.

X. Impotence. Impotence is common in diabetic dialysis patients. Autonomic neuropathy and peripheral vascular disease associated with diabetes are operative, as are the usual uremic causes. Management of impotence is discussed in Chapter 35.

XI. Referral for transplantation. In diabetic patients in whom no contraindication to transplantation exists, renal transplantation is the preferred method of managing ESRD. In such patients, dialysis should be considered as a temporary measure only. Diabetic patients with severe preexisting cardiac disease may not benefit from transplantation because in this group transplantation is associated with a high mortality rate (Philipson et al, 1986).

XII. Bone disease. Among diabetics with ESRD, adynamic bone disease is common (see Chapter 30). This bone disease is characterized by a low bone formation rate, which is presumably due to the high circulating levels of somatostatin inhibitors in affected patients. This low bone formation rate is believed to predispose diabetic patients to aluminum toxicity; diabetic patients on dialysis have been shown to accumulate bone aluminum at a faster rate than their nondiabetic counterparts (Andress et al, 1987). For this reason, every effort should be made to minimize the amount of aluminum-containing phosphate binders given.

XIII. Anemia. The response to erythropoietin is satisfactory for anemic diabetics treated with either hemodialysis or peritoneal dialysis. Dosage guidelines are the same as for nondiabetics (see Chapter 27).

XIV.   Conclusion. The care of diabetic patients is a demanding task. It requires intense attention to multiple details. In addition to members of the dialysis team, representatives of other specialties (e.g., vascular surgery, podiatry, ophthalmology, neurology) are needed. The existence of a diabetic team, with all of the subspecialties available, working under the coordination of a nephrologist acting as a primary care physician and a nurse-specialist in diabetes, who should provide continuous patient teaching, is highly desirable to provide the best care for this demanding and increasing dialysis population.

SELECTED READINGS

Al-Kudsi RR, et al. Extreme hyperglycemia in dialysis patients. *Clin Nephrol* 1982;17:228–231.

Amair P, et al. Continuous ambulatory peritoneal dialysis in diabetics with end-stage renal disease. *N Engl J Med* 1982;306:625–630.

Andress DL, et al. Early deposition of aluminum in bone in diabetic patients on hemodialysis. *N Engl J Med* 1987;316:292–296.

Beardsworth SF, et al. Intraperitoneal insulin: a protocol for administration during CAPD and review of published protocols. *Perit Dial Int* 1988;8:145.

Brownlee M. Advanced products of nonenzymatic glycosylation and the pathogenesis of diabetic complications. In: Porte D, Sherwin RS, eds. *Ellenberg and Rifkin's Diabetes Mellitus*, 5th ed. Stamford, CT: Appleton & Lange, 1997:229.

Brunner FP. End-stage renal failure due to diabetic nephropathy: Data from the EDTA registry. *HNO* 1989;3:127–135.

Collins AL, et al. Diabetic hemodialysis patients treated with a high Kt/V have a lower risk of death than with standard Kt/V. *J Am Soc Nephrol* 1991;2:318a (abst).

Daugirdas JT, et al. Hyperosmolar coma: cellular dehydration and the serum sodium concentration. *Ann Intern Med* 1989;110:855–857.

Eggers PW, et al. Nontraumatic lower extremity amputation in the Medicare end-stage renal disease population. *Kidney Int* 1999;56:1524–1533.

Fehmi H, et al. The insulin sparing effect of troglitazone in hemodialysis patients with type 2 diabetes. *J Am Soc Nephrol* 1998;9:114a (abstr).

Flynn CT. The Iowa Lutheran protocol. *Perit Dial Bull* 1981;1:100.

Ifudu O, et al. Interdialytic weight gain correlates with glycosylated hemoglobin in diabetic hemodialysis patients. *Am J Kidney Dis* 1994;23:686–691.

Kaldany A, et al. Reversible acute pulmonary edema due to uncontrolled hyperglycemia in diabetic individuals with renal failure. *Diabetes Care* 1982;5:506–511.

Khanna R, Leibel B. The Toronto Western Hospital protocol. *Perit Dial Bull* 1981;1:101.

Krepinsky JC, et al. Prolonged sulfonyl-urea induced hypoglycemia in diabetic patients in end-stage renal disease. *J Am Soc Nephrol* 1999:10:130a (abstr).

Legrain M, Rottembourg J. The "Pitie-Salpetriere" protocol. *Perit Dial Bull* 1981;1:101.

Lindblad AS, et al. A survey of the NIH CAPD registry population with end-stage renal disease attributed to diabetic nephropathy. *J Diab Compl* 1988;2:227.

Markel MS, Friedman EA. Care of the diabetic patient with end-stage renal disease. *Semin Nephrol* 1990;10:274.

Philipson JD, et al. Evaluation of cardiovascular risk for transplantation in diabetic patients. *Am J Med* 1986;81:630–634.

Popli S, et al. Acidosis and coma in diabetic maintenance dialysis patients with extreme hyperglycernia (abstract). *J Am Soc Nephrol* 1998;9:266a (abst).

Popli S, et al. Asymptomatic, nonketotic, severe hyperglycernia with hyponatremia. *Arch Intern Med* 1990;150:1962–1964.

Schomig M, et al. The diabetic foot in the dialyzed patient. *J Am Soc Nephrol* 2000;11:1153–1159.

Selgas R, et al. Comparative study of two different routes for insulin administration in CAPD diabetic patients: a multicenter study. *Adv Perit Dial* 1988;4:126.

Tzamaloukas AH. Avoiding the use of hypertonic dextrose dialysate in peritoneal dialysis. *Semin Dial* 2000;13:156–159.

Tzamaloukas AH, et al. Hypoglycernia in diabetics on dialysis with poor glycemic control: hemodialysis versus continuous ambulatory peritoneal dialysis. *Int J Artif Organs* 1992;15:390–392.

Tzamaloukas AH, et al. The relationship between glycemic control and morbidity and mortality in diabetics on dialysis. *ASAIO J* 1993;39:880–885.

Tzamaloukas AH. The use of glycosylated hemoglobin in dialysis patients. *Semin Dial* 1998;11:141.

Wens R, et al. Overestimation of blood glucose measurements by auto-analyser method in CAPD patients treated with icodextrin. *J Am Soc Nephrol* 1997;8:275a (abstr).

Windus DW, et al. Prosthetic fistula survival and complications in hemodialysis patients: effects of diabetes and age. *Am J Kidney Dis* 1992;19:448–452.

Yang C, et al. Low molecular weight heparin reduces triglyceride, VLDL, and cholesterol/HDL levels in hyperlipidemic diabetic patients on hemodialysis. *Am J Nephrol* 1998;18:384–390.

Internet Reference

Diabetes and ESRD links (http://www.hdcn.com/crf/diabetes)

Hypertension

Carmine Zoccali and George Dunea

Hypertension is considered to be a major cause of morbidity and mortality in dialysis patients. However, our estimate of the cardiovascular risk associated with arterial hypertension in the dialysis population is based on very few long-term studies. Most of the information comes from dialysis registries in which heart failure constitutes a major confounder. In a recent prospective study (Foley et al, 1996), low mean arterial pressure (MAP) was independently associated with mortality, and this association was a marker for a person's having cardiac failure prior to death. On the other hand, in this study, a 10 mm Hg rise in MAP was associated with an increased likelihood of developing left ventricular hypertrophy (LVH) and LV dilatation (+48%), cardiac failure (+44%), and ischemic heart disease (+39%), whereas a predialysis MAP ≤ 98 mm Hg minimized the occurrence and progression of LVH in patients without heart failure.

Hypertension is the main risk factor for LVH in dialysis patients, followed by age and anemia (Parfrey, 1996). There is now clear evidence that hypertension control has a beneficial effect on LVH (Cannella, 1993; London, 1994).

I. Definition and measurement. The "normal" arterial blood pressure in the general population is that associated with the minimum cardiovascular risk (less than 140/90 mm Hg). In dialysis patients, arterial pressure is measured by the nursing staff before, during and after dialysis. Which of these measurements should be taken as a measure of cardiovascular risk is scarcely defined. The average of several predialysis arterial pressure measurements is more strongly related to left ventricular mass than is the postdialysis arterial pressure (Conlon, 1996). For this reason, the average of several predialysis blood pressure values will give the best indication of whether antihypertensive drug therapy is required.

The value of 24-hour ambulatory monitoring as a guide to therapy in dialysis patients remains to be studied. Dialysis patients often fail to show the normal nocturnal drop in blood pressure, a phenomenon that has been attributed in part to nocturnal hypoxemia caused by sleep apnea (Zoccali et al, 1996). Available evidence indicates that the average 24-hour blood pressure does not represent a better predictor of LVH than the mean of several predialysis blood pressure measurements (Zoccali et al, 1999). The criteria for treatment are formulated in Table 26-1.

There may be seasonal variation in blood pressure in temperate climates, with systolic pressure being 10 mm Hg higher in the cold months than in the warm months. Apart from being temperature-related, the detailed mechanism of this variation is not known (Argiles et al, 1998).

II. Pathophysiology. Sodium and fluid retention are by far the main factors responsible for hypertension in dialysis patients.

Table 26-1. Indications for drug therapy of hypertension in dialysis patients

Definition

Hypertension: predialysis MAP > 106 mm Hg (i.e., about 140/90 mm Hg) when the patient is believed to be at so-called dry weight (see text).

Drug therapy mandatory

"Dry" predialysis MAP > 106 mm Hg.
"Dry" predialysis MAP = 98–106 mm Hg, and patient is anemic, scheduled to receive erythropoietin,[a] or patient has LVH.

Drug therapy recommended

"Dry" predialysis MAP 98–106 mm Hg, and patient already on erythropoietin and not anemic, with no LVH.
"Dry" predialysis MAP > 98 mm Hg and patient with LVH.

---

[a] The beneficial effect on left ventricular mass of a higher hematocrit during erythropoietin treatment may be in part counteracted by the erythropoietin-induced rise in arterial pressure.
MAP, mean arterial pressure; LVH, left ventricular hypertrophy.

A large proportion (50%–70%) of uremic patients become normotensive after hemodialysis treatment is initiated and the excess volume removed. In several studies, no relationship was found between arterial pressure and interdialytic weight gain, and on this basis, it was speculated that interdialytic weight gain, and on this basis, it was speculated that factors other than volume are responsible for hypertension in dialysis patients. However, analogous to the relationship between salt intake and arterial pressure in essential hypertension, the relationship between extracellular volume and arterial pressure in dialysis patients may be sigmoid rather than linear, so that in volume-expanded dialysis patients virtually no decrease in arterial pressure occurs until extracellular volume is reduced below the threshold value. In clinical practice, this threshold is often difficult to gauge; for example, certain patients who are thought to be "volume-resistant" eventually become normotensive with intensive ultrafiltration (Fishbane et al, 1996).

From a hemodynamic point of view, volume overload leads to an increase in blood pressure only when the vascular tone does not compensate for the volume excess (i.e., when physiologic autoregulation does not occur). The lack of a vasodilatory response to hypervolemia in dialysis patients may depend on an excess of vasoconstrictor factors or on a defect in vasodilatory factors.

III. Excess of vasoconstrictor factors. In uremic patients, the renin–angiotensin system is inappropriately activated in relation to volume status. Studies based on sympathetic microneurography have confirmed that sympathetic overactivity, possibly triggered by afferent signals originated in diseased kidneys, plays an important role in the pathogenesis of hypertension in such patients (Converse, 1992). Endothelin has been found to be markedly raised and directly related to arterial pressure in dialysis patients, but the link does not appear to be a causal one. The retention of digitalis-like sodium pump inhibitors, such as oubain and bufenolide, might be involved in the disturbed vasoregulatory response to hypervolemia in dialysis patients.

IV. Ischemic renal disease. In the elderly, ischemic renovascular disease is frequently associated with refractory hypertension and "flash" pulmonary edema during the pre–end-stage renal disease (pre-ESRD) phase. Ischemic renal disease is being increasingly recognized as a possible cause for renal failure in such patients. When ESRD supervenes, ischemic renovascular disease may continue to exacerbate hypertension, either via the renin–angiotensin axis or via enhanced renal sympathetic nerve activity. This potential cause of refractory hypertension in ESRD has not been well studied.

V. Lack of vasodilatory factors/inappropriate vasodilatory response. Whether accumulation of endogenous inhibitors of nitric oxide, such as asymmetric dimethylarginine, impairs endothelium-dependent vasodilatation in chronic renal failure remains controversial. The plasma concentrations of several vasodilatory peptides, such as atrial natriuretic factor (ANF), calcitonin gene–related peptide, and adrenomedullin, are markedly raised in dialysis patients, but it remains to be seen if these substances play a role in the disturbed regulation of vascular tone.

Although extracellular fluid volume and vascular tone control are intimately connected, the distinction between volume-dependent and volume-resistant hypertension is useful in clinical practice to the extent that it implies that chronic drug treatment should be considered only when careful attempts at correcting the body fluids excess have failed or were insufficient. The prevalence of hypertension was reduced to 5% with long dialysis in the Tassin, France, experience; this is a much lower prevalence than in the age-matched normal population. Extracellular volume, as measured by bioelectrical impedance analysis (BIA), was about 10% lower in patients treated by long dialysis in Tassin than in those treated with shorter dialysis (Luik, 1994). The hypothesis that long dialysis reduces arterial pressure by removing unknown vasoconstrictor substances still remains to be adequately tested.

VI. Treatment

A. Correction of overhydration and maintenance of dry weight. Ideally, dialysis treatment should bring patients back to a normal extracellular volume. In clinical practice, the "dry weight" is defined as the level below which further fluid removal would produce hypotension, muscle cramps, nausea, and vomiting. The weakness of this clinical definition is that the occurrence of these symptoms depends on the time at which ultrafiltration is performed, on the dialysis strategy (high sodium/ramped sodium dialysis, cold dialysis, bicarbonate dialysis), on the predialysis body fluid volume status, and on concomitant drug treatment. (Antihypertensive drugs of all sorts impair the reflex cardiovascular adjustments that physiologically occur during volume removal.) Achieving dry weight by following the above criterion allows the attainment of normotension in most cases.

When dialysis treatment becomes symptomatic and the patient remains hypertensive, an estimation of the body fluid volume status can be performed by BIA, which is an easy, safe, and reproducible technique of relatively low cost. We now have reliable reference frames for comparing results of BIA in dialysis patients and those in the general population (Piccoli, 1994). There are other methods for estimating the volume status in dialysis patients (such as inferior vena cava diameter and the measurement of ANF plasma concentration), but these methods are less reliable and costlier than BIA.

Another potentially useful method that remains to be validated is continuous recording of hematocrit during dialysis (Critline Monitor, In-Line Diagnostics, Riverdale, Utah) a "flat-line profile" indicating volume overload.

Once hypertensive dialysis patients attain a normal total-body water (TBW) value, antihypertensive drugs should be added. It is worth remembering that, virtually without exception, when hypertension recurs in a patient after having been well controlled by volume subtraction, volume excess is therefore again the cause of hypertension. Attempts to attain or reset the dry weight should be carefully conducted, keeping in mind that overzealous ultrafiltration may precipitate severe hypotension, with disastrous cardiovascular consequences (such as myocardial or cerebral infarction and mesenteric ischemia).

In symptomatic patients, the use of programmed "variable-sodium" dialysis, cold dialysis, or continuous blood volume monitoring during dialysis may be of value.

In about 14% of patients, there is a paradoxical postdialysis rise in arterial pressure (Cheigh, 1993). This is often interpreted as implying a state of relative dehydration. However, in these cases, no evidence of activation of the renin–angiotensin and sympathetic systems (the systems which physiologically counter-regulate volume deficiency) has been found. If TBW is increased, attempts to treat hypertension by fluid removal should be conducted with particular care in these cases.

Dry weight and nutritional status should be reevaluated at least four times per year because water retention can obscure important changes in body composition brought about by malnutrition. Hypertensive patients should be instructed not to gain more than 2.5%–3.0% of their body weight between dialysis sessions and to limit sodium intake to less than 100 mEq per day.

Although use of higher dialysis solution sodium levels is recently in vogue, lowering dialysate sodium levels for both hemodialysis and peritoneal dialysis (Enia et al, 1998) has been shown to reduce hypertension. Patients appear to maintain an individual sodium set point (Keen et al, 1997) and will ingest fluid after salt ingestion until this set point has been reached. Use of high dialysate sodium levels for patients with a naturally low serum sodium set point may induce thirst unnecessarily. On the other hand, use of a low-sodium dialysate in patients with a high set point may result in cramps and intradialytic hypotension.

It should be remembered that fluid ingestion normally is driven primarily by sodium ingestion via an intact thirst mechanism, and efforts to limit fluid ingestion in patients with high salt intakes will be fruitless. There may be a time delay (e.g., several weeks) between lowering extracellular fluid volume and a fall in blood pressure (Charra, 1998). For this reason, a blood pressure that does not fall initially after the dry weight has been lowered does not exclude hypervolemia as a cause of the hypertension.

In some patients, a thrice-weekly dialysis schedule using 3- to 4-hour session lengths will be insufficient to maintain euvolemia. In such patients, the choices are to increase the dialysis session length or to switch to a four times per week (or even a six times per week) dialysis schedule. Preliminary evidence suggests that more frequent dialysis not only reduces the blood pressure but also causes a reduction of LVH.

B.   Drug treatment. The indications for pharmacologic treatment are summarized in Table 26-1. In addition to the actual blood pressure reading, factors such as planned correction of anemia with erythropoietin therapy and presence of LVH must be considered. Also, patients with a tendency to congestive heart failure may benefit from afterload reduction when diastolic blood pressure is between 90 and 100 mm Hg.

1.   Calcium channel blockers. These drugs are the most frequently used for the treatment of volume-resistant hypertension in dialysis patients, dihydropyridines being the most popular. An early meta-analysis raised the concern that the short-acting formulation of the dihydropyridine drug nifedipine used at high doses might increase mortality in the hypertensive population (Furberg, 1995). This finding may be explained by "indication bias" (the decision to prescribe a calcium channel blocker for the treatment of hypertension may be determined by factors associated with coronary heart disease), and an ad hoc committee of the International Society of Hypertension concluded that "available evidence does not prove the existence of either beneficial or harmful effects of calcium antagonists on the risks of major coronary heart disease events." These drugs are efficacious for the treatment of hypertension in the dialysis patient, and recent evidence suggests that calcium antagonists do reduce cardiovascular events and mortality in nondialysis patients (INSIGHT and NORDIL Study Group Reports, 10th Eur Soc Hypertens Meeting, June, 2000). When using a calcium antagonist in a dialysis patient with volume-resistant hypertension, long-acting preparations should be used. The use of calcium antagonists for the treatment of hypertensive crisis is discussed separately (see below).

Verapamil can cause cardiac conduction problems, bradycardia, and constipation. Calcium channel blockers should be used with great caution in combination with β-adrenergic blockers because of the risk of congestive heart failure. Other side effects are ankle edema, headache, flushing, palpitations, and hypotension.

Calcium channel blockers are excreted primarily by the liver, their pharmacokinetic profile is unaltered in chronic renal failure and by dialysis (Table 26-2), and their dosage does not require any adjustment.

2.   Sympatholytic drugs (e.g., methyldopa, clonidine, guanabenz). There appears to be increased tonic sympathetic activity in dialysis patients. For this reason, use of central sympatholytic drugs, which inhibit sympathetic outflow by stimulating α-adrenoreceptors in the brain stem, is theoretically attractive. One side benefit of clonidine is its usefulness in the treatment of diarrhea due to autonomic neuropathy.

Table 26-2. Antihypertensive drugs in dialysis patients: dosages and removal during dialysis

Drug	Tablet Size (mg)	Initial Dose in Dialysis Patients (mg)	Maintenance Dose in Dialysis Patients (mg/d)	Removal During HD	% Renal Drug Excretion	% of Normal Dose to Prescribe in ESRD
Calcium antagonists						
Amlodipine	5	5 qd	5 qd	No	<10%	100%
Diltiazem, extended release	120, 180, 240, 300, 360	120 qd	120–300 qd	No	<4%	100%
Felodipine	5, 10	5 qd	5–10 qd	No	<0.5%	100%
Isradipine	5	5 qd	5–10 qd	No	0%	100%
Nifedipine XL	30, 60	30 qd	30–60 qd	No	<1%	100%
Verapamil	40, 80, 120	40 bid	40–120 bid	No	3–4%	100%
ACE inhibitors						
Captopril	25, 50	12.5 qd	25–50 qd	Yes[a]	80%	8–16%
Enalapril	2.5, 5, 10, 20	2.5 qd or qod	2.5–10 qd or qod	Yes[a] Yes[a]	100% (enalaprilat)	33–50%
Fosinopril	10, 20	10 qd	10–20 qd	Yes[a]	75%	50–100%
Lisinopril	5, 10, 20, 40	2.5 qd or qod	2.5–10 qd or qod	Yes[a] Yes[a]	100%	25–50%
Perindopril	4	2 qod	2 qod	Yes[a]	60–70%	10%/ avoid
Ramipril	1.25, 2.5, 5, 10	2.5–5 qd	2.5–10 qd	Yes[a]		33–66%
β-Blockers						
Acebutolol	200, 400	200 qd	200–300	Yes[a]	15–30%	33–50%
Atenolol	50, 100	25 qod	25–50	Yes[a]	75–85%	25–50%
Carvedilol	5	5 qd	5	Yes[a]	<2%	100%
Metoprolol	50, 100	50 bid	50–100 bid	Yes[a]	5–10%	100%
Nadolol	20, 40, 80, 120, 160	40 qod	40–120 qod	Yes[a]	60–75%	25%
Pindolol	5, 10	5 bid	5–30 bid	Yes[a]	36–39%	100%
Propranolol	10, 40, 80	40 bid	40–80 bid	Yes[a]	negligible	100%
Adrenergic modulators						
Clonidine	0.1, 0.2, 0.3,	0.1 bid	0.1–0.3 bid,	No	40–70%	50–75%
Clonidine (TTS) patch	0.2	weekly	weekly	No	40–70%	100%
Guanabenz	4, 8	4 bid	4–8 bid	No	<1%	100%
Guanfacine	1, 2	1 qod	1–2 qd	No	24–73%	100%
Labetalol	100, 200, 300	200 bid	200–400 bid	No	<5%	100%
Prazosin	1, 2, 5	1 bid	1–10 bid	No	<10%	100%
Terazosin	1, 2, 5	1 bid	1–10 bid	No	10–15%	100%
Vasodilators						
Hydralazine	10, 25, 50, 100	25 bid	50 bid	No	<10%	100%
Minoxidil	2.5, 10	2.5 bid	5–30 bid	Yes[a]	12–20%	50%
Angiotensin II antagonists						
Losartan	50	50 qd	50 qd	No	<13%	100%
Candesartan	4, 8, 16, 32	16 qd	4–32 qd	No	50%	50%

[a] Scheduling should be set up so that drugs that are removed by hemodialysis are administered after dialysis. No drug in the table undergoes substantial removal during CAPD.

HD, hemodialysis; CAPD, continuous ambulatory peritoneal dialysis; TTS, transdermal therapeutic system.

Moreover, methyldopa and clonidine are relatively inexpensive—often an important consideration. Side effects include sedation, dry mouth, depression, and postural hypotension. The last may be a particular problem in diabetic patients. Methyldopa may cause hepatotoxicity or a positive direct or indirect Coombs test, interfering with cross-matching of blood. Clonidine may cause rebound hypertension if it is abruptly withdrawn. This latter side effect is substantially reduced with the transdermal formulation (TTS). Guanabenz and guanfacine are less likely to cause rebound hypertension but are more expensive.

Methyldopa, clonidine, and guanfacine are excreted substantially by the kidneys, and dosage reductions may be required. Methyldopa is removed by hemodialysis to a substantial extent. Guanabenz is metabolized by the liver and requires no dosage adjustment in renal failure.

3. β-, α/β-, and α-adrenergic blockers. A theoretical case for the efficacy of peripheral adrenergic receptor blockers (β-blockers, α/β-blockers, and α-blockers) in dialysis patients also can be made, and these agents have documented efficacy. As angiotensin II may participate in causing high blood pressure in some dialysis patients, the use of β-blockers may be beneficial under such circumstances because these drugs can lower plasma renin activities. Finally, many β-blocking drugs have shown a documented cardioprotective effect in the setting of myocardial ischemia or infarction. Carvedilol, an α/β-blocker, reduces morbidity and mortality in patients with heart failure (Packer et al, 1996).

On the minus side, α-blockers may cause postural hypotension. Prazosin has been associated with first-dose syncope, so the first dose must be administered at bedtime. β-Adrenergic blockers have a high incidence of side effects, such as drowsiness, lethargy, and depression. β-Blockers need to be used cautiously in patients with a tendency toward pulmonary edema or asthma and in patients already being treated with some calcium channel blockers. β-Blockers have an adverse effect on serum lipids; they also may have an adverse effect on cell potassium uptake, thus tending to increase the serum potassium level. They can mask the symptoms of hypoglycemia and augment insulin-induced hypoglycemia. All may cause bradycardia and interfere with reflex tachycardia following volume depletion.

In mild to moderate essential hypertension, β-blockers have an efficacy similar to that of ACE inhibitors in the regression of LVH and are more efficacious than calcium channel blockers and α_1-receptor antagonists (Gottdiner et al, 1997).

Water-soluble β-blockers, such as atenolol and nadolol, are primarily excreted by the kidney and require dosage reduction when used in the treatment of renal failure patients. Atenolol and nadolol are removed substantially by hemodialysis, possibly contributing to paradoxical hypertension during dialysis. Recommended dosage in dialysis patients is given in Table 26-2.

4. ACE inhibitors. ACE inhibitors are well tolerated. The use of ACE inhibitors in dialysis patients is theoretically attractive. In dialysis patients, prekallikrein levels are low and ACE levels are high. The plasma renin activity level is overtly high in some dialysis patients and inadequately suppressed in certain volume-expanded patients. Angiotensin II in itself may contribute to LVH, and it has been shown that in dialysis patients the control of hypertension with the ACE inhibitor perindopril reverses LVH whereas the calcium antagonist netrendipine had no such effect (London, 1994). ACE inhibitors, but not amlodipine, have been shown to reverse increased muscle sympathetic nerve activity associated with chronic renal failure (Ligtenberg et al, 1999).

ACE inhibitors have been used with success in patients with congestive heart failure. In some dialysis patients, extreme thirst and large interdialytic weight gain have been linked to high plasma angiotensin II levels. Treatment with enalapril has been reported to reduce thirst and interdialytic weight gain, but this effect, if any, is small and of little help in clinical practice.

ACE inhibitors, by interfering with bradykinin breakdown, may be associated with an increased incidence of anaphylactoid reactions during dialysis. It appears that most of these reactions are associated primarily with one membrane, AN69. It has been shown that the AN69 membrane, due to its negative charge, can increase bradykinin formation from plasma. However, anaphylactoid reactions associated with ACE inhibitors have also been reported in patients being dialyzed with non-AN69 membranes in a reuse setting (Brunet et al, 1992). Interference with bradykinin breakdown by ACE inhibitors may amplify anaphylactoid dialyzer reactions via several different mechanisms. Concurrent administration of an ACE inhibitor and a β-blocker can further worsen an anaphylactic reaction due to any cause and can cause the patient to be refractory to therapy with epinephrine.

Other disadvantages of ACE inhibitors in a dialysis setting include the following: ACE inhibitors have been associated with hyperkalemia in patients with renal insufficiency. Other side effects are cough, skin rash, alteration of taste, and, rarely, agranulocytosis. Worsening of anemia and erythropoietin resistance is another purported side effect of ACE inhibitors, but a recent prospective crossover study failed to confirm this (Abu-Alfa et al, 1997). Because the plasma half-life of many ACE inhibitors (or of their active metabolites) is prolonged in renal failure, reduction in dosage is often required. The dosage in dialysis patients is given in Table 26-2.

5. Angiotensin II antagonists. Losartan is the first drug of this new class of antihypertensive agents. The efficacy of losartan in dialysis patients is comparable to that of ACE inhibitors. The drug is metabolized extensively by the liver and does not require dose adjustment .

6. Vasodilators (e.g., hydralazine, minoxidil). These drugs are used as second-line agents. They usually require addition of a sympatholytic or β-blocking drug because they tend to cause reflex tachycardia. Hydralazine is effective and inexpensive but must be combined with a β-blocker or central sympatholytic drug. Minoxidil is usually reserved for treatment of resistant hypertension. Side effects, related primarily to reflex tachycardia, include palpitations, dizziness, and worsening of angina pectoris. Hydralazine can cause a lupus-like syndrome at dosages of more than 200 mg per day. Because of diminished renal excretion of its active metabolite(s), the maximum allowable dosage should be reduced in dialysis patients. Minoxidil has been associated with pericarditis and is generally avoided in women because of the risk of hypertrichosis.

VII.   Hypertensive emergencies and urgencies. Hypertensive crises are now seen less frequently in dialysis patients. The term "hypertensive urgency" is reserved for patients who are at significant risk within a matter of days if left untreated [i.e., malignant hypertension without extraretinal (severe) organ damage and perioperative hypertension]. Hypertensive emergencies are defined as increases in arterial pressure that, if sustained for a few hours, would cause irreversible organ damage (Isles, 1994). Hypertensive encephalopathy, hypertensive left ventricular failure, hypertension associated with unstable angina/myocardial infarction, hypertension with aortic dissection, and cerebral hemorrhage/brain infarction are such emergencies. Malignant hypertension is defined as severe hypertension (diastolic blood pressure usually greater than 130 mm Hg) with bilateral retinal hemorrhages and exudates and is frequently diagnosed in patients presenting with hypertensive crises.

The ideal rate of reduction of blood pressure in *hypertensive urgencies* must represent a balance between the risks of inadequate and overly rapid reduction of blood pressure. In chronic hypertension, the range of cerebral autoregulation is reset upward so that patients may be less able to compensate for a sudden fall in pressure, which may precipitate cerebral infarction and blindness. For this reason, abrupt forms of therapy should be avoided in most cases. The short-acting formulation of nifedipine has been very frequently used as a first-line drug for severe hypertension in dialysis patients. There are now a number of reports documenting myocardial, cerebral, and retinal ischemia after use of such formulation. The long-acting preparation (or another long-acting calcium antagonist) or clonidine should be used instead as first-line therapy. If the patient is already on treatment with such drugs, a β-blocker or an ACE inhibitor or a combination thereof could be added. If oral therapy fails, parenteral drugs should be used (see below).

Hypertensive emergencies should be managed with parenteral drugs. Nitroprusside administered by continuous intravenous infusion (0.3–0.8 μg per kg per minute initially to a maximum of 8 μg per kg per minute) is particularly useful in heart failure and dissecting aneurysm but requires careful monitoring because its toxic metabolite (thiocyanate) is retained in renal failure. Cyanide levels should be monitored every 48 hours and should not exceed 10 mg per dL. The symptoms of thiocyanate toxicity are nausea, vomiting, myoclonic movements, and seizures. In general, the infusion should not be prolonged for more than 48 hours. Both nitroprusside and its metabolites are readily removed by dialysis. Intravenous labetalol may also be considered in patients without heart failure, asthma, or heart block (2 mg per minute to a total of 2 mg per kg). The slow intravenous administration of hydralazine (10–20 mg) is a well-tried alternative, but this drug should be avoided in ischemic heart disease.

A. The diabetic hypertensive patient. Diabetics compose almost one-third of dialysis patients. They usually have low-renin, volume-dependent hypertension. In diabetic patients, adrenergic blockers may aggravate orthostatic hypotension from autonomic neuropathy, clonidine may cause paradoxical hypertension, β-blockers may mask the symptoms of hypoglycemia or aggravate congestive heart failure, and vasodilators used alone may cause angina. Drug combinations may be used, and the ideal regimen must often be individualized on a trial-and-error basis.

SELECTED READINGS

Abu-Alfa A, et al. ACE inhibitors do not induce Epogen resistance in hemodialysis patients: a prospective, crossover study. *J Am Soc Nephrol* 1977;A1041.

Argiles A, Mourad G, Mion C. Seasonal changes in blood pressure in patients with end-stage renal disease treated with hemodialysis. *N Engl J Med* 1998;339:1364–1370.

Brunet P, et al. Anaphylactoid reactions during hemodialysis and hemofiltration: role of associating AN69 membrane and angiotensin I-converting enzyme inhibition. *Am J Kidney Dis* 1992;19:444–447.

Cannella G. Regression of left ventricular hypertrophy in hypertensive dialyzed uremic patients on long term anti-hypertensive therapy. *Kidney Int* 1993;44:881–886.

Charra B, Bergstrom J, Scribner BH. Blood pressure control in dialysis patients: importance of the lag phenomenon. *Am J Kidney Dis* 1998;32:720–724.

Cheigh JS, et al. Mechanism of refractory hypertension in hemodialysis patients. *J Am Soc Nephrol* 1993;4:340.

Conlon PJ. Predialysis systolic blood pressure correlates strongly with mean 24-hour systolic blood pressure and left ventricular mass in stable hemodialysis patients. *J Am Soc Nephrol* 1996;7:2658–2663.

Converse RL Jr, et al. Sympathetic overactivity in patients with chronic renal failure. *N Engl J Med* 1992;327:1912–1918.

Enia G, et al. Hypotensive effect of ultra-low sodium dialysate in CAPD patients: a double-blind, randomized, crossover study. 31st Ann Mtg Am Soc Nephrol. *J Am Soc Nephrol* 1998;99:282A.

Fishbane S, et al. Role of volume overload in dialysis-refractory hypertension. *Am J Kidney Dis* 1996;28:257–261.

Foley RN, et al. Impact of hypertension on cardiomyopathy, morbidity and mortality in end-stage renal disease. *Kidney Int* 1996;49:1379–1385.

Furberg CD, et al. Nifedipine. Dose related increase in mortality in patients with coronary heart disease. *Circulation* 1995;92:1326–1331.

Gottdiner JS, et al. Effect of single drug therapy on reduction of left ventricular mass in mild to moderate essential hypertension. Comparison of six antihypertensive agents. *Circulation* 1997;95:2007–2014.

Isles C. Hypertensive emergencies. In: Swales JD, ed. *Textbook of hypertension.* London: Blackwell Scientific, 1994:1233–1248.

Keen M, Janson S, Gotch F. Plasma sodium (CpNa) "setpoint": relationship to interdialytic weight gain (IWG) and mean arterial pressure (MAP) in hemodialysis patients (HDP). ASN 30th Annual Meeting, San Antonio. *J Am Soc Nephrol* 1997;8:241A.

Ligtenberg G, et al. Reduction of sympathetic hyperactivity by enalapril in patients with chronic renal failure. *N Engl J Med* 1999;340:1321–1328.

London GM, et al. Cardiac hypertrophy, aortic compliance, peripheral resistance, and wave reflection in end-stage renal disease. Comparative effects of ACE inhibition and calcium channel blockade. *Circulation* 1994;90:2786–2796.

Luik A, et al. Blood pressure control and fluid state in patients on long treatment time dialysis. *J Am Soc Nephrol* 1994;5:521.

Parfrey PS, et al. Outcome and risk factors for left ventricular disorders in chronic uraemia. *Nephrol Dial Transplant* 1996;11:1277–1285.

Packer M, et al. The effect of carvedilol on morbidity and mortality in patients with chronic heart failure. *N Engl J Med* 1996;334:1349–1355.

Piccoli A, et al. A new method for monitoring body fluid variation by bioimpedance analysis: the RXc graph. *Kidney Int* 1994;46:534–539.

Zoccali C, et al. Nocturnal hypertension and hypoxemia in dialysis patients. *J Am Soc Nephrol* 1996;7:1529.

Zoccali C, et al. Prediction of left ventricular geometry by clinic, predialysis, and 24h ambulatory BP monitoring in hemodialysis patients. *J Hypertens* 1999;17:1751–1758.

Internet Reference

Hypertension and cardiovascular disease in ESRD Patients: Links (http://www.hdcn.com/crf/hypertension)

Hematologic Abnormalities

Steven Fishbane and Emil P. Paganini

I. **Anemia**
A. **Etiologic factors.** Insufficient production of erythropoietin (EPO) is the predominant cause for anemia in patients with
end-stage renal disease (ESRD). EPO is normally produced by
endothelial cells in proximity to the renal tubules. As excretory
renal function is lost, there is a decline in the production of EPO
that correlates with the declining creatinine clearance. The
severity of the resulting anemia varies, but if untreated, then
hematocrit values of 18%–24% are typical. While the primacy
of EPO deficiency is indisputable, other factors may play important contributory roles. Also, patients with ESRD may develop
any of the other causes of anemia common in nonuremic subjects.
B. **Consequences**
  1. **Symptoms.** The manifestations of anemia may be due
  both to decreased oxygen delivery and to the compensatory
  change of increased cardiac output. The most prominent symptoms of anemia are fatigue and dyspnea. Sense of well-being is
  diminished. Less common symptoms include difficulty concen-
  trating, dizziness, sleep disorders, cold intolerance, and headaches. With severe anemia, there is an increase in cardiac output that may result in palpitations and a pounding pulse.
  There is left ventricular hypertrophy (LVH) and diminished
  exercise capacity. Other problems include deranged hemostatic function, impaired immune function, and diminished cognitive and sexual function. Exacerbations of angina, claudication, and transient ischemic attacks may also be observed.
  2. **Physical examination.** The primary physical examination finding of anemia is pallor, which may be best detected
  on the palms of the hands, the nailbeds, and the oral mucosa.
  A systolic ejection murmur due to increased cardiac flow may
  be heard over the precordium.
C. **Treatment**
  1. **Benefits**
    a. **Effect on outcome.** Cross-sectional and retrospec-
    tive studies have suggested that anemia in hemodialysis
    patients is associated with a decrease in life span, particu-
    larly when the hemoglobin concentration is less than 10 g
    per dL. A substantial part of this increased mortality may
    depend on increased cardiac disease due to anemia, includ-
    ing a higher incidence of LVH and dilatation as well as
    frank congestive heart failure (Foley et al, 1996). Recent
    analysis of a large payment database (US HCFA files) has
    shown that mortality, hospitalization rate, and hospital-
    ization days continue to decrease as hematocrit increases
    to 33%–36% (Ma et al, 1999).
    b. **Reduction in transfusion-related complications.**
    Prior to EPO therapy, up to 20% of patients on dialysis

required frequent transfusions with attendant risk of immediate transfusion reactions, viral infection, iron overload, and immune sensitization. The rate of blood transfusion has been greatly reduced by the use of recombinant human EPO (rHuEPO) therapy.

   c.   Improved quality of life and overall sense of well-being. Various assessment tools, such as Karnofsky's score, SF-36 values, and Sickness Impact Profiles, have documented an improved quality of life and functional status in ESRD patients treated with rHuEPO. Patients feel less fatigued, and their exercise capacity increases. There may be improvement as well in pruritus, sexual functioning, and leg cramps.

   d.   Regression of LVH. The left ventricle compensates for anemia by undergoing hypertrophy, a maladaptive change leading to an increased risk of morbidity and death. Within 3 months of starting rHuEPO therapy, regression of LVH may be demonstrable by echocardiography. In addition, ischemic electrocardiographic changes during exercise are significantly reduced.

   e.   Cognitive function. Cognitive function is improved after rHuEPO therapy both at a physiologic level (evoked somatosensory potential latencies) and at a clinical level (tests of cognitive function). Patients notice an improved ability to focus and concentrate.

   f.   Improved hemostasis. ESRD patients in whom hematocrit is less than 30% often have increased bleeding time that responds to correction of anemia. With rHuEPO therapy, serum fibrinogen and factor VIII concentrations increase and platelet aggregation is improved.

2.   Indications for EPO therapy and target hematocrit. EPO therapy should be initiated in the predialysis period when the creatinine clearance is less than 35 mL per minute and the hematocrit falls below 30%–33%. Certainly by the time patients reach dialysis, therapy should be initiated if the hematocrit is consistently below 33%. The optimal hematocrit for a patient with ESRD is not known. The National Kidney Foundation's Dialysis Outcomes Quality Initiative (NKF–DOQI) Anemia Guidelines (1997) recommend a target hematocrit for dialysis patients in the 33%–36% range. On the other hand, might raising the hematocrit to the normal range improve outcomes further? The recent Normal Hematocrit Cardiac Study (Besarab et al, 1998) involved the randomization of over 1,200 hemodialysis patients with cardiac disease to a hematocrit level of 30% versus a "normal" 42%. The study was terminated prematurely due to a trend toward more adverse outcomes in the higher hematocrit group (Besarab et al, 1998). Therefore, raising the hematocrit above the 33%–36% target range cannot be recommended at this time. However, similar studies are ongoing, and the optimum hematocrit level may yet turn out to be greater than 36%.

3.   Route of administration

   a.   Subcutaneous versus intravenous EPO. Subcutaneous injection is the preferred route of administration of rHuEPO for patients on either peritoneal dialysis or hemodialysis. The subcutaneous route improves the efficiency of therapy, resulting in a reduced dosing requirement for rHuEPO for a given hematocrit value.

Table 27-1 provides strategies adapted from the NKF-DOQI Anemia Guidelines for improving patient acceptance of subcutaneous dosing. EPO should be administered at the dialysis center (rather than administered by the patient at home) to ensure patient compliance. The use of very small-gauge needles is emphasized to reduce injection-related pain. In a recent multicenter study, patients reported minimal pain with subcutaneous injection of rHuEPO (Kaufman et al, 1998).

When converting a patient from intravenous to subcutaneous rHuEPO, the weekly intravenous dose should be divided initially as twice-weekly subcutaneous injections. A goal of therapy would be to decrease to once-weekly administration within several months as tolerated.

b. Intraperitoneal EPO. For patients on peritoneal dialysis for whom subcutaneous injection is not tolerated, intraperitoneal injection of rHuEPO may be used as a last resort. This route of administration results in relatively poor absorption and the need for higher doses. Injection into a dry abdomen improves absorption. An intraperitoneal EPO dosing protocol used at the University of Toronto has been described (Saohdeva et al, 1997).

c. Dosing

(1) Initial dose. A reasonable starting dose of rHuEPO for dialysis patients is 50–60 U per kg subcutaneously twice weekly. If a more rapid increase in hematocrit is needed, a starting dose of 75 units per kg may be used. If intravenous therapy is to be used, then the starting dose should be 50–75 units per kg thrice weekly. The goal of therapy is to achieve a target hematocrit within 3 months. An excessively rapid rise in the hematocrit

---

Table 27-1. Strategies for improving patient acceptance of subcutaneous recombinant human erythropoietin dosing

1. Initiate rHuEPO therapy among new patients with subcutaneous dosing. (If the patients have been on rHuEPO prior to initiating dialysis, then they have already been on subcutaneous dosing.)
2. Provide education for patients and staff regarding the improved efficacy of subcutaneous dosing.
3. When changing to subcutaneous dosing, establish a new unit-wide policy, and change all patients at the same time.
4. Use a very small-gauge needle (27 or 29 gauge).
5. Use the multidose rHuEPO preparation (contains benzyl alcohol).
6. Administer a single weekly injection if the dose is less than 4,000 units. (Smaller volume is associated with less discomfort.)
7. Rotate injection sites.

---

rHuEPO, recombinant human erythropoietin.
Adapted from the National Kidney Foundation Dialysis Outcomes Quality Initiative Guidelines.

should be avoided, as this may lead to an increased risk of hypertension or seizures.

(2) Initial response and plateau effect. During the initiation phase of therapy, hematocrit should be checked every 1–2 weeks, and the dose adjusted as needed. It is very common during the initiation of treatment for a "plateauing" of effect to occur; either the hematocrit stops increasing, or escalating doses of rHuEPO are required to reach therapeutic targets. This period of blunted response may be due to the induction of iron deficiency. Once the target hematocrit has been reached, the hematocrit should be checked every 2–4 weeks. During this maintenance phase of therapy, the dose of rHuEPO should be adjusted based on changes in hematocrit (Fig. 27-1).

The patient's responsiveness to rHuEPO should be reassessed on a continuing basis. A certain proportion of patients will be highly responsive, with hematocrit values consistently 33%–36%, and an rHuEPO dose of less than 5,500 U thrice weekly. At the other end of the spectrum, many patients will be somewhat resistant to therapy, with a blunted erythropoietic response. These patients need to be fully evaluated for causes of rHuEPO resis-

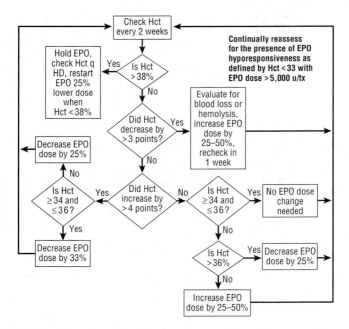

Fig. 27-1. Flow chart for adjusting the recombinant human erythropoietin (EPO) dose based on hematocrit (Hct) results. U/tx, units per treatment.

tance. The remaining patients will demonstrate intermediate responsiveness. The hematocrit of such patients will correlate with the rHuEPO dose prescribed and will increase in response to an increase in dose. The responsiveness to rHuEPO in all patients should be evaluated on an ongoing basis because the degree of responsiveness changes over time. In our experience, the development of resistance frequently develops after an increase in rHuEPO dose, probably reflecting the unmasking of iron deficiency.

d. Side effects of rHuEPO therapy

    (1) Worsening of hypertension. This is a common problem during the partial correction of anemia with rHuEPO therapy. In approximately 33% of patients, there will be a need to increase antihypertensive medication doses. However, it is rare for rHuEPO to be withdrawn because of uncontrollable hypertension. Risk factors include preexisting hypertension, a rapid increase in hematocrit, the presence of native kidneys, and severe anemia prior to treatment. The cause of the hypertensive effect is incompletely understood. Factors that may contribute include the partial reversal of hypoxic vasodilatation as the hematocrit rises, increased blood viscosity, a direct effect of rHuEPO on the vasculature, and increased cardiac output. rHuEPO induces a dose-dependent increase in the ratio of vasoconstrictive to vasodilatory prostanoids, increased vascular responsiveness to norepinephrine, and increased synthesis of endothelin-1 (Bode-Boger et al, 1996). Long-acting calcium channel blockers are very effective for treating hypertension associated with rHuEPO. In addition, recent evidence has suggested that antiplatelet therapy may be effective for blunting the hypertensive effect (Caravaca et al, 1994).

    (2) Seizures. These can occur in a small number of patients during periods of rapidly increasing hematocrit in association with hypertension. The risk of seizures is small using current rHuEPO dosing protocols.

    (3) Graft clotting. The increase in blood viscosity with higher hematocrit values on rHuEPO could theoretically cause increased dialyzer and arteriovenous graft clotting. Studies to date have not consistently demonstrated an increased risk of thrombosis when the hematocrit is raised to the 30%–36% range. In the Normal Hematocrit Cardiac Study described earlier, there was an increase in arteriovenous graft clotting among patients randomized to the 42% hematocrit group.

    (4) Effect on _Kt/V_. Dialysis urea clearance may decrease slightly as the hematocrit rises during rHuEPO therapy, due to a diminished proportion of plasma to red cell volume, but with hematocrit levels of less than 36%, the effect on urea clearance is of little clinical significance (See Chapter 2). The effect on creatinine clearance is somewhat greater.

    (5) Phosphorus balance. Control of the serum phosphate concentration may become more difficult during rHuEPO therapy. An improvement in appetite and dietary intake of phosphate in combination with a reduction in dialyzer clearance of phosphate at the higher hematocrit may explain this phenomenon.

(6) **Hyperkalemia.** This was occasionally seen in early studies of rHuEPO. Subsequent clinical experience has not demonstrated any increase in the risk for hyperkalemia during rHuEPO therapy.

e. **Causes of decreased response to rHuEPO therapy**

(1) **Iron deficiency.** The most important cause of a suboptimal response to rHuEPO therapy is iron deficiency. Iron deficiency can be present at the outset of therapy, but more commonly, it develops during therapy, either due to rapid utilization of iron to support erythropoiesis or as the result of blood loss (Table 27-2).

(a) **Blood loss.** Hemodialysis patients develop iron deficiency primarily because of chronic blood loss. Between retention of blood in the blood lines and dialyzer with each hemodialysis treatment, surgical blood loss, accidental bleeding from the access, blood sampling for laboratory testing, and occult gastrointestinal bleeding, iron losses may be substantial. Because of this increased blood loss, it is very difficult to maintain iron stores in hemodialysis patients using oral iron supplements only. Losses in peritoneal dialysis patients are substantially less, and these patients often can be maintained on oral iron therapy.

(b) **Functional iron deficiency.** In addition to a depleted iron supply, the demand for iron increases during rHuEPO treatment, leading to a further strain on depleted iron stores. After the intravenous injection of rHuEPO, there is an increase in the rate of erythro-

---

Table 27-2.   Causes of iron deficiency in hemodialysis patients

- Depletion of iron stores
- Chronic blood loss
    1. Blood retention by the dialysis lines and filter
    2. Blood sampling for laboratory testing
    3. Accidents related to the vascular access
    4. Surgical blood loss
    5. Occult gastrointestinal bleeding
- Decreased dietary iron absorption
    1. Phosphate binders inhibit iron absorption
    2. H2 blockers, proton pump blockers, and functional achlorhydria impair iron absorption
    3. Uremic gut does not absorb iron optimally
- Increased iron demand
    1. Due to increased rate of erythropoiesis induced by rHuEPO
    2. Impaired release of iron from storage tissues (reticuloendothelial blockade)

---

rHuEPO, recombinant human erythropoietin.

poiesis that leads to a greater immediate need for iron. In this setting, iron deficiency may occur even in the face of normal iron stores. This phenomenon has been termed "functional iron deficiency" and may be noted clinically by a low transferrin saturation despite a normal or elevated serum ferritin concentration.

(c) **Reticuloendothelial blockade.** Iron deficiency may also be exacerbated in patients with ESRD by the presence of reticuloendothelial blockade. In this condition, which may be common in patients on dialysis, the presence of low-grade chronic inflammation may lead to impaired release of iron from its storage sites.

(d) **Poor absorption of dietary iron.** Iron deficiency among patients on dialysis may be exacerbated by poor absorption of dietary iron. Hemodialysis patients who are iron-deficient absorb iron less efficiently than nonuremic subjects. In addition, the use of phosphate binders with meals reduces dietary iron availability.

(2) **Diagnosis**

(a) **Serum ferritin and transferrin saturation.** The serum ferritin concentration and the transferrin saturation percentage (TSAT) have been the two most widely used tests of iron status for dialysis patients. However, neither test is accurate for the assessment of iron deficiency in this patient population, and these tests provide only a rough estimate of iron status. Thus, patients should not be treated intensively with intravenous iron based only on the results of these indices. Instead, test results should be interpreted in the context of the response to rHuEPO therapy. Intensification of iron therapy should occur at a serum ferritin of less than 100 ng per mL or transferrin saturation of less than 20% in patients who are reasonably rHuEPO-responsive, and at a serum ferritin of less than 300 ng per mL or transferrin saturation less than 30% among patients with rHuEPO resistance. It is important to note that iron testing should always be delayed for 2 weeks after treatment with intravenous iron.

(3) **Treatment**

(a) **General principles.** Intensive iron therapy, particularly the regular use of parenteral iron in hemodialysis patients, results in higher hematocrit levels and lower dose requirements for rHuEPO. Intravenous iron may be administered on an episodic basis as needed when iron deficiency develops, or by the repeated administration of small doses to maintain iron balance.

A treatment flow chart is shown in Fig. 27-2. In general, all patients on dialysis require iron supplementation as long as they are not iron-overloaded (serum ferritin greater than 800 ng per mL).

(b) **Oral iron.** Oral iron preparations have been the mainstay of therapy because of their convenience and relatively low cost. However, these supplements are associated with inconsistent efficacy and troublesome

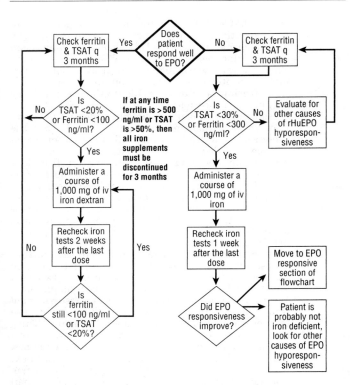

Fig. 27-2. Flow chart for iron management with iron dextran.

side effects, such as constipation, dyspepsia, bloating, or diarrhea. Gastrointestinal side effects due to iron may even impact adversely on nutritional status (Fishbane et al, 1988). NKF–DOQI guidelines state that oral iron may be used as initial iron therapy for hemodialysis patients, although they note that most patients will require the regular use of intravenous iron therapy.

Despite the limitations of oral iron therapy, it is clearly the most convenient route of administration for patients on peritoneal dialysis. They should be maintained on 200 mg per day of elemental iron, consumed 1 hour prior to meals. The serum ferritin and transferrin saturation should be checked every 3 months. Intravenous iron therapy should be used only when marked resistance to rHuEPO is present, and the serum ferritin is less than 150 ng per mL and the TSAT is less than 20%.

(i) Dosage and administration. Oral iron usually is given as ferrous sulfate, fumarate, or gluconate, in a dosage of 200 mg of elemental iron per day. The timing of the iron dose is important; ideally, iron should be taken 1 hour before meals to optimize efficacy. However, gastrointestinal side effects are increased when iron is taken on an empty stomach.

The primary sites of iron absorption are the duodenum and proximal jejunum, and gastrointestinal symptoms are proportional to the amount of elemental iron presented to the duodenum at a single time; reduction of symptomatology may require changing the oral preparation, using pediatric dosages at more frequent intervals, or even taking the iron dosage with food. Others have suggested giving the medication during dialysis sessions (e.g., at the beginning and the end of the session) to help ensure patient compliance. Yet another strategy is to give oral iron only at bedtime. A common problem with iron therapy is constipation. This can be managed with sorbitol. Some iron preparations contain small doses of ascorbic acid to enhance iron absorption, but the advantage of the added vitamin is not established. In addition to phosphorus binders, histamine-2 antagonists and proton pump inhibitors may all inhibit the absorption of oral iron supplements.

Readily available delayed-release preparations of iron (e.g., Ferro-Gradumet, Slow Fe, Ferro Sequels) minimize the release of iron in the stomach and theoretically cause less gastritis. Iron–polysaccharide complexes supply elemental iron rather than the iron salt (e.g., Niferex-150, Nu-Iron). Both delayed-release preparations and iron–polysaccharide complex–based tablets are substantially more expensive than the plain iron salts. It is not clear that any specific oral iron preparation causes fewer side effects than others.

(c) **Intravenous iron.** Three preparations are available and are widely used: iron dextran, iron gluconate and iron sucrose (approved in some European countries, undergoing trials in the United States at the time of this writing). Intravenous iron therapy has superior availability and efficacy when compared with oral iron therapy. In contrast, intravenous therapy costs more, and iron dextran is associated with occasional serious immediate anaphylactoid reactions (estimated to occur in 0.7% of patients treated). Reactions occur also with iron gluconate and sucrose, but severe reactions with iron gluconate or sucrose are much less commonly observed than with iron dextran.

The high efficacy of intravenous iron must be weighed against possible safety issues. Concerns relate to possible increases in risk for infection, oxidative effects on organs or the vasculature, and the risk for promoting atherosclerosis. The best studied problem is the risk for infection. Earlier studies noted higher serum ferritin levels to be associated with increased risk of infection. More recently, analysis of a claims database showed frequent low-dose intravenous iron use to be associated with an increase in the risk for infectious death. In contrast, a well-designed, large, prospective, multi-center study reported by (Hoen et al, 1998) found no relation between serum ferritin or treatment with iron with the risk for bacteremia. Other possible problems with iron treatment are theoretical and not well studied. One study, which needs confirmation, suggested that vitamin E may attenuate oxidative stress association with intravenous iron therapy (Roob et al, 2000). On balance, the benefit of intravenous iron in facilitating the achievement of higher hematocrit values (with an improvement in life span and quality of life) must be weighed against the risk of therapy.

(i)   Iron dextran. There are several dosing strategies. One is to give a 1,000-mg dose administered in divided doses over 10 consecutive hemodialysis treatments. Sometimes larger doses may be given at one time (e.g., up to 500 mg or even higher), as in the case of peritoneal dialysis patients in whom intravenous access is not regularly available. Another approach is to dose iron dextran on a weekly basis, giving 25–100 mg per week. When this approach is used, the dose should be held for at least 2 weeks prior to assessing iron stores with serum ferritin and iron binding studies. Dosing of intravenous iron administration on a regular basis has been associated with an increased risk of mortality due to infection. At this time, the causality of iron therapy in this relationship remains speculative (Collins et al, 1998).

Adverse effects of iron dextran. Iron dextran is supplied as a sterile liquid, containing 50 mg of elemental iron per milliliter. In nonuremic patients, immediate allergic reactions to intravenous iron dextran have been reported. These usually occur within 5 minutes of injection but may be delayed by 45 minutes or more. Anaphylactic reactions can cause hypotension, syncope, purpura, wheezing, dyspnea, respiratory arrest, and cyanosis. For this reason, epinephrine and other means to combat anaphylaxis must be at hand when intravenous iron dextran is administered. Milder immediate hypersensitivity reactions to iron dextran infusion include itching and urticaria. Delayed reactions can manifest as lymphadenopathy, myalgia, arthralgia, fever, and headache. Often delayed reactions can be controlled by limiting the size of each dose to 250 mg.

(ii)   Sodium ferric gluconate. Intravenous sodium ferric gluconate has been used in Europe for many years, with anecdotal reports suggesting good safety and efficacy profiles. The drug appears to have a clear advantage over iron dextran in that serious immediate reactions are probably markedly reduced. A recent study performed by (Nissenson et al, 1999) evaluated intravenous sodium ferric gluconate in iron-deficient hemodialysis patients. Patients were treated with 1,000 mg of sodium ferric gluconate given over eight dialysis treatments. Sodium ferric gluconate was effective, with peak hematocrit achieved by day 14 post treatment, with an acceptable safety profile.

Intravenous sodium ferric gluconate may be administered to hemodialysis patients in the amount of 1,000 mg given in divided doses over eight consecutive treatments (i.e., 125 mg per dose). At the time of this writing, this agent is approved in the United States to be administered only by intravenous infusion. A reasonable strategy is to dilute the drug in 200 mL normal saline and to infuse over 2 hours during the hemodialysis treatment. At the time of this writing, studies are under way in the United States to evaluate this drug for intravenous push dosing, which would improve convenience.

(iii) Iron sucrose. Intravenous iron sucrose has been in use in Europe for many years. Like sodium ferric gluconate, anecdotal reports indicate a good safety and efficacy profile. At the time of writing, studies of this agent are under way in the United States.

Both iron sucrose and sodium ferric gluconate bind their iron cores less avidly than iron dextran. This has raised some concern regarding possible oversaturation of transferrin in serum. This issue has been disputed by a recent study by (Seligman, 1999) who found that serum iron assays in common use measure not only transferrin-bound iron but also iron that had been bound to drug. Therefore, the assays may markedly overstate transferrin saturation unless 2 full weeks have passed since dosing with intravenous iron. It is likely that the "looser" iron binding of iron sucrose and sodium ferric gluconate are not of clinical significance, as evidenced by the excellent long-term safe use of these agents in Europe.

f.   Other causes of rHuEPO resistance

(1)   Hyperparathyroidism. Hyperparathyroidism is a well-documented and probably under-recognized cause of rHuEPO resistance. The degree of resistance is probably related most to the amount of marrow fibrosis, and it is unclear that the serum parathyroid hormone by radioimmunoassay (iPTH) level is a good marker for resistance. Nonetheless, in the rHuEPO-resistant patient who is found to have elevated iPTH levels, an intensification of the treatment of hyperparathyroidism is indicated. Among patients with severe hyperparathyroidism refractory to medical therapy, parathyroidectomy has been demonstrated to result in a significant improvement in erythropoiesis.

(2)   Infection. The release of cytokines during infection leads to a diminished bone marrow response to rHuEPO. A search for occult infection should be undertaken in patients with unexplained rHuEPO resistance. If infection is present, higher doses of rHuEPO may be effective by partially overcoming the temporary resistance.

(3) Inflammation. As with infection, states of sub-acute or chronic inflammation lead to an increased resistance to rHuEPO therapy. In patients on dialysis, inflammatory conditions may occasionally be occult or may be due to the bioincompatibility of the dialysis treatment itself. There is no perfect marker for occult inflammation, but C-reactive protein (CRP) is emerging as a valuable test for predicting rHuEPO hyporesponsiveness caused by inflammation (Gunnell et al, 1999).

(4) Inadequate dialysis. An association between the adequacy of hemodialysis and responsiveness to rHuEPO has been demonstrated (Ifudu et al, 1996). It is unclear whether the relationship is due simply to the degree of solute removal or to some other related factor, such as dialysis time, or the flux properties or biocompatibility of the dialyzer used. It is clear that when rHuEPO resistance is present, an effort to optimize the intensity of dialysis (and perhaps a change to a high-flux membrane) might be tried.

(5) Aluminum intoxication. Although problems with aluminum have become less common among dialysis patients, occasional problems may still occur, especially in patients who have been on dialysis for many years. The effect on erythropoiesis is a microcytic anemia associated with impaired iron utilization. Interestingly, intestinal aluminum absorption is significantly increased in patients with iron deficiency. A serum aluminum level provides a rough guide to aluminum status; if the results are suggestive, then either a deferoxamine stimulation test (see Chapter 31) or bone biopsy may be warranted.

(6) Bleeding. An important cause of an apparent hyporesponsiveness to rHuEPO is bleeding. Sometimes the bleeding may be occult as in gastrointestinal blood loss. Often the bleeding may be obvious, as in patients undergoing surgery, menstruating women, or those with accidents involving the vascular access. It is vitally important to limit blood loss by any means possible. In addition, fecal occult blood testing should be performed every 3–6 months when unexplained rHuEPO resistance is present.

(7) ACE inhibitors. ACE inhibitors may reduce EPO production in patients with chronic renal failure or following renal transplant. Among patients on dialysis, a reduction in rHuEPO responsiveness has not been uniformly demonstrated in association with these agents.

(8) Serum albumin. An association has been noted between hematocrit and serum albumin, suggesting a possible link between rHuEPO responsiveness and either covert inflammation or nutritional state. However, there is no evidence of causality in this relationship or that an improvement in nutrition would lead to an improvement in rHuEPO responsiveness.

(9) Other hematologic disease. Patients on dialysis are at risk for developing the same hematologic diseases as nonuremic subjects. Because of the emphasis on EPO deficiency, other hematologic diseases may go unrecognized. Among the potential causes are vitamin B_{12} or folic acid deficiency, hematologic malignancy, myelodysplastic syndromes, or hemolysis. Vitamin B_{12} and folic acid levels should be checked when unexplained rHuEPO resistance is present. When an exhaustive evaluation for causes of resistance is unrevealing, hematology consultation and a bone marrow biopsy may be considered as a last step in the process to rule out unexpected hematologic disease.

4. Androgen therapy. Androgens were occasionally utilized for anemia therapy in ESRD patients in the pre-rHuEPO era. The mechanism of the proerythropoietic effect is unclear but may simply be a manifestation of the overall anabolic effect of these agents. Virilization is a common side effect that limits the usefulness of androgens in women, and men occasionally suffer from priapism (more common among African American patients) or other side effects. With the introduction of rHuEPO, the use of androgen therapy has greatly decreased. There may still be a place for androgen therapy as an adjunct to rHuEPO therapy in older male patients. A study by Teruel et al (1996) in male hemodialysis patients older than 50 years found that nandrolone decanoate (200 mg per week intramuscularly) led to an increase in hematocrit equivalent to that induced by rHuEPO in other patient populations. In addition, there was less of a hypertensive effect with androgen than with rHuEPO therapy, and a beneficial anabolic effect as measured by increased serum albumin and dry weight. There were no significant side effects, other than an increase in serum triglycerides. Additional studies would be helpful in confirming these findings, but it would seem reasonable at this time to use nandrolone in older men who do not respond optimally to rHuEPO.

5. Red blood cell transfusions. Transfusion of packed red cells should be used in severely anemic patients who are experiencing symptoms. Transfusion should never be utilized without a subsequent evaluation for causes of bleeding.

6. Carnitine. It has been suggested that carnitine may enhance responsiveness to rHuEPO. As of this writing, there are few published data to support the use of this supplement for this purpose.

7. Ascorbic acid. Intravenous ascorbic acid has been reported to ameliorate EPO resistance in patients with serum ferritins >500 ng/mL (Tarng et al, 1998). These preliminary results need to be confirmed.

II. Hemolysis

A. General comments. Destruction of red blood cells, either intravascularly or extravascularly, may occasionally contribute to anemia in dialysis patients. Generally speaking, red cell survival appears to be shortened with chronic renal failure (mean 70 days versus 120 days in nonuremics). It is likely that this is due not to an inherent abnormality of the red cell but to an effect of the uremic environment. The survival of red cells from patients with chronic renal failure appears to be normal after transfusion into a nonuremic host.

B.   Diagnosis. Chronic hemolysis should be suspected when the patient develops high-grade rHuEPO resistance in the presence of increased serum LDH, unconjugated bilirubin, or a decrease in serum haptoglobin. The differential diagnosis of chronic hemolysis is broad, and includes all causes of hemolysis seen in nonuremic patients (Table 27-3), and several causes specific to patients treated with hemodialysis. Occasionally, hemolysis can be severe, associated with hypotension, back pain, and encephalopathy developing during the dialysis procedure. For some unknown reason, pancreatitis sometimes follows the acute hemolysis episode.

C.   Etiology

    1.   Chloramine. Chloramine is a rare but important cause of hemolysis, which may contaminate dialysate, resulting in oxidative stress to the red cell. Chloramine is used as a sterilant for some municipal water supplies, as it is believed to be more environmentally "friendly" than chlorine. Normally, chloramines are removed from the water source by the use of carbon filters. (Note that reverse osmosis does not remove chloramines.) Damage to the filters (usually two in series) may result in the release of chloramines into dialysate, oxidizing hemoglobin, causing the production of methemoglobin and Heinz bodies (oxidized clumps of hemoglobin). Product water should be tested before each hemodialysis shift for the presence of chloramine.

    2.   Hypotonic or overheated dialysate. Hemolysis has also been seen with the accidental use of hypotonic or overheated dialysate. The inadvertant use of hypotonic dialysate can lead to a brisk osmolar destruction of red cells.

Table 27-3.   Causes of hemolysis in dialysis patients

Related to the hemodialysis procedure
  Dialysis solution
    Contaminants
      Chloramine
      Copper, zinc
      Nitrates, nitrites
    Overheated
    Hypo-osmolar
  Reuse of sterilants (formaldehyde)
  Kinked or defective tubing—trauma to RBCs
  Needle trauma to RBCs
  Subclavian catheter (helmet cells, schistocytes)
Insufficient dialysis
Hypersplenism
Associated diseases
  Sickle cell anemia
  Other hemoglobinopathies
  Connective tissue diseases with vasculitis
Drug-induced
Hypophosphatemia

RBCs, reb blood cells.

3. Kinked blood line tubing. A clinical picture resembling microangiopathic hemolysis (schistocytes, triangle, and helmet cells) may occur due to damage of erythrocytes by kinked or defectively manufactured (narrowed) blood tubing, needle trauma, or catheter malfunction.

4. Copper. Hemolysis may also be caused by copper contaminating the dialysis water supply. The elimination of copper tubing has greatly reduced the risk of hemolysis due to this metal.

5. Formaldehyde. Excessive amounts of formaldehyde entering the circulation after dialyzer reprocessing may be an uncommon cause of hemolysis, due to a direct toxic effect through ATP depletion and to the induction of antibodies to erythrocytes.

D. Treatment. If acute, severe hemolysis is suspected, then the dialysis treatment should be terminated immediately. Circulatory support should be provided as needed, and an electrocardiogram must be obtained to determine if hyperkalemic changes are present and to assess for acute cardiac ischemia. A blood sample should be obtained for determination of hemoglobin, hematocrit, and serum chemistries.

III. Disorders of hemostasis

A. Introduction. The formation of a blood clot in response to vascular injury is a complex and highly conserved process in mammalian species. Disorders of platelet quantity or function lead to bleeding in superficial sites, such as the skin and mucous membranes. Disorders of the coagulation system usually lead to bleeding into deeper structures, such as muscle and joints. Prior to the introduction of dialysis, bleeding tendencies were long recognized among uremic subjects. Dialysis partially reverses the abnormal hemostasis, but ecchymoses, excessive access bleeding, and occasional severe bleeding episodes still occur.

B. Pathophysiology. Many factors contribute to the deranged state of uremic hemostasis, with disorders in platelet function (thrombasthenia) being most important. Platelet aggregation is abnormal, probably due to reduced intraplatelet ADP and serotonin levels, and defective thromboxane A_2 production. Platelet function may also be hindered in uremic patients by increased local nitric oxide production. An adhesion receptor, the glycoprotein (GP) IIb–IIIa complex, plays an important role in controlling the formation of platelet thrombi. In uremic patients, the activation of the GP IIb–IIIa receptor is impaired, but activation is partially restored by dialysis. There has been a suggestion that abnormalities of von Willebrand factor (important for maintaining platelet adhesion in rapid blood flow) may contribute to disordered uremic hemostasis, but study results have been inconsistent. Finally, anemia itself probably contributes significantly to uremic bleeding; abnormally prolonged bleeding time is significantly improved when the hematocrit is increased to greater than 30%.

C. Assessment. Disordered hemostasis should be evaluated in terms of clinical manifestations and by testing of skin bleeding time. Patients with ecchymoses, excessive access bleeding, or any clinically significant bleeding episodes (including hemorrhagic pericarditis) should have platelet count, prothrombin time, partial thromboplastin time, and bleeding time tested. The bleeding time becomes abnormal when the platelet count is decreased, when platelet function is impaired, or if the vascular wall is damaged. The risk for hemorrhage increases when the bleeding time is elevated to more than 10 minutes.

D.   Treatment. Intensive dialysis results in some improvement in bleeding tendency. However, the magnitude of the improvement is insufficient to result in a meaningful decrease in the risk for hemorrhage. The administration of cryoprecipitate (a plasma extract with high concentrations of von Willebrand factor) leads to a significant but temporary improvement in uremic platelet function. Desmopressin (a synthetic analog of antidiuretic hormone) leads to increased release of von Willebrand factor. A dose of 0.3 µg per kg body weight may be administered diluted in 50 mL of saline intravenously over 30 minutes. In a well-designed study, this regimen led to a reduction in bleeding time in 1 hour, which lasted for 8 hours. There were no significant side effects. Finally, repetitive intravenous infusions of conjugated estrogens may reduce bleeding time significantly. In contrast, one oral dose of 25 mg normalizes bleeding time for up to 10 days. This effect is in contrast to the relatively short period of action of cryoprecipitate or desmopressin. We would recommend the use of desmopressin and cryoprecipitate empirically for dialysis patients with severe acute bleeding. In contrast, conjugated estrogens may be helpful in correcting an abnormal bleeding time prior to planned surgery or to treat chronic gastrointestinal bleeding in patients with telangiectasia. Estrogens alone, PO, IV, or transdermally (Sloand and Schiff, 1995) or estrogen-progesteron combinations have all been used (Noris and Remuzzi, 1999). See internet references for detailed dosing protocols.

SELECTED READINGS

Bailie GR, et al. Special report: erythropoietin and iron use in peritoneal dialysis patients: report from the 1997 HCFA End-Stage Renal Disease Core Indicators Project. *Am J Kidney Dis* 1999;33: 1187–1190.

Besarab A, et al. The effects of normal as compared with low hematocrit values in patients with cardiac disease who are receiving hemodialysis and epoetin. *N Engl J Med* 1998;339:584–590.

Bode-Boger SM, et al. Recombinant human erythropoietin enhances vasoconstrictor tone via endothelin-1 and constrictor prostanoids. *Kidney Int* 1996;50:1255–1261.

Caravaca F, et al. Antiplatelet therapy and development of hypertension induced by recombinant human erythropoietin in uremic patients. *Kidney Int* 1994;45:845–851.

Collins A, et al. IV Iron dosing patterns and mortality. *J Am Soc Nephrol* 1998;9:988.

Fishbane S, et al. Reduced nPCR in patients with gastrointestinal side effects due to ferrous sulfate. *J Am Soc Nephrol* (Abstr.) 1998; 9:248A.

Fluck S, et al. Chloramine-induced hemolysis presenting as erythropoietin resistance. *Nephrol Dial Transplant* 1999;14:1687–1691.

Foley Rn, et al. A randomized controlled trial of complete vs partial correction of anemia in hemodialysis patients with asymptomatic concentric LV hypertrophy or LV dilatation. *J Am Soc Nephrol* (Abstr.) 1998;9:208A.

Foley RN, et al. The impact of anemia on cardiomyopathy, morbidity, and mortality in end-stage renal disease. *Am J Kidney Dis* 1996;28: 53–61.

Gunnell J, et al. Acute-phase response predicts erythropoietin resistance in hemodialysis and peritoneal dialysis patients. *Am J Kidney Dis* 1999;33:63–72.

Hoen B, EPIBACDIAL: a multicenter prospective study of risk factors for bacteremia in chronic hemodialysis patients. *J Am Soc Nephrol* 1998;9:869–876.

Ifudu O, et al. The intensity of hemodialysis and the response to erythropoietin in patients with end-stage renal disease. *N Engl J Med* 1996;334:420–425.

Kaufman JS, et al. Subcutaneous compared with intravenous epoetin in patients receiving hemodialysis. Department of Veterans Affairs Cooperative Study Group on Erythropoietin in Hemodialysis Patients. *N Engl J Med* 1998;339:578–583.

Macdougall IC, et al. Pharmacokinetics of novel erythropoiesis stimulating protein (NESP) compared with epoietin alfa in dialysis patients. *J Am Soc Nephrol* 1999;10:2392–2395.

Ma JZ, Ebben J, Collins AJ. Hematocrit level and associated mortality in hemodialysis patients. *J Am Soc Nephrol* 1999;10:610–619 (abst).

Ma JZ, et al. Hematocrit level and associated mortality in hemodialysis patients. *J Am Soc Nephrol* 1999;10:610–615.

Nissenson AR, et al. Sodium ferric gluconate complex in sucrose is safe and effective in hemodialysis patients: North American Clinical Trial. *Am J Kidney Dis* 1999;33:471–482.

NKF–DOQI. Anemia guidelines. *Am J Kidney Dis* 1997;30(4 Suppl 3): S192–S240.

NKF-DOQI clinical practice guidelines for the treatment of anemia of chronic renal failure. National Kidney Foundation-Dialysis Outcomes Quality Initiative. *Am J Kidney Dis* 1997;(4 Suppl 3):S192–S240.

Noris M, Remuzzi G. Uremic bleeding: closing the circle after 30 years of controversies? *Blood*. 1999;94:2569–2574.

Otti T, et al. Comparison of blood loss with different high flux and high efficiency hemodialysis membranes. *J Am Soc Nephrol* (Abstr.) 1998; 9:221A.

Roob JM, et al. Vitamin E attenuates oxidative stress induced by intravenous iron in patients on hemodialysis. *J Am Soc Nephrol* 2000; 11:539–549

Seligman PA, Schleicher RB. Comparison of methods used to measure serum iron in the presence of iron gluconate or iron dextran. *Clin Chem* 1999;45:898–901.

Sloand JA, Schiff MJ. Beneficial effect of low-dose transdermal estrogen on bleeding time and clinical bleeding in uremia. *Am J Kidney Dis* 1995;26:22–26.

Tarng DC, Huang TP. A parallel, comparative study of intravenous iron versus intravenous ascorbic acid for erythropoietin-hyporesponsive anaemia in hemodialysis patients with iron overload. *Nephrol Dial Transplant* 1998;13:2867–2872.

Teruel JL, et al. Androgen versus erythropoietin for the treatment of anemia in hemodialyzed patients: a prospective study. *J Am Soc Nephrol* 1996;7:140–144.

Van Wyck DB, et al. Safety and efficacy of iron sucrose in patients sensitive to iron dextran: North American Clinical Trial. *Am J Kidney Dis* 2000;36:88–97.

Xia H, et al. Hematocrit levels and hospitalization risks in hemodialysis patients. *J Am Soc Nephrol* 1999;10:1309–1316.

Internet References

NKF DOQI guidelines for anemia http://www.kidney.org

Anemia management protocols, links and updates http://www.hdcn.com/crf/anemia

Treatment of prolonged bleeding time: protocols http://www.hdcn.com/crf/bleeding

Infections

Joseph R. Lentino and David J. Leehey

I. Derangement of immune function in uremia

A. Etiology. In dialysis patients, there is impairment of several aspects of lymphocyte and granulocyte function. Unidentified uremic toxins are thought to be responsible; malnutrition or vitamin D deficiency can sometimes be a contributory factor. Much of the information about immune defects in chronic renal failure is based on research in hemodialysis patients. Some of the immune defects previously attributed to uremia may be due in part to periodic exposure of the blood to certain dialysis membranes. For example, granulocyte phagocytic ability, natural killer cell function, and lymphocyte interleukin-2 (IL-2) receptor density may be impaired to a greater extent when dialysis is performed using unsubstituted cellulose membranes than when using certain synthetic membranes (Himmelfarb and Hakim, 1994). Peritoneal neutrophil function is depressed due to removal of opsonins (immunoglobulin and complement) in the dialysate.

B. Inflammation, malnutrition, and outcome. A very interesting realization has developed over the past several years, namely, that markers of chronic inflammation, including serum amyloid A, interleukin-6 (IL-6), and C-reactive protein (CRP), are markers of atherosclerosis, cardiovascular disease, and poor outcome, not only in the dialysis population but in the elderly without apparent renal disease. Whether an infectious agent will ultimately be identified as an important cause of this syndrome remains speculative.

C. Clinical implications

1. Chronic inflammatory syndrome and poor outcome. To date, the cause of the chronic inflammatory syndrome associated with increased serum levels of acute phase proteins has not been identified, and it may be multifactorial. In dialysis patients in particular, low serum albumin levels and high death and hospitalization rates have been linked to high CRP levels. Elevations appear to be intermittent and have been associated both with infections and with use of indwelling venous catheters. One report that needs to be confirmed suggests that use of ultrapure dialysate results in lower plasma CRP levels (Panichi et al, 1998).

2. Increased susceptibility to infection

a. Frequency of bacterial infections. Bacterial infections occur more often in dialysis patients than in their nonuremic counterparts; the increase is probably related more to frequent violation of normal skin and mucosal barriers than to immune system dysfunction.

b. Severity of bacterial infections. Bacterial infections in dialysis patients appear to progress more quickly and to resolve less promptly than in nonuremic patients. However, formal documentation of this clinical impression is lacking. Whereas dialysis patients should not be considered as immunocompromised hosts in the same fashion as transplant recipients, initiation of antimicrobial therapy should be considered sooner and at a lower level of documentation of bacterial infection than in nonuremic patients.

c.   Morbidity and mortality as a function of dialyzer membrane. Whether the finding of immune defects present "chronically" (i.e., after 2 weeks of dialysis) in patients being dialyzed with unsubstituted cellulose membranes translates to increased infectious morbidity and mortality is not yet clear.

d.   Susceptibility to chronic hepatitis B and C infections. See Sections IV.B and IV.C.

3.   Reduced efficacy of vaccines. See Section V.

II.   Derangement of temperature control in uremia

A.   Baseline hypothermia in uremic patients. In 50% of hemodialysis patients, the predialysis body temperature is subnormal. The reason for this is unknown.

B.   Reduced pyrexic response associated with infections. Uremia per se does not appear to affect the temperature response to pyrogens. In addition, the degree of interleukin-1 (IL-1) production by stimulated uremic monocytes is normal. However, because of baseline hypothermia, and possibly because of frequently coexisting malnutrition, severe infections in some dialysis patients may not be associated with fever.

III.   Bacterial infections in dialysis patients

A.   Related to the access site

1.   Hemodialysis patients

a.   Incidence. The access site is the source of 50%–80% of bacteremias in hemodialysis patients. Bacteremia can lead to endocarditis, meningitis, osteomyelitis, paraspinal abscess or formation of septic emboli.

(1)   Temporary vascular access infections. Femoral venous catheter infections are rare when catheters are used for only a brief duration (no more than 72 hours). Some centers have used these catheters in ambulatory patients for more prolonged periods (Firek et al, 1987). However, our experience is that use of a femoral catheter for more than 3–7 days results in an unacceptably high infection rate. Internal jugular venous catheters are generally employed when access is required for longer periods. However, the incidence of serious infection increases with length of use, with a substantial incidence of bacteremia associated with catheters left in place for more than 3 weeks (Schwab et al, 1988). Strategies to minimize the risk of infection if the need for temporary hemodialysis access is expected to exceed 3 weeks include the following (in order of preference): (a) insertion of a cuffed catheter, (b) replacement of the catheter with a new catheter at a new site every 3 weeks, and (c) replacement of the catheter with a new one at the same site over a guide wire (providing there is no evidence of infection at the catheter exit site).

(2)   Permanent vascular access infections. Arteriovenous (AV) fistulas and grafts do not involve a skin exit site and hence are associated with lower rates of infection than venous catheters. The infection rate with AV fistulas is lower than with AV grafts.

b. Responsible flora. Local infections of the access site or those related to use of the access are usually secondary to common skin flora, such as staphylococci or streptococci. On occasion, other aerobic organisms, such as diphtheroids or gram-negative bacilli, and even anaerobes are the cause of infection.

c. Clinical presentation. The dialysis patient with bacteremia generally presents with chills and fever and may appear toxic. On occasion, however, symptoms and signs of infection are remarkably few or absent. Although redness, tenderness, or exudate at the access site may help to incriminate the site as the source of the infection, in many cases, an infected access site can appear normal. Fever and chills that occur shortly after catheter manipulation (e.g., commencement or cessation of dialysis) suggests catheter-associated bacteremia. Delayed treatment of sepsis in dialysis patients is an important cause of morbidity and mortality.

(1) Pyrogen reaction. Low-grade fever during hemodialysis may be related to pyrogens present in the dialysis solution rather than to actual infection. The time course of fever may be somewhat helpful in making the distinction between pyrogen reaction and infection. Patients with pyrogen-related fever are afebrile prior to dialysis but become febrile during dialysis; fever resolves spontaneously after cessation of dialysis. Patients with access site–related septicemia often are febrile prior to institution of dialysis and, in the absence of treatment, fever persists during and after dialysis. (An exception, as noted above, is that patients harboring infected hemodialysis catheters sometimes develop fever and chills only after commencement of dialysis.) Use of high-flux dialysis and dialyzer reuse are associated with an increased incidence of pyrogenic reactions. Blood cultures should always be obtained in any febrile hemodialysis patient, even when a pyrogen reaction is the suspected cause of the fever.

d. Management of presumed vascular access infection. In a febrile dialysis patient with a temporary (internal jugular, or femoral) catheter in place, if there is no obvious source of infection, then blood cultures should be obtained and the catheter removed. The tip of the catheter should be cultured as discussed in Chapter 4. Delay in removal of an infected catheter may result in otherwise preventable septic complications (e.g., endocarditis). If a permanent vascular access site (e.g., AV fistula or graft) appears to be infected, then antimicrobial therapy should be administered promptly, and dialysis should not be performed using the infected access; if response to treatment is not rapid, then early ligation or removal of the access should be considered. On the other hand, in the absence of obvious visual evidence of infection of a permanent access, it is generally safe to employ the access for hemodialysis while proceeding with antimicrobial therapy. We recommend the combination of vancomycin and an aminoglycoside pending culture results, but the initial choice of antimicrobials depends on the sensitivity of organisms prevalent in the patient's geographic region.

(1) Catheter-related bacteremia. The use of cuffed "permanent" hemodialysis catheters has increased in recent years. The presence of the cuff decreases the risk of infection; however, bacteremia associated with use of these devices remains a major problem. In a recent study (Marr et al, 1997), 40% of catheter-treated patients developed at least one episode of bacteremia over a 9-month period. Metastatic complications (osteomyelitis, septic arthritis, endocarditis) or death occurred in 22% of the infected patients. All complications were associated with gram-positive bacteremia. Attempted catheter salvage (antibiotic treatment without catheter removal) did not increase complications but was successful in only one-third of patients. It can be attempted in the absence of overt exit site or tunnel infection. Recent guidelines from the National Kidney Foundation Dialysis Outcomes Quality Initiative (NKF–DOQI) suggest removal of the catheter if the patient fails to improve within 36 hours of starting antibiotic therapy. Once bacteremia resolves, many clinicians prescribe long-term antibiotic therapy (4–6 weeks) in the hope of preventing recurrence. Possibly a better approach is to change the catheter over a guide wire (providing of course there is no exit site infection) followed by treatment with a shorter course of antibiotics (e.g., 2–3 weeks). This approach preserves venous access sites and may decrease the chance of recurrent infection (Shaffer, 1995).

Protocols for prevention of catheter-related infections in place at most dialysis units can decrease the incidence of bacteremia. These include use of sterile gauze (rather than occlusive dressings), wrapping of catheter caps with povidone–iodine solution–soaked gauze prior to cap removal, wiping of catheter hubs with povidone–iodine after cap removal, and appropriate use of masks (patient and staff) and gloves (staff). In a recent randomized study, the use of silver-impregnated catheters did not decrease infection rates (Treretola et al, 1998).

Recently, there has been interest in the "antibiotic lock" technique for prevention and treatment of catheter-related infections. This approach was shown to be useful in home-based parenteral nutrition patients (Messing et al, 1988). In hemodialysis patients, this procedure involves injecting a highly concentrated antibiotic solution (e.g., Vancomycin plus heparin) through the latex cap of the catheter. The antibiotic lock method has been recently employed to treat patients with an infected hemodialysis access device (Boorgu et al, 2000). It is important to note that high levels of certain antibiotics (e.g., gentamicin) are incompatible with heparin.

Another developing preventive strategy is to use antibiotic catheters impregnated with minocycline or rifampin (Darouiche et al, 1999) or with antiseptic compounds.

e. **Prophylactic antimicrobial administration**

(1) **Prophylaxis prior to an invasive procedure likely to result in bacteremia.** Although there is no definite evidence in the literature, it is our policy to administer antimicrobial prophylaxis to hemodialysis patients prior to invasive procedures associated with a substantial risk of bacteremia because of the abnormal vascular communication present. These include dental procedures (especially extractions), gastrointestinal procedures such as esophageal stricture dilation, sclerotherapy for esophageal varices, and endoscopic retrograde cholangiography with biliary obstruction (not necessary for routine endoscopy with or without biopsy) and genitourinary procedures including cystoscopy, urethral dilation, and transurethral prostate resection. The recommended antimicrobial is amoxicillin 2 g 1 hour before the procedure (or ampicillin 2 g IM or IV 30 minutes before the procedure). In penicillin-allergic patients, either clindamycin 600 mg PO or IV (dental or esophageal procedures) or vancomycin 1 g IV (other gastrointestinal and genitourinary procedures) can be substituted.

(2) **Long-term, continuous prophylaxis.** The skin and nasal carriage rate of *Staphylococcus aureus* in hemodialysis patients is about 50%. Prophylactic antimicrobial therapy with rifampin has been shown to be effective in decreasing infections due to this organism in such patients (Yu et al, 1986). Intranasal mupirocin calcium ointment is also effective in eradicating the carrier state and in uncontrolled studies has decreased the incidence of staphylococcal infection. Decision analysis suggests that weekly use of this agent in all patients without screening decreases infection rates and is cost-effective (Bloom et al, 1996). However, controlled trials in support of this contention need to be performed. A major concern is the development of mupirocin resistance with chronic use. Thus, most believe that nasal mupirocin is best reserved for patients with repetitive infections and nasal *S. aureus* carriage.

f. **Vancomycin-resistant gram-positive infections.** Concern about an increasing prevalence of vancomycin-resistant enterococci (VRE) in hospitalized patients has resulted in recommendations that vancomycin use be restricted in dialysis patients. Because of the relatively high incidence of staphylococcal organisms resistant to antistaphylococcal penicillins and cephalosporins, it is currently our policy to utilize vancomycin as initial therapy of life-threatening suspected *S. aureus* infections (e.g., catheter-related bacteremia). If possible, prolonged treatment with an alternative antibiotic can then be employed, depending on sensitivity results. Certain cephalosporins (e.g., cefazolin) have a very prolonged half-life in end-stage renal disease (ESRD) patients and can be dosed conveniently post dialysis.

  2. Peritoneal dialysis patients
  a. Incidence
  (1) Temporary peritoneal catheter infections.
  Temporary uncuffed catheters should not remain in place for more than 48 to 72 hours because more prolonged use is associated with an unacceptably high incidence of peritonitis.
  (2) Permanent access infection. Infection of the skin exit site of chronic peritoneal catheters or of the subcutaneous catheter tunnel can both cause and perpetuate peritonitis; catheter exit site and tunnel infections are important causes of morbidity and often necessitate catheter removal.
  b. Clinical manifestations and management. See Chapters 15 and 19.
  c. Antimicrobial prophylaxis. In the absence of other indications for prophylaxis, we do not routinely administer antibiotics prior to invasive procedures unless a vascular access is present. Long-term, continuous prophylaxis is discussed in Chapter 19.

B. Unrelated to the access site
  1. Urinary tract infection. In dialysis patients, the incidence of urinary tract infection is high, especially in those with polycystic kidney disease. In patients with a neurogenic bladder (e.g., diabetic patients), pyocystis (pus in the defunctionalized bladder) may be an unsuspected source of infection. See Chapter 35 for a full discussion of these topics.
  2. Pneumonia. Pneumonia is an important cause of mortality in this population; the possibility of gram-negative infection should be considered in patients dialyzed in a hospital setting. Dialysis patients may have unusual pulmonary infiltrates due to pulmonary calcification (now uncommon), which can resemble those due to pneumonia.
  3. Intra-abdominal infections. Diverticulosis and diverticulitis occur not uncommonly in dialysis patients and especially in those with polycystic kidney disease. In peritoneal dialysis patients, the differentiation between dialysis-associated peritonitis and peritonitis due to a disease process involving the abdominal viscera can be difficult (see Chapters 19 and 34). Acalculous cholecystitis has been reported. Intestinal infarction can occur as a complication of hypotension occurring during a dialysis session or between dialyses; bowel infarction should always be suspected in a dialysis patient with unexplained, refractory septic shock. Adrenal insufficiency may present with abdominal pain and hypotension, mimicking peritonitis. Since many patients are begun on peritoneal dialysis after a failed transplant and discontinuation of steroids, this possibility should be kept in mind.
  4. Tuberculosis. The incidence of tuberculosis has been estimated to be as much as 10-fold higher among hemodialysis patients than among the general population. Tuberculosis in hemodialysis patients is frequently extrapulmonary; disseminated disease may occur in the absence of chest x-ray

abnormalities. Difficulty in making the diagnosis is increased because delayed skin hypersensitivity to tuberculin reagent is often absent or diminished due to cutaneous anergy. A number of subtle, atypical presentations of tuberculosis can be encountered; for instance, patients may present with ascites and intermittent fever only, or with hepatomegaly, weight loss, and anorexia. The diagnosis of tuberculosis in extrapulmonary cases is usually made by demonstrating typical caseating granulomas on pleural or hepatic biopsy or by recovery of tubercle bacilli from culture of the biopsy material. When the index of suspicion for tuberculosis is high, presumptive therapy with antitubercular agents is sometimes warranted. Mortality in dialysis patients with tuberculosis has been reported to be as high as 40%.

    5. Listeriosis. Listeriosis, an unusual infection in the non-immunocompromised host, has been reported to occur in hemodialysis patients suffering from iron overload. The mechanism by which iron overload predisposes to listeriosis is speculative.

    6. *Salmonella* septicemia. In dialysis patients, severe *Salmonella* septicemia has been noted to occur; in nonuremic patients, *Salmonella* enteritis rarely progresses to sepsis.

    7. *Yersinia* septicemia. This infection has been reported in dialysis patients receiving deferoxamine chelation therapy. How deferoxamine administration increases the risk of severe *Yersinia* infection is unknown.

    8. Mucormycosis. This sometimes fatal infection is seen with unusual frequency in patients being treated with deferoxamine (see Chapter 31).

    9. *Helicobacter pylori*. Although patients with ESRD frequently have upper gastrointestinal complications, the prevalence of this infection appears to be the same in ESRD patients as in patients with normal renal function. Therapy is the same as in patients without ESRD.

IV. Viral infections

  A. Hepatitis A. The incidence of hepatitis A in dialysis patients is no greater than in the general population, given that transmission is usually by the fecal–oral route. The disease pursues the usual clinical course in dialysis patients. Chronic hepatitis as a result of hepatitis A infection is believed to occur rarely, if at all.

  B. Hepatitis B

    1. Epidemiology

      a. Hemodialysis patients. The incidence of infection with hepatitis B virus (HBV) has continued to decline; it was 0.06% among hemodialysis patients in 1995 (Tokars et al, 1998). The decreasing incidence of hepatitis B infection among hemodialysis patients in recent years is due to better screening of the blood supply for evidence of this infection and decreased transfusion requirements due to the availability of erythropoietin. However, recent outbreaks of hepatitis B in several hemodialysis units have occurred. Although hepatitis B vaccine should be administered to all susceptible hemodialysis patients, by 1995 only 35% of patients in the United States had been vaccinated (Tokars et al, 1998). Of note, only 50%–60% of vaccinated hemodialysis patients develop a protective antibody response.

b. Peritoneal dialysis patients. This group is at very low risk of acquiring hepatitis B infection. Nevertheless, HBV can be transmitted through exposure to peritoneal effluent.

2. Clinical presentation. Hepatitis B infection is largely asymptomatic in dialysis patients. Commonly, malaise is the only complaint. The occurrence of visible jaundice is rare. The only manifestation of infection may be an unexplained, mild (two- to threefold) elevation in the serum aspartate (AST) or alanine aminotransferase (ALT) level. The serum bilirubin and alkaline phosphatase concentrations may remain normal or be elevated only slightly.

3. Chronic hepatitis B infection. Hepatitis B infection in dialysis patients often runs a protracted course and in 50% of cases progresses to a chronic, HB_sAg-positive state. Development of clinically important persistent (or active) hepatitis is not nearly as common. Patients with high serum ferritin levels appear to be at increased risk for developing persistent hepatitis. At this time, treatment options are suboptimal; alpha-interferon may be helpful but results in seroconversion in less than one-third of patients.

4. Routine screening. Hemodialysis patients not known to be HB_sAb-positive should be screened periodically (usually every 3–6 months) for the presence of hepatitis B infection by determination of serum aspartate and alanine aminotransferases and HB_sAg values.

5. Prevention

a. Restricting the possibility of exposure to the virus. Epidemiologic principles can be utilized to decrease the risk of hepatitis B infection, both among patients and among dialysis staff. Table 28-1 lists the required precautions. Some centers recommend that patients with hepatitis B antigenemia be treated with either home hemodialysis or home peritoneal dialysis to decrease the chance of transmission to other patients and staff.

b. Vaccination. See Section V, below.

c. Hepatitis B immune globulin. This should be given after any exposure to the body fluids of a person known to be infected with HBV.

C. Hepatitis C. The prevalence of antibodies to hepatitis C virus (anti-HCV) in dialysis patients is higher than in healthy populations. Use of the second- and third-generation assays has increased the number of patients with positive tests. According to the U.S. Centers for Disease Control and Prevention (CDC), the prevalence of anti-HCV among hemodialysis patients in the United States in 1995 was 10.4% (Tokars et al, 1998). The high incidence and prevalence of HCV infection among dialysis patients can be attributed to several risk factors, including number of blood transfusions, duration of dialysis, mode of dialysis (lower risk in peritoneal dialysis patients), and a history of previous organ transplantation or intravenous drug abuse. Infection rates are declining, however, probably because of both decreased blood transfusions and improved

**Table 28-1.   Infection control practices
in the hemodialysis unit**

1. General Precautions for Staff and Patients
   a. Surveillance for HB_sAg and HB_sAb every 3–6 months
   b. Isolation of HB_sAg-positive patients (not necessary for HIV-
      and HCV-infected patients)
   c. Cleansing of dialysis machines and blood/body fluid–
      contaminated areas with 1% sodium hypochlorite (bleach)
      solution
   d. Dialyzer reuse prohibited for HB_sAg positive patients
   e. Universal precautions (see below)
   f. Protocol for exposure to blood/body fluids (see below)
2. Universal Precautions
   a. Staff must wear fluid-impermeable garments
   b. Gloves are to be used whenever there is potential for exposure
      to blood or body fluids
   c. Gloves must be changed and hands washed between patients
   d. Protective eyewear and face shields are worn when there is
      potential for splashing of blood (e.g., initiation and discontinu-
      ation of dialysis, changing the blood circuit)
   e. No recapping of contaminated needles; prompt disposal in
      appropriate container
   f. No eating or drinking in dialysis unit
3. Exposure to Blood
   a. Testing for HB_sAg and HB_sAb at time of incident and 6 wk
      later
   b. Testing for HIV (employee consent required) at time of inci-
      dent and 6 wk and 6 mo later
   c. If HB_sAg status of source patient is positive or unknown,
      administer hepatitis B immune globulin
   d. Test source patient for HIV (inform patient; consent may not
      be required)

HB_sAg, hepatitis B surface antigen; HB_sAb, hepatitis B surface antibody; HIV,
human immunodeficiency virus; HCV, hepatitis C virus.

infection control practices. Indeed, strict adherence to standard
infection control practice, such as changing gloves between patients, can prevent outbreaks. At the present time, there is no
evidence that sharing of dialysis machines, type of dialysis
membrane used, and dialyzer reprocessing are risk factors.
Therefore, the CDC does not recommend dedicated machines,
isolation of patients, or prohibition of reuse in hemodialysis
patients with anti-HCV.

Some dialysis units do not routinely test for HCV but reserve
testing for patients with biochemical evidence of liver disease.
This approach appears reasonable at the present time because
(a) HCV is not as infectious as HBV; (b) anti-HCV tests do not
distinguish between current and past infection; moreover, up
to 50% of tests may be falsely positive, and thus supplemental
assays (e.g., HCV RNA) are needed, (c) the average interval

between exposure and seroconversion is 8–10 weeks; thus, the anti-HCV test will be negative in recently infected patients.

The prevalence of anti-HCV among dialysis staff is similar to that of the general population (0%–6%). Immune globulin and/or α-interferon for postexposure prophylaxis of hepatitis C in health care workers is not recommended.

Hepatitis due to HCV occurs in less than 1.0% of hemodialysis patients. However, it is an important cause of liver disease in patients on dialysis. Treatment options are suboptimal. α-Interferon results in decreased transaminase levels and improved liver histology in most patients. However, relapses are common after cessation of treatment, and the incidence of side effects (myalgias, headache, fatigue, bone marrow suppression) is substantial. Treatment with this agent is probably most useful in patients in whom transplantation is planned. The combination of interferon plus ribavirin has been shown to decrease the rate of recurrence of infection in nondialysis patients. However, there has been concern raised with regard to the use of ribavirin in dialysis patients because the half-life of the drug is prolonged and it is not removed by hemodialysis.

D. Cytomegalovirus (CMV) and mononucleosis. These viral infections can mimic hepatitis due to B or C virus but occur uncommonly in dialysis patients.

E. Influenza. Dialysis patients are at increased risk for developing complications during influenza infection and should be vaccinated (see below). Use of antiviral agents for influenza prevention and treatment is discussed below (Section VI.B.14).

F. Acquired immunodeficiency syndrome (AIDS). Patients who were receiving hemodialysis prior to 1986 are at increased risk for developing human immunodeficiency virus (HIV) infection if they had received blood transfusions. Since that time, nearly all blood transfusions administered in the United States have been screened for antibody to HIV; the risk of transfusion-related infection with HIV has been greatly reduced.

1. Prevalence. The rate of HIV infection in hemodialysis patients is elevated slightly above that in the general population. Certain units will have higher percentages due to the demographics of their patient population. The prevalence is much higher in large urban areas serving minorities.

2. Clinical manifestations. Dialysis patients who are HIV-positive may be asymptomatic or may present with the full-blown AIDS syndrome. AIDS-related renal disease may be an important cause of renal failure in some patients. A rapidly progressive downhill course of dialysis patients with AIDS has been claimed, but whether the presence of renal disease accelerates the manifestations of AIDS is controversial. An overall survival rate of 50% over a 2-year period has been reported in one series of 32 patients. Prognosis of HIV-infected patients is dependent on the stage of HIV disease. Although the 6-month survival rate is only about 25% in patients with full-blown AIDS, patients who are HIV-positive without other clinical manifestations can live for many years on dialysis. Moreover, the use of combination chemotherapy, including protease inhibitors, is continuing to improve overall prognosis in this disease.

    3. Routine screening. There exists much controversy as to whether hemodialysis patients without clinical evidence of AIDS should be routinely screened for HIV positivity. The recommendation from the CDC is that routine screening not be performed. However, some dialysis units (especially those serving high-risk populations) are screening for HIV. Issues of confidentiality must be balanced against the risk to other patients and dialysis staff.

    4. Dialysis in patients who are HIV-positive. The CDC recommendation is that the choice between hemodialysis and peritoneal dialysis should not be affected by the finding of HIV positivity. However, home dialysis will lessen any possible risk to other patients and to dialysis staff. The peritoneal dialysate of HIV-positive patients should be considered infectious and handled appropriately. If hemodialysis is elected, the CDC guidelines maintain that only the usual body fluid precautions attendant to routine dialysis need be followed. The CDC does not recommend that a special dialysis machine be set aside for HIV-positive patients, and dialyzer reuse in HIV-positive patients is not forbidden.

    A number of dialysis units consider the CDC recommendations too liberal and are treating HIV-positive patients in the same manner as patients who are HB_sAg-positive (Table 28-1). Health care workers have developed HIV infection after skin or mucous membrane contact with HIV-infected blood, underscoring the importance of universal precautions during performance of dialysis.

    G. Hepatitis GB virus type C. A new hepatitis virus has recently been discovered. Evidence of infection with this virus was found in 3% of hemodialysis patients versus about 1% in a control population. About half of these patients had concomitant infection with HCV; none had active liver disease (Masuko et al, 1996).

    V. Vaccination. In dialysis patients, the antibody response to a number of commonly used vaccines is suboptimal. Nevertheless, vaccination against *Pneumococcus* infection, influenza, and hepatitis is believed to be indicated for almost all dialysis patients. Table 28-2 lists the recommended frequency of administration of commonly used vaccines. For all vaccines other than hepatitis B, the dosage is identical to that used in the general population.

    A. Vaccination against hepatitis B. All dialysis patients except those who are HB_sAg–positive or HB_sAb (antibody)–positive should receive the hepatitis B vaccine. To increase the chances of successful vaccination, the dosage of hepatitis B vaccine in dialysis patients should be twice the normal amount. A series of four intramuscular injections of 40 μg HB_sAg should be administered to the deltoid muscles at intervals of 0, 1, 2, and 6 months to complete the primary immunization series. Injection into the gluteal muscle is not recommended because gluteal injection has been associated with failure to develop antibody or with loss of antibody 6 to 12 months following immunization (in nonuremic as well as in uremic patients).

Table 28-2.   Immunizations recommended for dialysis patients

Vaccine	Frequency of Administration
Influenza A and B	Annually
Tetanus, diphtheria	Booster every 10 yr
Pneumococcus	Revaccination dependent on antibody response
Hepatitis B	For initial vaccination schedule give a total of four double doses with each injection split between the left and right deltoid muscles
	Consider intradermal vaccination for patients with low serum albumin values.
	Requirement for revaccination not yet known

Overall, the percentage of successful vaccinations against hepatitis B in dialysis patients is less than in the general population, and rates as low as 50%–60% have been reported. Some patients may not have responded because of gluteal vaccine administration or because of failure to complete the vaccination regimen. The response rate is low in patients with low serum albumin values. A new strategy that has been proposed is high-dose intradermal vaccination (Propst et al, 1998).

VI.   Antimicrobial usage in dialysis patients. Table 28-3 lists dosing guidelines for most commonly used antimicrobial, antifungal, and antiviral agents.

A.   General comments. An important trend has become manifest that can affect the way in which drugs are dosed in renal failure patients. Whereas in the past most such patients had minimal renal function and were dialyzed to a modest degree with low-flux membranes, the trend is to dialyze patients earlier, using high-flux membranes and larger amounts of dialysis (e.g., six-times-a-week schedules, high treatment Kt/V doses with thrice-weekly schedules). As a result, such patients with "end stage renal failure" receiving a drug that is completely renally excreted may require more frequent dosing than was previously recommended. This is particularly true for vancomycin, but it applies to many other drugs as well. For this reason, drug levels need to be measured, and in patients with residual renal function, the level of creatinine and/or urea clearance should be quantified when feasible.

B.   Comments pertaining to selected drug groups

1.   Tetracyclines. Use of tetracyclines is generally avoided in patients with renal insufficiency because of the antianabolic effect of these drugs; use of tetracyclines can lead to an increase in the serum urea nitrogen level and to worsening of acidosis. When a tetracycline is needed, doxycycline is often used. Although doxycycline also has antianabolic effects, the

Table 28-3. Antimicrobial, antiviral, and antifungal drug dosages for an adult dialysis patient (70 kgs)

Drug	Usual Nonuremic Dosage[a]	Half-life (h) Nonuremic Patient	Half-life (h) Dialysis Patient	Dialysis Patient Dosage as % of the Nonuremic Dosage	Usual Dialysis Patient Dosage[a]	Post-HD Supplement	Dosage for CAPD
Antimicrobial							
Amikacin	5–7.5 mg/kg q8–12h	3.1	86	10	See text	See text	See text
Amoxicillin	500 mg PO q8h	1.5	10–15	50–75	500 mg q12h	DAD	Same[b]
Ampicillin	0.5–2.0 g q4–6h	1.0	10–15	50	0.5–1 g q12h	DAD	Same
Ampicillin/ sulbactam	1.5 g q6h	See ampicillin			1.5 g q12h	DAD	Same
Azithromycin	500 mg qd × 1d 250 mg qd × 4d	68	?	100	500 mg qd × 1d 250 mg qd × 4d	DAD	Same
Azlocillin	3 g q4–6h	1.0	6	50	2 g q8–12h	DAD	Same
Aztreonam	0.5–2.0 g q8h	1.7	6	25–50	1 g q24h	500 mg	Same
Cefaclor	0.25–0.5 g PO q8h	0.75	2.8	33	250 mg q12h	250 mg	Same
Cefadroxil	0.5–1 g q12h	1.4	22	25–50	0.5–1 g q24–48h	0.5–1 g	Same
Cefamandole	0.5–2 g q4–6h	1.0	11	25	0.5 g q8–12h	500 mg	Same
Cefazolin sodium	0.5–1.5 g q8h	1.8	35	10–25	1.0–1.5 g q48–72h	DAD[c]	500 mg q24h
Cefepime	1–2 g q6–12h	2h	18h	25%	0.25–1.0 g qd	500 mg	?
Cefixime	200 mg q12h	3.6	13	50	200 mg q24h	200 mg	Same
Cefonicid sodium	1.0–2.0 g q24h	4.4	17–56	10	250 mg q72h	No	Same
Cefoperazone	2 g q12h	2.1	2.9	100	2 g q12h	1 g	Same

contin

Table 28-3. *Continued*

Drug	Usual Nonuremic Dosage[a]	Half-life (h) Nonuremic Patient	Half-life (h) Dialysis Patient	Dialysis Patient Dosage as % of the Nonuremic Dosage	Usual Dialysis Patient Dosage[a]	Post-HD Supplement	Dosage for CAPD
Cefotaxime sodium	1–2 g q6h	1.0	2.6	50	1–2 g q24h	1 g	0.5–1 g q24h
Cefotetan	1–2 g q12h	3.0	14–35	25	1–2 g q48h	DAD	1 g q24h
Cefoxitin	1–2 g q4–6h	0.7	18	15	0.5–1.0 g q24h	1 g	Same
Ceftazidime	0.5–2.0 g q8–12h	1.6	18–34	15	1 g q48h	DAD	0.5 g q24h
Ceftizoxime sodium	1–4 g q8–12h	1.4	30	10–25	1–2 g q48h	DAD	1 g q24h
Ceftriaxone	1–2 g q24h	8.0	15	50–100	1 g q24h	DAD	750 mg q12h
Cefuroxime	0.75–1.5 g q8h	1.7	17	33	750 mg q24h	DAD	Same
Cephalexin	0.25–1.0 g PO q6h	0.9	30	25	500 mg q12h	DAD	Same
Cephalothin sodium	0.5–2.0 g q4–6h	0.7	12	50	1 g q12h	DAD	Same
Cephapirin sodium	0.5–2.0 g q4–6h	0.7	2.6	50	1 g q12h	DAD	Same
Cephradine	0.5 g PO q6h	1.3	12	25	250 mg q12h	DAD	Same
Chloramphenicol	1 g q6h	4.0	4.0	100	1 g q6h	No	Same
Ciprofloxacin	500 mg q12h PO / 400 mg q12h i.v.	4.0	5.8	50	250 mg q12h PO / 200 mg q12h i.v.	No	Same
Clarithromycin	250–500 mg q12h	3–7	?	50	250 mg qd	DAD	Same

Drug	Normal dose			%	Dose in renal failure	Dialysis	Supplement
Clindamycin	600–900 mg q8h	2.7	4.0	100	600–900 mg q8h	No	Same
Dicloxacillin	0.25 g q6h	0.7	1.3	100	0.25 g q6h	No	Same
Doxycycline	100 mg q24h	18	21	100	100 mg q24h	No	Same
Enoxacin	200–400 mg q12h	3–6	?	50	200–400 mg ×1 dose; 100–200 mg q12h	No	Same
Erythromycin	500 mg q6h	1.6	4.5	100 (?)	See text	No	Same
Ethambutol hydrochloride	15 mg/kg q24h	3.1	9.0	60	15 mg/kg q48h	DAD	See text
Gentamicin sulfate	1.5 mg/kg q8h	3.1	60	10	See text	See text	Same
Imipenem	0.5–1.0 g q6–8h	1.0	3.7	50	125–280 mg q12h	DAD	Same
Isoniazid	300 mg qd	1.4, 5.2	2.3 (fast), 10.7 (slow)	66–100[d]	300 mg qd	DAD	Same
Levofloxacin	500 mg qd	6–7 h	35 h	25%	250 mg q48h	?	Same
Linezolid	400–600 mg BID	?	?	100% (ND)	?	DAD	?
Lomefloxacin	400 mg qd	8	45	50	400 mg ×1d; 200 mg qd	No	Same
Methenamine mandelate	1 g PO q6h	Avoid in renal failure					
Metronidazole IV	500 mg q6h	8.5	8.5	50	250 mg q6h	DAD	Same
Mezlocillin	3 g q4–6h	0.9	4.0	25	2.0 g q8h	DAD	Same
Moxalactam disodium	0.5–4.0 g q8–12h	2.3	21	25	1 g q24h	DAD	Same

continued

Table 28-3. *Continued*

Drug	Usual Nonuremic Dosage[a]	Half-life (h)		Dialysis Patient Dosage as % of the Nonuremic Dosage	Usual Dialysis Patient Dosage[a]	Post-HD Supplement	Dosage for CAPD
		Nonuremic Patient	Dialysis Patient				
Nafcillin sodium	0.5–1.0 g q4–6h	0.5	1.2	100	0.5–1.0 g q4–6h	No	Same
Nalidixic acid	1 g PO q6h	Avoid in renal failure					
Neomycin	6.6 mg/kg PO q6h	Avoid in renal failure					
Netilmicin sulfate	1.3–2.2 mg/kg q8h	2.7	40	10	See text	See text	See text
Nitrofurantoin	0.5–1.0 g PO q6h	Avoid in renal failure					
Ofloxacin	200–400 mg q12h	7.0	35	25	100–200 mg q24h	DAD	Same
Oxacillin sodium	0.5–1.0 g q4–6h	0.4	1.0	100	0.5–1.0 g q4–6h	No	Same
Penicillin G	0.3–5.0 mU q4–6h	0.5	10	25–50	1.5 mU q12h	DAD	Same
Penicillin V	250 mg q6h	1.0	4.0	50	250 mg q12h	250 mg	Same
Piperacillin	3–4 g q4–6h	1.2	4.2	50	3–4 g q8h	DAD	Same
Piperacillin/ tazobactam	3.375 g q6h	1.2	4.2	50	2.25 g q8h	DAD	Same
Rifabutin	300 mg qd	45 h	45h	100%	300 mg qd	?	?
Rifampin	600 mg qd	3.5	4.0	100	600 mg qd	No	Same
Sparfloxacin	400 mg load, then 200 mg qd	20 h	40 h	50%	200 mg q48h	?	?
Spectinomycin hydrochloride	2 g once	1.7	24	100	2 g once	No	Same
Streptomycin sulfate	500 mg q12h	2.5	70	15	See text	See text	See text

Ticarcillin	3 g q4–6h	1.5	15	25	1–2 g q12h	2 g	Same[e]
Ticarcillin/ clavulanate	3.1 g q6h	See ticarcillin			3.1 g load 2 g q12h	3.1 g	3.1 g q12h
Tobramycin	1.5 mg/kg q8h	3.1	70	10	See text	See text	See text
Trimethoprim (T)-sulfame-thoxazole (S)	See text	11(T) 11(S)	26(T) 35(S)	50	See text	See text	See text
Vancomycin hydrochloride	1 g q12h	5.6	200	< 10	1 g q7–10d	See text	See text
Antiviral							
Acyclovir IV	5–10 mg/kg q8h	3	19.5	15–20	2.5–5 mg/kg q24h	2.5 mg/kg	Same
Acyclovir PO	0.2–0.8 g 5 ×/d				0.2–0.8 g q24h	0.4 g	Same
Amantadine hydrochloride	100 mg q12h	24	500	< 10	100 mg q wk[f]	No	Same
Delavirdine	400 mg q8h	6 h	?	100% (ND)	?	?	?
Didanosine	200–300 mg bid	1.5	?	See text	See text	?	?
Famciclovir	125–500 mg q8-12h	2.3 h	19h	25%	125–250 mg q48h	?	?
Foscarnet sodium	60 mg/kg q8h × 3 wk then 90–120 mg/kg q24h	3.0	?	See text	See text	?	?
Ganciclovir	5 mg/kg q 12–24h	2.7	29	25	0.625–1.25 mg/kg thrice weekly	DAD	Same
Indinavir	800 mg q8h	1.8 h	?	100% (ND)	?	?	?
Lamivudine	150 mg q12h	5–11 h	20 h	12%	50 mg load 25 mg q d	?	?

continued

Table 28-3. *Continued*

Drug	Usual Nonuremic Dosage^a	Half-life (h) Nonuremic Patient	Half-life (h) Dialysis Patient	Dialysis Patient Dosage as % of the Nonuremic Dosage	Usual Dialysis Patient Dosage^a	Post-HD Supplement	Dosage for CAPD
Nelfinavir	750 mg q8h	2–3.5 h	?	?	?	?	?
Nevirapine	200 mg qd × 14, then 200 mg q12h	40 h	?	100% (ND)	?	?	?
Ribavirin	200 mg q8h	30–60	?	50%	200 mg q12h	DAD	Same
Rimantadine	100 mg q12h	32	50	50%	100 mg qd	No	?
Ritonavir	600 mg q12h	3.5 h	?	100% (ND)	?	?	?
Saquinavir	600 mg q8h	1–2 h?	?	100% (ND)	?	?	?
Stavudine	>60 kg; 40 mg q12h <60 kg; 30 mg q12h	1.2 h	7 h	12%	>60 kg; 20 mg qd <60 kg; 15 mg qd	?	?
Valacyclovir	0.5–1.0 g q8–12h	3 h	14 h	15%	500 mg qd	DAD	Same
Vidarabine	10–15 mg/kg/d	3.5^g	4.7^g	75	No data	DAD	Same
Zalcitabine	0.375–0.750 mg q8h	2	?	50%	0.75 mg q24h	?	?
Zidovudine (azidothymidine)	100 mg 5 ×/d	1.0	1.4	See text	See text	No	No

Antifungal

Drug							
Amphotericin B	24	24	35–70 mg qd	100	35–70 mg qd	No	Same
Fluconazole	30	?	400 mg qd × 1d 200 mg qd	100	200 mg qd	DAD	Same
Flucytosine	4.2	100	1.5 g q6h	10–25	0.5–1.0 g q48h	DAD	0.5–1.0 g q24h
Itraconazole	21	25	200 mg q12h	100	200 mg q12h	No	Same
Ketoconazole	8.0	8.0	200 mg q12–24h	100	200 mg q12–24h	No	Same
Miconazole nitrate	24	24	Variable	100	Variable	No	Same

HD, hemodialysis; PD, peritoneal dialysis (primarily CAPD); DAD, no post-HD supplement required, but on hemodialysis days schedule the usual dialysis patient dose after the dialysis session; ND, no or insufficient data, but probably no dose reduction.

Source: Data from *Goodman and Gilman's The Pharmacologic Basis of Therapeutics*, 8th ed. New York: Pergamon, 1990; *Physicians' Desk Reference*, 54th ed. Oradell, NJ: Medical Economics Co., 2000; J. P. Sanford, *Guide to Antimicrobial Therapy*. Dallas: Antimicrobial Therapy, Inc., 2000.

[a] Usual doses recommended for treatment of moderate-to-severe infections.

[b] Give usual HD patient dose.

[c] Prolonged half-life allows dosing thrice weekly post HD.

[d] No dosage reduction needed in patients known to be fast acetylators.

[e] Some recommend increasing the dose during PD to 3 g q12h.

[f] Long-term administration best avoided unless blood levels are followed.

[g] Half-life data are for the hypoxanthine metabolite: Ara-Hx.

percentage renal excretion for doxycycline (normally 40%) is lower than that for tetracycline (60%); no dosage adjustment for doxycycline is necessary in dialysis patients. Doxycycline is poorly removed by dialysis, and hence, the timing of the doxycycline dose relative to a dialysis treatment is not important. Minocycline and chlortetracycline are minimally excreted by the kidney and can be given in the usual dosages.

   2.   Erythromycin. Erythromycin, which has 12% renal excretion in nonuremic patients, requires no dosage adjustment in the presence of renal insufficiency.

   3.   Penicillins. Most penicillins are normally excreted by the kidney to a substantial extent (40%–80%) and are removed to a moderate degree by both hemodialysis and peritoneal dialysis. Therefore, both dosage reduction and posthemodialysis supplementation are generally recommended. From a practical standpoint, postdialysis supplementation is probably unnecessary; however, dosing should be timed so that a dose is given immediately after dialysis. Two exceptions to this general rule are nafcillin and oxacillin; because these drugs are substantially excreted by both the liver and the kidneys, dosage reduction is not necessary in the absence of concomitant hepatic functional impairment. Because of the high therapeutic index of penicillins, monitoring of serum levels is generally not necessary.

   4.   Cephalosporins. Most cephalosporins are normally excreted by the kidney to a large extent (e.g., 30%–96%), and dosage reduction is almost always necessary for dialysis patients. Most are removed to some extent by dialysis. Some of the newer long-acting cephalosporins (e.g., cefazolin, ceftazidime, ceftizoxime) can be administered thrice weekly (e.g., after each hemodialysis session in patients being dialyzed three times a week).

   5.   Aminoglycosides. Aminoglycosides should be administered carefully in dialysis patients. The percentage renal excretion is normally greater than 90%, and very substantial dosage reduction is necessary. Drug removal by dialysis is important, requiring a postdialysis supplement or addition of aminoglycoside to peritoneal dialysis solutions. The therapeutic index of these agents is low, with the major risk (in dialysis patients) being otovestibular toxicity. Loss of clinically important residual renal function may also occur.

   a.   Gentamicin and tobramycin

      (1)   Hemodialysis patients. The usual loading dose (1.5–2.0 mg per kg) is given; subsequently, 1 mg per kg is infused after each hemodialysis session. Although removal of gentamicin and tobramycin is primarily renal, extrarenal excretion of up to 20–30 mg per day has been reported in dialysis patients. Furthermore, many dialysis patients have some residual renal function, accounting for some renal drug removal. The postdialysis dose will have to replace drug lost during hemodialysis and drug removed due to nonrenal and residual renal excretion; thus, the amount of postdialysis dose may vary considerably from the suggested 1.0 mg per kg amount and should be adjusted based on the serum drug levels achieved (see below).

(2) Peritoneal dialysis patients. The easiest strategy for treating nonperitoneal infections in continuous ambulatory peritoneal dialysis (CAPD) and continuous cycling peritoneal dialysis (CCPD) patients is to give the usual loading dose intravenously and then to add 6 mg per L to the peritoneal dialysis solution. Although the strategy is simple, its efficacy and safety have not been evaluated. An alternative strategy for patients receiving CAPD or CCPD would be to give the usual loading dose followed by parenteral (intravenous or intramuscular) or intraperitoneal administration of additional small doses based on serum drug levels.

b. Amikacin. The strategy for amikacin is identical to that for dosing gentamicin or tobramycin. The loading dose should be 5.0–7.5 mg per kg. In hemodialysis patients, the posthemodialysis supplement should be in the range of 4.0–5.0 mg per kg. In peritoneal dialysis patients, the recommended amount of amikacin to add to the peritoneal dialysis solution was formerly 18–25 mg per L. Now there has been a trend to use lower doses of amikacin (e.g., for peritonitis, see Chapter 19).

c. Netilmicin. For netilmicin, the loading dose is 2 mg per kg, with a posthemodialysis supplement of 1–2 mg per kg. For patients receiving peritoneal dialysis, the strategy is similar to that described for gentamicin and tobramycin above.

d. Streptomycin. One-half of the normal (nonuremic) dose should be administered after hemodialysis. In CAPD patients, 20 mg per L should be added to the dialysis solution.

e. Monitoring of serum aminoglycoside levels. Serum drug levels should be monitored in all dialysis patients receiving aminoglycosides, except perhaps those being treated with intraperitoneal aminoglycosides for peritonitis. Monitoring of serum aminoglycoside levels is especially important in cases of serious infection where maximal efficacy is of paramount importance and during prolonged use where otovestibular toxicity is common.

(1) Peak aminoglycoside levels. The volume of distribution for aminoglycosides in dialysis patients is similar to that of nonuremic patients; therefore, peak serum levels should be similar to those in nonuremic patients given a similar dosage with a similar trough (predose) serum concentration.

(2) Trough aminoglycoside levels. In nonuremic patients, dosing is also adjusted based on the trough (predose) level because trough levels greater than 2 µg per mL (gentamicin, tobramycin, netilmicin) or 10 µg per mL (amikacin) are associated with toxicity. In dialysis patients, the altered pharmacokinetics of aminoglycosides may lead to difficulties in dosing if trough levels are taken into account. For example, when gentamicin is given post dialysis, the magnitude of the subsequent trough level will depend on the frequency of dialysis, as well as on the amount administered and the gentamicin half-life. With daily or even every-other-day dialysis, therapeutic peak levels (drawn 1 hour after the dose) of approximately 4.0–6.0 µg per mL may be associated with trough levels (drawn prior to the next dialysis) of greater than 2.0 µg per mL. Thus, (predialysis) trough levels higher than 2.0 µg per mL may need to be accepted if therapeutic peak levels are desired. Whether predialysis trough levels of greater than 2.0 µg per mL in a dialysis setting predisposes to otovestibular toxicity is unknown. This may be an important consideration with prolonged (more than 7–10 days) therapy.

Prolonged aminoglycoside therapy in peritoneal dialysis patients using intraperitoneal maintenance dosages results in random serum aminoglycoside levels of greater than 2 µg per mL (for gentamicin, tobramycin, netilmicin) or greater than 8 µg per mL for amikacin. For example, addition of 6 mg per L of gentamicin into the dialysate may result in a steady-state serum level of 3–6 µg per mL, which may result in otovestibular toxicity. Recommendations include administering intraperitoneal aminoglycoside once daily only or decreasing the concentration of intraperitoneal aminoglycoside when prolonged therapy is indicated (see Chapter 19).

(3) When the minimum inhibitory concentration (MIC) is known. When the organism is known, and the aminoglycoside MIC has been determined, the strategy should be to keep the peak serum drug level at least four times greater than the MIC value. Of course, one cannot exceed maximum safe peak drug levels; however, in some instances the MIC may be quite low, allowing a reduction in aminoglycoside dosage and serum drug levels without compromising treatment efficacy.

6. Trimethoprim–sulfamethoxazole. Trimethoprim may raise serum creatinine values in patients with renal impairment due to interference with tubular secretion of creatinine; this is not accompanied by a reduction in the glomerular filtration rate (as measured by the clearance of inulin). Trimethoprim is normally 80%–90% excreted by the kidney. Renal excretion of sulfamethoxazole is normally 20%–30%. Trimethoprim and sulfamethoxazole are removed well by hemodialysis but poorly by peritoneal dialysis.

For treatment of urinary tract infection, one single-strength tablet containing 80 mg of trimethoprim and 400 mg of sulfamethoxazole should be given twice daily. When giving high-dose intravenous trimethoprim–sulfamethoxazole (e.g., for treatment of *Pneumocystis carinii* pneumonia) in dialysis patients, 50% of the usual dose (the latter being 20 mg per kg per day based on the trimethoprim component) is given; the incidence of leukopenia may be increased when treating dialysis patients, and careful monitoring is essential. For hemodialysis patients, a large postdialysis supplement (e.g., 50% of the maintenance dosage) may be necessary to offset drug removal during dialysis.

7. Pentamidine. This potentially nephrotoxic drug is being increasingly used to treat *P. carinii* pneumonia in patients with AIDS. Renal excretion is minimal, and there is no removal by hemodialysis to speak of; the usual dosage of 300–600 mg can be given.

8. Vancomycin. Vancomycin is an extremely useful agent for the treatment of severe gram-positive infections in dialysis patients. Normally, vancomycin is excreted by the kidneys. Therefore, dosing intervals can be substantially increased in patients with renal failure, with dosing every 7–10 days generally necessary in patients with no renal excretory function. The amount of drug removal by hemodialysis is negligible when conventional dialyzers are employed. If a high-flux membrane is being used, a substantial reduction in vancomycin levels during dialysis may occur; the usual dosing of vancomycin (20 mg per kg initial dose with subsequent doses of 15 mg per kg every 7 days) may no longer be the best strategy. One group has had success giving 500 mg after each high-flux dialysis treatment (Barth et al, 1996). For patients with substantial residual renal function or for patients treated with continuous renal replacement therapies, vancomycin requirements may be substantially higher. Measurement of serum drug levels is necessary to assure adequate bactericidal levels and to avoid ototoxicity. Target peak and trough plasma concentrations are 30–40 µg per mL and 5–10 µg per mL, respectively. In hospitalized patients with life-threatening infection, we recommend administration of 20 mg per kg initial dose with measurement of the peak serum level (1 hour post dose); additional serum values are then obtained daily during the first week of therapy to guide subsequent dosing.

Vancomycin is removed to a minimal extent by peritoneal dialysis, and dosing is similar to that for hemodialysis patients dialyzed thrice weekly with a low-flux membrane.

9. Rifampin. Rifampin is a drug of increasing importance in dialysis patients, primarly because of its application to the treatment of *S. aureus* skin exit-site infections. Renal excretion of rifampin in nonuremic patients is only 7%; dosage need not be adjusted in dialysis patients.

10. Isoniazid, ethambutol, streptomycin. The percentage renal excretion of isoniazid varies depending on whether the patient acetylates the drug slowly (renal excretion = 30%) or rapidly (renal excretion = 7%). Isoniazid is well removed by dialysis. Dosage does not usually need to be adjusted in dialysis patients because decreased renal excretion is balanced by removal during dialysis. However, some authors recommend a small dosage reduction (e.g., 200 mg per day rather than 300 mg per day) because accumulation of isoniazid may occur at the 300 mg per day dosage in patients who are "slow acetylators."

Ethambutol and streptomycin are largely excreted by the kidney in nonuremic patients (80% and 40%, respectively); in dialysis patients, substantial reductions in dosages are required (Table 28-3).

11. Cilastatin. Cilastatin is an inhibitor of the renal dipeptidase enzyme that normally breaks down imipenem. Cilastatin half-life is prolonged from 1 hour to about 15 hours in renal failure, but cilastatin is dialyzable. Imipenem is available only with cilastatin and only in a 1:1 dosage ratio between the two compounds. The recommendations in Table 28-3 pertaining to imipenem apply to the imipenem–cilastatin combination.

12.   Clavulanate. Clavulanate is a β-lactamase inhibitor that slows bacterial breakdown of penicillins and cephalosporins. Clavulanate is popularly combined with amoxicillin or ticarcillin. The half-life of clavulanate increases from 0.075 to about 5.0 hours with renal failure, but clavulanate is dialyzable. The dosing recommendations for the parent antimicrobial in Table 28-3 usually apply as well to the antimicrobial–clavulanate combination.

13.   Fluoroquinolones. Currently, there are seven agents within this class available for use in the United States. Ciprofloxacin, levofloxacin, and trovofloxacin can be administered both orally and intravenously. Levofloxacin dosage in particular needs to be reduced in ESRD patients. Ofloxacin (a racemic mixture of dextro- and levofloxacin no longer used in the United States) also needs dosage adjustment.

14.   Anti-influenza agents. Amantadine, which can help prevent influenza A infection, should be used with great caution in hemodialysis patients because excretion of amantadine is almost exclusively renal. Because of its large volume of distribution, amantadine is removed very slowly by either hemodialysis or peritoneal dialysis. A better alternative is rimantidine, which is metabolized by the liver with less than 25% normally excreted unchanged by the kidney. Dosage is 100 mg daily for 5–7 days in dialysis patients and can be used for prophylaxis or treatment (especially if given within 48 hours of onset of symptoms). The drug is not removed by hemodialysis.

15.   Antiretrovirals. The first antiretroviral drug available for clinical use, zidovudine (azidothymidine), has now been used for more than a decade in patients with ESRD. It is predominantly hepatically metabolized to the inactive glucuronide metabolite 3′-azido-3′-deoxy-5′-O-β-D-glucopyranuronosyl thymidine (GZDV), with only about 20% normally excreted unchanged by the kidneys. However, in renal failure, alteration in elimination, possibly due to GZDV accumulation, necessitates dosage reduction (generally a 50% reduction) to avoid toxicity. We have observed that a 100-mg tid dosage can cause severe granulocytopenia in ESRD patients. There is no significant removal of the drug or its metabolite by either hemodialysis or peritoneal dialysis. Other nucleoside reverse transcriptase inhibitors (didanosine, zalcitabine, lamivudine) all require dosage adjustments in renal failure (Table 28-3). The non-nucleoside reverse transcriptase inhibitors nevirapine, delaviridine, and efavirenz are a heterogenous group with respect to renal clearance (Table 28-3). The majority of the protease inhibitors (ritonavir, indinavir, nelfinavir, and fortovase) require no dosage adjustment in renal failure. However, there are numerous drug–drug interactions with other medications metabolized by the hepatic cytochrome P450 isoenzyme system.

16. Acyclovir, famciclovir, and valacyclovir. These agents are all used to treat herpex simplex and varicella-zoster infections. Published literature and clinical experience suggest that commonly recommended dosages of oral acyclovir for the treatment of herpes zoster in dialysis patients (e.g., 800 mg q12h) are too high and may cause neurotoxicity, especially in CAPD patients (Davenport et al, 1992). The dosages recommended in Table 28-3 are safe in our experience. Both famciclovir and valacyclovir also require dosage reduction.

17. Other antiviral agents. Several antiviral agents are currently employed for the treatment of herpes viruses and CMV in immunocompromised patients (ganciclovir, foscarnet sodium, cidofovir). Ganciclovir dosage needs to be reduced by about 75%. Because hemodialysis results in substantial (50%) decreases in serum drug levels, doses should be administered after dialysis. Little information about dosing in ESRD patients is available for either didanosine or foscarnet sodium. The prolonged half-life of both drugs dictates a reduction in dose interval and total dosage. Foscarnet sodium given in a dosage of 60 mg per kg thrice weekly after hemodialysis appears to be safe (MacGregor et al, 1991). Cidofovir is utilized at a dosage of 5 mg per kg per wk for 2 weeks and then maintained at 5 mg per kg every 2 weeks for CMV disease in patients with normal renal function. With a creatinine clearance of less than 10 mL per minute, the dose is reduced by 90%. There are no data with regard to clearance of the drug via either hemodialysis or peritoneal dialysis. Patients should be closely observed for bone marrow toxicity.

C. Dosage reduction versus interval prolongation. In general, there is no advantage of one form of dosage modification over another (but see comments pertaining to the aminoglycosides above). Either method of reducing the amount of drug delivered over time can be used. The dosing schedules presented in Table 28-3 are, in our opinion, the most practical regimens.

D. Postdialysis supplements. Recommended post-hemodialysis supplements are listed in Table 28-3. These should be given in addition to the maintenance dosages listed. The post-hemodialysis supplements recommended here are geared for a conventional, 4-hour low-flux hemodialysis treatment only. In other instances, the amount of drug removed by hemodialysis is not sufficient to necessitate a posthemodialysis supplement, but timing of dosing so that a dose is given after dialysis is recommended. In general, peritoneal dialysis patients can be treated with usual hemodialysis patient doses. Drug dosing during continuous renal replacement therapy has been reviewed elsewhere (Joy et al, 1998) and is discussed in Chapter 10.

SELECTED READINGS

Barth RH, DeVincenzo N. Use of vancomycin in high-flux hemodialysis, experience with 130 courses of therapy. *Kidney Int* 1996,50: 929–936.

Bloom S, et al. Clinical and economic effects of mupirocin calcium on preventing *Staph. aureus* infection in hemodialysis patients. *Am J Kidney Dis* 1996;27:687–694.

Boorgu R, et al. Antibiotic lock in the treatment of infections associated with use of a subcutaneously implanted hemodialysis access device. *ASAIO J* 2000; in press.

Darouiche RO, et al. A comparison of two antimicrobial-impregnated central venous catheters. Catheter Study Group. *N Engl J Med* 1999;340:1–8.

Davenport A, et al. Neurotoxicity of acyclovir in patients with end-stage renal failure treated with continuous ambulatory peritoneal dialysis. *Am J Kidney Dis* 1992;20:647–649.

Deray G, et al. Pharmacokinetics of 3′-azide-3 deoxy-thymidine (AZT) in a patient undergoing hemodialysis. *Therapie* 1989;44:405–408.

Firek AF, et al. Reappraisal of femoral vein cannulation for temporary hemodialysis vascular access. *Nephron* 1987;47:227–228.

Himmelfarb J, Hakim RM. Biocompatibility and risk of infection in haemodialysis patients. *Nephrol Dial Transplant* 1994;9(Suppl 2):138–144.

Joy MS, et al. A primer on continuous renal replacement therapy in critically ill patients. *Ann Pharmacother* 1998;32:362–375.

MacGregor RR, et al. Successful foscarnet therapy for cytomegalovirus retinitis in an AIDS patient undergoing hemodialysis: rationale for empiric dosing and plasma level monitoring. *J Infect Dis* 1991;164:785–787.

Marr KA, et al. Catheter-related bacteremia and outcome of attempted catheter salvage in patients undergoing hemodialysis. *Ann Intern Med* 1997;127:275–280.

Masuko K, et al. Infection with hepatitis GB virus C in patients on maintenance hemodialysis. *N Engl J Med* 1996;334:1485–1490.

Messing B, et al. Antibiotic-lock technique: a new approach to optimal therapy for catheter-related sepsis in home-parenteral nutrition patients. *J Parenter Enter Nutr* 1988;12:185–189.

National Kidney Foundation. NKF–DOQI clinical practice guidelines for vascular access. *Am J Kidney Dis* 1997;30(4 Suppl 3):S150–S191.

Owen WF, Lowrie EG. C-reactive protein as an outcome predictor for maintenance hemodialysis patients. *Kidney Int* 1998;54:627–636.

Panichi V, et al. Plasma C-reactive protein is linked to backfiltration associated interleukin-6 production. *ASAIO J* 1998;44:M415–M417.

Pollard TA, et al. Vancomycin redistribution: dosing recommendations following high-flux hemodialysis. *Kidney Int* 1994;45:232–237.

Propst T, et al. Reinforced intradermal hepatitis B vaccination in hemodialysis patients is superior in antibody response to intramuscular subcutaneous vaccination. *Am J Kidney Dis* 1998;32:1041–1045.

Rodby RA, Trenholme GM. Vaccination of the dialysis patient. *Semin Dial* 1991;4:102.

Schwab SJ, et al. Prospective evaluation of a Dacron cuffed hemodialysis catheter for prolonged use. *Am J Kidney Dis* 1988;11:166–169.

Shaffer D. Catheter-related sepsis complicating long-term, tunnelled central venous dialysis catheters: management by guidewire exchange. *Am J Kidney Dis* 1995;25:593–596.

Swartz RD, et al. Hypothermia in the uremic patient. *Dial Transplant* 1983;12:584.

Tokars JI, et al. National surveillance of hemodialysis associated diseases in the United States, 1995. *ASAIO J* 1998;44:98–107.

Treretola SO, et al. Tunnelled hemodialysis catheter: use of a silver-coated catheter for prevention of infection—a randomized study. *Radiology* 1998;207:491–496.

Van Geelen JA, et al. Immune response to hepatitis B vaccine in hemodialysis patients. *Nephron* 1987;45:216–218.

Woeltje K, et al. Tuberculosis infection and anergy in hemodialysis patients. *Am J Kidney Dis* 1998;31:848–852.

Yu VL, et al. *Staphylococcus aureus* nasal carriage and infection in patients on hemodialysis: efficacy of antibiotic prophylaxis. *N Engl J Med* 1986;315:91–96.

Endocrine Disturbances

Raouf Sayegh and Victoria S. Lim

In dialysis patients, the various endocrine systems are deranged in subtle, often complex ways. Consequently, interpretation of standard tests of endocrine function and diagnosis of endocrine deficiency or excess can be difficult. Much of the information obtained has been based on hemodialysis patients; data on endocrine function in peritoneal dialysis patients are scant.

I. Insulin

A. Pathophysiology. The most prominent defect in carbohydrate metabolism in uremia is insulin resistance due to postreceptor defect. Insulin clearance by renal and extrarenal mechanisms is reduced and pancreatic β-cell response to hyperglycemia is blunted. All three disturbances are corrected by hemodialysis, but only partially.

B. Clinical issues. In nondiabetic uremic patients, insulin resistance results in a diabetic glucose tolerance curve; fasting blood glucose, however, is generally normal because insulin degradation is impaired. Hyperinsulinemia may stimulate very low-density lipoprotein synthesis, and insulin resistance impairs lipoprotein lipase activity, resulting in increased serum triglycerides. In peritoneal dialysis patients, the insulin requirement is markedly increased due to the exclusive use of glucose as the osmotic agent. The excessive glucose load may lead to obesity and aggravate existing hypertriglyceridemia.

How uremic derangements of insulin metabolism affect diabetic dialysis patients is discussed in Chapter 25.

II. Glucagon

A. Pathophysiology. Plasma glucagon levels are elevated in patients with renal insufficiency as a result of impaired glucagon and proglucagon degradation. Secretion of glucagon appears to be normal as plasma glucagon is appropriately suppressed by glucose administration and stimulated by arginine infusion.

B. Clinical issues. Glucagon augments gluconeogenesis. Hyperglucagonemia, by causing accelerated conversion of alanine to glycogen in the liver, might be partially responsible for protein hypercatabolism observed in some uremic patients.

III. Renin–angiotensin

A. Pathophysiology. Plasma renin activity is usually low in patients with renal insufficiency and undetectable in anephric subjects. In dialysis patients with intact kidneys, an increase in plasma renin activity does occur after volume contraction, assumption of upright posture, and adrenocorticotropic hormone (ACTH, corticotropin) stimulation, but the magnitude of response is blunted.

B. Clinical issues

1. Hypertension with hyperreninemia. In a small percentage of dialysis patients, severe hypertension persists after correction of hypervolemia. In some, but not all, such patients, the renin activity is increased. The mechanism is thought to be stimulation of renin release due to decreased renal perfusion.

Management of hypertension is discussed in Chapter 26.

2. Dialysis hypotension in anephric patients. Hypotension during hemodialysis occurs with greater frequency in anephric patients. The mechanism may in part be due to lack of renin release during ultrafiltration.

IV. Aldosterone

A. Pathophysiology. Plasma aldosterone levels are usually normal or reduced in dialysis patients. Aldosterone response to volume depletion, postural changes, ACTH and angiotensin infusion is generally blunted in hemodialysis patients but was normal in one study of peritoneal dialysis patients. Serum potassium appears to be the most important factor regulating aldosterone secretion. Aldosterone increases fecal potassium excretion and may enhance the transport of potassium intracellularly, protecting against hyperkalemia.

B. Clinical issues. In some dialysis patients, plasma aldosterone may be inappropriately low for the magnitude of hyperkalemia. Administration of fludrocortisone acetate (Florinef), a synthetic mineralocorticoid, has been reported to reduce serum potassium levels in anuric subjects. However, use of fludrocortisone in dialysis patients is probably not advisable because of the drug's substantial glucocorticoid effect.

V. Norepinephrine and epinephrine

A. Pathophysiology. Resting plasma catecholamine levels are generally elevated in patients with chronic renal failure. Increased synthesis appears an unlikely cause because both tyrosine hydroxylase and dopamine β-hydroxylase (DBH), the catecholamine-synthesizing enzymes, are reduced. Decreased renal excretion is well documented. Reduced catechol-O-methyltransferase activity impairs degradation of both norepinephrine and epinephrine. Decreased neuronal uptake as a potential cause is suggested by catecholamine depletion in the adrenergic nerve terminals of the salivary glands of uremic patients.

B. Clinical issues. Despite elevated plasma catecholamine levels, hypotension is a common problem during dialysis. This may be due in part to substantial clearance of norepinephrine during the procedure and in part to blunted end-organ responsiveness to norepinephrine. Whether the elevated catecholamine levels contribute to the hypertension observed in some dialysis patients is an unsettled question.

1. Pheochromocytoma. There is little published information about the diagnosis of pheochromocytoma in dialysis patients. Quantification of urinary catecholamine obviously is not useful. Because plasma norepinephrine levels may be moderately elevated in dialysis patients, the diagnosis of pheochromocytoma cannot be based primarily on plasma catecholamine values unless extremely high levels are found. The utility of a clonidine suppression test in this setting has not been evaluated. Other appropriate diagnostic tests should include computed tomography (CT) and/or magnetic resonance imaging (MRI) of the adrenal glands and abdomen.

Treatment of pheochromocytoma in dialysis patients includes α blockade first, then β blockade if needed. Due to vasodilatation, fluid replacement after tumor resection may be necessary to achieve adequate preload. Central venous pressure and pulmonary capillary wedge pressure measurement may help in the management during the postoperative period.

As continuous venovenous hemofiltration (CVVH) is now widely used in the intensive care setting for treatment of acute renal failure in hemodynamically less stable patients, it is important to note that plasma catecholamine concentrations do not change and that the amount of catecholamine loss is trivial during CVVH.

VI.   Cortisol

A.   Pathophysiology. Plasma cortisol half-life is prolonged in patients with renal insufficiency, and basal as well as integrated 24-hour plasma cortisol levels are not infrequently elevated in dialysis patients. Plasma free cortisol is increased to a greater extent than total cortisol, suggesting decreased binding to cortisol-binding globulin. Increased plasma cortisol levels may be offset to some degree by tissue resistance to glucocorticoid hormone action.

Elevated plasma cortisol levels may sometimes be a spurious finding due to cross-reactivity of some commercially available antisera with steroid metabolites that accumulate and reach higher than normal plasma concentrations in dialysis patients. For this reason, an unexpected high level should be rechecked with another assay procedure.

1.   Suppression and stimulation tests. In dialysis patients, plasma cortisol increases appropriately with ACTH stimulation. The suppressive effect of dexamethasone is demonstrable but blunted. The conventional 1-mg oral dose does not suppress cortisol secretion, but an 8-mg oral dose or a 1-mg intravenous dose will suppress plasma cortisol levels to about 2 μg per dL. In non-uremic patients with Cushing's syndrome, plasma cortisol remains about 10 μg per dL even after intravenous administration of 1 mg of dexamethasone. The blunted suppression of plasma cortisol by oral dexamethasone may represent abnormal pituitary–adrenal feedback or may be a consequence of decreased absorption or accelerated catabolism of dexamethasone.

B.   Clinical issues. Dialysis patients do not ordinarily present with signs or symptoms of Cushing's syndrome. If Cushing's syndrome is suspected, cortisol suppressibility should be evaluated using 1 mg intravenous dose. On the other hand, the diagnosis of primary hypoadrenocorticism in dialysis patients is primarily made on the basis of a low basal plasma cortisol coupled with a poor response to ACTH.

VII.   Thyroid function

A.   Pathophysiology. Serum total thyroxine (TT_4) is either normal or reduced in hemodialysis patients. The free thyroxine index (FT_4I), an indirect estimate of free T_4 derived from the product of TT_4 and the triiodothyronine (T_3) uptake ratio, usually changes in the same direction as TT_4, but to a lesser degree. The free fraction of T_4, measured by equilibrium dialysis, is increased and calculated levels of free T_4 are usually normal.

Serum thyroxine binding globulin (TBG) levels are normal. The discrepancy between T_3 uptake ratio and TBG binding capacity measurement suggests a displacement of T_4 from its binding sites by uremic toxins, inhibitors or drugs.

Serum total T_3 is frequently low; free T_3 index and free T_3 levels are likewise reduced. Serum levels of total reverse T_3 are normal, whereas the concentration of free reverse T_3 are elevated.

Serum thyroid-stimulating hormone (TSH) is normal. TSH response to thyrotropin-releasing hormone (TRH) is either normal or blunted; the peak value may be delayed, and TSH values may remain high for a longer time.

In patients undergoing peritoneal dialysis, significant amounts of TBG, T_4, and T_3 are lost in the peritoneal effluent. Despite these losses, serum TBG remained normal. Serum levels of TT_4 and TT_3 are either normal or reduced.

B. Clinical issues. Serum free T_4 increases transiently after hemodialysis, an effect attributed to heparin, which may compete with T_4 for its binding sites either directly or through raising serum levels of free fatty acids. Long-term hemodialysis is associated with a decrease in the serum levels of TT_4 and FT_4 index. By contrast, serum TT_3 either remained unchanged or increased modestly.

Most dialysis patients are euthyroid. A diagnosis of hypothyroidism should not be made on the basis of low circulating levels of T_4 and T_3 alone but requires the documentation of substantial elevation of serum TSH. Inappropriate thyroid hormone supplementation may result in excessive protein nitrogen wasting as low thyroid hormone in this situation is a protective adaptation for nitrogen conservation.

VIII. Testicular function

    A. Pathophysiology

        1. Gonadal function. Total and free serum testosterone levels are reduced. Decreased production of testosterone by the Leydig cells in the testis is believed to be the cause. The germinal epithelium is also adversely affected: Seminal fluid volume is small, and both the number and motility of sperm are decreased.

        2. Pituitary function. Pituitary function does not appear to be abnormal: plasma luteinizing hormone (LH) is either normal or slightly elevated. Plasma follicle-stimulating hormone (FSH) is normal. Plasma levels of both gonadotropins increased appropriately following administration of gonadotropin-releasing hormone or clomiphene (a nonsteroidal antiestrogen that stimulates gonadotropin secretion by blockade of estrogen-mediated negative feedback on the hypothalamus), suggesting intact pituitary function. Similarly, testosterone administration suppresses plasma LH appropriately.

        3. Hypothalamic function. The evidence supporting hypothalamic dysfunction includes sustained elevation of plasma FSH following restoration of renal function with transplantation and decreased LH pulsatile frequency. Children with renal failure have reduced gonadotropin pulsatility for their stage of pubertal maturation.

        4. Hyperprolactinemia. Serum prolactin levels are elevated in about 30% of dialysis patients; the magnitude of elevation is mild, about three to six times the levels found in control subjects. The presence of extreme degrees of hyper-prolactinemia (>100 ng per mL) is suggestive of concomitant pituitary disease and requires investigation. Increased serum prolactin levels are due to a combination of decreased meta-bolic clearance and increased pituitary secretion. The latter may be augmented by medication, such as methyldopa and phenothiazine.

Hyperprolactinemia in dialysis patients is rather resistant to inhibition by L-dopa or dopamine, but treatment with bromocriptine often can normalize the serum prolactin levels.

B.   Clinical issues. Decreased libido, impotence, and infer-tility are widely prevalent among dialysis patients. One should initially consider nonendocrine causes of impotence, including vascular insufficiency and autonomic neuropathy.

Testosterone administration normalizes plasma levels of the hormone but generally fails to improve uremic impotence. Plasma testosterone levels can also be raised by human chori-onic gonadotropin (hCG) and clomiphene administration. There are no long-term studies regarding these agents. In uncontrolled trials, suppression of hyperprolactinemia by bromocriptine has been reported to improve sexual function in men undergoing dialysis treatment.

In one double-blind study, zinc supplementation (zinc acetate or zinc gluconate tablets) resulted in increased plasma testos-terone level, reduced plasma LH and FSH concentrations, and improved libido and potency. However, many investigators failed to confirm the benefits of zinc treatment.

Treatment of anemia with recombinant human erythropoi-etin has been reported to improve sexual function in dialysis patients. One group of investigators found a reduction in plasma prolactin, normalization of the gonadotropins, and increased plasma testosterone. However, confirmation of these hormonal changes by others is still lacking.

IX.   Ovarian function

A.   Pathophysiology. In most female adult dialysis patients, the plasma estradiol levels are normal, suggesting relatively intact ovarian function. Estrogen normally exerts a negative feedback on pituitary gonadotropin secretion. In uremic patients, this negative feedback relation is intact as evidenced by in-creased plasma LH and FSH values following clomiphene admin-istration and during menopause. However, the positive feedback effect of estrogen on the hypothalamus, responsible for the mid-cycle LH and FSH surge, is lost. The latter was demonstrated by failure of LH and FSH to increase following exogenous estro-gen administration.

B.   Clinical issues. About half of the women on hemodialysis are amenorrheic. In those women who continue to menstruate, the menses are irregular and anovulatory. However, metromen-orrhagia may also occur, increasing the transfusion require-ment. Although infertility is very common, conception can take place, especially in well-dialyzed and well-nourished patients. Thus, contraception is advised in women who do not wish to become pregnant.

X. Growth hormone
A. Pathophysiology.
Renal failure patients have elevated fasting growth hormone (GH) levels. GH is not suppressible following glucose infusion and increases in an exaggerated fashion after arginine infusion. The high serum level is due to a combination of decreased degradation and increased secretion.

GH induces skeletal growth indirectly by inducing hepatic synthesis of somatomedins, which stimulates growth of the epiphyseal cartilage. Somatomedins are now identified as insulin-like growth factors (IGF) I and II. In chronic renal failure patients, circulating somatomedin activity, measured by bioassay, was shown to be reduced despite elevated levels by radioimmunoassay. Such discrepancy is attributable to the presence of somatomedin inhibitors in uremic plasma. Measurement of serum IGF-I and II by radioimmunoassay showed levels ranging from low to higher than normal values.

B. Clinical issues.
Statural growth is impaired in children with renal insufficiency; height age is usually more retarded than bone age. Delayed bone age and sexual maturation are beneficial in that the opportunity for statural growth is prolonged. Attempts to induce growth include adequate dialysis, increased nutritional intake, prevention of renal osteodystrophy, correction of metabolic acidosis, and recombinant human growth hormone (rhGH) administration.

As a result of rhGH treatment, children with renal failure exhibited a rise in growth velocity as well as an increase in body weight and midarm muscle circumference, suggesting a net anabolic effect. This salutary effect was achieved without any adverse effects on glucose tolerance and creatinine clearance. More importantly, the accelerated growth did not hasten bone age maturation, thus preserving growth potential.

XI. Parathyroid hormone (PTH)
A. Pathophysiology
1. Baseline PTH levels.
Plasma concentrations of PTH are elevated in dialysis patients due primarily to increased secretion caused by (a) a reduction in serum ionized calcium level and (b) an elevation in serum phosphorus value. Hypocalcemia in uremia is due to a combination of the following:

1. Phosphate retention and hyperphosphatemia
2. Reduced intestinal calcium absorption
3. Skeletal resistance to PTH

Hyperphosphatemia causes a reduction in plasma ionized calcium levels both by direct complexing with ionized calcium and by reducing residual renal production of 1,25-dihydroxyvitamin D_3. Factors 2 and 3 are, in part, caused by reduced serum levels of $1,25(OH)_2D_3$.

In uremia, the negative feedback between serum calcium and PTH secretion has a higher set point (i.e., a greater than normal level of serum calcium is needed to suppress PTH secretion). Thus, it is advantageous to keep the serum calcium at a slightly higher than normal level.

2. PTH assays.
Interpretation of the various PTH assays is discussed in Chapter 30.

B. Clinical issues.
The principal bone lesion of secondary hyperparathyroidism is osteitis fibrosa cystica. Extra-skeletal manifestations include the following:

1. Calcium deposition in the media of various arteries, sometimes resulting in ischemic necrotizing skin lesions
2. Periarthritis and myopathy
3. Pruritus
4. Anemia and bone marrow fibrosis

The association between hyperparathyroidism and impotence, neuropathy, encephalopathy, and impaired immune response is an interesting speculation and has not been firmly established.

Diagnosis of parathyroid-associated bone disease, and prevention and treatment of hyperparathyroidism, including when to recommend parathyroidectomy, are discussed in Chapter 30.

XII.   Vitamin D_3

A.   Pathophysiology. Vitamin D_3 is hydroxylated at the 25-position in the liver and at the 1-position in the kidney. The 1,25-dihydroxy form of D_3 is biologically the most active form. In dialysis patients, plasma concentrations of $1,25(OH)_2D_3$ are often low; the primary reason is reduced hydroxylation by the kidney. Such reduced hydroxylation may result from either intrinsic renal damage or hyperphosphatemia. The physiologic consequence of such a low 1,25-dihydroxyvitamin D_3 is decreased intestinal calcium and phosphorus absorption, reduced skeletal sensitivity to PTH, and impaired suppression of PTH secretion by serum calcium. The dihydroxy form of vitamin D_3 has been shown to bind directly to its receptors found in the parathyroid glands; binding with such receptors effectively suppresses PTH synthesis and secretion.

B.   Clinical issues. The dihydroxy form of vitamin D_3 is now widely used in the treatment of secondary hyperparathyroidism; it may be administered either orally or intravenously. It effectively suppresses PTH, but hypercalcemia is a common complication.

The administration and complications of vitamin D_3 treatment are discussed in Chapter 30.

XIII.   Calcitonin

A.   Pathophysiology. Calcitonin is produced mainly by the C cells or parafollicular cells of the thyroid gland. It inhibits bone resorption and therefore has a calcium- and phosphate-lowering effect. It is a sensitive marker for medullary thyroid carcinoma. Fractional rise in serum calcitonin following pentagastrin stimulation is similar in ESRD patients and normal subjects but markedly exaggerated in patients with medullary thyroid cancer.

B.   Clinical issues. The basal calcitonin level is modestly elevated in about 30% of ESRD patients.

SELECTED READINGS

Bommer J, et al. Improved sexual function in male haemodialysis patients on bromocriptine. *Lancet* 1979;2:496–497.

Campese VM, Iseki K, Massry SG. Plasma catecholamines and vascular reactivity in uremic and dialysis patients. *Contrib Nephrol* 1984;41:90–98.

DeFronzo RA, et al. Glucose intolerance in uremia: quantification of pancreatic beta cell sensitivity to glucose and tissue sensitivity to insulin. *J Clin Invest* 1978;62:425–435.

Guilloteau D, et al. Diagnosis of medullary carcinoma of the thyroid (MTC) by calcitonin assay using monoclonal antibodies: criteria for the pentagastrin stimulation test in hereditary MCT. *J Clin Endocrinol Metab* 1990;71:1064–1067.

Fine RN. Growth hormone and the kidney: the use of recombinant human growth hormone (rhGH) in growth-retarded children with chronic renal insufficiency. *J Am Soc Nephrol* 1991;1:1136–1145.

Handelsman DJ. Hypothalamic–pituitary gonadal dysfunction in renal failure, dialysis and renal transplantation. *Endocr Rev* 1985;6: 151–182.

Izzo JL Jr, et al. Sympathetic nervous system hyperactivity in maintenance hemodialysis patients. *Trans Am Soc Artif Intern Organs* 1982;28:604–607.

Lim VS, et al. Ovarian function in chronic renal failure: evidence suggesting hypothalamic anovulation. *Ann Intern Med* 1980;93:21–27.

Lim VS, et al. Protective adaptation of low serum triiodothyronine in patients with chronic renal failure. *Kidney Int* 1985;28:541–549.

Lim VS. Renal failure and thyroid function. *Int J Artif Organs* 1986;9: 385–386.

Lim VS, et al. Thyroid dysfunction in chronic renal failure: a study of the pituitary–thyroid axis and peripheral turnover kinetics of thyroxine and triiodothyronine. *J Clin Invest* 1977;60:522–534.

Mahajan SK, et al. Effect of oral zinc therapy on gonadal function in hemodialysis patients: a double-blind study. *Ann Intern Med* 1982;97: 357–361.

Nolan GE, et al. Spurious overestimation of plasma cortisol in patients with chronic renal failure. *J Clin Endocrinol Metab* 1981;52: 1242–1245.

Phillips LS, Kopple JD. Circulating somatomedin activity and sulfate levels in adults with normal and impaired kidney function. *Metabolism* 1981;30:1091–1095.

Ritz E, Bommer J. Discussion: zinc metabolism. *Contrib Nephrol* 1984;38:126.

Robey C, et al. Effects of chronic peritoneal dialysis on thyroid function tests. *Am J Kidney Dis* 1989;13:99–103.

Rosman PM, et al. Pituitary–adrenocortical function in chronic renal failure: blunted suppression and early escape of plasma cortisol levels after intravenous dexamethasone. *J Clin Endocrinol Metab* 1982;54:528–533.

Schaefer RM, et al. Improved sexual function in hemodialysis patients on recombinant erythropoietin: a possible role for prolactin. *Clin Nephrol* 1989;31:1–5.

Schaefer F, et al. Pulsatile gonadotropin secretion in pubertal children with chronic renal failure. *Acta Endocrinol* 1989;120:14–19.

Talbot JA, et al. Pulsatile bioactive luteinizing hormone secretion in men with chronic renal failure and following renal transplantation. *Nephron* 1990;56:66–72.

Weidmann P, et al. Dynamic studies of aldosterone in anephric man. *Kidney Int* 1973;4:289–298.

Bone Disease

James A. Delmez and Michael Kaye

I. Pathophysiology. Bone disease in dialysis patients is due primarily to the effects of secondary hyperparathyroidism. Hyperparathyroidism appears in many patients when the glomerular filtration rate (GFR) is in the range of 50–70 mL per minute. The causes of hyperparathyroidism include hypocalcemia, diminished circulating calcitriol levels, and phosphate retention. Low values of calcitriol are due to reduced 1-hydroxylation of 25-hydroxyvitamin D_3 in the kidney. Calcitriol inhibits parathyroid hormone (PTH) synthesis at the pre-pro-PTH messenger RNA (mRNA) level by acting on calcitriol receptors in parathyroid cells. In uremia, the calcitriol receptor density on parathyroid cells is reduced, making the cells less sensitive to this feedback inhibition. In addition, there is decreased sensitivity of the gland to calcium suppression, perhaps due to a decrease in the number of parathyroid cell calcium receptors (Gogusev et al, 1997). Also, hyperphosphatemia stimulates PTH secretion by a direct effect on the parathyroid gland (Silver et al, 1999). Eventually, chronically low calcium levels, lack of calcitriol inhibition, and hyperphosphatemia cause the parathyroid glands to increase to many times their original size through hypertrophy and hyperplasia.

Hyperparathyroidism is not present in all dialysis patients. In some, the serum PTH levels are slightly elevated, and the histologic bone picture is normal. In fact, an "adynamic" bone condition may develop, associated with few clinical manifestations but with a histologic picture of reduced bone activity.

In dialysis patients exposed to aluminum, toxic effects on bone can occur, either singly or superimposed on hyperparathyroidism. Aluminum-related bone disease is now far less common as the use of aluminum-containing phosphorus binders has dwindled and as dialysate water treatment standards have improved. Aluminum poisoning and hyperparathyroidism interact with each other at both the parathyroid glands and bone (Table 30-1).

II. Diagnosis

A. Bone biopsy

1. Indications and technique. Bone biopsy, essential for the characterization of bone disease in dialysis patients, should be performed for any of the indications listed in Table 30-2. Technical details are summarized in Table 30-3.

2. Information obtained. The following information is readily available from visual examination of the trabecular bone and marrow:

a. Histology

(1) Number of osteoclasts and resorption areas.

(2) Number and size of osteoblasts.

(3) Extent of marrow fibrosis.

(4) Amount and thickness of nonmineralized matrix (osteoid) covering the trabecular surface.

Table 30-1.   Interactions between aluminum poisoning and hyperparathyroidism

- Hyperparathyroidism appears to protect against bone aluminum toxicity. Patients with severe osteitis fibrosa cystica often have minimal aluminum staining on bone biopsy using the less sensitive aluminon stain because the aluminum is rapidly buried and is not visualized on the bone surface.
- Worsening of aluminum bone disease is often seen after parathyroidectomy. This is the reverse of hyperparathyroidism, with aluminum staying on the trabecular surface.
- Aluminum poisoning reduces the degree of hyperparathyroidism, probably by reducing the release of parathyroid hormone by the gland and by decreasing osteoblast activity.
- In severe aluminum poisoning, bone findings of hyperparathyroidism regress and may ultimately disappear.

    b.   Bone formation rate. This is estimated from tetracycline labeling. Because tetracyclines fluoresce, examination of the biopsy under the fluorescent microscope shows the deposited tetracycline and allows a determination of how much bone has been formed in the interval (usually 12 days) between two tetracycline administration periods.

    c.   Amount of surface aluminum staining.

    d.   Extent of marrow iron stores.

  3.   Interpretation

    a.   Hyperparathyroid bone disease. In hyperparathyroid bone disease (osteitis fibrosa), both formation and resorption of bone take place at an accelerated pace due to an increased number and activity of osteoblasts and osteoclasts. Another characteristic finding is increased marrow fibrosis. At times, bone is laid down so rapidly that it is not properly mineralized. In such cases, the amount of unmineralized bone (osteoid) is increased. The bone formation rate as calculated from sequential tetracycline labeling is accelerated. The degree of aluminum staining is usually mild. (Stain covers less than 30% of the trabecular surface.)

    b.   Aluminum-related bone disease. In pure aluminum-related bone disease, static bone histology can be completely normal or can present a picture of osteomalacia. In the latter, numbers of osteoblasts and osteoclasts are reduced, and there is an increased amount of osteoid, pointing to a defect in mineralization. Sometimes increased osteoid is not seen, consistent with an adynamic lesion. The

Table 30-2.   Indications for bone biopsy

- To assess the severity and amount of aluminum storage
- To investigate hypercalcemia
- Before proceeding with parathyroidectomy
- To assess bone pain and discomfort if other tests are inconclusive

Table 30-3.   Bone biopsy

Tetracycline labeling

Prior labeling with tetracyclines provides valuable information about the bone formation rate that would otherwise be unavailable.

1. A commonly used schedule is demeclocycline hydrochloride (declomycin) 150 mg twice daily for 3 days, 12 days without medication, and then tetracycline 250 mg twice daily for 4 days.
2. The biopsy is done 2–7 days after the last dose of tetracycline.

Biopsy technique

1. The usual biopsy site is a point 3 cm inferior and 3 cm posterior to the anterior superior iliac spine. A biopsy from the posterior iliac crest gives less precise information but is usually adequate for clinical purposes.
2. A Bordier-type trephine is used to obtain a transverse core (ideally at least 5 mm in diameter) through both cortices. Alternatively, the biopsy is taken vertically from the top of the crest 3 cm posterior to the anterior superior iliac spine using a trephine or drill.
3. The biopsy is immersed (fixed) in a suitable fluid, such as neutral phosphate-buffered formalin. Processing requires plastic embedding without decalcification and good-quality sectioning and staining followed by skilled interpretation.
   a. Stains used
   For histology: von Kossa, Masson-Goldner's, or modified trichrome
   For aluminum: acid solochrome azurine or aluminon
   For iron: Prussian blue
   b. Unstained sections, 8–20 mm thick, are examined for fluorescence. Sections are also examined under polarized light to determine the amount of woven bone present.
4. If the processing technique and a skilled interpreter are unavailable, the sample in fixative can be sent to a laboratory experienced in processing and interpretation.

---

bone formation rate, as measured by tetracycline labeling, is reduced.

In most instances, aluminon (triammonium salt of aurin tricarboxylic acid) stain covers more than 30% of the trabecular surface. Because the aluminon stain is not specific, false positives can result if there is marked iron overload, a condition readily excluded by staining for iron. False-negative aluminon staining as well as underestimation of the amount of aluminum present is a common problem. Acid solochrome azurine is a more sensitive stain for aluminum than aluminon and shows better correlation with indices of bone formation and bone resorption. Although some investigators have proposed measurement of bone aluminum content, this is not a routine test.

In many biopsies, a mixed lesion is seen with features of both hyperparathyroid bone disease and aluminum toxicity.

   c. Adynamic bone disease. In a considerable number of bone biopsies, an adynamic or aplastic lesion is found without evidence of surface aluminum staining. The osteoblast and osteoclast numbers are reduced, and the bone formation rate, as measured by tetracycline labeling, is abnormally low or zero. The osteoid thickness is normal or reduced, distinguishing it from osteomalacia.

Associated laboratory findings include a slightly elevated serum ionized calcium level and serum intact PTH values that are less than twice the upper limits of normal. The reason that there may be low bone turnover despite elevated levels of the hormone is that there is resistance of the bone to the biologic effects of PTH in renal failure. Low serum levels of bone-derived alkaline phosphatase may be a good predictive test for this condition. Associated skeletal abnormalities include a high incidence of vascular calcification. Vertebral and peripheral bone densities tend to be normal.

The cause of adynamic bone histology is unknown. The condition is associated with relatively low serum PTH levels, so that it may be due to overvigorous suppression of PTH in some patients. It is associated with peritoneal dialysis and may occur in more than 50% of biopsies in this population (Sherrard et al, 1993). It has been theorized that peritoneal dialysis causes better suppression of PTH because higher serum calcium levels are maintained in this population. Also, serum ionized calcium levels may be higher due to lower serum albumin levels. Adynamic bone disease also is seen in older patients and in patients with diabetes. Deficiency of insulin-like growth factors is a proposed etiologic explanation in these groups.

A dynamic bone disease is much more common in whites than in African Americans (Gupta et al, 2000). Adynamic bone histology can develop from, or change into, other histologic pictures. Because the condition is asymptomatic, the need for intervention (other than not overtreating hyperparathyroidism) is unclear. Reliance on the Aluminon stain alone will result in nonrecognition that aluminum is responsible for the low turnover state in some patients.

B. **Symptoms.** Mild to moderate bone disease in dialysis patients can be present without any symptoms. Once symptoms appear, the condition is already quite advanced.

1. **Hyperparathyroid bone disease.** The most prominent symptoms are bone pain, joint discomfort, and pruritus. Metastatic calcification with periarticular calcium deposits may lead to acute joint inflammation or pain and stiffness.

2. **Aluminum-related bone disease.** Aluminum toxicity is associated with bone pain that usually is more severe and incapacitating than that found with osteitis fibrosa. Fractures, commonly of the ribs but also of other bones, are not uncommon. (Fractures may occur with osteitis fibrosa, but they are less common than with aluminum intoxication.) Other symptoms of aluminum poisoning relate to anemia and central nervous system involvement (see Chapter 31).

C. **Signs**

1. **Hyperparathyroidism.** Bone tenderness is the most common finding. Rarely, enlarged parathyroid glands can be palpated on careful examination of the neck. Skin excoriation from scratching attests to pruritus due to metastatic calcification. In severe cases, metastatic calcification sometimes produces palpable calcium deposits under the skin and inflammation of the conjunctiva.

   2.   Aluminum poisoning. Bone tenderness may be present as well. Signs of aluminum-related neurologic involvement and anemia are discussed in Chapter 31.

D.   Laboratory findings

   1.   Hyperparathyroidism

   a.   Alkaline phosphatase. The serum level of bone-derived alkaline phosphatase will be uniformly elevated, at times reaching values 10 times the upper limit of normal. Alkaline phosphatase originates from sources in addition to bone (osteoblasts), the most important being liver, intestine, and kidney, and it is necessary to demonstrate normal liver enzyme values and exclude intestinal alkaline phosphatase elevation before assuming that an elevated total serum alkaline phosphatase level is of osseous origin (see Chapter 24).

   b.   Calcium. Serum total and ionized calcium concentrations are usually normal or slightly low. With advanced hyperparathyroidism associated with a large mass of autonomous parathyroid tissue, hypercalcemia may be present. Usually this is mild, not exceeding 12 mg per dL (3 mM). Hypercalcemia may also appear during treatment of hyperparathyroidism with calcium or vitamin D analogs.

   c.   Phosphorus. Serum inorganic phosphorus levels usually are elevated predialysis and commonly are 6–7 mg per dL (2–2.3 mM) or higher. Although PTH and phosphorus levels correlate, serum phosphorus values are a poor guide to the severity of the hyperparathyroidism.

   d.   Parathyroid hormone. Invariably, serum PTH levels are quite elevated. PTH is composed of 84 amino acids, with biologic activity present in the N-terminal region. There are several assays that measure only the intact hormone, and they usually correlate with the severity of osteitis fibrosa. Their use has reached worldwide popularity and acceptance. The assays are quickly performed, are reproducible, and measure biologically active hormone levels in plasma. Because the degradation rate of intact hormone is rapid (minutes), fluctuation in serum PTH levels over time can be readily detected. Normal values are 10–65 pg per mL, and levels higher than 250–300 pg per mL suggest the presence of hyperparathyroidism. Serum levels over 1,000 pg per mL are seen in patients with severe hyperparathyroidism and suggest that marked gland hyperplasia has occurred.

   Unlike the older assays, the measurement of intact PTH has shown that some dialysis patients have normal or even low levels. This usually is due to aluminum poisoning, but it can be seen following chronic calcium loading and is associated with adynamic bone histology.

   e.   Osteocalcin. Osteocalcin is derived from osteoblasts. Its serum levels are an indication of osteoblast activity and, indirectly, the level of PTH stimulation of bone formation. Standard osteocalcin assays give falsely high values because of the delayed metabolism of fragments. Nonetheless, there is usually a good correlation between osteocalcin and PTH levels.

2. Aluminum poisoning. Laboratory findings depend in part on the stage of aluminum-related bone disease. As the quantity of aluminum increases in the body, hyperparathyroidism tends to regress and may disappear, due in part to a direct inhibitory effect of aluminum on the parathyroid gland. For long periods, moderate aluminum storage and hyperparathyroidism may coexist, and only when substantial aluminum storage has taken place will signs of hyperparathyroidism lessen.

a. Alkaline phosphatase and serum PTH levels. In patients with longstanding aluminum toxicity, aluminum accumulation tends to induce regression of hyperparathyroidism. Then the serum concentrations of bone alkaline phosphatase and PTH are normal or only slightly elevated. In the past, when control of hyperparathyroidism was not well achieved for most dialysis patients, a normal or only mildly elevated serum PTH level was suggestive of aluminum-related bone disease. With recent advances in the control of hyperparathyroidism, the finding is less specific.

b. Calcium. Serum calcium values tend to be normal in aluminum-related bone disease, but frank hypercalcemia frequently develops when calcium salts or calcitriol are administered. Serum calcium levels rise because the absorbed calcium cannot be deposited into bone due to aluminum-related impairment of new-bone formation.

c. Serum aluminum levels. See Chapter 31.

d. Deferoxamine infusion test. See Chapter 31.

E. Radiologic findings

1. Hyperparathyroidism. Radiologic findings usually are absent in mild disease but always are present in severe hyperparathyroidism. The most reliable place to examine in determining hyperparathyroidism is the hands. The characteristic finding in osteitis fibrosa is bone loss (resorption) in the subperiosteal area, best seen on the radial side of the second and third phalanges. Associated erosion of the tuft of the distal phalanx also may be visible (use of a magnifying glass is helpful for recognition) and, when severe, may lead to blunting of the fingertip. The latter changes are pathognomonic of present or past osteitis fibrosa. Evidence of bone resorption also may be seen elsewhere in the skeleton, including the skull, giving it a "salt-and-pepper" appearance, and in the long bones, particularly the lesser trochanter of the femur. Disappearance of the lamina dura may be helpful when nondecayed teeth are present.

Disorganized, accelerated bone formation is associated with osteitis fibrosa and may be visible radiologically as osteosclerosis. Bone scanning using technetium radiopharmaceuticals will show increased skeletal uptake of isotope. The bone/soft tissue ratio of isotope uptake will be increased. Another radiologic finding is that of opacities in the soft tissues and blood vessels consistent with metastatic calcification.

2. Aluminum poisoning. Fractures, particularly of the ribs, are common, and signs of rickets may be seen in children. In some cases of aluminum-related bone disease, radiographic findings consistent with hyperparathyroidism are present, leading the unwary to an improper diagnosis. The most probable explanation is superimposition of the mineralization defect associated with aluminum toxicity on established osteitis fibrosa, retarding the healing of the erosive lesions. Under these circumstances, phalangeal erosions would be a sign of prior active osteitis fibrosa and do not necessarily mean that osteitis fibrosa is active. With progressive aluminum poisoning, the bone scan tends to revert to normal from the previous hyperparathyroid condition associated with a decrease of elevated bone/soft tissue ratios.

III.   Prevention and treatment. Prevention of uremic osteo-dystrophy hinges on minimizing the degree of secondary hyperparathyroidism and reducing the amount of bone aluminum accumulation.

    A.   Hyperparathyroidism. The pathogenesis of hyperparathyroidism in dialysis patients has been discussed in Section I. The primary causes are hypocalcemia, calcitriol deficiency, and phosphate retention. The sensitivity of the parathyroid glands to calcium suppression in renal failure is decreased, so that the serum calcium concentration required to inhibit PTH secretion needs to be 10–11 mg per dL (2.5–2.75 mM) instead of the usual 9–10 mg per dL (2.25–2.5 mM). Hyperphosphatemia can directly increase PTH secretion in renal failure even with normal calcitriol and ionized calcium levels (Lopez-Hilker et al, 1990). In addition, dietary phosphorus restriction prevents parathyroid hyperplasia in uremic rats independent of calcitriol or ionized calcium levels (Slatopolsky et al, 1996).

    There are three general approaches by which the serum calcium level can be maintained and the extent of secondary hyperparathyroidism minimized: calcium supplementation, control of the serum inorganic phosphorus level, and vitamin D therapy. Calcium supplementation and control of the serum phosphorus level are accomplished simultaneously by administration of calcium-containing phosphorus binders.

    1.   Calcium supplementation. Uremic patients may be in negative calcium balance because they often ingest 500 mg per day or less. Also, gut absorption of calcium may be reduced because of decreased serum calcitriol levels. The remedy is to prescribe oral calcium, in the form of calcium carbonate or acetate, and to maintain adequate dialysis solution calcium concentrations to prevent hypocalcemia. If the goal is solely to increase calcium absorption, calcium supplementation should be administered between meals or at night.

       a.   Dialysis solution calcium levels. The calcium level in the dialysis solution for hemodialysis should be between 5 and 7 mg per dL (1.25–1.75 mM). Lower calcium levels may exacerbate hypocalcemia and stimulate PTH secretion. For peritoneal dialysis, the standard dialysis solution calcium value of 7 mg per dL (1.75 mM) is usually adequate. However, low-calcium dialysis solutions (5 mg per dL) are useful to treat patients in whom hypercalcemia develops because of supplemental calcium administration or vitamin D therapy.

2. Control of serum inorganic phosphorus level

a. Rationale. Control of the serum inorganic phosphorus (Pi) level is important for several reasons.

(1) If the serum calcium concentration is to be maintained at the desired value of approximately 10 mg per dL (2.5 mM), a high serum Pi level can lead to an elevated calcium–Pi product. If the calcium–Pi product is greater than 60–70 (when both calcium and Pi are expressed in milligrams per deciliter), the risk of not only metastatic calcification but also of mortality is increased.

(2) High serum Pi concentrations will lower the serum ionized calcium level, resulting in stimulation of PTH secretion.

(3) High serum Pi values have an inhibitory effect on the enzyme that transforms 25-hydroxyvitamin D_3 into the much more active 1,25-dihydroxy derivative, causing or exacerbating vitamin D deficiency. This mechanism, however, is not applicable to severe renal failure.

(4) Lowering high serum Pi concentrations may reduce elevated serum PTH levels (Lopez-Hilker et al, 1990) and inhibit parathyroid gland growth (Slatopolsky et al, 1996).

Although desirable, it is not essential to lower the predialysis or, in the case of continuous ambulatory peritoneal dialysis (CAPD) patients, the average serum Pi level to 4 mg per dL (1.3 mM). An acceptable range is 4.0–5.5 mg per dL (1.3–1.8 mM).

b. Determinants of the serum Pi level (Table 30-4). During hemodialysis, typically 800 mg of Pi is removed per treatment, or about 2.5 g per week. Increasing the time on dialysis is of significant but limited benefit; usually the serum Pi level falls quickly during dialysis, reducing the Pi gradient across the dialyzer and impeding dialytic Pi removal.

Daily Pi intake is tied tightly to protein intake. Foods that have a particularly high Pi content are listed in Table 30-5. It is impractical to reduce daily Pi intake to below 800 mg per day, or about 5.6 g per week. From such an analysis it

---

Table 30-4. Determinants of the serum phosphorus level

Dietary Pi intake

Use of phosphorus binders

Pi absorptive capacity

Administration of vitamin D analogs, particularly calcitriol (vitamin D increases gut Pi absorption and increases Pi mobilization from bone)

Duration, frequency, and efficiency of the dialysis regimen

Residual renal function

Severity of hyperparathyroidism (Pi is mobilized from bone resorption)

Pi, serum inorganic phosphorus.

Table 30-5.   Foods especially high in phosphorus

Dairy products (milk, yogurt, cheese)
Liver, meat
Legumes
Nuts
Whole-grain breads and cereals
Many soft drinks (particularly colas)

is clear that use of phosphorus binders is essential if the serum Pi level is to be controlled. This does not mean that phosphorus need not be restricted. Phosphorus binders still allow up to 50% absorption of ingested phosphorus. If an unrestricted phosphorus intake is allowed (e.g., 1.4 g per day), 9.8 g of phosphorus would be ingested weekly. Even if only 50% were absorbed after phosphorus binding, 4.9 g would need to be removed by dialysis, or 1.6 g per hemodialysis session—twice the usual Pi loss. The result would be severe hyperphosphatemia. Phosphorus binders are indicated in almost all patients undergoing 3x/week dialysis schedules or short (6x/week) daily dialysis schedules. Those patients receiving 6x/week nocturnal dialysis require no phosphorus binders due to increased dialytic removal of phosphorus. No dietary phosphorus restriction is required, and in fact, patients receiving 6x/week nocturnal dialysis need to be supplemented with phosphorus either orally or by using a phosphorus-enriched dialysis solution.

c.   Phosphorus binders

(1)   Calcium-based. Calcium-containing phosphorus binders should be used initially for all patients. They also serve as a source of supplemental calcium. The calcium should be given with meals, in amounts proportional to the amount of phosphorus ingested, to maximize the degree of Pi binding. Administration with meals will reduce the degree of calcium absorption, but the amount of calcium absorbed is still substantial—usually sufficient and sometimes excessive. If the amount is excessive, the dialysate calcium concentration should be reduced.

Two compounds are widely used: calcium acetate and calcium carbonate. Per gram of calcium, calcium acetate is about twice as potent a phosphorus binder as calcium carbonate (Delmez et al, 1992). Thus, the usual dosage of calcium acetate is about half that of calcium carbonate. However, after the difference in dosage is taken into account, overall efficacy of the two drugs appears to be similar. Furthermore, because calcium carbonate is 40% calcium and calcium acetate is only 25% calcium, the number of tablets that must be taken daily is similar for the two drugs. It is important that the brand of calcium carbonate used meet U.S. Pharmacopoeia requirements and dissolve readily; some less expensive brands do not (Mason et al, 1992). Calcium citrate should not be used because citrate ingestion markedly increases gut aluminum absorption.

The dose of calcium-containing phosphorus binder required is highly variable and has to be titrated for each individual. For calcium acetate, a reasonable starting dosage is 600 mg of elemental calcium per day, equivalent to about 2.3 g of calcium acetate. For calcium carbonate, the starting dosage is about 1.5 g of elemental calcium per day. Up to twice these amounts (and sometimes more) may be necessary. The phosphorus content of typical meals should be analyzed by a dietician and the calcium administered in proportion to the estimated amount of phosphorus ingestion. For example, patients who routinely skip breakfast and eat a light lunch should take almost all of the tablets with the evening meal. Gas and abdominal discomfort can occur as unwanted side effects. Patients taking calcitriol or taking calcium compounds inappropriately at a time different from that of Pi ingestion are at greater risk of becoming hypercalcemic. The serum calcium levels of patients who are starting calcium-containing phosphorus binder therapy or whose medication is changing must be monitored weekly until the effect of any medication change has reached a plateau, which may take a month or more.

(2) Sevelamer. Sevelamer, a new Pi binder that does not contain calcium or aluminum (Renagel). The drug is a cationic polymer that binds Pi in the bowel through ion exchange and hydrogen bonding (Chertow et al, 1999). Sevelamer decreases Pi levels in hemodialysis patients and is well tolerated. The major advantage is a greatly reduced risk of hypercalcemia relative to use of calcium-containing phosphorus binders. A slight lowering of serum lipids due to a gut adsorptive effect may be a beneficial side effect (Chertow et al, 1999). Often it is necessary to prescribe 10–15 of the 440-mg capsules to ensure adequate phosphorus binding (Slatopolsky et al, 1999). 800 mg capsules are also available; however, to prevent negative calcium balance, the dialysate calcium should be 3.25–3.50 mEq per L if patients do not receive vitamin D analogs or oral calcium supplements.

(3) Aluminum-based. In general, aluminum-containing phosphorus binders should be avoided in dialysis patients. However, clinicians may find circumstances that they believe require their use. For patients with severe hyperparathyroidism and an elevated calcium–phosphorus product, vitamin D therapy for the control of hyperparathyroidism is contraindicated until the serum phosphorus level is controlled. Giving a calcium-containing phosphorus binder may be possible if the dialysate calcium level is reduced. Alternatively, aluminum-containing Pi binders could be used in such patients; in the short term, their use is unlikely to cause CNS symptoms or effects on bone, provided that concomitant ingestion of citrate (Shohl's solution, calcium citrate, fruit juices, Alka-Seltzer) is avoided. Once the phosphorus level is controlled, vitamin D therapy can be instituted to control the hyperparathyroidism. Subsequently, if the patient has been given aluminum, he or she should be converted to calcium-containing phosphorus binders as soon as possible. When use of an aluminum-containing phosphorus binder is being considered, a superior option is the administration of sevelamer.

Aluminum hydroxide in liquid or capsule form is used, providing approximately 1–4 g of aluminum hydroxide daily. The liquid form of aluminum hydroxide is a more potent binder than capsules, but it is also less well tolerated. Aluminum carbonate also can be used. Like calcium-containing binders, the aluminum salts should be taken with meals, the amount of aluminum ingested being proportional to the amount of food eaten. Constipation is a common side effect and can be combated by administering a stool softener and bulk laxative.

(4)   Mixtures of calcium-, aluminum-, or magnesium-based compounds. Occasionally such mixtures, individually tailored to a patient, may achieve control of the serum Pi level. Magnesium carbonate in conjunction with a 0.5 mEq per L magnesium dialysate was found to allow a decrease in the dose of calcium carbonate by 50% in hemodialysis patients. Despite a mean dose of 465 mg per day elemental magnesium, serum levels did not change nor did diarrhea develop (Delmez et al, 1996).

3.   Vitamin D therapy

a.   Rationale. There are several mechanisms for the beneficial effect of calcitriol in uremic bone disease.

(1) Provision of adequate calcitriol increases intestinal calcium absorption, increasing the serum calcium levels.

(2) Calcitriol therapy inhibits PTH secretion at the mRNA level and also may increase the sensitivity of the gland to the suppressant effects of calcium. Both mechanisms will result in lower serum levels of PTH and healing of osteitis fibrosa.

(3) A direct beneficial effect of vitamin D on bone mineralization in uremia has been alleged, but its existence is controversial.

b.   Indications. If dialysis is begun early and calcium-containing phosphorus binders are begun at the outset, some physicians do not initially treat routinely with calcitriol. If this strategy is employed, both the serum calcium level and the intact PTH concentration should be monitored regularly. Calcitriol therapy should be initiated if the serum calcium level cannot be maintained at 9–10 mg per dL or if the PTH level exceeds 250 pg per mL.

The alternative approach is to start calcitriol at the initiation of dialysis or even during the course of chronic renal insufficiency. The rationale for the alternative approach is to take advantage of the specific inhibitory effect of vitamin D on PTH production and the beneficial effects of vitamin D therapy on the sensitivity of the gland to calcium.

Calcitriol therapy increases gut phosphorus absorption and can exacerbate hyperphosphatemia. It also increases gut calcium absorption, and the combination of vitamin D therapy and calcium acetate or calcium carbonate commonly leads to hypercalcemia. In the past, before the availability of the intact PTH assay, the presence of early hyperparathyroidism was difficult to detect in the dialysis population, supporting empirical early vitamin D treatment. Now even modest elevations of PTH can be detected early, and some hold that treatment with vitamin D can be deferred until it is needed.

  c. Dosage. 1,25-Dihydroxyvitamin D, or calcitriol, is the recommended form. 1α-Hydroxyvitamin D is equally effective. Calcitriol can be given orally or intravenously. Intravenous administration is becoming more popular because compliance is assured and because high serum peak levels can be attained, resulting in effective suppression of PTH secretion and possibly shrinkage of hypertrophied parathyroid glands. Because higher dosages must be given orally to obtain parathyroid suppression, the oral route when employed daily is associated with a higher incidence of hypercalcemia. Intravenous calcitriol appears to be more effective than the oral drug given daily for causing PTH suppression. However, even with low-dosage intravenous calcitriol, hyperphosphatemia may be a troubling problem.

  Calcitriol is given orally starting with 0.25–0.5 µg per day, with the dosage increased by 0.25 µg per day every 1–2 months, provided that plasma calcium levels remain normal. Dosages in excess of 1.5 µg per day usually produce hypercalcemia eventually. Dosage requirements decrease once bone healing has occurred.

  An alternative strategy is to give "pulse" oral therapy of calcitriol. This may be especially useful for treating CAPD patients, for whom intravenous dosing is impractical. The dosing schedule varies considerably. One scheme is to give 1–3 µg twice a week. If hypercalcemia occurs, the dosage should be reduced or, preferably, the dialysate calcium concentration lowered. Pulse oral and intravenous calcitriol are probably equally effective in suppressing PTH and are associated with similar frequencies of hypercalcemia (Quarles et al, 1994). Oral calcitriol is less expensive.

  Pulse calcitriol may be useful in the treatment of moderate to severe hyperparathyroidism. To some extent, the dosage can be prescribed on the basis of the intact serum PTH levels. For PTH values of 250–600 pg per mL, giving 1–2 µg at the end of each hemodialysis session usually suffices. For patients with more severe disease in whom the glands are quite enlarged and with intact PTH levels 500–1,000 pg per mL, higher dosages (2–4 µg per dialysis session) may be required, sometimes for many months. For PTH levels higher than 1,000 pg per mL, 4–6 µg per treatment should be considered. Hypercalcemia and hyperphosphatemia often complicate high-dosage pulse calcitriol regimens. Use of low-calcium dialysate and or sevelamer may be helpful in limiting the incidence of hypercalcemia. Very large glands are unlikely to involute, and often surgical parathyroidectomy is required. However, a preoperative trial of calcitriol therapy helps to heal hyperparathyroid bone disease and reduces the extent of postoperative bone calcium uptake ("hungry bone syndrome").

In general, the goal should be to reduce the serum PTH level to about 150–200 pg per mL. Attempted reduction to the normal range (10–60 pg per mL) may lead to a histologic picture of adynamic bone, which, though asymptomatic, is neither desirable nor necessary.

d. **Problems**

(1) **High calcium-phosphorus product.** When the calcium–phosphorus product, defined as the product of the serum levels of these ions in milligrams per deciliter, exceeds 65, the risk of metastatic calcification is increased. Vitamin D therapy tends to increase further both calcium and phosphorus levels and can precipitate metastatic calcification. For this reason, the use of calcium-containing phosphorus binders, or (in some nephrologists' opinion) sevelamer, is mandatory when giving calcitriol, even in intravenous form.

(2) **Hypercalcemia.** Hypercalcemia is a relative but not an absolute contraindication to vitamin D therapy. Hypercalcemia may be a manifestation of severe hyperparathyroidism or reflection of decreased bone deposition of absorbed calcium due to aluminum-related bone disease.

If aluminum-related bone disease is not present, calcitriol therapy should be instituted. Hypercalcemia should be managed by use of low-calcium dialysis solution. Phosphorus binders must be continued to prevent hyperphosphatemia; if hypercalcemia worsens, the dosage of calcitriol should be reduced.

Patients who become hypercalcemic and have had past exposure to aluminum require bone biopsy to assess the extent of aluminum staining. If substantial aluminum is present, a course of deferoxamine therapy should be considered.

e. **Second generation vitamin D analogs.** One of the compounds being developed, 22-oxacalcitriol, appears to maintain an inhibitory effect on PTH secretion but to have less of a calcemic effect because gut calcium absorption is only mildly increased (Brown et al, 1999). Another analog of calcitriol, 19-*nor*-1,25-$(OH)_2D_2$ (paricalcitol, Zemplar), also possesses low calcemic and phosphatemic activity yet suppresses PTH (Slatopolsky et al, 1995) and is currently available in the United States in the intravenous form. The usual dose is approximately three to four times that of calcitriol. Another analog, a precursor of 1α-(OH)-vitamin D_2 (doxercalciferol, Hectorol) may also be efficacious in suppressing PTH in dialysis patients.

f. **Calcimimetic drugs.** Drugs which act directly on calcium receptors on parathyroid cells to inhibit PTH secretion are now being tested. One such drug, R-568, has been quite effective in lowering both PTH and serum calcium in preliminary trials (Goodman et al, 2000). More developmental work in this area is clearly required.

4. **Parathyroidectomy**

a. **Indications.** Failure of high-dosage intravenous calcitriol therapy to improve signs of hyperparathyroidism suggests the presence of large, poorly suppressible glands that require removal. Prolonged medical therapy of severe hyperparathyroidism risks raising the calcium–phosphorus product to a dangerous range, increasing the risk for metastatic calcification. For this reason, the argument can be made that surgical parathyroidectomy should be considered early rather than late if the hyperparathyroidism is severe.

The indications for parathyroidectomy are listed in Table 30-6. When parathyroidectomy is being contemplated for the treatment of refractory osteitis fibrosa or hypercalcemia, very high PTH levels would be expected, and it is important to document a high serum intact PTH level (e.g., usually more than 1,000 pg per mL) before contemplating surgery. A lower serum PTH level should be suppressible with calcitriol. Also, lower serum PTH levels should prompt one to question the diagnosis and look for aluminum-related bone disease. Bone biopsy should show marked osteitis fibrosa with many osteoclasts, increased tetracycline labeling, and minimal aluminum staining.

Pruritus often responds dramatically to parathyroidectomy that has been performed for other reasons. However, when parathyroidectomy is attempted principally for the purpose of relieving pruritus, the response rate is low. All other procedures, including ultraviolet light therapy, should be tried first. Disseminated skin necrosis (calciphylaxis) is of uncertain etiology, but this potentially lethal complication has been reported to improve after parathyroidectomy if serum PTH levels are high.

b. Relative contraindications. Recent studies have shown that accumulation of aluminum on the bone mineralizing surface increases markedly after parathyroidectomy and suggest that parathyroidectomy should not be done in patients who are aluminum-loaded. With optimum management, a bone biopsy should be performed prior to parathyroidectomy to exclude significant aluminum storage.

c. Surgical strategy. Parathyroid surgery is a complex endeavor and requires the services of a surgeon with expe-

Table 30-6. Indications for parathyroidectomy

- Severe progressive symptomatic osteitis fibrosa (skeletal pain and/or fractures) despite adequate medical management, including serum phosphorus control and calcitriol therapy
- Persistent hypercalcemia if other causes, particularly aluminum toxicity, have been excluded
- Severe intractable pruritus accompanied by evidence of hyperparathyroidism
- Persistent severe soft-tissue calcification despite attempts to control the serum phosphorus level
- Idiopathic disseminated skin necrosis (calciphylaxis) with high PTH levels
- Incapacitating arthritis, periarthritis, and spontaneous tendon ruptures

rience in head and neck surgery. Aberrantly located glands, and three, five, or even six rather than the usual four glands, may be present. An attempt may be made to localize the glands preoperatively using 10-MHz ultrasonographic scanning or thallium–technetium scanning, but this is usually not necessary. Large glands are expected when surgery is being contemplated to control refractory osteitis fibrosa or parathyroid-related hypercalcemia.

Until recently, the operation of choice has been subtotal parathyroidectomy: total resection of three glands and 75% of the fourth. The alternative approach has been total parathyroidectomy, with autotransplantation of some parathyroid tissue into the forearm or more recently, subcutaneously in the presternal area (Kinnaert et al, 2000). Both procedures entail some disadvantages, including the risks of permanent hypoparathyroidism and recurrence (or lack of resolution) of bone disease or hypercalcemia. Recurrence and failure to improve are troublesome problems; often it is uncertain whether the cause is hyperfunction of residual or transplanted parathyroid tissue or the unsuspected presence of an additional gland that was overlooked at the time of surgery.

For patients who are likely to remain permanently on dialysis, some clinicians perform total parathyroidectomy without autotransplantation. One advantage of total parathyroidectomy is that postoperative recurrence points to an overlooked gland. Also, subsequent medical management is simplified, requiring oral calcium carbonate (or acetate) only for phosphorus and calcium control after the initial postoperative period. The degree of postoperative hypocalcemia after total parathyroidectomy does not differ from that after the subtotal procedures, being primarily related to the severity of the osteitis fibrosa rather than the amount of parathyroid remnant. After healing, these patients will have a low bone turnover rate but a normal or increased bone mineral content (Kaye et al., 1993).

d.   Chemical ablation. Percutaneous injection of ethanol into the parathyroid glands of patients with severe secondary hyperparathyroidism has been used to cause regression of the glands and moderate parathyroid hormone secretion. It is performed using ultrasound or color Doppler flow mapping and may be considered in those who are poor surgical risks and in centers with the appropriate expertise (Kakuta et al., 1999). The risk of recurrent nerve palsy has been reported to be low .

e.   Postoperative hypocalcemia. Within several hours of parathyroidectomy, but especially during the first postoperative days, profound hypocalcemia can develop, the extent of which depends on the degree of osteitis fibrosa, which can be predicted by the extent of preoperative serum alkaline phosphatase elevation and bone histology. In addition to oral calcium supplements (2–4 g per day), large dosages of intravenous calcium (0.5–5.0 g per day) and oral or intravenous calcitriol (2–6 µg per day) may be required to maintain serum calcium levels in an acceptable range

(Dawborn et al, 1983). Some advocate starting calcitriol and oral calcium therapy a few days before the procedure even in hypercalcemic patients.

  f. Postparathyroidectomy aluminum exposure. After successful surgery, the danger of aluminum accumulation in bone is magnified, and every effort should be made to avoid aluminum-based phosphorus binders.

B. Aluminum poisoning. See Chapter 31.

IV. Calciphylaxis. There may be two separate syndromes: one in which there is ischemic necrosis affecting primarily the soft tissue of the legs and abdomen, and the other in which extremities are involved, such as the fingertips and penis. Diabetics may be at particular risk in this second group. We would restrict the term calciphylaxis to the first syndrome, in which necrosis may appear in the presence of good control of all parameters of mineral metabolism. Protein C or S deficiency has been suggested as an etiologic factor in some instances, but this has not been confirmed.

  Early signs and symptoms include livedo reticularis and painful, violaceous mottling of the skin, which becomes necrotic, producing boring ulcers with eschar formation and gangrene. The differential diagnosis includes vasculitis, cryoglobulinemia, and warfarin-induced skin necrosis.

  Treatment includes stopping of calcitriol and consideration of early parathyroidectomy. The condition is associated with a high mortality due to associated infection and sepsis. To date, one of us (JAD) has been uniformly pleased with the results following parathyroid gland removal if the PTH levels are very high. There is one case report where the oxygen tension of the tissues around an ulcer was quite low. Hyperbaric oxygen cured the ulcer (Vassa et al, 1994).

SELECTED READINGS

Alem AM, et al. Increased risk of hip fracture among patients with end-stage renal disease. *Kidney Int* 2000;58:396–9.

Bleyer AJ, et al. A comparison of the calcium-free phosphate binder sevelamer hydrochloride with calcium acetate in the treatment of hyperphosphatemia in dialysis patients. *Am J Kidney Dis* 1999;33: 694–701.

Brown AJ, Slatopolsky E. Vitamin D analogs: perspectives for treatment. *Miner Electrolyte Metab* 1999;25:337–41. Review.

Chertow GM, et al. Long-term effects of sevelamer hydrochloride on the calcium x phosphate product and lipid profile of haemodialysis patients. *Nephrol Dial Transplant* 1999;14:2907–14.

Clark OH, et al. Localization studies in patients with persistent or recurrent hyperparathyroidism. *Surgery* 1985;98:1083–1094.

Dawborn JK, et al. Parathyroidectomy in chronic renal failure. *Nephron* 1983;33:100–105.

Delmez JA, et al. Calcium acetate as a phosphorus binder in hemodialysis patients. *J Am Soc Nephrol* 1992;3:96–102.

Delmez JA, Slatopolsky E. Hyperphosphatemia: its consequences and treatment in patients with chronic renal disease. *Am J Kidney Dis* 1992;19:303–317.

Delmez JA, et al. Magnesium carbonate as a phosphorus binder: a prospective, controlled, crossover study. *Kidney Int* 1996;49:163–167.

de Vernejoul MC, et al. Increased bone aluminum deposition after subtotal parathyroidectomy in dialyzed patients. *Kidney Int* 1985;27: 785–791.

Dunlay R, et al. Direct inhibitory effect of calcitriol on parathyroid function (sigmoidal curve) in dialysis. *Kidney Int* 1989;36:1093–1098.

Gallieni M, et al. Low-dose intravenous calcitriol treatment of secondary hyperparathyroidism in hemodialysis patients. Italian Group for the Study of Intravenous Calcitriol. *Kidney Int* 1992;42: 1191–1198.

Gogusev J, et al. Depressed expression of calcium receptor in parathyroid gland tissue of patients with hyperparathyroidism. *Kidney Int* 1997;51:328–336.

Goodman WG, et al. A calcimimetic agent lowers plasma parathyroid hormone levels in patients with secondary hyperparathyroidism. *Kidney Int* 2000;58:436–45.

Gupta A, et al. Race is a major determinant of secondary hyperparathyroidism in uremic patients. *J Am Soc Nephrol* 2000;11:330–4.

Hampl H, et al. Long-term results of total parathyroidectomy without autotransplantation in patients with and without renal failure. *Miner Electrolyte Metab* 1999;25:161–70.

Hellman P, et al. Values of intact serum parathyroid hormone in different stages of renal insufficiency. *Scand J Urol Nephrol* 1991;25: 227–232.

Hutchinson AJ, et al. Low bone turnover disease. *Perit Dial Int* 1996;16:S295.

James LR, et al. Calciphylaxis precipitated by ultraviolet light in a patient with end-stage renal disease secondary to systemic lupus erythematosus. *Am J Kidney Dis* 1999;34:932–936.

Janigan DT, et al. Calcified subcutaneous arterioles with infarcts of the subcutis and skin ("calciphylaxis") in chronic renal failure. *Am J Kidney Dis* 2000;35:588-97. Review.

Kakuta T, et al. Prognosis of parathyroid function after successful percutaneous ethanol injection therapy guided by color Doppler flow mapping in chronic dialysis patients. *Am J Kidney Dis* 1999;33: 1091–1099.

Kaye M. Parathyroid surgery in renal failure: a review. *Semin Dial* 1990;3:86.

Kaye M, et al. Long term outcome following total parathyroidectomy in patients with end-stage renal disease. *Clin Nephrol* 1993;39: 192–197.

Kinnaert P, et al. Long-term results of subcutaneous parathyroid grafts in uremic patients. *Arch Surg* 2000;135:186–90.

Lopez-Hilker S, et al. Phosphorus restriction reverses hyperparathyroidism in uremia independent of changes in calcium and calcitriol. *Am J Physiol* 1990;259:F432–F437.

Martin KJ, et al. 19-Nor-1-alpha-25-dihydroxyvitamin D2 (Paricalcitol) safely and effectively reduces the levels of intact parathyroid hormone in patients on hemodialysis. *J Am Soc Nephrol* 1998;9: 1427–1432.

Martin KJ, et al. Pulse oral calcitriol for the treatment of hyperparathyroidism in patients on continuous ambulatory peritoneal dialysis: preliminary observations. *Am J Kidney Dis* 1992;19:540–545.

Mason NA, et al. Consumer vinegar test for determining calcium disintegration. *Am J Hosp Pharm* 1992;49:2218–2222.

Navarro JF, et al. Relationship between serum magnesium and parathyroid hormone levels in hemodialysis patients. *Am J Kidney Dis* 1999;34:43–48.

Oettinger CW, et al. The effects of calcium carbonate as the sole phosphate binder in combination with low calcium dialysate and calcitriol therapy in chronic hemodialysis patients. *J Am Soc Nephrol* 1992;3:995–1001.

Quarles LD, et al. Prospective trial of pulse oral versus intravenous calcitriol treatment of hyperparathyroidism in ESRD. *Kidney Int* 1994;45:1710–1721.

Sherrard DJ, et al. The spectrum of bone disease in end-stage renal failure—an evolving disorder. *Kidney Int* 1993;43:436–442.

Silver J, et al. Regulation of the parathyroid hormone gene by vitamin D, calcium and phosphate. *Kidney Int Suppl* 1999;73:S2–7. Review.

Slatopolsky E, et al. A new analog of calcitriol, 19-Nor-1,25-$(OH)_2D_2$ suppresses parathyroid hormone secretion in uremic rats in the absence of hypercalcemia. *Am J Kidney Dis* 1995;26:852–860.

Slatopolsky E, et al. Phosphorus restriction prevents parathyroid gland growth. High phosphorus directly stimulates PTH secretion in vitro. *J Clin Invest* 1996;97:2534–2540.

Slatopolsky E, et al. RenaGel, a nonabsorbed calcium- and aluminum-free phosphate binder, lowers serum phosphorus and parathyroid hormone. The RenaGel Study Group. *Kidney Int* 1999;55:299–307.

Sprague SM, Moe SM. Safety and efficacy of long-term treatment of secondary hyperparathyroidism by low-dose intravenous calcitriol. *Am J Kidney Dis* 1992;19:532–539.

Vassa N, Twardowksi ZJ, Campbell J. Hyperbaric oxygen therapy in calciphylaxis-induced skin necrosis in a peritoneal dialysis patient. *Am J Kidney Dis* 1994;23:878–881.

Web References

Uremic bone disease links: (http://www.hdcn.com/crf/bone)

Aluminum Toxicity

Patrick C. D'Haese and Marc E. DeBroe

In dialysis patients, the protective mechanisms against aluminum accumulation (renal excretion and the gastrointestinal barrier) are either absent or highly challenged by ingestion of pharmacologic doses of aluminum salts for the purpose of enteral phosphate binding. The clinical consequences of aluminum poisoning in dialysis patients include a neurologic syndrome, aluminum-induced bone disease, and anemia. At the present time, due to the availability of adequate procedures for water treatment and the almost universal replacement of aluminum hydroxide by calcium-containing phosphate binders, frank aluminum overload is rarely seen. Notwithstanding this, acute intoxications occasionally are reported in centers from various parts of the world. Furthermore, low-level accumulation of aluminum in some patients may lead to subtle disorders at the level of the parathyroid gland, osteoblast function, and hematopoiesis.

Hence, knowledge of patient risk factors, recognition of early signs and symptoms, and regular monitoring of serum aluminum levels (at least twice a year) is still recommended to limit the occurrence of aluminum toxicity in dialysis patients.

I. Risk factors. All dialysis patients who are ingesting aluminum-containing phosphate binders (e.g., aluminum hydroxide or carbonate) are at risk for aluminum poisoning. In the past, aluminum intoxication was also caused by aluminum absorption from dialysis solutions contaminated with high concentrations of the element. With modern production and testing methods, the aluminum concentration in dialysis solutions should not exceed 5 µg per L. Apart from dialysis solutions, certain intravenous preparations (e.g., albumin, hyperalimentation solutions, and some medications) may also contain substantial amounts of aluminum; frequent administration of such preparations may exacerbate aluminum overload in dialysis patients.

A. Hyperparathyroidism protects against aluminum overload. Patients with secondary hyperparathyroidism appear to be relatively resistant to aluminum-associated bone disease, possibly because aluminum accumulation in bone is inhibited in the presence of osteoclast activity. Conversely, after parathyroidectomy, patients are unusually susceptible to aluminum-induced osteomalacia and should be protected vigorously from aluminum exposure. Because aluminum poisoning of the parathyroid glands may suppress the release of parathyroid hormone (PTH), aluminum-related bone disease can occur eventually, even in initially hyperparathyroid patients.

B. Iron depletion. Patients with relative iron depletion constitute a growing fraction of the dialysis population due to the introduction of erythropoietin for the correction of the anemia. With iron depletion, there is increased binding of aluminum to transferrin together with an up-regulation of transferrin receptors in tissues such as the parathyroid gland, which results in an increased uptake of aluminum.

C. Diabetes. Diabetic patients also appear to be sensitive to aluminum-induced bone disease as a result of a low rate of bone formation and an increased rate of whole-body aluminum accumulation.

D. Children. Children are believed to have an increased gut absorptive capacity for aluminum and should not be treated with aluminum-containing phosphate binders if at all possible.

E. Citrate. Ingestion of citrate (e.g., as Shohl's solution or even with citrate-containing juices) along with aluminum in any form can greatly increase gut aluminum absorption and lead to acute aluminum-induced encephalopathy.

II. Signs and symptoms. Signs and symptoms of brain, bone, and blood involvement may or may not occur concurrently, and absence of findings in one organ system does not preclude severe involvement in the others.

A. Neurologic syndrome. Although encephalopathy is now rare, it is the most dramatic and severe manifestation of aluminum toxicity. Symptoms and signs are listed in Table 31-1. The electroencephalographic findings consisted of multifocal bursts of slow or delta waves, often accompanied by spikes. Onset or exacerbation of neurologic symptoms has been observed during deferoxamine (DFO) therapy, presumably because of redistribution of mobilized aluminum into the brain. Also, as noted above, the neurologic syndrome may be precipitated by concomitant ingestion of aluminum-containing antacids or phosphorus binders and citrate.

B. Bone disease. The manifestations of aluminum-related bone disease, discussed in detail in Chapter 30, are summarized in Table 31-2. The definitive diagnosis is established by bone biopsy. Overt bone aluminum accumulation has disappeared over the past few years, but the issue of clinically overt bone disease has switched to interferences with parathyroid gland function and bone turnover.

Table 31-1. Symptoms and signs of aluminum-related neurologic toxicity

Early
Intermittent disturbances (stuttering, stammering)
Dyspraxia

Late
Constant speech disturbances
Apraxia[a]
Asterixis
Myoclonic jerks
Seizures
Personality changes
Global dementia

[a] Apraxia is the inability to perform learned movements on demand.

**Table 31-2. Manifestations of
aluminum-related bone disease**

Symptoms and signs
Severe and diffuse bone pain
Muscle weakness (especially upper legs)
Spontaneous fractures

Laboratory findings
Slightly elevated serum calcium value, which may rise dramatically
    after vitamin D administration
Normal or slightly elevated serum PTH level (i.e., low for the degree
    of renal failure)
Normal serum alkaline phosphatase concentration
Persistence of hypercalcemia after parathyroidectomy
Elevated serum aluminum levels and/or positive DFO test

Bone biopsy findings (see Chapter 30)
Either adynamic lesions or increased amount of unmineralized bone
    (osteomalacia)
Reduced bone formation rate by double tetracycline labeling
Positive aluminum staining at the trabecular surface (however,
    there may be falsely positive staining if iron is in excess)
Elevated bone aluminum content (not as good an indicator as
    aluminum staining)

PTH, parathyroid hormone; DFO, deferoxamine.

C. Anemia. The signs and symptoms of aluminum-related
anemia at the patient level are the same as those of any other
anemia. The anemia is typically microcytic, and the presence of
microcytosis with normal serum ferritin levels suggests that
aluminum intoxication may be the causative factor. Aluminum
might induce a defect in iron utilization or interfere with the
bioavailability of stored iron for erythropoiesis. Aluminum
accumulation has also been associated with a resistance to
erythropoietin therapy.
III. Diagnosis of aluminum overload
  A. Serum aluminum levels
    1. Measurement. Because aluminum is ubiquitous in
nature, special attention should be paid to avoid contamination of the serum sample during handling and preparation
for aluminum determination (Table 31-3). Electrothermal
atomic absorption spectrometry is the method of choice for
determination of the element.
    2. Indications. The serum aluminum concentration is no
longer checked routinely in many parts of the world where oral
aluminum-containing salts are no longer used as phosphorus
binders. However, the possibility of inadvertent contamination of dialysis solution concentrate or feed water must always
be remembered. Some units continue to routinely check serum
aluminum levels every 6–12 months. Of course, serum aluminum levels should be checked promptly in any patient suspected of suffering from aluminum-related involvement of
brain, bone, or blood. Also, unexplained hypercalcemia, espe-

Table 31-3. Serum aluminum levels: prevention of contamination during sampling and aluminum determination

Sampling
Sample should be obtained before heparinization
Use syringes and needles without detectable aluminum release
Use no glassware
Samples must be stored in stoppered plastic tubes pretested for the amount of aluminum that they release

Determination
Use only double-distilled water with aluminum level of <1.0 μg/L
Minimal number of manipulation
Minimal number of reagents
Use pretested plastic sample tubes and sample cups
No pipettes with metallic bodies
Dust-free environment

cially with a low serum PTH, should lead to consideration of possible aluminum toxicity. Determination of aluminum is difficult and should be performed by a qualified laboratory.

3. Interpretation and normal values. In nonuremic patients, the serum aluminum concentration is normally less than 2 μg per L. In most dialysis patients who have been receiving oral aluminum compounds, serum aluminum concentrations being monitored regularly will range between 10 and 60 μg per L. Within this general range, the relationship between the serum aluminum value and the extent of aluminum accumulation is poorly predictable (Table 31-4). Evidence has been presented that in the current dialysis population a threshold serum aluminum level of 30 μg per L is a reliable index for the detection of aluminum overload [defined as a bone aluminum level greater than 15 μg per gram wet weight and/or a positive (more than 0%) aluminon staining]. It has recently been shown that cessation of ingestion of aluminum-containing phosphate binders can quickly (over several days) reduce the serum aluminum concentration. In the data relating baseline serum aluminum levels to aluminum overload that have been generated by many investigators, aluminum-containing medications were usually not stopped prior to measurement of serum aluminum levels. Thus, for the present, if a patient is taking aluminum-containing phosphate binders, then these should probably be continued during measurement of baseline serum aluminum levels, as well as during performance of the DFO test (described below). Recently, an inverse relationship was repeatedly demonstrated between a patient's serum aluminum and iron status.

B. DFO test

1. Rationale. In some patients, particularly those with iron depletion or iron overload or in whom aluminum hydroxide has recently been withdrawn, the serum aluminum level poorly predicts the bone/tissue aluminum deposition. DFO is a chelating compound that liberates aluminum from its body

Table 31-4. Serum aluminum levels: Diagnostic value[a]

Serum aluminum level (µg/L)	Implications
<2	Normal range (subjects with normal renal function)
<30	Aluminum-related bone disease unlikely but possible particularly when patients are iron-overloaded. In these subjects DFO testing is recommended.
30–60	Aluminum-related bone disease quite possible, especially if serum PTH levels are low or low-normal. A DFO test is recommended.
>60	Aluminum-related bone disease probable, but not invariably present, especially if serum PTH levels are high, iron-transferrin saturation is low, or the DFO-test is negative.
>100	Aluminum-related bone disease most probable unless patient is iron-deficient and/or the DFO test is negative. Neurologic disorders should be checked for by taking the patient's electroencephalogram.

[a] Serum aluminum levels are a useful indicator of toxicity when determined at regular intervals (every 6 mo). Monitoring should be performed in all dialysis patients.
DFO, deferoxamine; PTH, parathyroid hormone.

stores (e.g., in bone, liver), causing DFO–aluminum (i.e., aluminoxamine) to enter the blood from these sites. The diagnostic value of serum aluminum monitoring can be enhanced when used in combination with a DFO test.

2. Method. A DFO dose of 5 mg per kg should be used. The DFO test should be performed under strictly standardized conditions as listed in Table 31-5.

3. Interpretation. An increment in the serum aluminum level (ΔSAl) of 50 µg per L as determined 44 hours after DFO (5 mg per kg given intravenously during the last hour of a dialysis session) points to the presence of aluminum overload [bone aluminum greater than 15 µg per g and/or a positive (greater than 0%) aluminon staining]. Moreover, in combination with a serum immunoreactive PTH (iPTH) measurement, a ΔSAl threshold of 50 µg per L will allow one to differentiate between (a) aluminum overload, (b) increased risk for toxicity (aluminon staining greater than 0%), and (c) aluminum-related bone disease (greater than 15% Aluminon positivity and a bone formation rate below 220 µm^2 per mm^2 per day) (Table 31-6).

Table 31-5. The deferoxamine test

Hemodialysis patients
1. A baseline serum aluminum value is obtained prior to a hemodialysis session.
2. Five mg/kg DFO in 150 mL of 5% glucose water is infused into the venous blood line during the last 60 min of the same hemodialysis session; vital signs are closely monitored during DFO infusion.
3. At the start of the next hemodialysis session (44 h after DFO administration), a second serum aluminum level is determined.

Peritoneal dialysis patients
1. A baseline serum aluminum concentration is measured at any time during the day.
2. Five mg/kg DFO in 150 mL of 5% glucose water is given intravenously during the last 60 min of a CAPD exchange. Alternatively, the same amount of DFO is added to the nocturnal exchange for CAPD patients or to the long daytime exchange for CCPD patients.
3. The serum aluminum value is determined in a second sample drawn 44 h after termination of the DFO infusion or the DFO-containing exchange.

Side effects
Hypotension can occur during DFO infusion; treat by temporarily stopping the infusion, and administering a volume expander if required.

Continuation of aluminum-containing phosphate binders throughout the test
This is controversial. If these medications are stopped, then an acute decrease in the serum aluminum level can be expected.

DFO, deferoxamine; CAPD, continuous ambulatory peritoneal dialysis; CCPD, continuous cycling peritoneal dialysis.

a. How serum iPTH levels affect interpretation of a positive DFO test. Using the 5 mg per kg DFO test, patients with a ΔSAl greater than 50 µg per L have a positive test and may have aluminum overload. However, if the serum iPTH is greater than 650 ng per L, then the high PTH levels may protect them against the deleterious effects of the element at the bone mineralization front. Aluminum toxicity is more likely when a positive DFO test is accompanied by a serum iPTH lower than 650 ng per L. There is a great chance for aluminum-related bone disease to be present in patients with a positive DFO test when the serum iPTH has decreased to below 150 ng per L (Table 31-6). A serum aluminum increment of less than 50 µg/liter after DFO administration suggests that aluminum-associated bone disease is unlikely to be present; if bone-related symptoms are present, then the workup should focus on excluding hyperparathyroidism as a possible cause.
4. Indications (Fig. 31-1). The DFO test should be performed in all dialysis patients who have signs or symptoms

**Table 31-6. Serum aluminum increment
after 5 mg/kg deferoxamine diagnostic value**[a]

Serum aluminum increment (ΔSAl)	Implications
<50 µg/L	Aluminum overload unlikely to be present.
>50 µg/L and iPTH >650 ng/L	Aluminum *overload* likely to be present; however, the risk for aluminum *toxicity* is minimal.
>50 µg/L and iPTH 150–650 ng/L	Increased risk for toxicity most probable. PTH levels should be followed intensively.
>50 µg/L and iPTH <150 ng/L	Aluminum-related bone disease most probable. Confirm by bone biopsy and consider 5 mg/kg DFO treatment.
>300 µg/L	Neurologic disorders and side effects most probable. Check by taking the patient's electro-encephalogram. Use the alternative schedule for DFO therapy.

[a] Using a 5 mg/kg DFO dose.
DFO, deferoxamine; iPTH, inorganic parathyroid hormone.

(related to bone, brain, or blood) suggestive of aluminum toxicity.

In patients with a normal iron status and a basal serum aluminum level below 30 µg per L, the DFO test in general will not add much information to regular serum aluminum monitoring. In iron-overloaded patients, however, DFO testing will correct for false negatives because in these subjects low basal serum aluminum levels may be accompanied by an increased body burden. In patients treated for hyperparathyroidism with vitamin D and/or parathyroidectomy, the aluminum status should be reevaluated since hypoparathyroidism holds an increased risk for aluminum toxicity.

IV. Treatment of aluminum overload. Once aluminum overload has been identified, treatment should be initiated, especially in symptomatic patients.

A. Discontinuation of aluminum-containing medications

1. General. In all patients, the first line of therapy is to discontinue the use of aluminum-containing phosphate binders or with sevelamen if hypercalcemia is present. The latter can be replaced with calcium-containing preparations or with sevelamer if hypercalcemia is present. Control of the serum phosphate level can often be improved by reducing dietary phosphate intake and by augmenting removal of phosphate by use of a large surface area dialyzer and a longer dialysis session length. If frequent albumin infusions or hyperalimen-

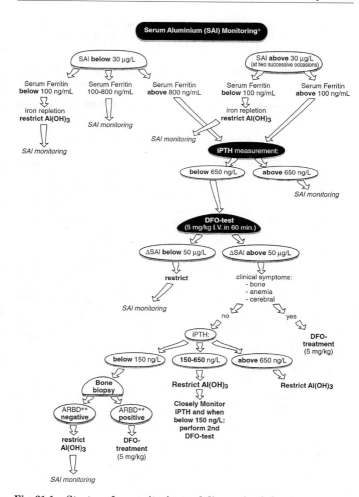

Fig. 31-1.   Strategy for monitoring and diagnosis of aluminum over-load. SAl, serum aluminum; δ SAl, increase in serum aluminum; ARBD, aluminum-related bone disease. [Adapted from DeBroe ME, Drüeke TB, Ritz E. Consensus conference on the diagnosis and treatment of aluminum overload. *Nephrol Dial Transplant* 1993; 8(Suppl 1). D'Haese PC, et al. Diagnostic value of low dose DFO test. *Nephrol Dial Transplant* 1995;10:1874–1884.]

tation supplements are being given, the aluminum content of these solutions should be determined; if high, the risk–benefit ratio of continuing these preparations should be assessed. In asymptomatic patients, there is preliminary evidence to suggest that simply stopping aluminum-containing medications can result in improved bone histology and an increased bone formation rate.

2. Hypercalcemia on switching to calcium-containing phosphate binders. A common problem encountered when attempting to partially or completely change a patient's phosphate-binding regimen from aluminum- to calcium-based medication is the prompt induction of hypercalcemia. Because of the risk of hypercalcemia, vitamin D analogs should initially be withheld. Calcium must be given with meals to maximize the amount of phosphate binding and to limit the amount of calcium absorption. Despite all of these measures, hypercalcemia often occurs because of defective bone mineralization induced by aluminum poisoning. In such cases, a course of low-dose DFO therapy should be considered, as it will improve bone mineralization; one can then expect less hypercalcemia during administration of calcium-containing phosphate binders. Use of a low-calcium dialysis solution may also be of benefit. Sevelamer hydrochloride (Renagel) is an effective phosphorus binder that contains neither calcium nor aluminum. Where available and financially affordable, use of sevelamer hydrochloride obviates the problem of hypercalcemia on making the initial switch from aluminum-containing phosphorus binders. After the bone recovers and aluminum toxicity recedes, calcium-containing phosphorus binders can be given with caution.

B. DFO therapy

1. Rationale. Aluminum in the blood is about 80%–90% protein-bound; protein binding is the primary reason for aluminum being poorly removed during dialysis, even when serum values are high. After DFO administration, the absolute serum aluminum concentration is increased, and most of the increase is in the form of a dialyzable DFO–aluminum complex (MW 583 daltons). The latter (i.e., aluminoxamine) is removable by hemodialysis (with or without concomitant hemoperfusion) or by peritoneal dialysis. DFO administration may also increase markedly the fecal excretion of aluminum.

2. Indications (Fig. 31-2). DFO therapy should be considered for patients with clinically suspected or biopsy-proven aluminum-related bone disease. If bone aluminum staining is negative and the bone formation rate is not reduced, but the DFO test is positive (or baseline serum aluminum values are high), then DFO therapy should be deferred and the patient treated conservatively by stopping aluminum-containing phosphate binders and using calcium salts instead. High PTH levels are protective, and as long as they are high, chelation therapy should be deferred.

3. Risks of precipitating or exacerbating aluminum-related encephalopathy. During DFO therapy, a neurologic syndrome similar to aluminum-related encephalopathy has been reported. The exact mechanism is unknown but is

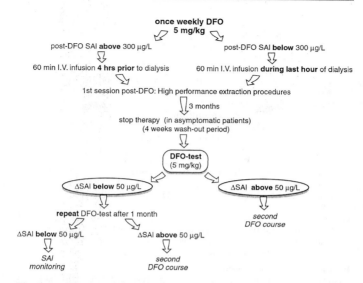

Fig. 31-2. Strategy for treatment of aluminum overload. SAl, serum aluminum; δSAl, increase in serum aluminum. [Adapted (*) from DeBroe ME, Drüeke TB, Ritz E. Consensus conference on the diagnosis and treatment of aluminum overload. *Nephrol Dial Transpl* 1993;8(Suppl 1). (*) Barata JD, et al. Low dose DFO treatment. *Nephrol Dial Transplant* 1996;11:125–132.]

theorized to be due to redistribution of aluminum mobilized by DFO into the brain. The risk of encephalopathy will be lessened if low DFO doses are used to limit the rise in the serum aluminum levels as described in Table 31-7.

In severely intoxicated patients in whom the serum aluminum level after DFO may rise to above 300 µg per L, worsening of patients' neurologic state has been observed even when doses as low as 5 mg per kg were administered in the conventional fashion (i.e., during the last hour of dialysis followed by removal of the chelates 44 hours later). These side effects were not found when the chelator was given via an alternative schedule (4–5 hours before the start of the dialysis session). Patients with central nervous system manifestations of aluminum toxicity should undergo DFO therapy because there is no other method for removal of aluminum from the body.

4. Other DFO side effects. A number of side effects, including retinal and auditory toxicity, have been reported when DFO is used. These are listed in Table 31-8. Even though the risk for these side effects is greatly reduced by using a 5 mg per kg dose, it may be wise to obtain a baseline audiogram and funduscopic examination in all patients scheduled to undergo DFO treatment and to repeat these examinations periodically while therapy is in progress. The use of DFO has

Table 31-7.   Deferoxamine treatment in hemodialyzed patients

Hemodialysis patients

A. Starting dose: 5 mg/kg DFO (dissolved in 150 mL of 5% glucose water) is administered IV (into the venous blood line) during the last 60 min of a hemodialysis session; vital signs are monitored closely during DFO infusion.

   1. If the baseline serum aluminum level is greater than 300 μg/L, then initial therapy should consist of discontinuation of aluminum-containing phosphate binders. DFO should not be given until the baseline concentration falls below 300 μg/L.

   2. If the post-DFO serum aluminum level increases to above 300 μg/L, then the chelator should be administered 4–5 h before the start of the dialysis session (alternative method).

B. Frequency of administration: DFO should be administered once a week.

C. The DFO test is repeated every 3 mo after a 4-wk washout period. If the serum aluminum increment 48 h after DFO administration is less than 50 μg/L at two successive tests (1 month interval), further DFO treatment is not recommended.

Peritoneal dialysis patients

In general, the strategy is as for hemodialysis patients. DFO is given once a week. It may be given intraperitoneally in the same dose as listed for hemodialysis patients, added to the longest dwelling exchange of the day (nocturnal exchange in CAPD patients, daytime exchange in CCPD patients). The long-term safety of intraperitoneal DFO administration has not been established.

Duration of therapy and follow-up

DFO treatment may be continued for 6–12 mo. Expect serum calcium levels to fall, alkaline phosphatase and PTH levels to rise, signs of hyperparathyroidism to increase, and erythrocyte mean corpuscular volume and hematocrit to rise slightly.

DFO, deferoxamine; CAPD, continuous ambulatory peritoneal dialysis; CCPD, continuous cycling peritoneal dialysis; PTH, parathyroid hormone.

Table 31-8.   Hazards of chronic deferoxamine administration[a]

Susceptibility to *Yersinia* sepsis and to mucormycosis
High-frequency sensorineural hearing loss
Decrease in visual acuity
Loss of color vision
Maculopathy
Acute mental changes?

---

[a] Acute side effects (e.g., hypotension) can occur during deferoxamine infusion.

been associated with the development of often fatal sepsis with *Rhizopus*. This is most likely due to the fact that the complex of iron and DFO (i.e., feroxamine) is used as a source of iron by these non–siderophore-producing germs. DFO-treated dialysis patients, particularly those with hemosiderosis, are exposed to increased levels of circulating feroxamine, which may represent an increased risk for *Rhizopus* infection. As the amount of feroxamine that is formed after DFO is highly dose-dependent, the risk for this side effect should be reduced by using the 5 mg per kg dose.

5. Method of DFO therapy. One method of DFO administration is described in Table 31-7. Dose-finding studies have offered a growing body of evidence that sufficient aluminum chelation is obtained with lower DFO doses, thus providing a rationale for the use of a 5 mg dose per kg body weight in the treatment of aluminum overload. Recent clinical studies have demonstrated the latter dose to be efficient in the removal of aluminum, as well as in the reduction of side effects. DFO should be given once weekly. In subjects with post-DFO serum aluminum levels above 300 µg per L, the DFO should be given 4–5 h before the dialysis session. This will ensure maximal aluminum chelation while limiting exposure to circulating aluminoxamine, ferrioxamine, and unchelated DFO.

6. Accelerated removal of the DFO–aluminum complex using high-performance extraction procedures. DFO therapy will only be successful when the DFO–aluminum complex is effectively removed during dialysis. The DFO–aluminum clearance of conventional dialyzers is modest and varies with the type of membrane used. However, with high-flux dialyzers or by using the AluKart charcoal cartridge in combination with a conventional dialyzer, the clearance of DFO–aluminum is increased substantially. One strategy is to use these high-extraction devices once a week, during the dialysis session that follows DFO administration. When hemoperfusion is used, the cartridge is usually inserted proximal to the dialyzer and maintained in the extracorporeal circuit throughout the dialysis session.

7. Follow-up and response to DFO therapy. In most cases, clinical improvement of aluminum-related bone disease begins several weeks after initiation of DFO therapy. The rapid response can be explained by the preferential removal of aluminum from critical sites. As therapy is continued for a 6- to 12-month period, the following laboratory changes can be expected: (a) serum PTH concentrations may increase; this is probably due to the fact that secretion of PTH is no longer inhibited by aluminum. Concomitantly, the serum alkaline phosphatase values may rise. (b) The serum calcium levels may fall due to increased mineralization of bone. The amount of calcium supplement may be increased and vitamin D may be restarted to keep the serum calcium concentrations high and prevent hyperparathyroidism. (c) The serum ferritin levels may decrease as a result of concomitant removal of DFO-chelated iron. The decrease is usually to the normal range only; ordinarily, iron supplementation is not needed. (d) The erythrocyte mean corpuscular volume and hematocrit may both increase.

A repeat bone biopsy after 6 months of DFO therapy should reveal decreased aluminum staining, an increased bone formation rate, and evidence of increased osteoblast and osteoblast activity.

V. Prevention. Water used for making dialysis solution should be analyzed periodically for its aluminum concentration to ensure that the water treatment system in use is functioning properly.

Administration of aluminum in any form to the patient groups identified at the outset of this chapter as being at increased risk for aluminum toxicity should be avoided whenever possible. Use of calcium-containing phosphorus binders is now the universal standard of care. For patients with gastrointestinal intolerance or hypercalcemia associated with calcium-containing agents, use of sevelamer hydrochloride (Renagel) should be the alternative of choice. However, this drug is not universally available and is expensive, so in a fast-diminishing minority of patients, use of aluminum-containing phosphate binders continues to be necessary to achieve adequate control of the serum inorganic phosphorus concentration.

SELECTED READINGS

Andress DL, et al. Bone histologic response to deferoxamine in aluminum-related bone disease. *Kidney Int* 1987;31:1344–1350.

Barata JD, et al. Low-dose (5 mg/kg) desferrioxamine treatment in acutely intoxicated haemodialysis patients using two drug administration schedules. *Nephrol Dial Transplant* 1996;11:125–132.

Cannata JB, et al. Serum aluminum transport and aluminum uptake in chronic renal failure: role of iron and aluminum metabolism. *Nephron* 1993;65:141–146.

DeBroe ME, et al. New insights and strategies in the diagnosis and treatment of aluminium overload in dialysis patients. *Nephrol Dial Transplant* 1993;8(Suppl 1):47–50.

DeBroe ME, et al. Consensus conference: diagnosis and treatment of aluminium overload in end-stage renal failure patients. *Nephrol Dial Transplant* 1993;8(Suppl 1):1.

D'Haese PC, et al. Use of the low-dose desferrioxamine test to diagnose and differentiate between patients with aluminum-related bone disease, increased risk for aluminum toxicity, or aluminum overload. *Nephrol Dial Transplant* 1995;10:1874–1884.

D'Haese PC, Couttenye MM, DeBroe ME. Diagnosis and treatment of aluminium bone disease. *Nephrol Dial Transplant* 1996;11 (Suppl 3):74–79.

Froment DP, et al. Site and mechanism of enhanced gastrointestinal absorption of aluminum by citrate. *Kidney Int* 1989;36:978–984.

Ihle BU, Becker G, Kincaid-Smith PS. Clinical and biochemical features of aluminum-related bone disease. *Kidney Int* 1986;29(Suppl 18):S80–S86.

Ittel TH, et al. Effect of iron status on the intestinal absorption of aluminum: a reappraisal. *Kidney Int* 1996;50:1879–1888.

Mazzaferro S, et al. Relative roles of intestinal absorption and dialysis-fluid–related exposure in the accumulation of aluminum in haemodialysis patients. *Nephrol Dial Transplant* 1997;12:2679–2682.

Olivieri NF, et al. Visual and auditory neurotoxicity in patients receiving subcutaneous deferoxamine infusions. *N Engl J Med* 1986;314:869–873.

Rosenlöf K, Fyhrquist F, Tenhunen R. Erythropoietin, aluminium, and anaemia in patients on haemodialysis. *Lancet* 1990;335:247–249.

Smans KA, et al. Transferrin; mediated uptake of aluminum by human parathyroid cells results in a reduced parathyroid hormone secretion. *Nephrol Dial Transplant* 2000;15:in press.

Van Landeghem GF, et al. Competition of iron and aluminum for transferrin: the molecular basis for aluminum deposition in iron-overloaded dialysis patients? *Exp Nephrol* 1997;5:239–245.

Van Landeghem GF, de Broe ME, D'Haese PC. Al and Si: their speciation, distribution, and toxicity. *Clin Biochem* 1998;31:385–397.

Vasilakakis DM, et al. Removal of aluminoxamine and ferrioxamine by charcoal hemoperfusion and hemodialysis. *Kidney Int* 1992;41:1400–1407.

32

Dialysis in Infants and Children

Susan R. Mendley, Richard N. Fine, and Amir Tejani

Choices in dialysis treatment for infants and children are wide and include the full range of therapies utilized in adult patients. Theoretical considerations of clearance, kinetic modeling, and adequacy of dialysis apply equally in pediatric dialysis, although they are less well studied in this population than in adults. There are important technical considerations in performing dialysis on patients whose weights may vary by as much as 50-fold. Furthermore, there are indications for and complications of the dialysis procedure that are unique to children. Finally, chronic care of children receiving dialysis is complex and requires attention to growth and development, age-specific nutritional interventions, consequences of metabolic disturbances, and psychosocial adjustment to achieve the goal of complete rehabilitation.

I. Acute dialysis

A. Indications. The indications for acute dialysis in an infant, child, or adolescent are similar to those in adults and include:

1. Oliguric acute renal failure where optimal nutritional and medical support will require fluid and/or electrolyte removal.

2. Volume overload with congestive heart failure, pulmonary edema, or severe hypertension not manageable with diuretics or conservative measures.

3. Hyperkalemia with electrocardiographic abnormalities.

4. Metabolic acidosis that cannot be safely corrected with sodium bicarbonate administration because of risk of sodium or volume overload.

5. Symptoms of uremic encephalopathy, with particular attention to seizures.

6. Uremic pericarditis.

7. Tumor lysis syndrome or severe hyperuricemia complicating chemotherapy for malignancy.

8. Progressively rising blood urea nitrogen (BUN) level in a situation where imminent recovery is not anticipated and uremic consequences are likely. The BUN level where concern arises will vary with the age of the child; 35–50 mg per dL (12–18 mmol per L) is potentially dangerous in an infant, whereas 150 mg per dL (54 mmol per L) in an adolescent may necessitate initiation of dialysis.

9. Inborn error of metabolism with severe organic acidemia or hyperammonemia.

10. Toxic ingestion. Guidelines for extracorporeal therapy for poisoning are found in Chapter 12.

B. Choice of acute dialysis modality

1. Acute peritoneal dialysis is most often used in this age group and has several advantages. It does not require sophisticated equipment or technical expertise. One can avoid the need for vascular access, blood priming, and anticoagulation; hemodynamic instability is uncommon. Continuous peritoneal dialysis provides efficient clearance in small children. However, severe hyperammonemia, hyperphosphatemia, or hyperkalemia often requires more rapid correction; in such situations, hemodialysis (sometimes in combination with continuous arteriovenous or venovenous hemofiltration) may be more appropriate. Furthermore, volume removal by ultrafiltration in peritoneal dialysis is often unpredictable and may not be rapid enough in some patients with congestive heart failure or pulmonary edema. Dialysate leakage with risk of peritonitis may limit acute peritoneal dialysis.

There are no guidelines as to what constitutes adequate peritoneal dialysis in acute renal failure (ARF), and one attempts maximum possible clearance to compensate for catabolic stress, utilizing continuous exchanges. The initial prescription may include hourly exchanges; more frequent exchanges can be performed, although a greater fraction of total time is then spent in filling and draining, rather than in solute exchange. An automated cycler facilitates this process, limiting nursing effort and repeated opening of the catheter. When a cycler is unavailable, a modification can be made for small patients by hanging a large dialysis solution bag attached to a Buretrol device (a sterile graduated cylinder) connected to the patient's peritoneal dialysis catheter either by a stopcock or a Y set. A drainage line is attached to the other limb of the Y or the stopcock. One periodically measures the desired volume into the Buretrol and infuses it into the patient. The effluent dialysate is drained via the other limb of the Y set, measured, and the process repeated without opening the system. The availability of cyclers that can deliver small exchange volumes has largely supplanted the manual acute procedure in infants and young children.

Exchange volumes are targeted at 40 mL per kg or greater, but immediately after catheter placement, it is prudent to limit volumes to half or three-fourths of this volume to avoid leakage, which predisposes to peritonitis. Hourly exchanges usually result in obligate ultrafiltration even when 1.5% dextrose concentration is used, so that parenteral or enteral fluid intake is needed to avoid volume depletion and prolongation of ARF.

2. Acute hemodialysis in infants and small children requires experience and technical expertise, as well as size-appropriate dialyzers, blood lines, and vascular catheters. Very small patients may require blood priming of the hemodialysis circuit. Small patient size allows efficient and rapid solute clearance where appropriate (i.e., ammonia) but must be approached with caution where overly rapid osmolar shifts could precipitate seizures (reportedly more common in children than in adults). Dialyzers are available in a wide range of sizes for neonates through older adolescents (see Table 32-1);

Table 32-1.   Characteristics of dialyzers suitable for pediatric use

Dialyzer	Priming volume (mL)	Surface area (m²)	Urea clearance ($Q_B = 200$)	B_{12} clearance	KoA	Membrane	Manufacturer
Mini minor, Minor	20, 43	0.23, 0.41	51 ($Q_B = 100$) 76 ($Q_B = 100$)	8, 13	151, 316	Cellulose	Cobe
CA50, 70, 90	35, 45, 60	0.5, 0.7, 0.9	128, 153, 169	26, 34, 42	245, 333, 426	Cellulose acetate	Baxter
CA-HP90	60	0.9	213 ($Q_B = 300$)	59	512	Cellulose acetate	Baxter
100-HG, 200-HG, 300-HG	18, 34, 44	0.2, 0.6, 0.8	82 ($Q_B = 100$), 150, 167	19, 39, 48	384, 343, 465	Cellulosynthetic (Hemophan)	Cobe
B3 0.5A, B3 1.0A	35, 61	0.5, 1.0	137, 175	45, 70	278, 550	PMMA	Toray
F3, F4, F5	28, 42, 63	0.4, 0.7, 1.0	125, 155, 170	20, 32, 45	231, 374, 494	Polysulfone	Fresenius
F40, F50, F60A/B	42, 63, 82	0.7, 1.0, 1.3	165, 176, 185	75, 110, 118	447, 562, 709	Polysulfone	Fresenius
CF-1211	61	0.8	160	34	408	Cellulose	Baxter
C061, C081, C101	50, 61, 71	0.6, 0.8, 1.0	144, 160, 171	41, 49, 54	311, 408, 504	Cellulose	Terumo

PMMA, polymethylmethacrylate.

however, the choices for very small dialyzers are limited. Acute hemodialysis is performed when peritoneal dialysis is contraindicated because of an intra-abdominal process (including diaphragmatic hernia, omphalocele, gastroschisis, or the presence of a ventriculoperitoneal shunt) or respiratory limitation.

3. Continuous therapies. Continuous arteriovenous hemofiltration (CAVH) or continuous venovenous hemofiltration (CVVH) with or without dialysate (CAVHD, CVVHD) has been utilized in pediatric patients, ranging from preterm infants to older adolescents. The physiologic principles are unchanged from those in adults (see Chapter 10); because of small patient size, clearance can be extremely efficient, replacing a large fraction of endogenous renal function. In particular, continuous therapies permit better phosphorus clearance than intermittent hemodialysis or peritoneal dialysis and are thus frequently employed in the tumor lysis syndrome in children with Burkitt's lymphoma or acute lymphoblastic leukemia.

Maintaining vascular access with adequate flow in small vessels can be problematical (Table 32-2) and is often the limiting factor in both CAVH and CVVH. We have found pump-driven CVVH to perform more reliably and maintain circuit patency, although others have reported equal success with CAVH. As in acute hemodialysis, the entire circuit volume must be considered and a blood prime used if it is greater than 10% of the patient's blood volume. Cooling of the blood circuit is a concern in slow-flow systems in infants; a blood warmer may be used in-line, although it increases the circuit volume. Hemofilters appropriate for pediatric use are listed in Table 32-3. Ultrafiltration is controlled by volumetric pump or automated weighing to avoid errors in replacement fluid which, if compounded over days of therapy, could be dramatic in a small, anuric patient. The Baxter BM11/BM14, the Gambro, Prisma,

Table 32-2. Catheters for use in pediatric extracorporeal renal replacement therapy

Patient size	Catheter size	Access location
Neonate	UVC—5.0F UAC—3.5, 5.0F *or* 5.0 single lumen *or* 6.5, 7.0F dual lumen	Umbilicus Femoral vein(s) UVC?, femoral vein
3–15 kg	6.5, 7.0F dual lumen	Femoral/ subclavian vein
16–30 kg	7.0, 9.0F dual lumen	Femoral/ int jugular/ subclavian
>30 kg	9.0, 11.5F dual lumen	Femoral/ int jugular

UVC, umbilical vein catheter; UAC, umbilical artery catheter.

Table 32-3.   Hemofilters appropriate for pediatric use

Hemofilter	Priming volume (mL)	Surface area (m²)	Ultrafiltration rate (mL/min, $Q_B = 100$)	Membrane	Manufacturer
Minifilter, Minifilter Plus	8, 15	0.2, 0.8	0.5–1.5, 1–8	Polysulfone	Renal Systems
HF 400, 700	28, 53	0.3, 0.7	20–35, 35–45	Polysulfone	Renal Systems
Multiflow 60	47	0.6	14–29	AN69	Hospal
PAN-03, -06	33, 63	0.3, 0.6	15–28, 28–43	PAN	Asahi
PRISMA M60 set	90			AN69	Gambro

AN69, acrylonitrile and sodium methallyl sulfonate; PAN, polyacrylonitrile.

the Braun Biopact, and the Fresnius 200 BH have been used in pediatric patients. Although the reported precision of the pumps in most systems is merely ±10%, clinical experience suggests that the delivered volumes are considerably closer to target. There are a few reports demonstrating the safety of these systems in infants. Ultrafiltration rates in infants and small children may be as low as 5–30 mL per hour without replacement fluids (slow continuous ultrafiltration) or as high as 100–600 mL per hour; larger children can tolerate ultrafiltration and replacement rates near those of adults. In choosing replacement solutions, we favor coadministration of a bicarbonate-based solution with a calcium-containing solution; commercially available lactate-based replacement solutions could present an excessive lactate load to a small patient.

II. Chronic dialysis

A. Indications. Optimal management of chronic renal failure (CRF) avoids some of the historical indications for initiation of dialysis. Anemia, acidosis, hyperparathyroidism and growth delay can usually be managed medically, so nephrologists must be attuned to subtle indications of uremia, i.e., diminished energy (less vigorous play), resumption of napping, anorexia (with failure of usual expected weight gain) and inattentiveness at school or failure to attain expected developmental milestones. Guidelines from the National Kidney Foundation-Dialysis Outcomes Quality Initiative (NKF–DOQI) for adults recommend dialysis initiation when glomerular filtration rate (GFR) falls below a weekly Kt/V-urea of 2.0 unless there is strong evidence of stable or improving nutritional status; there are no studies in children to support or refute this recommendation, and measurement of residual GFR in small children can be problematical. Nonetheless, we consider that pediatric patients require at least as much or more renal function as adults and support dialysis initiation prior to symptomatic uremia. Chronic dialysis is often an interim measure to allow time to prepare for kidney transplantation or to permit a period of growth enhanced by recombinant human growth hormone prior to steroid use with transplantation.

B. Choice of chronic dialysis modality

1. Chronic peritoneal dialysis is the therapy of choice for pediatric patients. Peritoneal surface area is correlated with body surface area; therefore, small children have a relatively large surface for solute exchange compared with adults. Also, transperitoneal solute movement in younger patients is as efficient as, or more efficient than, in adults, further increasing the efficiency of the modality. Peritoneal equilibration testing (PET) shows young children more likely to fall in the category of high or high-average transport. Since these characteristics result in enhanced glucose absorption, there will be relatively rapid attainment of osmotic equilibrium between dialysate and plasma, limiting ultrafiltration on long dwells. For this reason, automated forms of peritoneal dialysis utilizing short dwells are most commonly employed in this population.

Peritoneal dialysis offers additional benefits as a chronic dialysis modality. It is technically simple and avoids the need for chronic vascular access (which is particularly difficult in infants and small children). Blood pressure and volume status are usually better controlled with peritoneal dialysis than with hemodialysis. Less time is spent in the hospital and in the dialysis unit, with more time spent at school and engaged in other age-appropriate activities. Parents often feel they have greater control over their child's care when they perform peritoneal dialysis. Language barriers are usually not insurmountable with translators and pictorial teaching aids.

  a.   Limitations to peritoneal dialysis. Previous abdominal surgery may result in intra-abdominal adhesions that make peritoneal dialysis impossible, particularly repair of complex urogenital anomalies, which are often a cause of ESRD in children. The presence of a ventriculoperitoneal shunt is usually a contraindication to peritoneal dialysis because of the risk of central nervous system involvement with peritonitis, although there are reports of successful peritoneal dialysis in this situation. The presence of a ureterostomy, pyelostomy, or loop ileostomy is not an absolute contraindication to performance of peritoneal dialysis, although anecdotally the risk of exit site infection and peritonitis with urinary organisms is increased.

  b.   Transplantation in peritoneal dialysis patients. Peritoneal dialysis is continued up to the time of renal transplantation without increased risk of infection. The peritoneal dialysis catheter is often removed at the time of living-donor transplantation (assuming immediate graft function), but sometimes it is left in place if a cadaver transplantation is performed. The catheter is removed electively once graft function is stable; delay in catheter removal has been associated with posttransplantation peritonitis in the dry abdomen.

  c.   Complications of peritoneal dialysis. The complications of pediatric peritoneal dialysis include those already described in adults (see Chapters 19–21). Peritoneal dialysis presents particular problems for children and families. Months or years of a demanding regimen may result in "burnout" or caregiver fatigue, which exacerbates underlying family conflicts; noncompliance becomes common, particularly among adolescents. The presence of a peritoneal dialysis catheter may adversely affect body image. Children have a higher rate of peritonitis than adults, which further complicates therapy. Eradication of nasal *Staphylococcus aureus* carriage leads to decreased exit site infection and peritonitis in adults; no similar studies have been performed in children. Congenital defects in the diaphragm have been discovered that result in communication between the pleural and peritoneal spaces. In some cases, a change to automated peritoneal dialysis (APD) with empty periods may permit continuation of peritoneal dialysis. Some children become obese from excessive glucose absorption from dialysate; this presents additional problems for body image as well as adversely affecting blood lipid levels and an already increased risk of cardiovascular disease. Chronic hypoalbuminemia develops in some patients, particularly with repeated peritonitis; its long-term consequences for growth in stature and lean body mass are unknown.

C. Apparatus for acute and chronic peritoneal dialysis

1. Peritoneal dialysis solutions are available in bags of 250, 500, 750, 1,000, and 1,500 mL appropriate for small patients, in addition to standard adult exchange sizes of 2, 2.5, and 3 L. Calcium concentrations of 1.25 mM and 1.75 mM are used depending on the required dose of calcium-based phosphorus binder. (Aluminum binders are strictly avoided because of the greater risk of aluminum encephalopathy and bone disease in children.) Five- and 10-L bags for APD are available in both calcium concentrations.

Standard dextrose concentrations (1.5%, 2.5%, and 4.25%) are utilized depending on the need for ultrafiltration. Enhanced glucose absorption in small children occasionally warrants higher glucose concentration to maintain ultra-filtration, although short-dwell dialysis is usually preferred in that situation. Amino acid–containing peritoneal dialysis solutions have been utilized only to a limited degree in under-nourished pediatric peritoneal dialysis patients (perhaps because of a greater reliance on supplemental nasogastric tube feeding). Solutions of higher lactate concentrations (40 mEq per L) are generally preferred for better control of acidosis.

2. Peritoneal dialysis catheters are available in neonatal and pediatric sizes of almost any configuration used in adults, including Tenckhoff (curled and straight), swan-neck, and Toronto Western, usually with a choice of one or two cuffs. Most commonly placed in children is a one-cuff, curled Tenckhoff catheter with a straight tunnel and a laterally oriented exit site; recent North American Pediatric Renal Transplant Coop-erative Study data suggest a benefit to double-cuffed catheters and downward-oriented exit sites in decreasing peritonitis rates. The column disk catheter is avoided in infants and chil-dren because the bowel may become entrapped between the columns of the device.

a. **Implantation.** Chronic catheters are almost invari-ably implanted surgically in pediatric patients under gen-eral anesthesia. There is little experience with laparoscopic placement in this population. Several technical points have been alleged to be important:

(1) Sealing the peritoneum around the catheter (to prevent leakage) by use of a purse-string suture, which is also affixed to the cuff. The exit site should be directed caudally, as shown in Fig. 32-1, to facilitate drainage and to minimize the risk of exit site infection.

(2) Use of a second purse-string suture to seal the pos-terior rectus sheath opening and fix the posterior rectus sheath to the upper part of the cuff (to prevent leakage and displacement; this is not shown in Fig. 32-1).

(3) Performance of a partial omentectomy (to prevent obstruction).

(4) Intraoperative search for and closure of associated hernial defects, especially a patent tunica vaginalis.

We try to allow two weeks for healing of the abdomen before using the catheter. It can be used immediately for acute peritoneal dialysis or unanticipated clinical deteri-

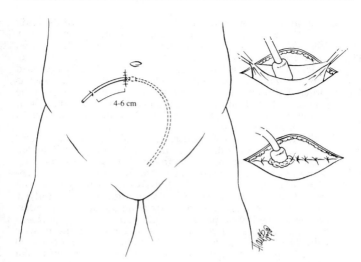

Fig. 32-1.   One method of implanting a peritoneal catheter in children. The purse-string suture used to seal the peritoneum includes the catheter cuff. A second purse-string suture (not shown) may also be used as described in the text to seal the posterior rectus sheath. (Modified from Alexander SR, et al. *Clinical parameters in continuous ambulatory peritoneal dialysis for infants and children. CAPD update.* New York: Masson, 1981.)

oration in chronic renal failure, but one risks early leakage. Small exchange volumes and performance of APD in the supine position may help avoid dialysate leakage.

   b.   Acute "temporary" catheters can be placed after prefilling the abdomen with dialysate as in adults (see Chapter 15 for description of the technique in adults). However, the temporary catheters are stiffer, conferring a greater risk of bowel injury. Therefore, immobilization is needed while the catheter is in place, which is particularly difficult in children. Furthermore, temporary catheters have a high rate of infection if left in place for more than 3 days and a greater risk of dialysate leakage than chronic catheters. For these reasons, we prefer to utilize a surgically implanted chronic peritoneal dialysis catheter for acute peritoneal dialysis. In unstable patients, the procedure can be performed at bedside in the intensive care unit.

   3.   APD cyclers have facilitated peritoneal dialysis in young patients, and nearly all available cyclers permit sufficiently small exchange volumes to be used even in infants. Pediatric cycler tubing is available for some models of cyclers; it helps reduce dialysis inefficiency due to dead space in the tubing, which is an important consideration with very small dwell volumes (less than 200 mL).

D. Chronic peritoneal dialysis prescription

1. CAPD. The technique for performing CAPD in the pediatric patient is similar to that in adults. Fill volumes are determined by patient comfort, but most children can tolerate 40 mL per kg without discomfort or leakage once their catheter exit-site is well healed. The choice of glucose concentration depends on ultrafiltration needs (fluid intake minus urine output and insensible losses).

a. Kinetic modeling of CAPD as Kt/V-urea and creatinine clearance has been performed in children; however, adequate clearance has not been defined. The NKF–DOQI recommendation for adequate CAPD in adults is a weekly Kt/V-urea of 2.0 and creatinine clearance of 60 L per week per 1.73 m^2. These values should be viewed as minimum clearances in light of the larger dietary protein intake recommended for growing children and the potential for long-term neurocognitive consequences of underdialysis. Long-term studies that would define adequate peritoneal dialysis clearance in children using age-appropriate end points, such as growth and neurocognitive development, have not yet been performed.

Regular collections of effluent dialysate and residual urine output (in continent patients with normal bladder function) are used to ensure that target clearance values are being achieved and that loss of kidney function is not compromising the adequacy of therapy. Even very diminished residual GFR (0.5 mL per minute or less) may significantly impact on the dialysis prescription in small patients; a limitation arises in how one can reliably measure such a small GFR. In practice, urea and creatinine clearance are regularly calculated (approximately every 4 months) and incorporated into the total weekly clearance. Those patients unable to perform urine collections should be assumed to have no residual GFR to avoid inadvertent underdialysis.

Many patients can achieve acceptable clearance and ultrafiltration with four exchanges per day; some will require more. The risk of non-compliance with the dialysis prescription and missing exchanges increases as the task of dialysis becomes more burdensome and intrudes on usual family activities.

2. APD is well suited for chronic peritoneal dialysis in children, accommodating their efficient solute exchange and higher risk of peritonitis. APD can be performed without a daytime dwell (nightly intermittent peritoneal dialysis, NIPD), with a daytime dwell (continuous cycling peritoneal dialysis, CCPD), or with a daytime dwell and midday exchange if solute clearance or fluid removal necessitate. NIPD may allow improved nutritional intake and decrease the risk of hernia formation, but clearance will likely be adequate only in patients with high or high-average transport as measured by PET. The day dwell of CCPD may allow one to shorten nightly treatments (desirable in older children) or improve clearance for low and low-average transporters; yet high transporters usually absorb most of their long dwell if it is left in all day.

The initial prescription is guided by transport characteristics determined by PET, typically ranging from five to nine exchanges per night with dwell times of 45 minutes to 2 hours.

   a. Kinetic modeling. Although kinetic modeling of peritoneal dialysis delivery has been performed in children treated by CCPD and NIPD, adequate clearances have not been defined. Dialysate and urine collections are performed to assess the actual delivered dialysis dose at a given prescription. Collections are repeated whenever the prescription is changed and at regular intervals to assess changes in residual renal function and peritoneal transport function. We strive to exceed NKF–DOQI recommendations for weekly Kt/V-urea and creatinine clearance (2.1 per week and 63 L per week per 1.73 m^2, 2.2 per week and 66 L per week per 1.73 m^2, for CCPD and NIPD, respectively). In our practice, young children with PET-defined high or high-average permeability peritoneal membranes can almost always exceed these values, particularly if there is residual renal function. Older children with low-average permeability peritoneal membranes and without residual renal function often require a midday exchange to achieve acceptable clearances.

   3. Tidal dialysis has been performed in children, although published reports have only included adolescents. It can enhance clearance in patients with borderline values for Kt/V and creatinine clearance who would otherwise need to change modalities. Also, children with abdominal pain at the end of a drain may be more comfortable if left with fluid in the abdomen at all times.

E. Chronic hemodialysis. Chronic hemodialysis is the appropriate modality for children and families not capable of providing reliable home care. Furthermore, large adolescents with low-permeability peritoneal membranes may not achieve adequate clearance on peritoneal dialysis without a burdensome exchange schedule, and such adolescents are appropriate candidates for hemodialysis. Because hemodialysis treatments take children out of usual activities (school and play), a hemodialysis unit must provide intensive nursing, tutoring, play therapy, age-appropriate toys, as well as occupational and physical therapy during dialysis treatments.

   1. Hemodialysis equipment
   a. Vascular access. Vascular access remains a major limitation to successful hemodialysis in small children. Placing and maintaining permanent accesses in small vessels requires experienced and dedicated surgeons and radiologists. Vascular catheters can be placed by interventional radiologists or surgeons depending on the best experience available in an institution. A conservative strategy for permanent access is critical because of the lifelong need for renal replacement therapy. Many young adults leave pediatric dialysis units after 15 years of dialysis (with interval failed renal transplants), and one must ensure they have not depleted all options for long-term dialysis access.

      (1) Catheters (Table 32-2). Currently available double-lumen hemodialysis catheters range in size from 7F to 12F in lengths appropriate for small children. Both temporary and permanent catheters are available, and precurved models for internal jugular cannulation are available in larger sizes. The catheter tip should be radiologically positioned in the junction of the superior vena cava and right atrium.

In small infants and neonates, single-lumen catheters may be more appropriate considering vessel size. In neonates, a catheter can be inserted into the vena cava through the umbilical vessel if the vessel is still patent. Most of these catheters can be left in place for several weeks.

(2) Fistulae and grafts. In older children, creation of an arteriovenous fistula between the radial artery and cephalic vein in the nondominant arm with an end-to-side anastomosis is a common mode of vascular access. When blood vessel size is too small for constructing an adequate fistula, a polytetrafluoroethylene (GoreTex or Impra) graft can be placed between an extremity artery and vein. Children with myelomeningocele may prefer a graft placed in the thigh because of absent sensation. Lower-extremity grafts allow unimpeded play or school-work during dialysis treatments but risk leg edema and hypertrophy.

(3) Blood flows. Desired blood flow rate is calculated from urea clearance specifications for the chosen dialyzer with an initial target urea clearance of 3 mL per minute per kg to avoid symptomatic disequilibrium. Higher urea removal rates are usually tolerated after the first few treatments when the patient is no longer acutely uremic. Smaller blood vessels cause higher venous resistance than in adults, which eventually limits flow, typically in the range of 40–120 mL per minute in small children and 150–300 mL per minute in older children. Small catheters often limit flow to 25–100 mL per minute because of limited arterial inflow. When using a single-needle system, set the blood pump speed to a rate that will deliver an effective blood flow as computed from the stroke volume and cycle time.

b. Dialyzers. A limited listing of dialyzers that may be appropriate for small patients is provided (Table 32-1).

c. Blood lines. Appropriately sized blood lines allow control of circuit volume. If the volume of the entire extracorporeal circuit exceeds 10% of the patient's blood volume (more than 8 mL per kg), a warmed blood (or albumin) prime is usually given to ensure hemodynamic stability. Blood lines are available in a range of sizes: neonatal (20 mL), infant (40 mL), and pediatric (73 mL). It is important that the blood pump be properly calibrated for infant blood lines. Neonatal lines are not compatible with many currently available volumetric dialysis machines; thus, one must choose between the risk of a large blood prime and the risk of less than perfect control of ultrafiltration.

d. Dialysate. Bicarbonate dialysate is standard for pediatric hemodialysis; it provides better hemodynamic stability and fewer intradialytic symptoms. Patients with small muscle mass will be unable to metabolize a large acetate load quickly.

   e.   Dialysis machines. Dialysis machines that provide volumetric ultrafiltration control are required. Small errors in ultrafiltration volume (of a few hundred milliliters) may cause symptomatic hypotension or chronic volume overload. Blood flows must be accurate within the range of 30–300 mL per minute and the blood pump calibrated to different size lines.

2.   Hemodialysis prescription. A cautious approach to avoiding disequilibrium involves use of a target urea clearance of 3 mL per minute per kg, which is calculated from the specifications of the chosen dialyzer and the blood flow attainable through the patient's access. Early treatments may be programmed even more slowly if the patient is very uremic; repeated short treatments are usually advisable during initiation of hemodialysis when the BUN is extremely elevated. Once a stable, chronic dialysis prescription is attained, more efficient urea clearance is usually well tolerated and fluid removal is more often a cause of intradialytic symptoms. With conditioning and distraction, most children can tolerate hemodialysis sessions lasting 3–4 hours.

   a.   Anticoagulation. The strategy for heparin administration to infants and children is similar to that for adults. Clotting is minimal when the activated clotting time (ACT) is prolonged to approximately 150% of the population baseline value. A "lowdose" heparin protocol would be used to prolong the clotting time to 125% of the population baseline value. The initial loading dosage is usually 10–20 units per kg, with lower dosages being used for infants and children weighing less than 15 kg. The initial maintenance heparin infusion rate (for the first 20–30 minutes) can be set at 0.3–0.5 units per kg per minute, with further adjustments based on changes in the ACT. Low molecular weight heparin has been used in children receiving chronic hemodialysis, but published reports are very limited.

   In older children, heparin-free dialysis can be performed successfully. Different dialyzer membrane types have not been systematically compared with regard to clotting. Clotting will be more likely in smaller children, in whom the blood flow rate is usually low relative to the size of the dialyzer.

   b.   Kinetic modeling of hemodialysis. Formal three-point urea kinetic modeling of hemodialysis has been performed in children, and results are useful in assessing the efficiency of the dialysis treatment as well as dietary protein intake (as a function of urea generation rate) during the interdialytic period. Recommended dietary protein intake in children is greater than that in adults, and the long-term effects of inadequate intake on growth and neurologic development are of even greater concern. The technical aspects of kinetic modeling are discussed in Chapter 2 and are applied similarly in children. The slow-flow technique for blood sampling is important for accurate measurement and the duration of slow flow is determined by the volume of the blood line from the needle or catheter to the sampling port. Pediatric blood lines can be adequately cleared by a slow-flow rate (60 mL per minute) for 17 seconds; we predict infant lines will require 12 seconds at a slow-flow rate of 20 mL per minute. The greater reliance on catheters in pediatric dialysis raises concern that recirculation will diminish treatment efficiency; this can be measured as discussed in Chapters 2 and 4.

Although there is some experience with single-pool kinetic modeling in pediatric dialysis, it may be inappropriate in this population. In particular, when small patients receive efficient clearance (i.e., relatively high K/V), there is a greater chance of postdialysis urea rebound with reequilibration of urea from either the intracellular space or relatively underperfused tissues. Thus, single-pool modeling would significantly overestimate dialysis efficiency and urea generation rate, and double-pool modeling may more accurately describe therapy. The latter requires either a 60-minute postdialysis (equilibrated) BUN or an intradialytic value that can be extrapolated to the equilibrated value using published formulas (Smye et al, 1992).

c.   Adequacy of hemodialysis. As is the case for peritoneal dialysis, guidelines for adequate hemodialysis therapy have not been specifically tested in children with end points appropriate for this population, such as growth and neurocognitive development. The NKF–DOQI recommendation in adults for a minimum delivered dose of dialysis of $Kt/V = 1.2$ (single pool, variable volume) or urea reduction rate (URR) of 65% is a useful reference point. Residual renal function can significantly impact on the hemodialysis prescription, especially in very small patients. Regular measurements are needed to assure overall treatment adequacy as the GFR falls. If patients are unable to perform urine collections, they should be assumed to have no residual GFR to avoid inadvertent underdialysis.

As described above, urea rebound may be significant in small patients receiving efficient clearance, which may render an adult-defined target Kt/V inadequate. Because of a concern for subtle effects of inadequate dialysis and the larger dietary protein needs of children, most pediatric dialysis units attempt to achieve a significantly higher Kt/V. In practice, it is relatively easy to achieve single-pool Kt/V values well in excess of 1.4 in small children. Although double-pool modeling appears to be relevant in this population, as yet one cannot propose an appropriate double-pool Kt/V.

d.   Complications

(1)   Disequilibrium and seizures. Infants and small children develop seizures as a manifestation of the disequilibrium syndrome more commonly than adults. For this reason, the blood flow rate and session length are usually limited for the first few treatments. Overly rapid urea removal is generally avoided by choosing an appropriately sized dialyzer to provide 3 mL per minute per kg urea clearance for the initial treatments; often, blood flows are limited by the caliber of the dialysis access. Other measures sometimes utilized to help prevent disequilibrium syndrome include keeping the dialysate sodium at or slightly above the plasma level, and the prophylactic infusion of mannitol (0.5–1.0 g per kg body weight) during the hemodialysis session.

(2) Hypotension. Intradialytic hypotension and cramping with fluid removal greater than 5% of body weight are common, yet interdialytic weight gains can be large in anuric children on largely liquid diets and in noncompliant adolescents, resulting in sustained interdialytic hypertension. Volume removal must be closely monitored because blood pressure is normally lower and there is a narrower margin to hypotension. Infants and very young children are prone to precipitous falls in blood pressure with no warning and no ability to communicate distress. Isolated ultrafiltration or lower dialysate temperature may make fluid removal more tolerable. If hypoalbuminemia is present, intravenous albumin infusion (0.5–1.5 g per kg) will increase oncotic pressure and may permit ultrafiltration. Repeated treatments may be the only way to remove fluid safely, and many children require more than three treatments per week for fluid and blood pressure management.

(3) Hypothermia with isolated ultrafiltration. If warmed dialysis solution is not circulated, then the extracorporeal blood circuit will function as a radiator, cooling the blood and the infant. Core body temperature should be continually monitored throughout dialysis, especially during isolated ultrafiltration.

III. Care of the pediatric ESRD patient
A. Nutrition. Comprehensive nutritional management is important for the achievement of growth and physical development through ESRD. The recommended energy intakes for pediatric dialysis patients depend on their ages and should be the same as the recommended dietary allowances (RDAs) for their nonuremic counterparts. For infants, the RDA for energy is approximately 100 kcal per kg per day. Such high intakes may require supplementation, either orally or by gavage feeding, which can be performed at night concomitantly with CCPD. Attempts to provide calories well in excess of the RDA to further enhance growth are usually not effective and induce obesity. However, failure of expected weight gain is an indication for increased energy intake. In older children, the recommended energy intake ranges from 40 to 70 kcal per kg per day, depending on age and activity level.

Protein requirements for children depend on their age and are greater than adult RDA. The recommended dietary protein intake (DPI) for pediatric hemodialysis patients is 0.4 g per kg per day above their RDA for age. The recommended DPI for peritoneal dialysis patients is greater to compensate for anticipated peritoneal losses, which are more significant in infants and toddlers; such very young pediatric peritoneal dialysis patients should consume 0.7–0.8 g per kg per day above their RDA with close monitoring of the adequacy of protein stores.

There is limited experience with the use of amino acid–containing peritoneal dialysis fluids, although individual patients have been treated for up to a year.

Supplementation of water-soluble vitamins is routine practice for children treated with chronic peritoneal dialysis or hemodialysis. Fat-soluble vitamins should not be supplemented as clearance of vitamin A metabolites are impaired, risking hypervitaminosis A; an appropriate multivitamin must be selected. Dietary intake of zinc and copper appears to be inadequate in pediatric peritoneal dialysis patients, and supplementation may be necessary in those with evidence of trace metal deficiency.

It is difficult to impose fluid, sodium, and potassium restrictions on pediatric patients; however, such restrictions are usually unnecessary when peritoneal dialysis is the treatment modality. For hemodialysis patients, restrictions depend on the amount of residual urinary output and become more onerous for anuric patients. In the latter group, relatively stringent sodium, phosphorus, potassium, and fluid restrictions are necessary. For example, daily fluid intake in an anuric infant on hemodialysis should be limited to 400–500 mL per m^2, and formula should be concentrated and appropriately supplemented to achieve nutritional goals.

Enteral feeding supplements designed for adults should be used cautiously in young children. For example, hypermagnesemia has been reported due to a relative excess of magnesium in some of these preparations (Sherbotie et al, 1999).

B.   Hypertension. Hypertension in children undergoing peritoneal dialysis is usually the result of incorrect dialysate glucose concentrations chosen at home coupled with excessive sodium intake; it is usually managed with dietary counseling and parent education regarding appropriate dialysate solutions and monitoring of weight and blood pressure at home. In hemodialysis patients, hypertension is not uncommon and in most cases is related to inadequate fluid removal during dialysis and noncompliance with sodium and fluid restrictions. In patients who continue to remain hypertensive despite increased dialysis time, lowered dialysate temperature or isolated ultrafiltration may make volume removal more tolerable. Dietary and psychological counseling for patient and family are advisable in cases of repeated noncompliance as noncompliance may reflect more serious difficulties on the part of the patient in coping with the chronic disease process. If modifications in the dialysis prescription are not adequate for blood pressure control, antihypertensive medications are indicated. All antihypertensive agents typically prescribed for adults have been used successfully in pediatric dialysis patients, and doses should be titrated to age-appropriate blood pressure targets and reassessed frequently.

C.   Anemia. Children undergoing hemodialysis tend to become anemic more frequently than adults. Children respond quite well to erythropoietin; the indications, route of administration, and potential complications are similar for children and adults. Some centers have used intraperitoneal erythropoietin and have reported good results (Kausz et al, 1999). Dosage per kilogram is often higher in children than in adults. Iron deficiency and repeated episodes of peritonitis adversely affect the erythropoietin response, and noncompliance with home therapy is occasionally a problem. Iron supplementation, either intravenous or oral, is usually necessary in pediatric ESRD patients; blood loss in the hemodialysis circuit is an important cause of iron deficiency in very small patients, especially when more than three treatments per week is prescribed. Androgen therapy, while rarely used in adults, is contraindicated in prepubertal children because it may lead to premature closure of epiphyses.

D.   Growth. Few longitudinal studies describing growth in pediatric patients undergoing CAPD or APD have been undertaken. Initial data comparing growth with CAPD or APD to that obtained with hemodialysis seemed to favor the peritoneal dialysis approach; however, definitive controlled studies have not been performed. In children undergoing CAPD or APD, improvement in growth has been linked to a reduction in the degree of secondary hyperparathyroidism. Others have attributed better growth with CAPD or APD to improved nutritional intake, but, as noted above, increasing energy intake much above the RDA will not usually be of benefit.

1.   Recombinant human growth hormone (rhGH) therapy. There is evidence that rhGH treatment increases growth rate in children receiving chronic dialysis, although not as effectively as in children with chronic renal insufficiency not yet receiving dialysis. The usual dosage is 0.05 mg per kg per day or 30 IU per m^2 per week as a nightly subcutaneous injection, although other dosing strategies have been used including intraperitoneal administration and alternate-day injections. The administration of rhGH after renal transplantation is somewhat controversial; some have suggested that it may induce an increase in renal transplant rejection rates.

2.   Acidosis. Metabolic acidosis is common in children with ESRD and is more problematic in those receiving hemodialysis than those treated with peritoneal dialysis. Chronic acidosis may impair growth by affecting the growth hormone/insulin-like growth factor–1 axis, as well as exerting a catabolic effect on lean body mass. Some pediatric patients would benefit from higher dialysate bicarbonate concentrations and oral sodium bicarbonate or sodium citrate therapy to maintain a serum bicarbonate concentration ≥22 mEq per L.

E.   Renal osteodystrophy. Renal osteodystrophy can be largely prevented or treated in pediatric patients undergoing CAPD or CCPD by assiduous attention to the serum calcium, phosphorus, parathyroid hormone, and alkaline phosphatase levels. Serial adjustments in the calcium and calcitriol dosage until the serum calcium level is in the upper range of normal are needed to effect healing of osteitis fibrosa. Hyperphosphatemia should be controlled by dietary counseling and by oral administration of phosphate binders to an age-appropriate level. Phosphorus restriction is particularly difficult to achieve in infants and children because of the higher recommended protein intakes, and we rely on low-phosphorus infant formula and avoidance of milk. Phosphorus intake should be restricted to 300–400 mg per day in infants and to 500–1,000 mg per day in children. Calcium carbonate and calcium acetate are used as phosphate binders. The use of aluminum-containing phosphate binders is best avoided because infants and children with chronic renal failure appear to be quite prone to develop aluminum toxicity. The serum alkaline phosphatase levels vary with age, and normal age-related values should be consulted whenever test results are being interpretated.

SELECTED READINGS

Coppo R, et al. Providing the right stuff feeding children with chronic renal failure. *J Nephrol* 1998;11:171–176.

Donckerwolcke R, et al. Renal replacement therapy in children. In: Jacobs C, et al, eds. *Replacement of renal function by dialysis*, 4th ed. Dordrecht: Kluwer Academic, 1996.

Ellis EN, et al. Use of pump-assisted hemofiltration in children with acute renal failure. *Pediatr Nephrol* 1997;11:196–200.

Fine RN, Alexander SR, Warady BA. *CAPD/CCPD in children*, 2nd ed. Boston: Kluwer Academic, 1998.

Kari JA, et al. Outcome and growth of infants with severe chronic renal failure. *Kidney Int* 2000;57:1681–1687.

Kausz A, et al. Intraperitoneal erythropoietin in children on peritoneal dialysis: A study of pharmacokinetics and efficacy. *Am J Kidney Dis* 1999;34:651–656.

Lieberman KV. Pediatric continuous arteriovenous hemofiltration. In: Nissenson AR, et al, eds. *Clinical dialysis*, 3rd ed. Norwalk, CT: Appleton & Lange, 1995.

Lilien M, et al. Hyperhomocyst(e)inaemia in children with chronic renal failure. *Nephrol Dial Transplant* 1999;14:366–368.

Mendley SR, et al. Measurement of peritoneal dialysis delivery in children. *Pediatr Nephrol* 1993;7:284–289.

Mendley SR, Majkowski NL. Peritoneal equilibration test results are different in infants, children, and adults. *J Am Soc Nephrol* 1995;6:1309–1312.

North American Pediatric Renal Transplant Cooperative Study (NAPRTCS) 1999 Annual Report, EMMES Corp, Potomac, MD, 1999.

Schaefer F, et al. Peritoneal transport properties and dialysis dose affect growth and nutritional status in children on chronic peritoneal dialysis. Mid-European Pediatric PD Study Group. *J Am Soc Nephrol* 1999;10:1786–1792.

Sherbotie JR, Terrill C. Risk of hypermagnesemia in children with chronic renal insufficiency receiving enteral feedings formulated for adults with renal failure. *J Am Soc Nephrol* 1999;10:88 (astr).

Smye SW, et al. Paediatric haemodialysis: estimation of treatment efficiency in the presence of urea rebound. *Clin Phys Physiol Meas* 1992;13:51–62.

Warady BA, et al. Optimal care of the pediatric end-stage renal disease patient on dialysis. *Am J Kidney Dis* 1999;33:567–583.

Zempsky WT, et al. Lidocaine iontophoresis for topical anesthesia before intravenous line placement in children. *J Pediatr* 1998;132:1061–1063.

Internet references

ESRD in children. Links and guidelines. (http://www.hdcn.com/crf/kids)

V

Special Problems Pertaining to Various Organ Systems

Heart and Circulation

Anthony J. Nicholls

I. Scope of the problem. The prevalence of cardiovascular disease in the dialysis population is elevated, primarily because of an increased presence of the usual risk indicators for atherosclerosis, especially hypertension and diabetes. Factors specifically associated with uremia, such as hypertriglyceridemia, hyperparathyroidism, vascular calcification, abnormal calcium and phosphorus metabolism, and elevated serum levels of hemocysteine, urate, and oxalate, may also play a role. Many dialysis patients have high serum levels of inflammatory mediators such as C-reactive protein that have been associated with cardiovascular risk and atherosclerosis. Left ventricular hypertrophy (LVH) is endemic in dialysis patients, and LVH is a strong risk factor for cardiovascular mortality. Well-designed comparisons of peritoneal dialysis and hemodialysis patients with regard to cardiovascular risk have yet to be undertaken. However, dialysis registries in North America and Europe document that cardiovascular events are the prime cause of death in both hemodialysis and peritoneal dialysis patients.

II. Hypertension. Hypertension is found in 80% or more of patients with renal failure at the time of beginning regular dialysis and is a prime contributor to both atherosclerosis and heart failure. Management of hypertension is described in Chapter 26.

III. Hyperlipidemia (see also Chapter 21)
  A. Hypertriglyceridemia
   1. Incidence and etiologic factors. Around one-third of dialysis patients have hypertriglyceridemia, with values usually ranging from 200 to 300 mg per dL and occasionally up to 600 mg per dL. The predominant underlying cause is a deficiency of lipoprotein lipase, resulting in reduced lipolysis of triglyceride-rich lipoproteins (very low-density lipoproteins, or VLDLs). Enrichment of low-density lipoprotein (LDL) particles with triglycerides suggests partial deficiency of hepatic lipase also. These basic defects are exaggerated by the use of β-adrenergic blockers, high-carbohydrate diets, absorption of glucose from peritoneal dialysate, the use of acetate dialysate, the use of heparin, and decreased hepatic blood flow from cardiac insufficiency. Associated abnormalities include a reduction in high-density lipoproteins (HDLs), increased chylomicron remnants and intermediate-density lipoproteins, and reduced apolipoprotein A-I (apoA-I) levels.
   2. Diagnosis. Blood for measurement of serum triglyceride levels should be obtained prior to heparin administration (heparin stimulates the action of lipoprotein lipase) after a fast of at least 12 hours. In peritoneal dialysis patients, the presence of glucose in the abdomen prior to blood sampling does not result in a true fasting determination, but for practical reasons, dialysis is not stopped routinely prior to blood sampling.

3. Treatment

   a. Indications. An elevated plasma triglyceride concentration is an independent (albeit weak) risk factor for coronary artery disease in the normal population and, by extrapolation, may be of some relevance in the dialysis patient. However, hypertension and cigarette smoking are more potent risk factors, and undue emphasis on the role of hypertriglyceridemia (which is usually mild in degree) is unlikely to be rewarding. The enthusiasm for treatment should increase in proportion to the degree of serum triglyceride elevation.

   b.   Diet. For all dialysis patients, the dietary recommendations listed in Chapter 23 should be followed. The recommendations include consumption of a diet with a 1:1 ratio of polyunsaturated to saturated fat, mild restriction of total carbohydrate intake, and limitation of the use of refined carbohydrate. Alcohol ingestion in any amount should be strongly discouraged. Despite the slightly malnourished status of many dialysis patients, an important minority, especially among those receiving peritoneal dialysis, will be obese, and in this subgroup, caloric restriction may be necessary to achieve ideal body weight.

   The administration of fish oil supplements (omega-3 fatty acids) reduces both triglyceride levels and platelet aggregability. However, long-term compliance is poor, and benefits remain speculative.

   c.   Drugs. There is no evidence to support the use of triglyceride-lowering drugs in dialysis patients, but most physicians feel more comfortable attempting to reduce extreme levels. The fibrate drugs (clofibrate, bezafibrate, gemfibrozil, fenofibrate) enhance lipoprotein lipase activity and are the logical agents to use for triglyceride reduction. Clofibrate is particularly toxic in renal failure and is almost obsolete in any case. Bezafibrate, fenofibrate, and gemfibrozil have a major renal route of excretion and in dialysis, patients need dose reduction to 25% of usual. Even then myopathy may occur, so that muscle enzyme monitoring is essential. Although a modest elevation of HDLs will accompany reduction of triglyceride levels, a reduction in heart disease has not been demonstrated.

   d.   Exercise. Physical training and regular exercise are highly recommended for dialysis patients; they result in reduced serum triglyceride concentrations and an improved sense of well-being.

   e.   Avoiding drugs known to exacerbate hyperlipidemia. The most important offenders are the β-adrenergic blocking drugs. In dialysis patients with hypertriglyceridemia, β-blockers can be replaced with alternative agents that do not increase the serum lipid levels.

   f.   Sodium and fluid restriction in patients receiving peritoneal dialysis. The use of high-glucose dialysis solution necessary to effect ultrafiltration increases the amount of glucose absorbed, exacerbating hypertriglyceridemia in susceptible patients. In such patients, a lower intake of fluid results in a lower need for ultrafiltration, permitting the use of a lower average dialysis solution glucose concentration.

g. Other. Several preliminary studies suggest that use of a high-flux dialyzer membrane may result in lower serum triglyceride levels (Josephson et al, 1991); if so, the mechanism is unknown. Not all investigators find this (House et al, 2000). Changing from regular to low molecular weight heparin has been reported to cause a fall in serum cholesterol levels and beneficial effects on serum apolipoprotein levels (Schneider and Schmidt, 1991).

B. Serum apolipoprotein concentrations. The lipoprotein profile in dialysis patients may be abnormal even in those with normal serum cholesterol and triglyceride levels. ApoA-I and apoA-II are reduced, whereas apoB, apoC-I, apoC-II, apoC-III, and apoE are increased. Serial measurements in patients progressing from renal impairment to dialysis show that apolipoprotein abnormalities precede lipid disturbance; ideally, therapy should target normalization of the protein moieties as well as lipids.

C. Lipid peroxidation. Increased lipid peroxidation is believed to accelerate atherosclerosis. In dialysis patients, the degree of lipid peroxidation is increased. This may be due in part to the fact that activities of antioxidant enzymes in the blood are low, as are intracellular levels of ascorbic acid and tocopherols.

D. Hypercholesterolemia. Dialysis patients usually have normal total cholesterol levels. Low serum cholesterol levels are predictive of poor nutritional status and are associated with an elevated mortality. Even when total cholesterol is normal, HDL cholesterol tends to be low. Fewer than 10% of patients have hypercholesterolemia worth treating with drugs, but following a diet rich in polyunsaturated fatty acids and restricted in saturated fat and cholesterol is prudent for all patients. Bile acid sequestrants are of little value in dialysis patients; they may aggravate hypertriglyceridemia, interfere with drug absorption, and cause bloating and constipation. The hydroxymethylglutaryl coenzyme A reductase inhibitor, simvastatin, has been evaluated in dialysis patients; the usual dosage of 10–40 mg per day can be used. Apart from elevation of transaminase levels in some patients, side effects are few. A 25% reduction in triglyceride levels with elevation of HDL and apoA-I levels is to be expected, as is a reduction in serum total cholesterol values.

IV. Ischemic cardiac disease

A. Risk factors and prevention. A number of risk factors for atherosclerosis operate in uremic patients (Table 33-1). The message for prevention is clear: treat hypertension as vigorously as possible, discourage smoking, control plasma phosphorus rigidly with phosphorus binders and dietary manipulation, consider parathyroidectomy early rather than late when calcitriol treatment fails to control progressive biochemical evidence of hyperparathyroidism, and encourage healthy eating habits and exercise. There is no known treatment to reduce elevated serum levels of C-reactive protein and other inflammatory mediators. A diet containing soy proteins is anti-atherogenic in animal studies. Mortality in United States Asian dialysis patients is relatively low. Whether this is due to a soy-protein-containing diet is

**Table 33-1.   Risk factors for
atherogenesis in end-stage renal failure**

Hypertension
Cigarette smoking
Diabetes mellitus
Insulin resistance (in nondiabetic renal failure)
Lipid disorders
       Hypertriglyceridemia
       Reduced high-density lipoprotein–cholesterol
       Reduced apoenzyme A-I
       Hypercholesterolemia in patients with past nephrotic syndrome
Vascular calcification
       Diabetes
       Hyperparathyroidism
       Increased calcium phosphate product
Elevated serum homocysteine
Elevated serum C-reactive protein
?Elevated plasma urate and oxalate
?Free oxygen radicals
?Polyamines

completely speculative. Vitamin E administration may reduce the extent of LDL-oxidation in dialysis patients (Islam et al, 2000), and it also may reduce the oxidative damage associated with iron therapy (see Chapter 27). However, vitamin E is not widely prescribed for this purpose. Serum homocysteine elevations are only partially normalized by treatment with folic acid, pyridoxine, or vitamin B12. Studies suggest that doses of folic acid about 2.5 mg/day do not provide additional benefit. A most promising strategy to lower homocysteine in ESRD patients was reported using intravenous folinic acid and pyridoxine. This lowered homocysteine in most dialysis patients into the range of 12 µmoles per L in 37 HD patients, and 78% of the patients achieved a normal Hcy level (Touam et al, 1999). The study requires confirmation, and outcomes data need to be obtained. See Yeun and Kaysen (2000) for an excellent review of the topic of lipid oxidation, inflammatory markers, and homocysteine in end stage renal disease.

   B.   Management of angina pectoris. The pharmacologic approach to angina in dialysis patients is similar to that in the normal population. The progressive introduction of sublingual nitrates, oral long-acting nitrates, β-blockers, and calcium entry blockers is appropriate. The usual dosages of sublingual and oral nitrates can be given to dialysis patients.

     1.   Role of anemia. Coronary artery disease is commonly unmasked when angina develops as the hemoglobin falls below a critical value. Such patients will need recombinant human erythropoietin therapy or regular blood transfusion to maintain hematocrit above the individual level at which angina is disabling.

     2.   Angina during the hemodialysis session. For patients whose angina manifests primarily during the hemodialysis session, a number of therapeutic options are available. Nasal oxygen should be given routinely. If the anginal episode is associated with hypotension, then initial treatment should be to raise the blood pressure by elevating the feet and by cautiously administering saline. Sublingual nitroglycerin can be given as soon as the blood pressure has increased to a clinically acceptable value. The blood flow rate should be reduced and ultrafiltration stopped until the anginal episode subsides. If the blood pressure is not substantially reduced when angina manifests, then sublingual nitroglycerin should be administered as initial therapy. However, a fall in blood pressure can then be anticipated, and the patient should be placed in a reclining position.

Predialysis administration of 2% nitroglycerin ointment may be of benefit when applied 1 hour prior to a hemodialysis session. Predialysis administration of β-blockers, oral nitrates, or calcium channel blockers may be of benefit but must be done cautiously because the risk of hypotension during the dialysis session may be increased. When giving a calcium channel blocker prior to hemodialysis, diltiazem may be preferred over verapamil or nifedipine because diltiazem has less effect on cardiac conduction and contractility than verapamil and less peripheral vasodilatory effects than nifedipine.

C.   Coronary artery bypass surgery and angioplasty. Patients whose angina fails to respond to medical treatment need not be precluded from consideration for revascularization procedures because of renal failure. Although there are no data showing increased survival in renal failure patients treated surgically for angina, symptomatic benefit can readily be attained. However, recent reports indicate perioperative mortality rates up to 20% in dialysis patients with severe heart disease (New York Heart Association Class IV). If noninvasive investigations show severely impaired left ventricular function, surgery probably is inappropriate.

The results of percutaneous transluminal coronary angioplasty in dialysis patients are disappointing. Early success nears 100%, but angina commonly recurs by 6 months, with angiographic evidence of aggressive restenosis.

Routine exercise stress testing is not indicated, as candidates for revascularization select themselves by virtue of symptoms alone. Asymptomatic transplant candidates with a previous history of angina or myocardial infarction should have treadmill testing, as renal transplantation is associated with a high perioperative myocardial infarction rate.

The risk of coronary arteriography is no greater in the dialysis patient than in the nonuremic population. Dialysis is usually scheduled promptly after arteriography to accelerate removal of osmotically active radiographic contrast media, although the benefits of this are controversial. Pre- and postoperative management of dialysis patients undergoing cardiac surgery is similar to that for any other major operation.

D.   Dialysis of patients after acute myocardial infarction. Hemodialysis should be done using all of the methods described in Chapter 17 to minimize the possibility of hypotension during dialysis. If the hematocrit is low, then transfusion up to approximately 33%–36% is reasonable to increase the reserve capacity of the blood to carry oxygen.

V.   Pericardial disease. Pericarditis accounts for 3%–4% of all deaths in dialysis patients, as a result of tamponade, cardiac arrhythmias, or heart failure. Pericarditis is most conveniently classified as either uremic or dialysis-associated.

A.   Uremic pericarditis. Uremic pericarditis is defined as disease in patients not yet on maintenance dialysis therapy. With the widespread strategy of early dialysis of patients with renal failure, uremic pericarditis is not commonly seen today. Its presence is an absolute criterion for the prompt initiation of dialysis treatment.

B.   Dialysis-associated pericarditis. Dialysis-associated pericarditis is defined as disease appearing in a patient who has been following a maintenance dialysis program.

    1.   Etiology. Intercurrent bacterial or viral infection, hypercatabolism, volume overload, hyperparathyroidism, hyperuricemia, and malnutrition have all been proposed as etiologic factors. Some of these factors may act as triggering agents, but most of them are markers of inadequate dialysis, which can usually be partially incriminated in causing pericarditis in a regular dialysis patient.

    2.   Diagnosis. The diagnosis is usually established by the finding of a pericardial friction rub in a patient with chest pain. Less commonly, dialysis-associated pericarditis may manifest as frequently recurring hypotension during dialysis or, in an asymptomatic patient, as an occult pericardial effusion detected on echocardiography.

    3.   Treatment

      a.   Monitoring. Small asymptomatic pericardial effusions (less than 100 mL) are not uncommon in hemodialysis patients. These effusions have no clinical importance and should be left alone. What is problematic is the diagnosis of impending cardiac tamponade. Patients with symptomatic pericarditis need to undergo repeated echocardiography to quantify any increase or decrease in the size of the pericardial effusion. Echocardiography does not permit a definitive diagnosis of tamponade per se. Pulsus paradoxus may be absent in tamponade, but unexplained hypotension during dialysis may be a vital clue to impending hemodynamic decompensation.

      b.   Intensification of dialysis. Initially, the dialysis schedule should be intensified, usually by increasing the frequency of dialysis to five to seven times weekly for 2–4 weeks. In contrast to the response of uremic pericarditis to the initiation of regular dialysis (where 90% of patients improve rapidly), dialysis-associated pericarditis responds less predictably to intensive dialysis. Hydration should be rigidly controlled and nutrition maintained. The regular dialysis schedule should be revised and then assessed by some measure of urea kinetics. Some patients may benefit from a switch to peritoneal dialysis.

      c.   Drugs. Controlled trials of indomethacin and other nonsteroidal anti-inflammatory drugs show no benefit for pain relief and no impact on effusion; these drugs are not indicated. Similarly, no benefit can be shown for systemic or intrapericardial corticosteroid therapy.

d. Surgical drainage. Failure to recognize the need for timely surgical drainage of large pericardial effusions may have dire consequences for the patient; the onset of tamponade may be rapid and without premonitory signs. Hence, regular echocardiographic monitoring of the size of an effusion is vital. Surgical drainage by subxiphoid pericardiostomy should be performed whenever the effusion size is estimated by echocardiography to exceed 250 mL (posterior echo-free space larger than 1 cm) even when hemodynamic compromise is absent. Surgical drainage is mandatory when overt tamponade appears.

(1) Subxiphoid pericardiostomy. The surgical drainage procedure of choice is subxiphoid pericardiostomy (i.e., insertion under local anesthesia of a large-bore tube into the pericardial space). The tube is left in place to closed drainage for several days until drainage ceases. Instillation of locally acting steroids (e.g., triamcinolone) has not been proven necessary and increases the risk of infection.

(2) Pericardiocentesis using a blindly inserted needle is dangerous and never indicated except as an emergency therapy for patients with life-threatening tamponade. Hemorrhagic effusions are poorly evacuable through the needle, and the risk of coronary artery or cardiac puncture and arrhythmia is substantial.

(3) Anterior pericardiectomy has been favored by some, but general anesthesia and thoracotomy are unnecessary risks given the uniformly successful response to drainage by subxiphoid pericardiostomy.

C. Constrictive pericarditis. Constrictive pericarditis can appear as an unusual complication of dialysis-associated pericarditis or as the first manifestation of pericardial disease. Constrictive pericarditis may masquerade as congestive cardiac failure; the best means of differentiation is by right heart catheterization. Even then, the diagnosis may be in doubt and can be proved only by a favorable response to total pericardiectomy.

D. Purulent pericarditis. Occasionally, patients are found to have purulent pericarditis as a complication of septicemia, often as a result of access site infection. These patients often require anterior pericardiectomy in addition to antimicrobial therapy.

E. Risks of dialysis therapy in patients with pericarditis. Pericarditis increases the risks of bleeding, arrhythmia, hypotension, and tamponade during hemodialysis, and intensive (daily) hemodialysis subjects the patient to the additional dangers of dehydration, hypokalemia, and hypophosphatemia.

1. Bleeding. Heparin-free dialysis should be used, because of the risk of precipitating pericardial bleeding and tamponade.

2. Arrhythmia. The increased risk of arrhythmia during hemodialysis is presumably due to irritation of cardiac pacemaker zones by the overlying inflammation. Management strategy includes monitoring of the cardiac rhythm during hemodialysis and ensuring that an adequate dialysis solution potassium concentration is present.

3.   Hypotension and cardiac tamponade. The risk of hypotension is increased only if effusion is present; hypotension in this setting may reflect cardiac tamponade precipitated by decreased cardiac filling attendant to intravascular volume depletion.

4.   Dehydration. Dehydration is common with daily, intensive dialysis schedules. An ultrafiltration controller should be used and set to prevent the patient from going below a clinically determined target dry weight.

5.   Hypokalemia and hypophosphatemia. These disturbances are completely preventable by supplementing the dialysis solution with potassium (up to 4.0 mEq per L) and/or phosphorus (about 1.3 mmol per L) whenever predialysis serum levels of these minerals are in the low or low-normal range.

6.   Metabolic alkalosis. Daily dialysis may precipitate metabolic alkalosis unless the dialysis solution bicarbonate level is appropriately reduced. Most modern dialysis machines can deliver dialysates with bicarbonate levels of 25 mM or less.

VI.   Left ventricular dysfunction and hypertrophy

A.   Left ventricular hypertrophy. In dialysis patients, left ventricular hypertrophy (LVH) is strongly associated with premature death, cardiac events, dialysis hypotension, and arrhythmias. Increased left ventricular volume is the most common abnormality, but more subtle disorders of both systolic and diastolic function may be detected. The hypertrophic response to chronic chamber enlargement may be inadequate, possibly due to hyperparathyroidism or vitamin D deficiency. LVH is probably a more important determinant of survival than coronary artery disease in the dialysis population and may be more amenable to therapeutic intervention.

B.   Heart failure versus fluid overload. Fundamental to an appreciation of the problem of left ventricular dysfunction in dialysis patients is the differentiation between heart failure and fluid overload. In extreme cases, the distinction is simple; for example, after acute massive myocardial infarction, the rapid onset of pulmonary edema without change in body weight is clearly due to heart failure, whereas its development in a young anuric patient after excessive fluid ingestion is most likely due to fluid overload. In practice, these factors combine in an individual patient. Attempts have recently been made to use ultrasonography of the vena cava and measurement of circulating atrial natriuretic peptide to aid in assessment of appropriate circulating volume, but neither method has supplanted clinical judgment. A lack of increase in the hematocrit during dialysis (measured using an on-line optical or ultrasound sensor) despite fluid removal is a more reliable clue to the existence of an overhydrated state.

C.   Pathogenesis of left ventricular dysfunction. The potential causative factors of left heart dysfunction in dialysis patients are listed in Table 33-2.

D.   Diagnosis. Echocardiography is a much more sensitive measure of LVH than radiography or electrocardiography. Increased ventricular stiffness leading to impaired diastolic function can be demonstrated by pulsed Doppler studies.

Table 33-2. Factors leading to left ventricular dysfunction and/or hypertrophy in dialysis patients

Hypertension
Fluid overload
Anemia
Ischemic heart disease
Arteriovenous fistula
Myocardial calcification
Systemic disease (e.g., amyloidosis, polyarteritis, scleroderma)
Uremia

E. Prevention of left ventricular dysfunction and hypertrophy
   1. Control of blood pressure and fluid balance. Aggressive treatment of hypertension from the earliest phases of renal impairment is mandatory. In the anuric patient, the target dry weight should be constantly reviewed to minimize the chronic effects of subtle degrees of fluid overload. In hemodialysis patients, excessive interdialysis weight gain (more than 3–4 kg) is clearly associated with an elevated cardiovascular mortality. If patients are unable to restrict sodium and fluid intake between dialysis sessions, a switch from hemodialysis to peritoneal dialysis may be necessary.
   2. Arteriovenous (AV) fistulas and grafts. Although forearm fistulas occasionally lead to a high output state, this problem is more often encountered with upper arm brachial fistulas, and close attention to the size of the AV fistula is essential during surgical construction. Bradycardia during fistula or graft occlusion (by finger pressure) suggests that the AV shunt is importantly and pathologically contributing to an increased cardiac output (Branham's sign). The test is specific, but absence of bradycardia on fistula or graft occlusion by no means exonerates the AV communication as a cause of the heart failure.
   3. Anemia. The role of anemia in LVH and subsequent heart failure has been clarified since the introduction of erythropoietin. Only if blood pressure is adequately controlled will maintenance of hemoglobin at 10 g per dL or more eventually lead to a reduction in left ventricular mass and volume, and the cardiothoracic ratio on chest radiograph will shrink. It is likely that regression of LVH will confer long-term cardiac benefit with reduction in mortality from heart failure, and both death risk and hospitalization rates are reduced when the hemoglobin is high (Ma et al, 1999).
F. Management
   1. Acute pulmonary edema. Acute pulmonary edema in the dialysis patient usually results from fluid overload on the background of often covert left ventricular dysfunction. The role of volume overload is readily evidenced from inspection of the patient's dialysis weight chart. Less commonly, pulmonary edema appears without excess weight gain and is then more likely to be due to acute myocardial infarction, pericarditis, or,

occasionally, endocarditis. The immediate management is initially along conventional lines. In patients with an obvious increase in cardiac afterload (as assessed by cold, cyanosed peripheries), vasodilatation with transdermal, oral, or intravenous nitrates is indicated unless the systolic blood pressure is below 100 mm Hg. The patient will need urgent ultrafiltration. In the peritoneal dialysis patient, the use of high-dextrose dialysis solution delivered by a peritoneal dialysis cycler usually produces a rapid loss of fluid. For the hemodialysis patient, ultrafiltration, either as isolated ultrafiltration (see Chapter 10) or ultrafiltration during dialysis, is indicated.

Reassessment of the patient's target dry weight is necessary after the acute drama of pulmonary edema has passed. Often acute pulmonary edema occurs in the clinical setting of a recent catabolic illness when flesh weight has been lost, but total weight remains constant, with consequent hidden overhydration.

2.   **Chronic heart failure**
   a.   **General guidelines.** The management of chronic heart failure in dialysis patients is fraught with difficulty. The tightrope between dehydration with symptomatic hypotension on the one hand and fluid overload with overt pulmonary edema on the other becomes ever trickier to negotiate, and symptomatic hypotension at the initiation of hemodialysis becomes ever more problematical. It becomes almost impossible to maintain many patients with intractable heart failure on hemodialysis successfully; for such patients, peritoneal dialysis should be considered because maintenance of a constant body weight becomes a simpler matter.
   b.   **Drug therapy.** Cardiac glycosides may benefit some patients, but their use is associated with an increased risk of arrhythmia. The loading dosage of digoxin should be halved, with an initial maintenance dosage of 62.5 µg (0.0625 mg) on alternate days. Therapy should be monitored by 12-hour postdose blood levels. Angiotensin-converting enzyme (ACE) inhibitors and other vasodilators may be employed to ameliorate symptoms of heart failure in dialysis patients, but their use is often attended by hypotension, and they are less efficacious in dialysis patients than in patients with normal renal function. The possible impact of ACE inhibitors on mortality in the dialysis population is unknown but their use has been associated with a reduction in the degree of LVH (Cannella et al, 1997). The dosage schedules in uremia for these agents are discussed in Chapter 26. Vasodilators may need to be withheld before a hemodialysis session if blood pressure falls abruptly during dialysis.
   c.   **Other.** Hemoglobin should be maintained at 11–12 g per dL with the use of erythropoietin. The consequent slight rise in blood pressure that commonly accompanies a rise in hemoglobin is often useful in heart failure patients and improves tolerance to both vasodilator drug therapy and the hemodialysis procedure itself. AV fistulas may need to be closed if a patient successfully transfers to peritoneal dialysis.

VII. Endocarditis

A. Incidence and etiologic factors. Whereas infective endocarditis is an unusual infection in peritoneal dialysis patients, it is not rare in hemodialysis patients, being the result of dissemination of infection from the vascular access site.

B. Prevention

1. Avoidance of access site infection. The widespread use of internal jugular venous dialysis catheters for medium-term vascular access has led to an increase in bacteremic episodes in the dialysis population. Routine microbiologic surveillance of catheter exit sites is unhelpful, but catheters associated with clinically infected exit sites need early removal if local suppuration does not rapidly clear with antimicrobial therapy. The importance of planned early permanent access cannot be overemphasized. Eradication of infection from infected vascular prostheses may be impossible without removal of the devices themselves.

2. Prolonged antimicrobial therapy for staphylococcal bacteremia. In many patients, acute bacterial endocarditis will complicate an already recognized episode of *Staphylococcus aureus* bacteremia, and the latter infection should be treated as a presumed endocarditis with two anti-staphylococcal agents (floxacillin, erythromycin, gentamicin, vancomycin), given for 4–6 weeks. Such prolonged antimicrobial therapy should avoid the complication of valvular sequestration of infection in most patients with bacteremia diagnosed at an early stage.

C. Diagnosis. Symptoms and signs of endocarditis are in general similar to those in patients without renal failure. However, the clinical evaluation of murmurs may prove difficult because cardiac murmurs are common in the ordinary dialysis population owing to anemia, valvular calcification, and the presence of AV fistulas. Because a substantial percentage of dialysis patients are normally hypothermic, the body temperature with infection may be elevated to only slightly above the normal range or not at all. Often the only clinical manifestation of endocarditis may be orthostatic dizziness in a patient with positive blood cultures, occasionally accompanied by mild neurologic manifestations, which may be misinterpreted as being due to the disequilibrium syndrome or to uremia.

D. Management. Due to the frequent occurrence of a blunted immune response in uremic patients, endocarditis may occur with greater than usual severity in the dialysis patient, with early development of valvular and myocardial abscesses. Although appropriate antimicrobial therapy should be the first line of management, renal failure should not in itself exclude consideration of cardiac surgery. Indications for valve replacement are the same as those in the general population, including progressive valvular destruction, progressive heart failure, recurrent embolization, or a fever unresponsive to well-selected antimicrobial therapy.

VIII. Arrhythmias

A. Etiology and incidence. There are many reasons that cardiac arrhythmias are common in dialysis patients. These patients often suffer from LVH or ischemic heart disease. Serum levels of a number of ions that can affect cardiac conduction, including potassium, calcium, magnesium, and hydrogen, are often abnormal or may undergo rapid fluctuations during hemodialysis. Hypoxemia may accompany the hemodialysis procedure. Hypophosphatemia, recently linked with arrhythmias, may also occur in dialysis patients. Calcific cardiomyopathy may involve the conducting tissues.

Nonetheless, whereas some workers have reported a high incidence of cardiac arrhythmias, including self-terminating ventricular tachycardia, atrial fibrillation, and frequent premature ventricular contractions in dialysis patients, others have not found the incidence of arrhythmias to be increased.

B. Clinical settings

    1. Arrhythmias occurring primarily during the hemodialysis session

        a. Associated with use of digitalis preparations. This group is at the highest risk of arrhythmia, partly from the drug itself but also due to underlying heart disease. Hence, digitalis preparations should be used only with good indication and the patient monitored closely. Electrolyte shifts during hemodialysis should be minimized, ensuring that serum potassium does not fall below 3.5 mEq per L. Dialysis solution potassium may need to be increased to 3.0–3.5 mEq per L, restricting dietary potassium to avoid predialysis hyperkalemia. Intracellular shifting of potassium during dialysis may be minimized by reducing both dialysis solution glucose (from 200 to 100 mg per dL) and, when acid–base status permits, bicarbonate (from 35–38 to 20–30 mEq per L). Persistent ventricular arrhythmias associated with digitalis may be suppressed by oral quinidine therapy, but if the digoxin had been prescribed to control the ventricular rate in patients with atrial fibrillation, a switch to amiodarone is preferable.

        b. Not associated with digitalis preparations. Pericarditis, LVH, ischemic heart disease, and amyloidosis predispose to arrhythmias during hemodialysis. Hypotension, frequently due to silent myocardial ischemia, often triggers the event. Myocardial ischemia may be revealed by ambulatory electrocardiographic monitoring, with ST segment analysis in addition to standard arrhythmia evaluation. In such patients, antianginal prophylaxis may be necessary in addition to alterations in dialysis solution potassium and calcium levels. Finally, maintenance of an adequate blood hemoglobin level is vital.

        c. Drug dosing for management of acute arrhythmias. In the event that a serious arrhythmia supervenes during a hemodialysis treatment, the dialysis session should be terminated and the blood returned cautiously. Prompt pharmacologic management of the arrhythmia and/or cardioversion can proceed in the usual fashion. The loading dosages of selected agents used in emergency management of arrhythmias are listed in Table 33-3.

    2. Management of chronic arrhythmias in dialysis patients. Chronic arrhythmias that may require treatment in dialysis patients include recurrent atrial tachyarrhyth-

Table 33-3. Loading dosages of selected antiarrhythmic drugs (for emergency treatment only)

Drug	Usual loading dosage in nonuremic patients	Loading dosage in dialysis patients	Comments
Adenosine	6–12 mg IV by rapid bolus	Same	Not for chronic therapy
Amiodarone	800–1600 mg/d PO for 1–3 wk	Same	Hepatic excretion; not dialyzable
Bretylium tosylate	5 mg/kg IV	Same	Over 20 min; may cause hypotension
Digoxin	0.75–1.0 mg IV	Reduce by 50%	Infuse over 24h; watch serum potassium level, dialysis solution potassium level
Disopyramide	300 mg PO	Reduce by 50%	
Flecainide acetate	Loading dosage not recommended	Same	
Lidocaine	1–3 mg/kg IV	Same	Infusion rate >7 mg/min may cause hypotension
Phenytoin	1,000 mg IV	Same	Rapid infusion may cause arrhythmia; max. safe infusion rate: 50 mg/min
Procainamide hydrochloride	100 mg q5min IV to max. 1,000 mg	Same	IV loading hazardous; safer PO
Propafenone	Loading dosage not recommended	Same	New drug: caution
Propranolol hydrochloride	1–3 mg IV	Same	Max. infusion rate: 1 mg/min
Quinidine sulfate	600 mg PO	Same	
Verapamil	5–10 mg IV	Same	Max. infusion rate: 2 mg/min

mias, frequent ventricular ectopic beats with recurrent ventricular tachycardia, and bradyarrhythmias. Beyond simple measures such as cessation of smoking and caffeine intake, the management strategy is often complex and can comprise drug therapy, cardioversion, pacemaker insertion, and electrophysiologic evaluation of pharmacologic agents with the aid of cardiac catheterization and provocation of the arrhythmia. While a detailed discussion of arrhythmia management is beyond the scope of this book, some points regarding drug pharmacokinetics in dialysis patients deserve emphasis (Tables 33-4 and 33-5).

   a.   Class I drugs (membrane stabilizers)
      (1)   Ia drugs. Ia drugs (quinidine, procainamide, and disopyramide) prolong the action potential duration (APD). All of these drugs have significant renal excretion; early toxicity may manifest with prolongation of the QT interval, and severe toxicity results in torsades de pointes.
      (2)   Ib drugs. Ib drugs (lidocaine, mexiletine, tocainide, phenytoin) reduce the APD. Toxicity is unusual in dialysis patients except with tocainide.
      (3)   Ic drugs. Flecainide, encainide, lorcainide, and propafenone are membrane stabilizers devoid of effect on the APD. The first three of these drugs share pharmacologic properties, are negatively inotropic, and are predominantly renally excreted. In view of excess deaths associated with the use of these drugs in some nonrenal populations, they should be used, if at all, with extreme caution in dialysis patients and with close monitoring of drug levels. There is yet little experience with propafenone in renal failure, but it appears to be the safest class Ic drug at present. It has weak β-blocking properties, which may be valuable in patients with underlying ischemic heart disease. No dosage modification for propafenone is necessary.
   b.   Class II drugs (antisympathetic agents). The starting dosages of β-blockers are given in Table 26-2. In general, the dosage can be titrated against the heart rate. Bretylium has important antisympathetic activities as well as class III actions (increased APD). Although bretylium is purely renally excreted without significant metabolism, patients can be given the usual loading dosage of 5 mg/kg (as a fast intravenous bolus) for resistant ventricular fibrillation. The maintenance dosage, however, must be sharply reduced Table 33-4.
   c.   Class III drugs (increase in the APD alone). Amiodarone is the only important agent in this group. No special problems are attached to its use in dialysis patients.
   d.   Class IV drugs (calcium channel blockers). None of these agents has significant renal excretion, so they can be given in normal dosage. The cardiac depressant effect of verapamil may be more obvious in hemodialysis patients with poor left ventricular function.
   e.   Digoxin. See Section VI.F.2.b.

Table 33-4. Selected cardiac drugs in dialysis patients: maintenance dosages

Drug	Tablet size (mg)	Nonuremic maintenance dose range (mg/day)	Dialysis patient dose (% nonuremic patient dose)	Suggested initial dose for dialysis patients (mg)	Plasma half-life (h) Nonuremic patients	Plasma half-life (h) End-stage renal disease	Renal excretion (%)
Amiodarone	100, 200	100–600	Same	Same	25–50 d	?	<1
Bretylium[a]	IV only	5–10 mg q6h	25	0.5–2 mg/hr	9	30+	75
Digoxin	0.125, 0.25	0.125–0.50	25	0.0625 qod	40	80–120	60
Disopyramide[b]	100, 150	400–800	25	50 q12h	6	10–18	55
Flecainide	100	200–400	25	50 q12h	16	10–60	30
Lidocaine	IV only	1–4 mg/min	100	Same	2	2	2
Mexiletine	150, 200, 250	600–900	?Same	200 q8h	10	16	15
Procainamide[c]	250, 375, 500	2,000–4,000	25	250 q12h	3	6–14	70
N-acetylprocainamide					6	40–70	80
Propafenone	150	450–900	100	Same	6	6	1
Quinidine	200, 300, 324	800–1,600	75	200–324 q8h	6	4–14	20
Tocainide	400, 600	1,200–2,400	50	600 q24h	13	17–27	40

[a] See Adir J. et al. Nomogram for bretylium dosing in renal impairment. *Ther Drug Monit* 1985;7:265.
[b] Atropinic side effects are common in dialysis patients.
[c] N-Acetylprocainamide metabolite is largely renally excreted.
qod, once every other day.

Table 33-5.   Dialysability of selected cardiac drugs

	Substantially removed by	
Drug	Hemodialysis	Peritoneal dialysis
Amiodarone	No	No
Atenolol	Yes[a]	Yes
Bretylium	No	No
Digitoxin	No	No
Digoxin	No	No
Diltiazem	No	No
Disopyramide	No	No
Flecainide	Yes[a]	Yes
Lidocaine	No	No
Mexiletine	No	No
Phenytoin	No	No
Procainamide	Yes[a]	No
Propafenone	No	No
Propranolol	No	No
Quinidine	Not usually	No
Tocainide	Yes[a]	Yes
Verapamil	No	No

[a] A dosage supplement may be necessary after a dialysis session.

  f. Adenosine. This has a specific role in the treatment and diagnosis of junctional tachycardia. The drug is totally removed from the circulation in minutes, and the dosage is unchanged in renal failure.

  g. Dialyzability of antiarrhythmic drugs. This information is given in Table 33-5. With those drugs that are dialyzable, a small supplemental dose may be needed after a hemodialysis session.

 3. Sudden death in dialysis patients. Cardiac events associated with hyperkalemia are believed to be responsible for an significant number of deaths of dialysis patients each year. The patients at risk are often young and unwilling to accept a rigidly restricted diet and need frequent counseling and advice. The prevention and management of hyperkalemia in dialysis patients are discussed further in Chapter 5. Noncompliant dialysis patients with severe hyperkalemia often present with severe weakness, sometimes in association with fluid overload. An electrocardiogram should be obtained at once. When severe electrocardiographic findings are present, the treatment should usually include, in addition to emergency hemodialysis, the intravenous infusion of calcium chloride or calcium gluconate, and/or infusion of glucose plus insulin. Calcium infusion brings about a prompt effect and is preferred by many. Intravenous albuterol infusion is as effective and safe as glucose plus insulin. Albuterol therapy and glucose/insulin infusion can be combined for a synergistic effect. Frequently, the above antihyperkalemic measures are used in various combinations simultaneously.

SELECTED READINGS

Bostom AG, et al. Controlled comparison of L-5-methyltetrahydrofolate versus folic acid for the treatment of hyperhomocysteinemia in hemodialysis patients. *Circulation* 2000;101:2829–2832.

Cannella G, et al. Inadequate diagnosis and therapy of arterial hypertension as causes of left ventricular hypertrophy in uremic dialysis patients. *Kidney Int* 2000;58:260–268.

Cannella G, et al. Prolonged therapy with ACE inhibitors induces a regression of left ventricular hypertrophy of dialyzed uremic patients independently from hypotensive effects. *Am J Kidney Dis* 1997;30:659–664.

Cheung AK, et al. Atherosclerotic cardiovascular disease risks in chronic hemodialysis patients. *Kidney Int* 2000;58:353–362.

Daugirdas JT, et al. Subxiphoid pericardiostomy for hemodialysis-associated pericardial effusion. *Arch Intern Med* 1986;146:1113–1115.

Deighan CJ, et al. Atherogenic lipoprotein phenotype in end-stage renal failure: origin and extent of small dense low-density lipoprotein formation. *Am J Kidney Dis* 2000;35:852–862.

Foley RN, et al. Serial change in echocardiographic parameters and cardiac failure in end-stage renal disease. *J Am Soc Nephrol* 2000; 11:912–916.

Gehr TWB, Sica DA. Antiarrhythmic medications: practical guidelines for drug therapy in dialysis. *Semin Dial* 1990;3:33.

Herzog CA, et al. Long-term outcome of dialysis patients in the United States with coronary revascularization procedures. *Kidney Int* 1999;56:324–332.

House AA, et al. Randomized trial of high-flux vs low-flux haemodialysis: effects on homocysteine and lipids. *Nephrol Dial Transplant* 2000 Jul;15(7):1029–1034.

Huting J, et al. Abnormal diastolic left ventricular filling by pulsed Doppler echocardiography in patients on continuous ambulatory peritoneal dialysis. *Clin Nephrol* 1991;36:21–28.

Islam KN, et al. Alpha-tocopherol supplementation decreases the oxidative susceptibility of LDL in renal failure patients on dialysis therapy. *Atherosclerosis* 2000;150:217–224.

Khaitan L, et al. Coronary artery bypass grafting in patients who require long-term dialysis. *Ann Thorac Surg* 2000;69:1135–1139.

Leunissen KM, et al. Plasma alpha–human atrial natriuretic peptide and volume status in chronic hemodialysis patients. *Nephrol Dial Transplant* 1989;4:382–386.

Ma JZ, et al. Hematocrit level and associated mortality in hemodialysis patients. *J Am Soc Nephrol* 1999;10:610–619.

Nicholls A, Edward N, Catto GR. Staphylococcal septicaemia, endocarditis, and osteomyelitis in dialysis and renal transplant patients. *Postgrad Med J* 1980;56:642–648.

Raj DS, et al. Advanced glycation end products: a Nephrologist's perspective. *Am J Kidney Dis* 2000;35:365–380.

Schneider H, Schmitt Y. Low molecular weight heparin: how does it modify lipid metabolism in chronic hemodialysis patients? *Klin Wochenschr* 1991;69:749–756.

Touam M, et al. Effective correction of hyperhomocysteinemia in hemodialysis patients by intravenous folinic acid and pyridoxine therapy. *Kidney Int* 1999;56:2292–2296.

Ventura SC, Garella S. The management of pericardial disease in renal failure. *Semin Dial* 1990;3:21.

Wong JS, et al. Survival advantage in Asian American end-stage renal disease patients. *Kidney Int* 1999;55:2515–2523.

Yeun JY, Kaysen GA. C-reactive protein, oxidative Stress, homocysteine, and troponin as inflammatory and metabolic predictors of atherosclerosis in ESRD. *Current Opinion Nephrol and Hypertens* 2000:(Fall). in press.

Zebe H. Atrial fibrillation in dialysis patients. *Nephrol Dial Transplant.* 2000;15:765–768.

Internet Reference

Cardiovascular disease in ESRD (http://www.hdcn.com/card)

The Digestive Tract

Susie Q. Lew, Beat von Albertini,
and Juan P. Bosch

I. Common gastrointestinal (GI) symptoms

A. Anorexia. Anorexia is a nonspecific symptom that may be a manifestation of uremia or due to a number of other causes associated with uremia and the dialysis process.

B. Nausea and vomiting. Nausea and vomiting are nonspecific symptoms that may be manifestations of uremia or due to fluid and electrolyte changes during the dialysis treatment.

Prior to the initiation of dialysis, patients may complain of nausea and vomiting. These symptoms usually disappear with dialysis and removal of uremic toxins. Once patients are on maintenance dialysis, nausea and vomiting may be symptoms associated with inadequate dialysis. Check the fractional urea clearance *(Kt/V)* to ensure adequate dialysis.

During the dialysis treatment, nausea and vomiting are associated with hypotension. Hypotension may be due to rapid fluid removal in patients with large interdialytic weight gain or due to the presence of acetate when its metabolism is compromised during a treatment using acetate bath. Patients with large interdialytic weight gain need dietary counseling to limit salt and fluid intake. Hemodialysis techniques, such as sequential isolated ultrafiltration or sodium modeling, may relieve these symptoms during rapid fluid removal.

Nausea and vomiting may not be related to uremia or to the dialysis treatment itself. If these symptoms persist after the aforementioned possibilities have been addressed, a thorough evaluation of cerebral or GI abnormalities is necessary.

C. Dyspepsia. Dyspepsia is defined as persistent or recurrent abdominal discomfort centered in the upper abdomen (epigastrium). Dyspepsia and indigestion are terms that are frequently interchangeable. Symptoms may include epigastric pain or discomfort, bloating, belching, eructations, and flatulence. Dyspepsia may be due to a true GI pathologic process, such as peptic ulcer disease, gastroesophageal reflux disease, gastritis, duodenitis, or gastroparesis, as seen in diabetic patients. Alternatively, dyspepsia may be related to medications that dialysis patients are required to take, such as phosphate binders (e.g., calcium carbonate or aluminum salts) or iron supplements. Evaluation for organic lesion is warranted if the history and physical examination are suggestive of such lesions. Prokinetic agents, antacids, and histamine H2 receptor antagonists are the most widely used agents in the management of dyspepsia. Dosing of these drugs in renal failure is discussed below in Section II.A.3. (prokinetic drugs) and Section II.B.3. (H_2-blockers).

D. Constipation. Constipation is not an uncommon complaint among dialysis patients. The causes of constipation are multifactorial. Patients' fluid intake is limited. Dietary restriction of high-potassium fruits and vegetables decreases the fiber content of ingested food. Medications such as calcium- or aluminum-containing phosphate binders and iron supplements cause constipation. Patient inactivity and underlying medical conditions may contribute to constipation. Narcotics given as an analgesic, such as codeine and meperidine, can cause constipation, as well as mental status change in patients with end-stage renal disease (ESRD).

Constipation may result in obstipation with obstruction, fecal impaction, and even bowel perforation. Long-term complications of constipation are thought to contribute to the etiologic process of diverticular disease, as well as hemorrhoids. In patients treated with peritoneal dialysis, decreased bowel motility can cause dialysate outflow obstruction through the peritoneal catheter.

Dietary changes to increase the fiber content in food usually corrects constipation. If constipation persists, the following agents may be used: *Emollient:* docusate sodium (Colace) 100 mg PO qd to tid prn, casanthranol and docusate sodium (Peri-Colace) 1–2 capsules or 1–2 tablespoons PO qhs prn; *Stimulant:* bisacodyl (Dulcolax) 1–3 tablets PO qd prn; and *Hyperosmotic:* sorbitol 70% 30 mL PO qhs, lactulose (Chronulac) 30 mL PO qhs. Sodium polystyrene sulfonate resin plus sorbitol (Kayexalate) has been associated with intestinal necrosis in ESRD patients, either given by enema or by the oral route (Dardik et al, 2000). It is not clear if the sorbitol component alone is equally dangerous. Whereas the combination is still widely used to treat hyperkalemia, use of sorbitol to treat constipation, where there are alternatives available, may not be wise. Soap suds, mineral oil, and tap water enemas or bisacodyl or glycerin suppositories once daily may be used for more immediate results. Colyte or GoLYTELY may be used for bowel preparation for endoscopy or radiology studies despite the high electrolyte content and the large volume ingested.

Medicinal fiber in the form of psyllium (Metamucil) should be avoided. Both sodium and potassium are present in the preparation, and a large volume of liquid is required in preparation. Laxatives containing magnesium, citrate, or phosphate should be avoided (e.g., milk of magnesium, magnesium citrate, and Fleet's products containing phosphate). Magnesium is poorly handled by patients with ESRD. Hypermagnesemia can result in development of neurologic disorders. Citrate, in general, should be avoided in patients with ESRD because it increases absorption of aluminum from the GI tract. Hyperphosphatemia from phosphate intake can upset the delicate calcium/phosphorus balance and contribute to the sequela of secondary hyperparathyroidism.

E.   Diarrhea. There are four major mechanisms of diarrhea:

1. Osmotic diarrhea due to the presence in the gut lumen of unusual amounts of poorly absorbable, osmotically active solutes
2. Secretory diarrhea due to intestinal ion secretion or inhibition of normal active ion absorption
3. Deranged intestinal motility

4. Exudation of mucus, blood, and protein from sites of inflammation

An episode of diarrhea on an occasional basis is not uncommon and may be related to bowel irritability associated with dietary intake or viral GI disorder.

Diarrhea following a period of constipation may signal fecal impaction. Treatment is focused on constipation.

An acute episode of bloody diarrhea associated with abdominal pain, fever and signs of sepsis, and hypotension, especially during hemodialysis, may suggest ischemic bowel disorder or bowel infarction. ESRD patients are prone to this disease because of their atherosclerosis-associated risk factors such as hypertension, diabetes mellitus, and dyslipidemia.

Diarrhea associated with fever suggests an infectious cause. Blood and stool specimen for culture and sensitivity are required. *Clostridium difficile* enteritis may occur after prolonged antimicrobial therapy. Oral vancomycin or metronidazole is used in the treatment of *C. difficile* enteritis.

Persistent diarrhea requires a workup similar to that in patients without ESRD. Suspect autonomic neuropathy in patients with diabetes mellitus. Endoscopy is required to diagnose inflammatory bowel disorders. Malabsorption is suspected if food fibers or fat are found in the stool. Dietary adjustment or digestive enzyme replacement may help or correct malabsorption.

In noninfectious diarrhea, loperamide hydrochloride (Imodium) or diphenoxylate hydrochloride and atropine sulfate (Lomotil) may be used for temporary relief.

F. Hiccups. Hiccups are inspiratory sounds associated with abrupt rhythmic involuntary contractions of the diaphragm and closure of the glottis. Diaphragmatic irritation, hyponatremia, or other metabolic derangements, such as uremia, may result in intractable hiccups. Those due to uremia can be corrected with dialysis. Medications that have been reported as successful in controlling hiccups include chlorpromazine, metoclopramide, quinidine, phenytoin, valproic acid, baclofen, and nifedipine.

G. Others. Dysgeusia, metallic taste in the mouth, and a peculiar odor to the breath are sometimes noted by uremic patients. Uremic stomatitis is a peculiar oral inflammation that some patients manifest. Parotitis and sicca syndrome are commonly present, thus limiting compliance with fluid restriction. Such oral and gustatory complications may exacerbate decreased nutritional intake in some uremic patients. The use of zinc supplementation and intensified dialysis may be helpful in decreasing these symptoms. Finally, it should be noted that the concomitant administration of sodium polystyrene sulfonate and a nonabsorbable antacid such as magnesium or aluminum hydroxide can engender a metabolic alkalosis.

II. Upper GI diseases
A. Gastritis, duodenitis, and peptic ulcer disease
1. **Gastric acid production and gastric intestinal hormone levels.** The pathogenesis of uremic GI lesions is not understood. Fasting serum gastrin is commonly elevated in chronic renal failure. Levels of gastrin correlate with the degree of renal insufficiency, as gastrin is removed by the kidney.

There appears to be no correlation between gastrin level, gastric acid secretion, or the presence of upper GI lesions. GI hormones, including secretin, gastric inhibitory polypeptide, and cholecytokinin, may be elevated in uremic patients. Their contribution to GI dysfunction and symptoms is uncertain.

Neither *Helicobacter pylori* infection, hypergastrinemia, nor hyperacidity appears to play a major role in the pathogenesis of uremic gastroduodenal lesions. Upper endoscopy of stable dialysis patients reveals abnormalities in up to 51% of cases. Gastritis, duodenitis, and mucosal erosions are most commonly seen.

Gastritis and duodenitis in dialysis patients can be treated with ranitidine 150 mg q24h at bedtime.

2. Infection with *H. pylori*. *H. pylori* is present in almost all cases of nonerosive chronic active gastritis and in some cases of chronic gastritis without the active component. *H. pylori,* which displays abundant urease activity, appears not to be increased in uremic patients.

Current techniques used to detect *H. pylori* include (a) culture, (b) serology, (c) rapid urease tests, (d) urea carbon breath tests and (e) detection of antigen in the feces.

Treatment for *H. pylori* includes one to three antibiotics given in combination with a proton-pump inhibitor or H_2-receptor antagonist. For dosing of these agents in renal failure see Section II.B.3., below. Use of bismuth-based regimens should be avoided because of accumulation of bismuth due to impaired renal excretion (Gladziwa et al, 1994). Treatment has been reported to reduce gastric ammonia levels (Tamura et al, 1997) and partially normalize elevated serum gastrin levels (Gur et al, 1999).

3. Gastric retention. Gastroparesis is frequently encountered in patients with diabetes mellitus. This is associated with autonomic neuropathy. Diagnosis can be made with an isotopic gastric emptying study. Prokinetic drugs block dopaminergic receptors in the upper alimentary tract, stimulating motility of the esophagus, stomach, and upper small intestine. Prokinetic agents include domperidone and metoclopramide. In nonuremic patients, both were equally efficacious, but central nervous system side effects were less with domperidone (Patterson et al, 1999). There is little information about pharmacokinetics of domperidone in renal failure patients (Lauritsen et al, 1990). Metoclopramide is renally excreted to a large extent, and the usual dose of 10–15 mg qid should initially be reduced by at least 50% in patients with minimal renal function. Metoclopramide is normally given 30 minutes before meals and at bedtime. Cisapride, which in some hands was a more efficacious drug than either domperidone or metoclopramide, is no longer sold in the United States because of the regular occurrence of a QT-interval prolongation, worsened by coadministration of many other common drugs, and occasional occurrence of fatal arrhythmia.

Gastric retention is uncommon in nondiabetic dialysis patients but does occur, and its correction results in improved nutritional status (Ross et al, 1998). Patients on CAPD may complain of symptoms of gastric retention when dialysate is present in the peritoneum and is relieved with draining of the dialysate.

B. Upper GI bleeding

    1. Incidence and etiology. According to one study, the sources of upper GI bleeding are gastritis (38%), duodenal ulcer (24%), duodenitis (14%), gastric ulcer (9.5%), esophageal varices (9.5%), and Mallory–Weiss tear (5%). Proposed mechanisms for upper GI hemorrhage with chronic renal failure include disturbances in serum gastrin, in gastric acid secretion, in the mucosal barrier, and in the clotting process; the use of ulcerogenic drugs, such as anti-inflammatory drugs that inhibit prostaglandin synthesis (nonsteroidal anti-inflammatory drugs, or NSAIDs, and aspirin); and infection associated with *H. pylori.*

    However, in another study by Zuckerman et al (1985), angiodysplasia was the most common source of upper GI bleeding, as well as recurrent bleeding in the patients with renal failure. Causes for upper GI bleeding in patients with chronic renal failure are as follows: angiodysplasia of the stomach or duodenum (24%), erosive gastritis (18%), duodenal ulcer (17%), erosive esophagitis (17%), gastric ulcer (12%), Mallory–Weiss (8%), and erosive duodenitis (3%). It is possible that angiodysplastic lesions in both the upper and lower tract in these patients are no more common than in the general population. However, they are discovered more frequently because of their greater tendency to bleed. It has been suggested that renal failure plays a role in the pathogenesis of these lesions. One theory states that functional failure of the precapillary sphincter due to volume overload and submucosal venous obstruction leads to vascular ectasia. Another theory states that a low blood flow state during dialysis followed by reactive hyperemia results in eventual angiodysplasia. Finally, others suggest that potassium or gastrin, agents known to reduce precapillary arteriolar tone, have a causative role in the development of these lesions. Angiodysplastic lesions in patients with chronic renal failure are more likely to bleed than such lesions in patients without renal failure. Uremic platelet dysfunction may play a contributory role.

    2. Diagnosis. Esophagogastroduodenoscopy (EGD) is more likely to provide an accurate diagnosis than a single-contrast barium meal radiograph in patients with upper GI bleeding.

    3. Management. Treatment of upper GI bleeding is the same as for nonuremic patients. It consists of nasogastric aspiration, transfusion, and the administration of acid secretion inhibition with histamine H2 blockers or pump inhibitor and antacids.

    H_2 blockers include Cemetidine (Tagamet), ranitidine (Zantac), famotidine (Pepcid), and nizatidine (Axid). All of these drugs are partially excreted renally, and their usual dosage should be reduced by at least 50% in chronic renal failure. For nizatidine, the recommendation is to give 150 mg every other day (versus the usual 150 mg twice a day dosing in nonuremic patients).

Omeprazole (Prilosec) 20 mg PO qd has antisecretory action based on inhibition of the parietal cell H,K-ATPase, the pump responsible for acid secretion. Dosing is unchanged in renal insufficiency.

Antacids containing aluminum and magnesium hydroxide effectively heal ulcers, but should be avoided in dialysis patients to avoid aluminum toxicity and hypermagnesemia. Sucralfate (Carafate) is a sulfated polysaccharide, sucrose octasulfate, complexed with aluminum hydroxide. Sucralfate should not be used in dialysis patients because of the risk of intestinal aluminum absorption (Robertson et al, 1989).

Risk factors for ulcer formation (NSAIDs and aspirin ingestion, smoking, etc.) should be eliminated if possible.

For the management of angiodysplasia, see below in lower GI bleeding.

C. Gallbladder disease. Chronic cholecystitis and cholelithiasis are common in dialysis patients. In one study, gallstone disease was detected in 33% of the dialysis population, of whom 82% were asymptomatic. The stones were radiolucent in 88% of cases, radiopaque in 8%, and mixed in 4%. The prevalence of gallstone disease in dialysis patients correlated significantly with age only. In patients with polycystic kidney disease, dilation of the common bile duct is unusually common (Ishikawa et al, 1996). Symptomatic patients can be treated with laparoscopic cholecystectomy or traditional cholecystectomy. Asymptomatic patients usually undergo cholecystectomy if they are renal transplant candidates.

III. Lower GI diseases

A. Diverticulosis and diverticulitis. Right-sided diverticular disease is more common in the dialysis population than in the general population. Constipation due to dietary restriction of fluid, fruits, and vegetables and due to the use of certain phosphate binders predisposes dialysis patients to diverticular disease. Colonic diverticula are increased among those suffering from polycystic kidney disease. These large diverticula are prone to perforate. Complications of diverticulosis include diverticulitis and colonic perforation. Diverticulitis is a relative contraindication for peritoneal dialysis. In renal transplant candidates with recurrent diverticulitis, segmental resection of the lesions prior to transplantation may prevent subsequent perforation when high-dose steroid therapy is initiated after renal transplantation.

B. Spontaneous colonic perforation. Spontaneous colonic perforation may be seen in patients with increased risk, such as those with diverticular disease, amyloidosis, constipation, post-transplantation immunosuppressive treatment, and infections. Spontaneous perforation may occur in the absence of an obvious cause or risk factor. A vasculitic pathogenesis has been proposed. When a patient receiving dialysis presents with abdominal pain, consider impending or actual colonic perforation. If perforation occurs, the mortality rate is extremely high.

C. Discrete colonic ulceration. A patient with ESRD who is receiving hemodialysis and who presents with symptoms similar to those of appendicitis or carcinoma of the colon, or even with rectal bleeding, may have discrete, nonspecific single ulcers of the cecum or ascending colon. The pathogenesis of such lesions is unknown. Treatment is oriented towards symptoms.

D. Intestinal necrosis. Necrosis of the small and large intestines has been reported in renal failure patients receiving oral or rectal sodium polystyrene sulfonate in sorbitol. Whether the culprit is the exchange resin or sorbitol is under investigation.

E. Colonic carcinoma. With regard to colonic carcinoma, vigilance should be exercised in their detection. At a minimum, the official clinical practice guidelines for their detection in the general population should also apply to ESRD patients.

F. Angiodysplasia. Angiodysplasias are thought to be acquired lesions of the GI tract affecting the submucosal and mucosal blood vessels. These lesions, usually multiple and small (measuring less than 5 mm), are usually located in the cecum and right colon. The diagnosis is best made by angiography or endoscopy. Angiodysplasia can cause acute and chronic blood loss in ESRD patients and presents predominantly in patients over the age of 50. In addition to correcting platelet dysfunction and decreasing the dose of heparin used during dialysis treatments, conservative therapy with low-dose estrogens (i.e., oral conjugated estrogen therapy, 0.3–0.625 mg per day), have been shown to stop the bleeding, whereas bowel resection did not help because of the presence of multiple lesions. If the lesion is seen, electrocautery can also be used to control bleeding.

G. Ischemic bowel disease. The combination of atherosclerosis involving the intestinal vasculature and prolonged episodes of hypotension, especially during and after hemodialysis treatments, predisposes patients to ischemic bowel disease and bowel infarction. Nonocclusive mesenteric ischemia is a serious complication of long-term hemodialysis. Patient risk factors include generalized atherosclerosis, congestive heart failure, multiple medications, and the need to remove large volumes of fluid from the intravascular space, resulting in relative hypovolemia and hypotension. Some patients present with abdominal pain, hypotension, and bloody diarrhea, whereas others present with signs and symptoms of sepsis without an obvious cause. Nonocclusive mesenteric ischemia of intestinal vasculature can be diagnosed with arteriography.

H. Peritonitis. See Chapter 19.

I. Hernia. See Chapter 20.

IV. Ascites

A. Hemodialysis-associated ascites. The diagnosis of ascites of ESRD or idiopathic dialysis ascites is made when ascites exists without evidence for a causative underlying disease, such as congestive heart failure, cirrhosis of the liver, or abdominal malignancy. The cause of the hemodialysis-related ascites is not clear. It is associated with persistent volume overload, cachexia, or low serum albumin levels. It has been hypothesized that the pathogenesis of idiopathic dialysis-related ascites might be multifactorial: the increased capillary hydrostatic pressure caused by volume overload and the decrease of oncotic pressure by hypoalbuminemia, together in the face of abnormal peritoneal permeability, promotes the formation of ascites.

The treatment for ascites of ESRD revolves around adequate dialysis. Volume status can be controlled with better fluid balance by the patient and adequate removal during dialysis treatments (including isolated ultrafiltration). Patients should be encouraged to eat well in order to maintain adequate nutritional status in light of the catabolic process of dialysis. Patients who are dialyzed adequately have a lower incidence of the common GI symptoms described above to interfere with adequate nutritional intake.

The ascitic fluid can be difficult to remove by dialysis due to (a) continued patient noncompliance with fluid restriction, (b) increased intra-abdominal pressure caused by the ascites interfering with cardiac function and venous return, and (c) high oncotic pressure of the ascitic fluid if the protein content is high. (Protein concentration tends to be low initially.)

Other methods for the removal of dialysis-associated ascites include placing the patient on peritoneal dialysis, inserting a LeVeen peritoneovenous shunt, or performing a renal transplantation.

Chylous ascites associated with acute pancreatitis has been seen in a patient undergoing continuous ambulatory peritoneal dialysis.

V.   Liver disease
A.   Hepatitis. See Chapter 28.

B.   Hemosiderosis. Hemosiderosis (iron overload) is now rarely seen in dialysis patients compared with the pre-erythropoietin era when blood transfusion, and therefore iron loading, was given to maintain hematocrit. If hemosiderosis is detected, it is better to use erythropoietin to consume iron rather than to use iron-chelating agents. The chelating agent, deferoxamine, has been associated with cerebral, pulmonary, and intestinal mucormycosis in nondiabetic dialysis patients.

VI.   Pancreatitis.
Acute pancreatitis is suspected when a patient complains of left upper quadrant pain with elevated serum amylase and lipase levels. The serum amylase level is often elevated in dialysis patients. However, the level rarely exceeds two to three times the upper limit of normal. The diagnosis of pancreatitis in dialysis patients is made by clinical assessment and laboratory tests. The use of laboratory tests to diagnose peritonitis is discussed in Chapter 24.

The usual causes for pancreatitis should be considered. Hyperparathyroidism and hypercalcemia may be seen more frequently in dialysis patients than in the general population because calcium-containing antacids are often used as phosphate binders. An acute episode of hemolysis due to blood line trauma to erythrocytes during hemodialysis can present as pancreatitis. Why hemolysis causes pancreatitis in this setting is unknown.

Acute pancreatitis occurs at a rate of 0.03 per patient-year in peritoneal dialysis patients and 0.01 per patient-year in hemodialysis patients. The mortality rate is 21%. Acute pancreatitis follows organ transplantation (renal, hepatic, and cardiac transplantation) in 2%–9% of patients. About half of these attacks occur beyond the sixth postoperative month. The mortality rate varies between 20% and 70% (Padilla et al, 1994). Contributing factors to posttransplantation pancreatitis include secondary hyperparathyroidism, hyperlipidemia, viral infections, vasculitis, and immunosuppressive therapy with corticosteroids, L-asparaginase, or azathioprine. The overall aim or medical therapy is to stop pancreatic autodigestion by reducing pancreatic enzyme synthesis and secretion ("putting the pancreas at rest") or by inactivating pancreatic hydrolases. The second aim is to prevent potentially disastrous infectious complications, such as pancreatic abscess, ascending cholangitis, and bacterial pneumonia. There is no specific treatment regimen or prophylactic antibiotic therapy that has been shown to have clinical benefit for either goal. Therefore, the mainstays of the management of mild pancreatitis are good general supportive care and watching for development of severe disease and localized complications. The treatment is the same as for nonuremic patients. Supportive care of acute pancreatitis consists of analgesia for pain control, restoration and maintenance of intravascular volume, and frequent monitoring of physical findings and vital signs. To minimize pancreatic secretions, patients should be given nothing by mouth. Nasogastric suction is indicated for symptomatic relief of vomiting, severe nausea, and developing or complete paralytic ileus. Once the pain has subsided, small feedings of a diet high in carbohydrate but low in protein and fat are begun, with increments to regular food several days later as tolerated but avoiding large meals. The use of H_2 blockers is controversial.

VII. Bowel preparation for surgery, radiography, or colonoscopy. Electrolyte solutions containing ethylene glycol polymers (e.g., Colyte, GoLYTELY) may be used in bowel preparation procedures. Four liters of Golytely or Colyte, containing approximately 236 g polyethylene glycol 3350, 23 g sodium sulfate, 7 g sodium bicarbonate, 6 g sodium chloride, 3 g potassium chloride, is ingested 4–12 hours prior to the procedure. Because of the osmotic properties of the polyethylene glycol, little if any of the administered solution is absorbed. The solution is promptly evacuated by rectum, thus cleansing the bowel. Other effective preparations include castor oil, extract of senna fruit, or bisacodyl tablets or suppositories. Dosage for these need not be adjusted for renal function.

SELECTED READINGS

Araki H. Significance of serum pepsinogens and their relationship to Helicobacter pylori infection and histological gastritis in dialysis patients. *Nephrol Dial Transplant* 1999;14:2669–2675.

Badalamenti S, et al. High prevalence of silent gallstone disease in dialysis patients. *Nephron* 1994:22:225–227.

Bender JS, et al. Acute abdomen in the hemodialysis patient population. *Surgery* 1995;117:494–497.

Bruno MJ, et al. Acute pancreatitis in peritoneal dialysis and haemodialysis: risk, clinical course, outcome, and possible aetiology. *Gut* 2000;46:385–389.

Chang JJ, Yeun JY, Hasbargen JA. Pneumoperitoneum in peritoneal dialysis patients. *Am J Kidney Dis* 1995;25:297–301.

Dardik A, et al. Acute abdomen with colonic necrosis induced by Kayexalate-sorbitol. *South Med J* 2000;93:511–513.

Fontan MP, et al. Chylous ascites associated with acute pancreatitis in a patient undergoing continuous ambulatory peritoneal dialysis. *Neprhon* 1993;63:458–461.

Gur G, et al. Impact of helicobacter pylori infection on serum gastrin in hemodialysis patients. *Nephrol Dial Transplant* 1999;14:2688–2691.

Gladziwa U, Koltz U. Pharmacokinetic optimisation of the treatment of peptic ulcer in patients with renal failure. *Clin Phamacokinet* 1994;27:393–408.

Ishikawa I, et al. High incidence of common bile duct dilatation in autosomal dominant polycystic kidney disease patients. *Am J Kidney Dis* 1996;27:321–326.

Lauritsen K, et al. Clinical pharmacokinetics of drugs used in the treatment of gastrointestinal diseases (Part I). *Clin Pharmacokinetic* 1990;19:11–31.

Lillemoe KD, et al. Intestinal necrosis due to sodium polystyrene (Kayexalate) in sorbitol enemas: clinical and experimental support for the hypothesis. *Surgery* 1987;101:267.

Marcuard SP, Weinstock JV. Gastrointestinal angiodysplasia in renal failure. *J Clin Gastroenterol* 1988;10:482–484.

Matsuo H, et al. A case of hypermagnesmia accompanied by hypercalcemia induced by a magnesium laxative in a hemodialysis patient. *Nephron* 1995;71:477–478.

Melero M, et al. Idiopathic dialysis ascites in the nineties: resolution after renal transplantation. *Am J Kidney Dis* 1995;26:668–670.

Negri AL, et al. Upper gastrointestinal bleeding in patients in chronic hemodialysis. *Nephron* 1994;67:130.

Padilla B, et al. Pancreatitis in patients with end-stage renal disease. *Medicine* 1994;73:8–20.

Patterson D, et al. A double-blind multicenter comparison of domperidone and metoclopramide in the treatment of diabetic patients with symptoms of gastroparesis. *Am J Gastroenterol* 1999;94: 1230–1234.

Richardson JD, Lordon RE. Gastrointestinal bleeding caused by angiodysplasia: a difficult problem in patients with chronic renal failure receiving hemodialysis therapy. *Am Surg* 1993;59:636–638.

Robertson JA, et al. Sucralfate, intestinal aluminum absorption, and aluminum toxicity in a patient on dialysis. *Ann Intern Med* 1989;111:179–181.

Ross EA, Koo LC. Improved nutrition after the detection and treatment of occult gastroparesis in nondiabetic dialysis patients. *Am J Kidney Dis* 1998;31:62–66.

Rutsky EA, et al. Acute pancreatitis in patients with end-stage renal disease without transplantation. *Arch Intern Med* 1986;146: 1741–1745.

Scheff RT, et al. Diverticular disease in patients with chronic renal failure due to polycystic kidney disease. *Ann Intern Med* 1980;92: 202–204.

Schroeder ET. Alkalosis resulting from combined administration of a "nonsystemic" antacid and a cation-exchange resis. *Gastroenterology* 1969;56:868.

Tamura H, et al. Eradication of Helicobacter pylori in patients with end-stage renal disease under dialysis treatment. *Am J Kidney Dis* 1997;29:86–90.

Ventrucci M, et al. Alterations of exocrine pancreas in end-stage renal disease: do they reflect a clinically relevant uremic pancreopathy? *Dig Dis Sci* 1995;40:2576–2581.

Vreman HJ, et al. Taste, smell and zinc metabolism in patients with chronic renal failure. *Nephron* 1980;26:163–170.

Genitourinary Tract and Male Reproductive Organs

Petras V. Kisielius and Anthony J. Schaeffer

I. General considerations

A. Imaging studies. The sensitivity and specificity of various imaging modalities for detecting lesions in end-stage kidneys have never been established by large autopsy or surgical series. Renal imaging studies may be less accurate in the presence of advanced adult polycystic kidney disease or acquired renal cystic disease.

1. Ultrasonography. The noninvasiveness, absence of side effects, and relatively low cost of ultrasonography make it an ideal screening study, especially when serial examinations are needed.

2. Computed tomography (CT). CT may be more effective than ultrasonography in demonstrating small cysts and parenchymal lesions in cystic kidneys. Intravenous infusion of contrast during CT scanning can produce mild to moderate parenchymal enhancement in end-stage kidneys. Contrast-induced fluid overload is avoided by dialyzing the patient after the study although the clinical necessity of this approach has been questioned, especially when low osmolality contrast dye is used. CT is also the test of choice for detecting calculi. Nevertheless, because of its use of radiation, frequent need of contrast, and greater cost, CT is a second-line test to be used when ultrasonography is inconclusive.

3. Other imaging modalities. Excretory urography frequently fails to image end-stage kidneys. Thus far, the ability of magnetic resonance imaging (MRI) to define pathology in the cystic kidneys of dialysis patients is not as promising as expected; however, it can be considered when CT and ultrasonography are not diagnostic. Angiography is usually not helpful in defining masses that are indeterminate on ultrasonography and CT.

II. Acquired renal cystic disease (ARCD)

A. Etiology and incidence. Acquired renal cystic disease is a disorder characterized by the development of bilateral cortical and medullary cysts in previously noncystic kidneys in hemodialysis and peritoneal dialysis patients. ARCD has been described in uremic patients without a history of dialysis. The exact pathogenesis of ARCD remains unknown. Its overall incidence of ARCD in dialysis patients is about 50%. The incidence increases with the duration of dialysis regardless of the underlying renal pathology. Approximately 80% of patients have ARCD after 3 years of dialysis therapy, whereas up to 90% have it after 8 years of dialysis. ARCD has been described in children. Renal transplantation appears to halt further progression and may cause regression of the disorder in some.

B.   Symptoms and complications. Usually, ARCD is asymptomatic and diagnosed incidentally on ultrasonography, CT, or MRI. However, patients with ARCD may develop secondary polycythemia [due to production of erythropoietin (EPO) by the cysts], cyst infections, cyst hemorrhage, spontaneous rupture of the kidney, nephrolithiasis, and renal cell carcinoma. Associated symptoms, such as flank or abdominal pain, hematuria, fever, weight loss, or an unexplained drop in hematocrit, warrant investigation with imaging studies. Occasionally, ARCD kidneys will increase markedly in size, such that inherited polycystic kidney disease is simulated (Bakir et al, 1999).

C.   Management. Asymptomatic patients with ARCD need to be screened periodically for renal cell carcinoma as described below. Management of each of the complications of ARCD is discussed in the appropriate section below.

III.   Flank pain (Table 35-1)

A.   Etiology and workup. The differential diagnosis is listed in Table 35-1. Flank pain occurs in up to 36% of hemodialysis patients with adult polycystic kidney disease as opposed to 2% of hemodialysis patients with end-stage renal disease (ESRD) due to other causes. In general, the diagnostic workup of flank pain proceeds in the same fashion as for nonuremic patients.

B.   Management

1.   Analgesic treatment. Morphine is the drug of choice in the management of colic or flank pain in dialysis patients, but

---

Table 35-1.   Approach to flank pain in dialysis patients

Etiology
Cyst-related
    Subcapsular hemorrhage
    Perirenal hemorrhage
    Hemorrhage into a cyst
    Enlarging cyst
    Extrinsic ureteral obstruction by a cyst
    Cyst infection
Pyelonephritis
Renal cell carcinoma
Acute ureteral obstruction (colicky pain)
    Stone
    Blood clot
    Sloughed papilla

Diagnosis
    CT and/or ultrasonography
    Retrograde pyelography

Management
    Pain control
    Codeine (give q24h instead of q6h); beware of constipation
    Morphine can be used cautiously (initially 50% of the usual
        dosage) for severe pain
    Treat the underlying disorder

CT, computed tomography.

it should be used with caution. Although morphine is metabolized mostly by the liver, the clearance of morphine metabolites is reduced in renal failure, resulting in a prolonged sedative effect. Codeine's half-life is prolonged in dialysis patients; therefore, the dosing interval for the drug should be raised from 6 to 24 hours. Aspirin should be avoided because of its effects on the bleeding time. Acetaminophen can be used in the usual dosage. Meperidine and propoxyphene should be avoided because their toxic nor-derivatives have prolonged half-lives in dialysis patients.

    2. Specific treatment. Specific treatment for flank pain depends on the underlying cause and follows standard urologic principles.

IV. Bleeding (Table 35-2)

    A. Etiology and workup. Bleeding from the collecting system or renal parenchyma can manifest as microscopic or gross

---

Table 35-2. Approach to bleeding in dialysis patients (into the urinary tract, a cyst, or retroperitoneum)

Etiology
Urinary tract bleeding
    Urinary tract infection
    Nephrolithiasis
    Subcapsular or perinephric hematoma from a hemorrhagic cyst
    Renal cell carcinoma
    Transitional cell carcinoma
    Bladder amyloidosis
    Bilateral renal papillary necrosis
    Hematologic derangement
    Flank or retroperitoneal bleeding
    Cyst hemorrhage
    Spontaneous rupture of the kidney

Diagnosis
Complete peripheral blood count
Coagulation profile, bleeding time
Urine culture
Ultrasonography or CT scan
Urine cytology, cystoscopy, retrograde pyelography if hematuria present
Angiographic localization of brisk bleeding site

Management
Correction of any associated coagulopathy
Treatment of hemorrhage or shock if present
Correction of bleeding time if abnormal, using desmopressin, cryoprecipitate, or estrogens as described in Chapter 27
Angiographic embolization of a bleeding vessel for persistent or severe bleeding
Endoscopic coagulation of bleeding sites in the calyces of the renal pelvis if possible
Surgical nephrectomy if required

CT, computed tomography.

hematuria. Etiologic factors are listed below. Up to one-third of hemodialysis patients with adult polycystic kidney disease experience hemorrhage into cysts. Acute perinephric hematoma leading to a "Page kidney" with secondary accelerated renal hypertension has been reported in a hemodialysis patient. Intracystic bleeding can manifest as dull flank or abdominal pain. Orthostatic hypotension or even shock may supervene if hemorrhage is severe. Dissection of a hemorrhagic cyst into the collecting system is a common cause of microscopic and gross hematuria in patients with adult polycystic kidney disease and is the cause of gross hematuria in 5% of patients with ARCD.

   B.   Management. Management of bleeding is contingent on the underlying cause. Heparin-free or regional citrate methods should be used to perform hemodialysis if bleeding is active.

V.   Urolithiasis. The incidence of urolithiasis in hemodialysis and continuous ambulatory peritoneal dialysis (CAPD) patients is about 5%–11%, compared with 3% in the general population. The incidence is even higher in patients with adult polycystic kidney disease. Most stones are composed of protein matrix, amyloid material, calcium oxalate, or a combination of the three. Aluminum–magnesium urate stones have also been reported in hemodialysis patients on long-term therapy with oral aluminum-containing phosphate binders. The symptoms of urolithiasis in hemodialysis patients are similar to those in nonuremic patients. Standard urologic management of symptomatic urolithiasis (with the exception of high fluid volume ingestion) is employed. The use of extracorporeal shock wave lithotripsy to pulverize upper tract stones in dialysis patients has not been fully explored. Hemodialysis patients with recurrent calcium oxalate stones secondary to primary hyperoxaluria type I should be treated with high-flux dialysis and, ultimately, combined renal and hepatic transplantation to halt and reverse ongoing systemic complications of the disease.

VI.   Urinary tract infections. Maintenance hemodialysis patients, especially those with underlying adult polycystic kidney disease, have an increased risk of developing urinary tract infections (UTIs). UTIs are more common in female dialysis patients, and the incidence increases with age in both sexes. Gram-negative organisms, notably *Escherichia coli,* predominate.

   A.   Cystitis
      1.   Clinical presentation. In oliguric patients, the symptoms of cystitis are similar to those in nonuremic individuals. However, gross hematuria is unusually common and occurs in up to one-third of cases. Anuric patients may present with suprapubic discomfort or foul-smelling urethral discharge and progress to pyocystis (see below).
      2.   Diagnosis. Voided urine samples from oliguric patients, even from those voiding only a few milliliters per day, are usually sufficient for diagnosis. Urethral catheterization and bladder lavage may cause infection and should be reserved for the symptomatic anuric patient.
      The presence of pyuria is not always indicative of infection (Eisinger et al, 1997). Absence of visible bacteria does not rule out UTI. A urine culture is essential to make the diagnosis. As in nonuremic patients, we consider a colony count greater

than 10^3 in a properly collected urine specimen to be suggestive of infection but there are no good studies in this area in
dialysis patients.

3. Treatment

   a.   Antimicrobials to use. Optimally, antimicrobial
   therapy should be based on sensitivity testing of the organism involved. If empirical therapy is warranted, penicillin,
   ampicillin, cephalexin, a fluoroquinolone, or trimethoprim
   should be used because they are safe and may attain
   adequate urine levels in ESRD patients. The dosing of these
   agents in dialysis patients is given in Table 28-3. In female
   dialysis patients, trimethoprim–sulfamethoxazole is generally chosen over ampicillin for treatment of recurrent UTIs;
   trimethoprim–sulfamethoxazole is less likely to be associated with the emergence of resistant organisms in the fecal
   flora, the source of most uropathogens in women.

   b.   Treatment schedule. The most appropriate treatment schedule for dialysis patients with cystitis has not been
   determined. We usually repeat a urine culture on the third
   or fourth day of treatment, document that the urine shows
   no growth, and continue therapy for a total of 5–7 days. Ten
   days of antimicrobial therapy is warranted in patients with
   adult polycystic kidney disease because of their increased
   susceptibility to pyogenic complications of UTIs. A follow-up
   urine culture should be obtained 7–10 days after completing
   therapy.

   It is difficult to achieve adequate urinary drug levels of
   ticarcillin, doxycycline, sulfisoxazole, and the aminoglycosides in dialysis patients; hence, these agents are not
   recommended for treatment of cystitis. However, when
   the responsible uropathogen is resistant to trimethoprim–
   sulfamethoxazole, cephalexin, fluoroquinolones, and the
   penicillins, one of these alternative drugs can be employed
   if its use is supported by the results of sensitivity testing.
   The use of nalidixic acid, nitrofurantoin, tetracycline, and
   methenamine mandelate is generally contraindicated in
   anuric patients due to the prolonged half-lives of these
   agents and the accumulation of toxic metabolites.

4.   Problems

   a.   Unresolved infection occurs when urine cultures
   remain positive during therapy. Causes include:

      (1)   Bacterial resistance.

      (2)   Selection of a resistant mutant while on therapy.

      (3)   Presence of a second unsuspected resistant bacte-
      rial species with resulting overgrowth.

      (4)   Inability of the diseased kidney to achieve bacte-
      riostatic or bactericidal antimicrobial concentrations in
      the urine.

      (5)   Excessive mass of bacteria, such as with a staghorn
      calculus, an infected communicating renal cyst, or a blad-
      der stone.

      If reculture and sensitivity testing show bacterial resis-
   tance, then the antimicrobial therapy should be adjusted.
   If the original infecting organism is still sensitive to the
   initial therapy, the dosage should be increased if possible
   or intravesical antimicrobial therapy should be adminis-

tered. If a source of bacteria, such as a staghorn calculus, is identified, it must be removed to cure the UTI.

b. Bacterial persistence is a recurrent infection from a source within the urinary tract. It is suspected if infections with the same bacteria return immediately after treatment is completed. Causes include:

(1) Infected cysts, as in adult polycystic kidney disease or ARCD.

(2) Infection stones (e.g., staghorn calculus).

(3) Bacterial prostatitis.

c. Reinfection is a recurrent infection caused by the same or different species of bacteria entering the urinary tract at varied intervals. Reinfection is not usually due to an identifiable anatomical lesion but rather to reintroduction of bacteria from a source outside the urinary tract, most frequently the rectal flora. Vesicoenteric or vaginal fistulas are a rare cause of reinfection.

d. Diagnostic procedures. All patients with recurrent infection should be evaluated for residual urine and urethral stenosis or stricture or bladder outlet obstruction. A renal ultrasonographic study and plain film tomograms of the kidney should be obtained in dialysis patients with possible bacterial persistence. CT with and without contrast infusion may be used if ultrasonographic findings are indeterminate. Cystoscopy is recommended if hematuria occurs or to help rule out enterovesical fistula in patients with pneumaturia. Ureteral catheter localization studies should also be performed if bacterial persistence is suspected. Patients found to have a congenital or acquired anatomical abnormality responsible for their infections should have the focus removed surgically.

5. Antimicrobial prophylaxis. The safety of long-term antimicrobial prophylaxis in dialysis patients with frequent reinfections is not known. Low-dose trimethoprim–sulfamethoxazole and cephalexin would probably be the safest drugs to use.

B. Pyocystis

1. Definition. Pyocystis, the accumulation of pus in a nonfunctioning bladder, occurs with increased frequency in hemodialysis patients. The pathogenesis of pyocystis is not clearly known.

2. Presentation. Pyocystis should always be suspected in an anuric dialysis patient with fever of unknown origin. Symptoms can include suprapubic or abdominal pain, foul-smelling urethral discharge, or sepsis. On examination, suprapubic tenderness and a distended bladder may be found.

3. Diagnosis. A complete peripheral blood count often shows leukocytosis. Blood cultures may or may not be positive. Catheterization reveals pus, culture of which usually grows a mixed flora.

4. Management. Treatment consists of adequate drainage via an indwelling urethral catheter, followed by intermittent catheterization and bladder irrigations with antimicrobial solutions until the infection clears. Parenteral antimicrobials, chosen according to culture and sensitivity reports, should be administered if systemic manifestations are present. Cystourethroscopy and possibly cystometrography should be performed to rule out a bladder outlet obstruction, a large bladder diverticulum, or a neurogenic bladder. Rarely, surgical drainage procedures or even simple cystectomy may be necessary in refractory cases.

C. Prostatic abscess. Hemodialysis has been reported to be a risk factor for the development of prostatic abscess. Diagnosis should be suspected in a male patient with a febrile UTI associated with irritative and obstructive voiding symptoms, as well as perineal discomfort. Rectal examination will reveal a tender and boggy prostate that often harbors a fluctuant mass. Transrectal ultrasonography or CT should be used to confirm the diagnosis. Standard urologic management should be employed.

D. Upper urinary tract infections and pyogenic complications

   1. Etiology and incidence. Upper tract infections in dialysis patients occur most commonly as a result of retrograde ascent of uropathogens in the urinary tract. Patients with cystic kidneys and especially those with adult polycystic disease are particularly susceptible to upper tract infection and its complications. Infected cysts, pyonephrosis, and renal and perirenal abscesses may develop.

   2. Clinical presentation. A patient with an infected cyst or renal or perirenal abscess usually presents with dysuria, recurrent UTIs, fever, night sweats, abdominal or flank pain, or sepsis. Occasionally, the patient may be asymptomatic. A tender, tense mass may be palpable in the flank or abdomen.

   3. Diagnosis. Leukocytosis is commonly present. Urine culture will identify the responsible organism if the parenchymal infection communicates with the collecting system. However, culture results can be negative when the infected cyst does not communicate with the urinary tract, or with pyonephrosis due to a cyst or stone that completely obstructs a ureter.

   Ultrasonography or CT may identify infected cysts and provide a point of reference for determining response to antimicrobial therapy. The use of indium-111 (^{111}In) leukocyte imaging and gallium-67 (^{67}Ga) citrate single photon emission computed tomography (SPECT) transaxial imaging in localizing infected cysts has been described and may be considered when ultrasonography or CT is inconclusive.

   4. Antimicrobial therapy. In patients with cystic kidneys, antimicrobial therapy of upper tract infection should be continued for at least 3 weeks. Many antimicrobials penetrate renal cysts poorly, and the degree of antimicrobial penetration depends on whether the cysts are derived from the proximal tubule or the distal nephron. Lipid-soluble trimethoprim, ciprofloxacin, metronidazole, clindamycin, erythromycin, and doxycycline have been shown to achieve good bactericidal levels in the fluids of both types of cysts, and should be good choices, depending on the suspected organism. Ciprofloxacin has been shown to sterilize infected cysts in some patients. Non–lipid-soluble antimicrobials, such as the aminoglycosides, the third-generation cephalosporins, and the penicillins, have generally failed to cure infections in polycystic kidneys, presumably because of their poor penetration into cysts derived from the distal nephron.

5.   Treatment of recurrent upper tract infection.
Patients with adult polycystic kidneys with bacterial persistence localizing to one side (as documented by ureteral catheter localization studies) should have the source of infection
removed surgically. Pyonephrosis and renal and perirenal
abscesses cannot be cured by antimicrobial therapy alone
and require immediate surgical intervention. Percutaneous
drainage of an infected cyst under radiographic control may
be appropriate in medically unstable patients, but surgical
intervention currently remains the procedure of choice for
most localized abscesses. Laparoscopic unroofing of an infected
cyst may be considered if clearly identifiable. Nephrectomy is
indicated when an infected cyst is unresponsive to antimicrobial therapy or cyst drainage. Delay in nephrectomy is associated with increased morbidity and mortality.

VII.   Screening for malignancy
  A.   Renal cell carcinoma
    1.   Incidence. Most authors report that the incidence
of renal cell carcinoma in dialysis patients is increased
(Maisonneuve et al, 1999), and especially in those with adult
polycystic kidney disease or with acquired renal cystic disease
(ARCD). Cases of renal cell carcinoma have been reported with
pediatric hemodialysis patients with ARCD. Transplantation
may lower the malignant potential of native kidneys with
ARCD but does not prevent the development of cancer in all.
    2.   Presentation. The manifestations of renal cell carci-
noma include anorexia, weight loss, unexplained fever, hematuria, flank pain, and palpable mass.
    3.   Screening. Ultrasonography or CT is required to estab-
lish the diagnosis. Because of the possibility of malignancy, we
recommend a baseline renal ultrasound at the onset of maintenance hemodialysis or peritoneal dialysis and annually
thereafter. Ultrasound also should be performed in all patients
with any suggestive symptoms or with unexplained polycythemia. The presence of enlarged kidneys (in which the risk
of malignant transformation is higher) mandates more frequent ultrasound scanning (e.g., every 4–6 months). CT is
obtained to confirm the finding of a mass on ultrasound or to
investigate inconclusive sonographic findings.
    4.   Treatment. Solid masses greater than 3 cm in diameter
or with CT attenuation numbers greater than 20 Hounsfield
units should be considered to be malignant and treated by rad-
ical nephrectomy. Though lesions less than 3 cm are traditionally considered to be benign adenomas, such tumors have
been known to metastasize and should be followed carefully
with serial ultrasound or CT examination.
    In addition to the tumor criteria described above, radical
nephrectomy should be considered for any tumor with unexplained liver function abnormalities, polycythemia or hypercalcemia. Nephrectomy should also be considered in patients
with rapidly enlarging kidneys and possibly in candidates for
renal transplantation. Whereas in the past, prophylactic
nephrectomy for ARCD was rarely considered, the idea is
more attractive today with the availability of EPO.
  B.   Carcinoma of the renal pelvis. Up to 40% of dialysis
patients with analgesic nephropathy ultimately develop cancer

of the renal pelvis, although transitional cell carcinoma is more common, squamous cell carcinoma may occur. Hematuria is the most frequent presenting complaint. Screening is described in Table 35-2. In patients with renal failure due to Chinese herb nephropathy, the prevalence of urothelial carcinoma is extremely high, leading some to propose prophylactic removal of native kidneys and ureters (Nortier et al, 2000).

C. Adenocarcinoma of the prostate. The incidence has been reported to be significantly increased in hemodialysis patients. An annual prostate-specific antigen (PSA) blood level and digital rectal examination should be obtained in male patients 50 years of age or older, and in those 40 years of age or older who have a family history of prostate cancer or who are of African American descent. Annual PSA screening is appropriate in patients with a life expectancy of 10 years or more. The accuracy of total PSA as a marker of prostatic disease appears to be the same in hemodialysis patients as in nonuremics, but the ratio of free PSA to total PSA is non-specifically increased (Sasagawa et al, 1998).

D. Other. An increased incidence of bladder cancer in hemodialysis patients also has been suggested.

VIII. Erectile dysfunction

A. Incidence and etiology. More than 50% of male hemodialysis patients have partial or complete erectile dysfunction as documented by nocturnal penile tumescence studies. Various theories have been proposed to explain the cause of erectile dysfunction in these patients; however, the exact pathogenesis has not been proven. In ESRD patients, vascular causes probably predominate.

B. Diagnostic plan

   1. History. First, one must distinguish organic from functional impotence. Aspects from the history suggesting an organic cause include the absence of erections upon awakening or with masturbation; the use of cimetidine or antihypertensive, antipsychotic, antidepressant, or anticholinergic medication; diabetes; atherosclerotic vascular disease (claudication, angina); and a history of alcohol abuse, myocardial infarct or stroke, smoking, pelvic trauma, surgery, exposure to radiation, or long-distance bicycling (which may cause penile vascular compromise). Functional impotence is suggested by the presence of erections upon awakening, complaints of premature ejaculation, successful sexual activity with other partners or in other situations, abrupt onset of the dysfunction, and temporally related social stresses. Interview of the sexual partner is usually helpful in assessing the problem.

   2. Physical examination. The examiner should note the presence or absence of secondary male sexual characteristics and gynecomastia; the presence, size, and consistency of the testes and prostate; whether Peyronie's plaques of the penis are present; the quality of femoral pulses; and the presence or absence of femoral bruits. The integrity of the somatic afferents of the erection reflex arc is assessed by testing of the bulbocavernosus reflex. The integrity of the sacral dermatomes is checked by assessing sensation to pin prick in the perineal region. Penile biothesiometry is a good screening test to rule out somatic afferent neuropathies of the penis.

3. **Routine laboratory tests.** Determination of morning testosterone and prolactin levels helps in excluding endocrine causes of impotence. Plasma levels of 17β-estradiol may be checked in selected cases. A fasting blood glucose concentration, serum cholesterol, high-density lipoproteins, and triglyceride levels also are measured.

4. **Other tests.** Numerous other diagnostic tests are available to further define the cause of erectile dysfunction; however, their usefulness in evaluating a particular patient is best left to the urologist.

5. **Therapy**

a. **Antihypertensive drugs and EPO.** Changing the antihypertensive medication may be of benefit. Angiotensin-converting enzyme inhibitors, calcium channel blockers, α-adrenergic blockers, hydralazine, and minoxidil are associated with a low incidence of impotence and should be substituted for methyldopa, reserpine, clonidine, and β-adrenergic blocking drugs (all of which have been linked to impotence). Anemia, if present, should be corrected with recombinant human EPO. EPO administration has resulted in reversal of impotence in some patients.

b. **Sildenafil (Viagra) and apomorphine (Uprima).** The type V phosphodiesterase inhibitor sildenafil (Viagra) has become a widely used treatment for impotence. Two preliminary reports suggest that sildenafil is useful in dialysis patients (Rosas et al, 1999; Macdougall et al, 1999). The usual doses (50 mg) were employed. Use in patients who are also taking long-acting nitrates is contraindicated because of increased cardiovascular risk. Apomorphine works by stimulating central release of dopamine. Apomorphine side effects include nausea and severe hypotension, the latter worsened by ingestion of nitrates and/or alcohol. There is no published experience with use of apomorphine in dialysis patients. Metabolism of both sildenafil and apomorphine is by the liver, and no dose adjustment in renal failure should be required based on pharmacokinetic considerations.

c. **Testosterone.** Experience with testosterone replacement in dialysis patients with biochemically proven hypogonadism is not encouraging (Lawrence et al, 1998).

Testosterone replacement therapy (as testosterone enanthate) or chronic human chorionic gonadotropin therapy can be attempted in impotent dialysis patients with 8 a.m. serum testosterone values below 300 ng per dL. A prostate and rectal examination along with a baseline PSA determination should be performed prior to starting hormonal replacement therapy. A recent study suggests that men with hypotestosteronism are more likely to harbor occult prostate cancer with a "normal" PSA, and ultrasonographically guided prostate biopsy might be considered before starting hormonal therapy in these patients.

d. **Vacuum–constriction devices** create a vacuum over the shaft of the penis after a constricting band has been placed at the base of the penis. This causes pooling of blood in the penis distal to the band and an erection. Side effects include blocked ejaculation, temporary changes in penile sensation, blue discoloration of the penis, and a cool-feeling penis. The band should not be left on for more than 30 minutes. Reasonable success rates in dialysis patients have been reported (Lawrence et al, 1998). If this form of treatment is unsuccessful, the patient should be referred to a urologist for consideration of other treatment options.

  e. Autoinjection therapy. Selected patients can be taught to self-inject at home with alprostadil (prostaglandin E_1), papaverine, or a combination of papaverine and phentolamine to achieve erections for intercourse. Teaching should be performed by a urologist, who is best able to deal with the possible complications. The use of autoinjection therapy in dialysis patients has not been well studied.

  f. Alprostadil urethral suppository (medicated urethral system for erection, or MUSE). Some patients are candidates for self-administration therapy with this medication. Though the medication is Food and Drug Administration–approved, its use in dialysis patients has not been well documented. Relative contraindications include sickle cell anemia or trait, leukemia, and multiple myeloma. Complications include temporary pain in the penis, urethra, or perineum; urethral injury; incidence of hypotension, light-headedness, dizziness (3%); syncope (0.4%); priapism (0.1% or less). The first administration of MUSE should be given in the office under supervision of a urologist to monitor for potential complications. The medication is not to be used more than twice in a 24-hour period in nonuremic patients.

  g. Surgery. The surgical procedure most commonly used to treat impotence in dialysis patients is implantation of a penile prosthesis. Its success rate, operative mortality, and morbidity in the dialysis population have not been reported; however, among nonuremic patients the satisfaction rate has been high. Potential complications include infection, erosion, and mechanical failure.

  There are few data concerning the success of venous or arterial surgery for the treatment of impotence in dialysis patients.

  h. Transplantation. Early renal transplantation has been reported to improve sexual function in some patients, possibly because (a) hormonal imbalances of uremia are ameliorated and (b) the development of penile vasculopathy may be prevented or delayed.

IX. Male subfertility
  A. Incidence and etiology. Subfertility is a common problem in male hemodialysis patients. Fifty percent have diminished sperm counts, impaired sperm motility, and abnormal sperm forms. Hemodialysis patients have an increased incidence of testicular atrophy, interstitial fibrosis, and Leydig cell dysfunction. The pathogenesis is not fully known; hypothalamo-pituitary dysfunction/gonadotropin deficiency or resistance, discussed in Chapter 29, may play a role.

  The diagnostic workup of subfertility is the same as that in nonuremic patients. Readily treatable causes, such as varicocele, retrograde ejaculation, hyperprolactinemia, hypogonadotropic hypogonadism, vas deferens obstruction, infection, and presence of antisperm antibodies, should be ruled out. Specific therapy depends on etiologic factors. The use of zinc, clomiphene, chronic human chorionic gonadotropin treatment, or recombinant EPO treatment to restore fertility in dialysis patients is controversial. Transplantation appears to offer the best chance for cure.

X. Priapism. Priapism has been reported to occur in maintenance hemodialysis patients. The cause is unknown. The development of priapism for more than 4–6 hours requires prompt aspiration of blood from the corpora cavernosa. If the penis remains rigid, α-adrenergic agonists should be administered intracavernosally. Immediate surgical intervention is mandatory if the above measures fail. The successful use of 1–5 mg of metaraminol injected intracavernosally, as well as a single incident involving use of continuous bupivacaine–fentanyl epidural anesthesia to reverse spontaneous priapism have been described in hemodialysis patients. Cardiovascular monitoring should be conducted while these agents are administered.

XI. Peritoneal dialysis and genital/penile edema. Three to four percent of patients receiving peritoneal dialysis, especially CAPD, develop genital edema due to the seeping of dialysate into the genital area through a patent processus vaginalis, a ventral hernia, a defect at the catheter insertion site, or a peritoneal defect from previous surgery. Diagnosis and treatment are discussed in Chapter 20.

SELECTED READINGS

Bakir AA, et al. Dialysis-associated renal cystic disease resembling autosomal dominant polycystic kidney disease: a report of two cases. *Am J Nephrol* 1999;19:519–522.

Chaudhry A, et al. Occurrence of pyuria and bacteriuria in asymptomatic hemodialysis patients. *Am J Kidney Dis* 1993;21:180–183.

Converse RL, et al. Sympathetic overactivity in patients with chronic renal failure. *N Engl J Med* 1992;327:1912–1918.

Dalal S, et al. Penile calcification in maintenance hemodialysis patients. *Urology* 1992;40:422–424.

Daudon M, et al. Urolithiasis in patients with end stage renal failure. *J Urol* 1992;147:977–980.

Dunn MD, et al. Laparoscopic nephrectomy in patients with end-stage renal disease and autosomal dominant polycystic kidney disease. *Am J Kidney Dis* 2000;35:720–725.

Eisinger RP, et al. Does pyuria indicate infection in asymptomatic dialysis patients? *Clin Nephrol* 1997;47:50–51.

Fornara P, et al. Laparoscopic nephrectomy: comparison of dialysis and non-dialysis patients. *Nephrol Dial Transplant* 1998;13:1221–1225.

Gibson P, Watson ML. Cyst infection in polycystic kidney disease: a clinical challenge. *Nephrol Dial Transplant* 1998;13:2455–2457.

Gupta S, et al. CT in the evaluation of complicated autosomal dominant polycystic kidney disease. *Acta Radiol* 2000;41:280–284.

Handelsman DJ, Dong Q. Hypothalamo—pituitary gonadal axis in chronic renal failure. *Endocrinol Metab Clin North Am* 1993;22:145–161.

Handelsman DJ, Liu PY. Androgen therapy in chronic renal failure. *Baillieres Clin Endocrinol Metab* 1998;12:485–500.

Ishikawa I, et al. Ten-year prospective study on the development of renal cell carcinoma in dialysis patients. *Am J Kidney Dis* 1990;16:452–458.

Jensen J, et al. The prevalence and etiology of impotence in 101 male hypertensive outpatients. *Am J Hypertens* 1999;12:271–275.

Lawrence IG, et al. Correcting impotence in male dialysis patients: experience with testosterone replacement and vacuum tumescence therapy. *Am J Kidney Dis* 1998;31:313–319.

Macdougall IC, et al. Randomized placebo-controlled study of sildenafil (Viagra) in peritoneal dialysis patients with erectile dysfunction. *J Am Soc Nephrol* 1999;10:318a (Abstr.).

Maisonneuve P, et al. Cancer in patients on dialysis for end-stage renal disease: an international collaborative study. *Lancet* 1999; 354:93–99.

McVary KT, et al. Topical prostaglandin E1 SEPA gel for the treatment of erectile dysfunction. *J Urol* 1999;162:726–730.

Malavaud B, et al. High prevalence of erectile dysfunction after renal transplantation. *Transplantation* 2000;69:2121–2124.

Nortier JL, et al. Urothelial carcinoma associated with the use of a Chinese herb. *N Engl J Med* 2000;342:1686–1692.

Ou JH, et al. Transitional cell carcinoma in dialysis patients. *Eur Urol* 2000;37:90–94.

Palmer BF. Sexual dysfunction in uremia. *J Am Soc Nephrol* 1999;10: 1381–1388.

Rodriguez-Antolin A, et al. Treatment of erectile impotence in renal transplant patients with intracavernosal vasoactive drugs. *Transplant Proc* 1992;24:105–106.

Rosas SE, et al. Sildenafil treatment for erectile dysfunction (ED) in dialysis patients. *J Am Soc Nephrol* 1999;10:267a (Abstr.).

Sasagawa I, et al. Serum levels of total and free prostate specific antigen in men on hemodialysis. *J Urol* 1998;160:83–85.

Sobh MA, et al. Effect of erythropoietin on sexual potency in chronic haemodialysis patients. A preliminary study. *Scand J Urol Nephrol* 1992;26:181–185.

Terasawa Y, et al. Ultrasonic diagnosis of renal cell carcinoma in hemodialysis patients. *J Urol* 1994;152:846–851.

Truong LD, et al. Renal neoplasm in acquired cystic kidney disease. *Am J Kidney Dis* 1995;26:1–12.

Watanabe K, et al. Amyloid urinary-tract calculi in patients on chronic dialysis. *Nephron* 1989;52:334–337.

36

Obstetrics and Gynecology

Susan Grossman and Susan Hou

In women with end-stage renal disease (ESRD), the hypothalamic–pituitary–ovarian axis is deranged, giving rise to subfertility, loss of libido, and dysfunctional uterine bleeding. Treatment of several gynecologic infections may have to be modified because of altered drug metabolism.

I. Birth control
A. Indications. Forty percent of women younger than 55 treated with dialysis menstruate, but anovulatory periods and infertility are the rule. There is some suggestion that the use of erythropoietin (EPO) and the increasing intensity of dialysis resulting from increased target fractional urea clearance *(Kt/V)* may have changed the hormonal abnormalities described in dialysis patients and that the frequency of pregnancy may have increased. Dialysis patients may have occasional ovulatory periods, and when pregnancies occur, patient management is enormously complicated. Birth control is advisable for women who do not wish to conceive. It is difficult to identify women at higher risk for pregnancy. Women who become pregnant once on dialysis frequently conceive again. Women who have become pregnant with renal insufficiency prior to starting dialysis and women with regular menses are at increased risk, but pregnancies have occurred in women following years of amenorrhea while being treated with dialysis.

B. Methods of contraception. Diaphragms and condoms can be used as in individuals with normal renal function. Oral contraceptives can be used but are contraindicated in women with a history of thrombophlebitis or hypertension, and relatively contraindicated in women whose underlying renal disease is systemic lupus erythematosus. The provision of estrogen offers the theoretical benefit of protecting bones from the effects of hypoestrogenemia seen in dialysis patients.

Many women on dialysis have prolonged periods of anovulatory bleeding, associated with the unopposed effect of estrogen on the endometrium. Estrogen–progesterone cycling might reduce the risk of endometrial cancer, which is associated with unopposed estrogen. Use of intrauterine devices (IUDs) is associated with increased bleeding during hemodialysis as a result of heparinization and a risk of peritonitis in continuous ambulatory peritoneal dialysis (CAPD) patients, so that the use of IUDs is discouraged.

II. Pregnancy
A. Frequency and outcome. Pregnancy occurs in women of childbearing age treated with dialysis at a rate of about 0.5% per year. For reasons that are unclear, conception occurs two to three times more frequently in hemodialysis patients than in CAPD patients. Approximately 40% of pregnancies in women

who conceive after starting dialysis result in surviving infants. Fifty-six percent of unsuccessful pregnancies end in spontaneous abortion, 11% in stillbirth, 14% in neonatal death, and 18% in therapeutic abortion. Approximately 40% of spontaneous abortions occur in the second trimester.

B. Diagnosis. The average gestational age at which diagnosis of pregnancy is made is 16.5 weeks. Amenorrhea is common, and symptoms of early pregnancy such as nausea are often attributed to metabolic or gastrointestinal problems. A blood-based pregnancy test [serum levels of the β subunit of human chorionic gonadotropin (hCG)] should be done prior to gastrointestinal x-ray studies for abdominal complaints. Urine pregnancy tests are not reliable even if the patient is not anuric. Even with blood tests, false positives and false negatives occur. The small amounts of hCG produced by somatic cells may be excreted slowly enough in renal failure for blood levels to be borderline positive for pregnancy. During pregnancy, hCG levels are more elevated than expected for gestational age, and gestational age should be determined by ultrasonography. The reasons for false-negative test results are unclear.

C. Management

    1. Management of hypertension. The major maternal risk associated with pregnancy in dialysis patients is severe hypertension. Eighty percent of pregnant dialysis patients have some degree of hypertension (blood pressure greater than 140/90 mm Hg). Forty percent have severe hypertension with diastolic blood pressures greater than 110 mm Hg or systolic blood pressures greater than 200 mm Hg. Seventy-five percent of severe hypertension occurs before the third trimester. Intensive care unit admissions for control of accelerated hypertension are required in 2%–5% of pregnant dialysis patients. Patients should be trained to take their blood pressure daily and report any increases promptly. Hypertension, even when severe, may not require the termination of pregnancy. The first step toward blood pressure control, as in the nonpregnant patient, is to make sure that the woman is euvolemic.

        a. Drug therapy. If the blood pressure remains higher than 140/90 mm Hg when the patient is euvolemic, there are several first-line drugs that can be used safely, including methyldopa, β blockers, and labetalol. There is less experience with calcium channel blockers, clonidine, and α blockers, but these are probably safe. Hydralazine can be added to any of these but does not work as a single agent when given orally. Angiotensin-converting enzyme inhibitors are contraindicated in pregnancy. In animal studies, they have been associated with a fetal loss rate of 80%–93%. In humans, their use has been associated with an ossification defect in the skull, dysplastic kidneys, neonatal anuria, and death from hypoplastic lungs.

        b. Superimposed preeclampsia and hypertensive crisis. Women treated with chronic dialysis are at increased risk for superimposed preeclampsia, but the diagnosis is almost impossible to make in the absence of findings of the HELLP syndrome (Hemolysis, Elevated Liver enzymes, and

Low Platelet count), such as thrombocytopenia, elevated liver enzymes, or microangiopathic hemolytic anemia.

(1)   Antihypertensive drugs. Intravenous hydralazine is the drug of first choice for hypertensive crisis in pregnant women and should be given in doses of 5–10 mg every 20–30 minutes. Labetalol is a good alternative. Rarely, if a patient must be transported, diazoxide, which has a long duration of action, can be used in doses of 30 mg. Nitroprusside should be avoided. Cyanide toxicity has been described in the infants of normal women, and the risk would be increased in women with renal disease.

(2)   Magnesium. Magnesium is superior to other anticonvulsants for seizure prophylaxis in women with preeclampsia, but it must be used with extreme caution in dialysis patients. A loading dose can be given safely. Additional magnesium should not be given until after dialysis or until after a drop in serum magnesium level has been demonstrated. Magnesium potentiates the hypotensive effects of calcium channel blockers, and the two should not be used together.

2.   Dialysis regimen during pregnancy

a.   Modality. Although the previous edition of this book suggested that peritoneal dialysis was preferable to hemodialysis, more extensive data have shown no difference in outcome between hemodialysis patients and peritoneal dialysis patients, as measured either by infant survival or by mean gestational age of live-born infants. Dialysis modality should not be changed because of pregnancy. The choice of modality should be made on the basis of the usual factors. Placement of a peritoneal catheter is possible at any stage of pregnancy.

b.   Amount of dialysis. There are no firm guidelines for dialysis regimens in pregnant patients but increasing dialysis to ≥ 20 hours per week appears to improve outcome. Daily dialysis decreases the fluid removal requirement at each treatment, decreasing the risk of hypotension during dialysis. Daily dialysis also allows the patient to eat a high-protein diet to ensure that the needs of pregnancy are met. Increasing the amount of dialysis in peritoneal dialysis patients is difficult. Late in pregnancy, women have difficulty with severe abdominal distention, and exchange volume has to be decreased. It becomes necessary to increase the frequency of exchanges even to maintain the same level of dialysis. A combination of daytime exchanges and nighttime cycling is often necessary. As of this writing, we still recommend six-times-weekly dialysis in hemodialysis patients with a target Kt/V of 1.5–1.7 for each treatment and 6–8 exchanges per 24 hours in peritoneal dialysis patients.

c.   Dialysis bath. When a bath containing 3.5 mEq per L calcium is used, the patient receives almost 1 g of calcium with each hemodialysis treatment. With daily dialysis, there is a risk of hypercalcemia. With calcium-containing phosphate binders, the use of a 2.5 mEq per L calcium bath has become more common, but there is some production of calcitriol by the placenta, which may increase serum calcium. Predialysis serum calcium levels should be checked weekly. The fetus needs a total of 25–30 g of calcium for calcification of the fetal skeleton. Orally, the patient will require 2 g per day if a 2.5 mEq per L calcium bath is used, and calcium-containing phosphate binders should provide enough calcium.

With a standard bath (e.g., containing 35–40 mEq per L of bicarbonate), daily dialysis carries a risk of alkalosis. Metabolic alkalosis carries an increased risk in pregnant women who have a concurrent respiratory alkalosis; however, in the few instances where arterial blood gases have been done, compensatory hypercapnia has occurred in women with severe metabolic alkalosis. A dialysis bath containing 25 mEq per L of bicarbonate may be necessary. When this is not available, bicarbonate can be removed by increasing ultrafiltration and replacing the losses with saline.

d. Heparinization. Clotting of the extracorporeal circuit and the dialysis access occurs frequently during pregnancy. Heparin does not cross the placenta, and unless there is vaginal bleeding, it is not necessary to lower the dose.

3. Anemia. Dialysis patients who become pregnant usually experience a worsening of anemia. It has become the usual practice to continue EPO during pregnancy. Congenital anomalies have not been reported in infants of the small number of women who took EPO during organogenesis. In animals, congenital anomalies have been seen only at dosages of 500 units per kg. There is little information on whether or not EPO crosses the placenta in humans. EPO has been associated with hypertension in nonpregnant patients but does not appear to aggravate the hypertension seen in pregnant dialysis patients. Women treated with EPO prior to pregnancy require markedly increased doses during pregnancy. The hematocrit has usually dropped by the time the pregnancy is recognized. We recommend doubling the dose of EPO when pregnancy is diagnosed. Pregnancy in normal women requires 700–1,150 mg of iron. We have found an increase in iron requirements during pregnancy and have given intravenous iron. Folate requirements are increased in normal pregnant women. Folate deficiency is associated with an increase in neural tube defects. Folate losses increase with intensive dialysis, and folate supplementation should be doubled.

4. Labor and delivery. Eighty percent of infants born to dialysis patients are premature. Reasons for prematurity include premature labor, maternal hypertension, and fetal distress. Home contraction monitoring can be used so that premature labor can be identified promptly. Premature labor has been successfully treated with terbutaline, magnesium, nifedipine, and indomethacin. Magnesium has been given intravenously in hemodialysis patients and has been added to the peritoneal dialysis solution in peritoneal dialysis patients. Magnesium must be used with extreme care in women with renal failure, as discussed above. Blood levels should be monitored frequently. A loading dose can be given, but additional doses should only be given when the level is low. Magnesium should not be used with nifedipine because the combination can cause profound hypotension. Indomethacin has also been used with success, but patients must be monitored for oligohydramnios, and the fetus must be monitored for right heart dilatation. In women with residual renal function, indomethacin may result in further deterioration in glomerular filtration rate and the need for increased dialysis.

Infants of dialysis patients are frequently small for gestational age, but it is not clear whether their growth restriction is the result of azotemia per se or of maternal hypertension. There is an increased risk of stillbirth in dialysis patients, and antenatal monitoring should be started as soon as there is a chance of survival outside the mother (26 weeks). Contraction stress tests using oxytocin should be avoided because of the risk of precipitating premature labor.

In CAPD patients, cesarean section can be done extraperitoneally, with the catheter left in place, and CAPD can be resumed 24 hours after delivery, starting with small exchange volumes and increasing over a 48-hour period. If there is leakage from the incision, the patient can be hemodialyzed for 2–4 weeks.

Even a normal-appearing infant should be monitored in a high-risk nursery. At birth, the infant, whose kidneys are normal, has a BUN and serum creatinine similar to the mother's, and the infant experiences a solute diuresis requiring careful monitoring of electrolytes and volume status.

There does not appear to be any increased risk of congenital anomalies, but the information on growth and development is sketchy.

III.   Estrogen replacement therapy

   A.   Premenopausal women. Given the recent interest in the antiatherosclerotic effect of estrogens and replacement therapy in postmenopausal women, some investigators have investigated use of estrogens, usually by the transdermal route, in dialysis patients. In one study, women on hemodialysis with low estrogen levels were treated with transdermal estradiol with cyclic addition of a progesterone derivative. Regular menses were induced, and improvement in libido and sexual activity was reported (Matuskiewicz-Rowinska et al, 1999). There also was an improvement in lumbar bone density in the estrogen-treated group at 1 year.

   B.   Postmenopausal women. There are very few studies in this area. In one small, short-term (8-week) trial, postmenopausal women with ESRD treated with 2 mg per day of oral, micronized estradiol had a substantial increase in high-density lipoprotein (HDL) cholesterol levels (Ginsburg et al, 1998). In another study (Modena et al, 1999), the use of antihypertensive therapy plus transdermal estradiol with oral norethisterone acetate in hypertensive postmenopausal women resulted in a greater reduction of left ventricular mass after 18 months than use of antihypertensive therapy alone. The effects of postmenopausal estrogens on preservation of bone mass in ESRD patients have not been studied. At this point, the benefits of routine treatment of postmenopausal dialysis patients need further study.

IV. **Dyspareunia.** Some women dialysis patients may experience dyspareunia because of estrogen deficiency and resulting vaginal dryness. Dyspareunia resulting from atrophic vaginitis from low estrogen levels can be corrected by intravaginal conjugated estrogens (Premarin) 2–4 g daily or oral estrogen/progesterone compounds. A daily dose of 0.625 mg of conjugated estrogen and 2.5 mg of medroxyprogesterone provides enough estrogen to prevent dyspareunia. If there is breakthrough bleeding on this combination, progesterone can be increased to 5 mg. As substantial amounts of estrogen are absorbed from intravaginal estrogens, these women should receive progesterone as well.

V. **Sexual dysfunction**

A. **Incidence and etiology.** Fifty percent of female dialysis patients under the age of 55 are sexually active. A majority of women on dialysis experience some sexual dysfunction. They suffer from both decreased libido and decreased ability to achieve orgasm. Treatment with EPO appears to be associated with an improvement in sexual function, but most of the data collected have been in men. Various reasons for sexual dysfunction have been proposed, including hyperprolactinemia, gonadal dysfunction, depression, hyperparathyroidism, and change in body image.

B. **Hyperprolactinemia.** Of female dialysis patients, 75%–90% are hyperprolactinemic. The mean serum prolactin levels in women with sexual dysfunction are higher than in patients with normal sexual function. Treatment of hyperprolactinemia with the dopamine agonist bromocriptine has been reported (in limited uncontrolled studies) to improve sexual function in both men and women on dialysis. However, bromocriptine has not come into widespread use because hemodialysis patients may be particularly susceptible to the hypotensive effects of this drug. Bromocriptine should be started at a dose of 1.25 mg, and the first dose should be taken at night. Subsequent doses can be increased gradually. Doses of 2.5 mg bid should be adequate to suppress prolactin secretion. When correctable physical problems cannot be found, dialysis patients should be referred for sex therapy, as would patients without renal failure.

VI. **Dysfunctional uterine bleeding**

A. **Incidence.** Many women develop amenorrhea when the glomerular filtration rate falls to less than 10 mL per minute. Menstruation often returns once dialysis is started in as many as 50% of patients. Over half of women with ESRD who menstruate report hypermenorrhea. Women on hemodialysis and CAPD report similar menstrual abnormalities. Because many women on dialysis (approximately 60% of those who menstruate) have irregular cycles, dysfunctional uterine bleeding is common and is of concern because it may be an early sign of endometrial cancer. Blood loss may lead to severe anemia even in women treated with EPO, although the introduction of EPO has made the management of dysfunctional uterine bleeding substantially easier.

B. **Management**

1. **Screening for malignancy.** Management depends on age and whether menses have ceased.

    a.   Women older than 40 years of age with no menses for a year prior to the bleeding episode. Cancer risk is high, and dilatation and curettage should be performed.

    b.   Women older than 40 years; menstruation has not ceased for a year prior to bleeding. The cancer risk is moderate. Dilatation and curettage is not routinely necessary, and performance of several endometrial biopsies is probably sufficient to screen for malignancy.

    c.   Women younger than 40 years. The cancer risk is relatively small, and a yearly Papanicolaou (Pap) smear is usually sufficient screen for tumor.

  2.   Anticoagulation. The lowest possible dosage of heparin should be used to perform hemodialysis when a woman is menstruating. Heparin-free techniques and citrate anticoagulation also are available, as described in Chapter 9.

  3.   Bloody peritoneal fluid during peritoneal dialysis. During menstruation or ovulation, the peritoneal fluid can become bloody. There is no specific management, except perhaps to avoid addition of heparin to the peritoneal dialysis solution. In some cases, frank hemoperitoneum may occur, requiring suppression of ovulation (Harnett et al, 1987). An aseptic peritonitis picture during menstruation or ovulation has also been reported (Poole et al, 1987).

  4.   Management of anemia. Anemia should be managed with EPO, as in other dialysis patients (see Chapter 27). Heavy uterine bleeding will result in increased iron requirements, and it may be necessary to give iron intravenously.

  5.   Hormonal therapy. Recent advances in therapy have facilitated the management of dysfunctional uterine bleeding in women with ESRD.

    a.   Oral contraceptives remain the safest therapy and the first-line treatment, although they should not be used if blood pressure control is a problem. The theoretical benefits of using estrogen/progesterone combinations to prevent uterine cancer and osteoporosis have been discussed above.

    b.   Medroxyprogesterone acetate (Depo Provera). The usual dosage is 100 mg given intramuscularly once a week for 4 weeks and then once a month. This drug is best reserved for patients with chronic hypermenorrhea who do not respond to oral hormonal therapy. Because many patients on dialysis have a bleeding tendency, intramuscular injections on a regular basis are undesirable. Moreover, the half-life of intramuscular medroxyprogesterone acetate is unpredictable.

    c.   Gonadotropin-releasing hormone agonists. These can be used in patients who continue to have excessive menstrual bleeding and do not respond to oral contraceptives and progestins. The monthly dosage is 7.5 mg of long-acting leuprolide acetate intramuscularly. This drug is extremely expensive. There is one report of ovarian hyperstimulation in a patient on chronic dialysis who received two doses of leuprolide acetate (Hampton et al, 1991). The authors postulate that women with ESRD may be at risk for this complication due to decreased excretion of gonadotropin-releasing hormone agonists.

   d. High-dose intravenous estrogens. In the case of acute excessive blood loss, high-dose estrogen therapy can be used, giving 25 mg of conjugated estrogens intravenously every 6 hours. Bleeding usually subsides within 12 hours.

   e. Deaminoarginine vasopressin (DDAVP). In setting of acute blood loss when bleeding time is prolonged, DDAVP, in a dosage of 0.3 μg per kg in 50 mL of saline, should be given every 4–8 hours for 3–4 doses.

6. Nonsteroidal anti-inflammatory agents have been shown to be effective in women who ovulate. Since most women with ESRD are anovulatory, these agents may be less effective in this setting. Also, women with ESRD are at increased risk of gastrointestinal complications. Nonsteroidal anti-inflammatory agents should probably be reserved for women who have occasional slightly increased bleeding associated with menstrual cramps.

7. Laser ablation. The neodymium:yttrium-aluminum-garnet (Nd:YAG) laser now offers a safe and effective alternative to hysterectomy. With this technique, the endometrial lining is ablated by vaporizing all three of its layers. Patients are pretreated with either danazol 200 mg four times daily for 4–6 weeks or with gonadotropin-releasing hormone agonists. The technique requires a surgeon trained and experienced in operative hysteroscopy and the use of Nd:YAG laser. The procedure leads to permanent infertility.

8. Hysterectomy. For postmenopausal women with significant dysfunctional uterine bleeding, hysterectomy may be the approach of choice. The proposed operation should be carefully discussed with the patient, and concomitant medical problems and the risks of surgery should be taken into consideration. With the advent of endometrial ablation with laser, hysterectomy will now probably be reserved for women who have bleeding secondary to uterine fibroids or to other uterine or pelvic pathology that in itself warrants the surgery. Hysterectomy should be done only as a life-saving procedure in a premenopausal woman who is a candidate for renal transplantation because the latter frequently restores fertility.

VII. Gynecologic neoplasms

   A. Benign. Uterine fibroids, or leiomyomata, are extremely common, occurring in approximately 25% of women older than 30 years. There is no information about their incidence in chronic renal failure. Uterine fibroids usually present with either menometrorrhagia or symptoms related to the enlarging uterus pressing on nearby organs (i.e., pain, pressure, constipation). Small, asymptomatic leiomyomata can be managed with observation. Indications for therapy include size over 12 weeks gestation, symptomatic bleeding, pain or pressure, urinary retention, torsion, degeneration with acute abdominal pain, prolapse through the cervix, and increase in size after menopause. Women still of childbearing age who are potential candidates for transplantation should have myomectomy performed rather than hysterectomy, if surgically feasible, to preserve childbearing potential. Hysterectomy is the treatment of choice for women who are postmenopausal. In the past, vaginal hysterectomy was thought to have more complications than abdominal hysterectomy. With the advent of prophylactic antibiotics, abdominal hysterectomy now has more postoperative complications than vaginal. If the patient's leiomyomata are less than 10–14 weeks gestational size, vaginal hysterectomy is the preferred approach. If the leiomyomata are not small enough to be removed vaginally, a trial of gonadotropin-releasing hormone agonists for approximately 8 weeks may allow as many as 76% of women with fibroids too large for vaginal hysterectomy to shrink enough to allow that mode of surgery.

B. Incidence of malignant tumors. Although it was previously believed that the incidence of endometrial carcinoma is increased in adult female dialysis patients, several recent studies suggest that breast, endometrial, and ovarian cancers may not be increased in this population.

C. Screening. Women with ESRD should be screened for breast cancer according to guidelines for nonuremic women. Pap smears should be done yearly to screen for cervical cancer in dialysis patients. Women who have had immunosuppressive therapy, either because of previous transplantation or underlying renal disease, or women with AIDS should have Pap smears every 6 months because of the increased incidence of cervical cancer in these populations. Endometrial cancer usually presents as dysfunctional uterine bleeding, the investigation and management of which have been discussed above. Ovarian cancer usually presents with vague abdominal symptoms and later as an ovarian mass. Abdominal discomfort, nausea, and weight loss induced by ovarian cancer may initially be misinterpreted as symptoms of uremia or underdialysis. In patients on peritoneal dialysis, ovarian cancer may present as bloody peritoneal fluid, an abnormal peritoneal cell count, or a change in the color of the fluid. A high index of suspicion is necessary to detect ovarian cancer at an early and potentially curable stage.

D. Diagnostic procedures

1. Lower gastrointestinal series. Use of laxatives and purgatives to prepare the bowel for x-ray examinations is discussed in Chapter 34. When actually performing the lower gastrointestinal examination, the amount of water used to dilute the contrast material can be reduced to one-fourth of the normal amount.

2. Computed tomography. Intravenous contrast infusion, if needed to perform a computed tomography (CT) scan or angiography, is not contraindicated in the dialysis patient. Although the administration of contrast involves increasing intravascular volume and osmolality, immediate dialysis following the study can be performed if deemed necessary. A patient on peritoneal dialysis requiring an abdominal CT scan can present for the examination with dialysis fluid in the abdomen.

3. Pelvic and abdominal ultrasonography. The patient on peritoneal dialysis with a suspected pelvic or ovarian lesion should undergo ultrasonographic scanning of the involved area. In those instances where pelvic pathologic changes cannot be visualized without distending the bladder, the latter can be filled via a Foley catheter.

4. Transvaginal ultrasonography. It is possible to delineate pelvic abnormalities more clearly using transvaginal ultrasonography because of the proximity of the probe to the pelvic organs and the relatively thin vaginal vault, which enables the use of higher sound frequencies and therefore higher resolution. On the other hand, the transabdominal probe gives a more panoramic view of the pelvis, showing the interrelationship of the major anatomical structures in the pelvic organs and their possible pathology. The transvaginal probe is able to furnish a more focused image of the organ of interest but only permits effective imaging to 7–10 cm in depth. Unlike transabdominal pelvic ultrasonography, it is best for the patient to have the transvaginal ultrasonographic study done while her bladder is empty. Since many patients on dialysis are not able to fill their bladders unless a Foley catheter is placed and fluid instilled into the bladder, it makes sense to first perform transvaginal ultrasonography if the pelvic pathology is suspected and proceed to transabdominal pelvic ultrasonography if the information needed cannot be obtained with the transvaginal approach. CAPD patients should have the abdomen full for transabdominal ultrasonography and empty for transvaginal ultrasonography.

E. Management. The management of gynecologic cancers and nonmalignant tumors in women with chronic renal failure includes surgical excisions and chemotherapy.

1. Surgery. Several points pertaining to gynecologic procedures can be emphasized. In patients with peritoneal catheters undergoing pelvic or abdominal operations, we leave the catheter in place unless there is bacterial contamination of the peritoneal cavity. When there is a low but measurable risk of peritoneal contamination as in a vaginal hysterectomy, we administer 1.0 g vancomycin hydrochloride and 1.0 g cefoxitin prophylactically intravenously just prior to surgery. If the patient is known to be colonized with *Pseudomonas*, tobramycin 2.0 mg per kg intravenously should be added to the prophylactic regimen. Postoperatively, the catheter is irrigated with 500 mL of peritoneal dialysis solution three times daily to maintain patency. Irrigations are decreased to once daily when the fluid is no longer bloody. We wait 10 days to 2 weeks before using the catheter again, maintaining the patient by hemodialysis during the interim.

2. Chemotherapy. Use of chemotherapeutic agents in dialysis patients is beyond the scope of this handbook.

F. Transplantation after curative resection of gynecologic neoplasms. Because immunosuppression increases the risk of tumor, most transplantation centers wait 2–5 years before transplanting a patient who has had a malignancy. Early stage cervical cancer does not contraindicate transplantation, but transplantation after "curative" treatment of other tumors must be individualized according to prognosis.

VIII. Gynecologic infections. Adult female dialysis patients are subject to the same infections that occur in women without renal disease. Some changes in treatment are required because of the effect of renal failure and dialysis on drug metabolism.

A. *Candida*. *Candida albicans* is the most common cause of vulvovaginitis. Treatment is not affected by either renal failure or dialysis. A 7-day course of vaginal suppositories containing miconazole nitrate, nystatin, or clotrimazole usually eradicates the infection. If the infection recurs, a 2-week repeat course of therapy may be necessary. Women with recurrent infections may be able to prevent them by using one intravaginal suppository of a topical antifungal agent once a month. In addition, the patient may benefit from sodium bicarbonate douching (2 tablespoonfuls of sodium bicarbonate per liter of lukewarm water) every 2 days for a week because *Candida* grows best in an acidic environment. Systemic therapy, consisting of one 150-mg oral dose of fluconazole, is now available and has been shown to be an effective therapy for *Candida* vulvovaginitis. The one-time-dose therapy does not need to be changed in patients on hemodialysis or CAPD. Patients on hemodialysis should take the fluconazole after a dialysis treatment.

B.   *Trichomonas.* Treatment of *Trichomonas* vaginal infection is unchanged from the usual regimen: administration of metronidazole 250 mg PO tid for 7 days. Metronidazole is dialyzable, and the medication should not be taken immediately before dialysis. All sexual partners should be treated as well.

C.   Nonspecific vaginitis. *Gardnerella vaginalis* is the most common organism implicated in nonspecific vaginitis. Usually a number of anaerobic and aerobic bacteria are recovered from cultures obtained from the vaginal secretions. Several therapeutic regimens are currently approved by the US Centers for Disease Control and Prevention: metronidazole, 500 mg PO bid for 7 days; 0.75% intravaginal metronidazole gel, 5 g twice daily for 7 days; 2% clindamycin vaginal cream 5 g once daily for 7 days. The short-term cure rates for each regimen appears similar. All can be used unchanged in the dialysis patient, although, as discussed above, metronidazole doses should be taken after hemodialysis. Sexual partners should also be treated if vaginitis recurs.

D.   *Chlamydia* and *Mycoplasma.* These organisms are often the cause of nonspecific vaginitis that does not respond to metronidazole therapy. In addition, they are major causes of infertility and pelvic inflammatory disease. Seventy percent of women with *Chlamydia* infection have no symptoms. It may produce subtle vaginal discharge, increase in vaginal bleeding with menses, mild lower abdominal pain, or dysuria. Diagnosis can be done through culture or antigen detection with monoclonal antibodies or DNA probes. Some antigen detection tests can be applied effectively to urine samples in patients who are not anuric. Treatment is to administer doxycycline 100 mg daily for 14 days. Other tetracyclines should be avoided in dialysis patients for reasons discussed in Chapter 28. Alternative regimens include a single 1-g dose of azithromycin, ofloxacin 150 mg daily for 7 days, or erythromycin 500 mg PO qid for 14 days. Only ofloxacin and doxycycline also treat gonorrhea. Sexual partners should also be treated.

E.   Genital herpes. Oral acyclovir has been shown to shorten the intensity and duration of first-time infections with genital herpes. Acyclovir is normally excreted by the kidney and is dialyzable. When herpetic infection is severe enough to warrant use of acyclovir, the drug should be given in a reduced dosage of 200 mg PO bid, with the doses scheduled in such a way that one is normally given after a dialysis session.

Symptomatic treatment with sitz bath, providone–iodine compresses, and lidocaine jelly should be done in the usual manner. Patients should refrain from intercourse when they have visible lesions, although viral shedding is known to occur even in their absence. Patients with recurrent episodes of genital herpes (more than six episodes per year) can decrease or prevent recurrences by taking at reduced dosages either acyclovir (200 mg PO bid) or famciclovir (125 mg every 48 hours).

F. Gonorrhea. In many locations, ceftriaxone has become the initial drug of choice because of the increased incidence of penicillin-resistant gonococci. The one-time 250 mg IM dosage is not changed for dialysis sessions. Treatment with penicillin follows usual dosage regimens. Probenecid, included in the usual regimen to retard renal excretion of penicillin, need not be given when treating dialysis patients. If the patient is allergic to penicillin, doxycycline in the usual dosage can be administered. Therapy of resistant strains should be guided by local information and sensitivity results.

G. Syphilis. The treatment of syphilis is unchanged in the dialysis patient. Staff should be aware that secondary syphilis is highly contagious through blood contact. Dialysis machines should be cleaned with formaldehyde or sodium hypochlorite solution after use in a patient with secondary syphilis.

H. Hepatitis. Types B and C hepatitis have been shown to be transmitted through sexual intercourse, although there is probably only low-level sexual transmission of hepatitis C, which is facilitated by concomitant HIV infection. Sexual partners of patients with type B hepatitis should be given hyperimmune globulin and the hepatitis vaccine if they are not already hepatitis B surface antibody–positive. After the partner has been vaccinated, there is no reason for the patient and her partner to refrain from sexual intercourse once sufficient serum titers of hepatitis B antibody have been induced in the partner. Sexual partners of patients with hepatitis C should be tested for hepatitis C antibody. If antibodies are present in the partner, there is no reason to refrain from sexual intercourse. A partner who does not have the antibodies should be warned of the risk of transmission of the infection and advised to abstain from sexual intercourse until the other's serum liver enzyme values have returned to the normal range. If sexual abstinence is not acceptable to the patient, use of a condom, although not completely protective, is strongly advised as long as the risk of infection exists.

I. Human papillomavirus. Human papillomavirus infection has become one of the most common sexually transmitted diseases in the United States. Patients may present with venereal warts or with an abnormal Pap smear. There is no difference in therapy of this infection for dialysis patients. None of the treatments is entirely satisfactory, but the lesions may resolve spontaneously. Frequently used therapies include cryosurgery, electrodesiccation, caustic agents, surgical excisions, and ablation with laser. Topical podophyllin is often used as a first line of therapy; however, it has a cure rate of less than 50% and has been associated with bone marrow suppression. Cryosurgery or laser ablation is preferable. Sexual partners of patients with human papillomavirus infection should be referred to a urologist experienced in detection and management of asymptomatic human papillomavirus infection. The infection may be markedly aggravated by immunosuppression.

J. HIV. Patients who are HIV-positive should be counseled regarding potential transmission of the virus to their sexual partners. If the nephrologist does not feel competent to discuss the risks of various sexual practices or to take a detailed sexual history, the patient should be referred to someone who is experienced in HIV safer-sex counseling (see Chapter 28 for further discussion of dialysis of the patient who is HIV-positive).

SELECTED READINGS

Buccianti G, et al. Cancer among patients on renal replacement therapy: a population based survey in Lombardy, Italy. *Int J Cancer* 1996;66:591–593.

Chertow GM, et al. Cost effectiveness of cancer screening in end stage renal disease. *Arch Intern Med* 1996;156:1345–1349.

Ginsburg ES, et al. Effects of estrogen replacement therapy on the lipoprotein profile in postmenopausal women in ESRD. *Kidney Int* 1998;54:1344–1350.

Hampton HL, Whitworth NS, Cowan BD. Gonadotropin-releasing hormone agonist (leuprolide acetate) induced ovarian hyperstimulation syndrome in a woman undergoing intermittant hemodialysis. *Fertil Steril* 1991;55:429–431.

Harnett JD, et al. Recurrent hemoperitoneum in women receiving continuous ambulatory peritoneal dialysis. *Ann Intern Med* 1987;107:341–343.

Holley JL, et al. Gynecologic and reproductive issues in women on dialysis. *Am J Kidney Dis* 1997;29:685–690.

Hou S. Frequency and outcome of pregnancy in women on dialysis. *Am J Kidney Dis* 1994;23:60–63.

Hou S. Pregnancy in chronic renal insufficiency and end-stage renal disease. *Am J Kidney Dis* 1999;33:235–245.

LeBrun CJ, et al. Life expectancy benefits of cancer screening in the end stage renal disease population. *Am J Kidney Dis* 2000;35:237–243.

Matuszkiewicz-Rowinska J, et al. The benefits of hormone replacement therapy in pre-menopausal women with estrogen deficiency on hemodialysis. *Nephrol Dial Transplant* 1999;14:1238–1243.

Modena MG, et al. Double-blind randomized placebo-controlled study of transdermal estrogen replacement therapy on hypertensive postmenopausal women. *Am J Hypertens* 1999;12(1O Pt 1):1000–1008.

Nakamura Y, Yoshimura Y. Treatment of uterine leiomyomas in premenopausal women with gonadotropin-releasing hormone agonists. *Clin Obstet Gynecol* 1993;36:660–667.

Poole CL, et al. Aspectic peritonitis associated with menstruation and ovulation in a peritoneal dialysis patient. In: Khanna R, et al, eds. *Advances in continuous ambulatory peritoneal dialysis.* Toronto: Peritoneal Dialysis Bulletin, 1987.

Toma H, et al. Pregnancy in women receiving renal dialysis or transplantation in Japan: a nationwide survey. *Nephrol Dial Transplant* 1999;14:1511–1516.

Musculoskeletal and Rheumatic Diseases

Jonathan Kay and Jessie E. Hano

Joint pain is a relatively common symptom among patients undergoing maintenance dialysis for chronic renal failure. More than 70% of patients receiving hemodialysis report joint symptoms. The prevalence of these symptoms increases with longer duration of hemodialysis. Over 95% of patients undergoing hemodialysis for 19 years or longer have shoulder pain and carpal tunnel syndrome. Joint inflammation has been observed in over half of the patients in one cohort receiving peritoneal dialysis.

β_2-Microglobulin amyloid deposits are prevalent among patients receiving long-term dialysis therapy and may cause pain and limitation of joint motion. Several different intra-articular crystals (calcium pyrophosphate, monosodium urate, hydroxyapatite, and calcium oxalate) may induce joint inflammation in the patient with chronic renal failure. Septic arthritis occurs more frequently among individuals undergoing hemodialysis than in the general population. Osteonecrosis develops as a musculoskeletal complication of chronic renal failure, usually in patients who have undergone renal transplantation or taken corticosteroids for another reason. Tendons may rupture spontaneously in patients receiving hemodialysis. Olecranon bursitis may develop in patients undergoing hemodialysis. Joint pain in the patient receiving dialysis may also be associated with the underlying disease process that led to renal failure, such as diabetes mellitus, systemic lupus erythematosus, primary (AL) amyloidosis, scleroderma, or rheumatoid arthritis complicated by secondary (AA) amyloidosis. Multiple factors may contribute to the development of muscle weakness in some patients undergoing dialysis. Secondary hyperparathyroidism and aluminum-related osteomalacia (discussed in Chapters 30 and 31) also may be associated with musculoskeletal symptoms.

I. β_2-microglobulin amyloidosis. Signs and symptoms of β_2-microglobulin amyloidosis are infrequently observed in patients with chronic renal failure who have not yet received dialysis treatment (Table 37-1). The prevalence of musculoskeletal β_2-microglobulin amyloid deposition increases with duration of hemodialysis from 21% within 2 years to 100% after more than 13 years following the initiation of hemodialysis. Among patients undergoing continuous ambulatory peritoneal dialysis (CAPD), the prevalence of β_2-microglobulin amyloid deposition is similar to that in patients receiving chronic hemodialysis.

   A.   Pathophysiology. β_2-Microglobulin is the subunit protein in the amyloid associated with long-term dialysis. This nonglycosylated, 11,800-d protein is normally present in most biologic fluids, including serum, urine, and synovial fluid. It is filtered by glomeruli and catabolized after proximal tubular reabsorption.

Table 37-1.   Musculoskeletal manifestations of β_2-microglobulin amyloidosis

Upper extremities
    Scapulohumeral periarthritis
    Carpal tunnel syndrome
    Flexor tenosynovitis
Spine
    Destructive spondyloarthropathy
    Periodontoid pseudotumor
    Extradural amyloid deposits
Bone cysts
Pathologic fractures

Serum β_2-microglobulin concentrations range up to 2.7 mg per L in healthy individuals with normal renal function. Because the rate of β_2-microglobulin synthesis (1,400–2,300 mg per week) exceeds the rate of its removal by different dialysis modalities (400–1,000 mg per week), serum β_2-microglobulin levels are elevated up to 60-fold in patients undergoing dialysis. The degree of residual renal function appears to be the most important factor in determining serum β_2-microglobulin levels. However, when GFR is less than 2.1 mL per minute, the markedly elevated predialysis serum β_2-microglobulin levels are 20%–40% lower in patients treated with CAPD or high-flux hemodialysis using polysulfone dialyzers than in patients treated with low-flux hemodialysis using cellulose-based dialyzers .

Current theories regarding the pathogenesis of β_2-microglobulin amyloidosis implicate the role of advanced glycation end product (AGE) modification of proteins, which confers on the proteins resistance to proteolysis, increased affinity for collagen, and the ability to stimulate activated mononuclear leukocytes to release proinflammatory cytokines such as tumor necrosis factor–α (TNF-α), interleukin-1β (IL-1β), and interleukin-6 (IL-6). AGE-modified proteins are poorly cleared by dialysis modalities. Thus, patients undergoing dialysis have elevated levels of these modified proteins as compared with individuals with normal renal function or functioning renal allografts. AGE-modified β_2-microglobulin has been identified in amyloid deposits of patients receiving long-term hemodialysis and may play a significant role in the development of β_2-microglobulin amyloidosis. The propensity for β_2-microglobulin amyloid to deposit in osteoarticular tissue may be due to the enhanced binding of AGE-modified proteins to collagen.

B.   Clinical manifestations. The presence of shoulder pain, carpal tunnel syndrome, and flexion contractures of the fingers in a patient undergoing long-term hemodialysis is highly suggestive of β_2-microglobulin amyloidosis (Table 37-1).

    1.   Shoulder pain. Shoulder pain, often bilateral, occurs in up to 84% of patients receiving hemodialysis for 10 years or longer. Patients receiving chronic hemodialysis often report anterolateral shoulder pain that is worse when they are in a supine position, especially during dialysis treatments and at night, and may improve when they assume a sitting or standing position. The coracoacromial ligament and the bicipital groove are sometimes tender to palpation. Range of shoulder motion may be limited, especially in abduction, and adhesive capsulitis of the shoulder may be present.

2. Carpal tunnel syndrome. Carpal tunnel syndrome results from compression of the median nerve at the wrist where it passes through a narrowed carpal tunnel. It occurs frequently in patients undergoing either hemodialysis or peritoneal dialysis. The prevalence increases with duration of dialysis treatment, with carpal tunnel syndrome occurring in up to 73% of patients receiving hemodialysis for 10 years or longer.

The pathogenesis of carpal tunnel syndrome in patients undergoing dialysis is probably multifactorial. Deposits of β_2-microglobulin amyloid may compress the median nerve as it passes through the carpal tunnel. However, although β_2-microglobulin amyloid deposits can be detected in the carpal tunnel of most affected cases, amyloid is not present in all biopsy specimens. Patients may report exacerbation of their symptoms during hemodialysis, perhaps due to a fistula-induced arterial steal phenomenon causing median nerve ischemia in the narrowed carpal tunnel. The increase in extracellular fluid volume between dialysis treatments may lead to edema in the carpal tunnel and median nerve compression.

a. Symptoms. Most often, patients complain of numbness, tingling, burning, or a sensation of "pins and needles" in the fingers of the affected hand. The hand may feel stiff or swollen. Although symptoms usually are present in the distribution of the median nerve (over the thumb, index, and middle fingers, and radial aspect of the ring finger), patients sometimes complain of sensory disturbance over the entire hand. Aching pain also may be referred to the forearm. Symptoms of carpal tunnel syndrome often are worse at night or during hemodialysis and are exacerbated by activities involving repeated flexion and extension at the wrist. They occur more frequently on the side of the longest functioning vascular access. However, some patients have developed symptoms of carpal tunnel syndrome in an arm that had not been used for vascular access.

b. Examination. In early cases of carpal tunnel syndrome, there may be no objective loss of sensation or muscle strength. Symptoms can often be provoked by tapping over the palmar aspect of the carpal tunnel (Tinel's sign) or by having the patient hold his or her wrists in a flexed position for 1 minute (Phalen's sign). In more advanced cases, perception of light touch, pinprick, temperature, or two-point discrimination may be diminished in the distribution of the median nerve. The abductor pollicis brevis muscle may be weak and, in longstanding cases, there may be atrophy of the thenar eminence.

c. Diagnosis. The differential diagnosis of carpal tunnel syndrome includes spondylosis of the lower cervical spine, thoracic outlet syndrome, sensorimotor polyneuropathy or mononeuropathy, and radial arterial steal syndrome in patients with an arteriovenous fistula. Except in early cases of carpal tunnel syndrome, median nerve compression at the carpal tunnel can usually be established definitively by electromyography (EMG) and nerve conduction velocity studies.

d. Treatment. Splinting the affected wrist in a neutral resting position, especially at night and during dialysis treatments, may relieve symptoms temporarily. If splinting is unsuccessful or poorly tolerated, injection of the carpal tunnel with microcrystalline corticosteroid esters will provide about 30% of patients with permanent relief of symptoms. If symptoms improve inadequately after injection or if there is significant objective loss of motor or sensory function, surgical decompression of the carpal tunnel yields improvement in more than 90% of patients. However, despite surgery, carpal tunnel syndrome symptoms generally recur within 2 years in patients with β_2-microglobulin amyloidosis.

3. Finger flexion contractures. Individuals receiving long-term hemodialysis frequently develop irreducible flexion contractures of the fingers caused by deposition of β_2-microglobulin amyloid along the flexor tendons of the hands. These deposits may make the digital flexor tendons of the hand adhere to one another, creating a subcutaneous soft tissue mass in the palm.

4. Destructive spondyloarthropathy. β_2-Microglobulin amyloidosis affects the axial skeleton in about 10% of patients undergoing long-term hemodialysis. Axial skeletal involvement presents as a destructive spondyloarthropathy, the radiographic features of which include narrowing of the intervertebral disk spaces and erosion of the vertebral end-plates without appreciable formation of osteophyte. The lower cervical spine is most often affected; however, similar changes may also occur in the dorsal and lumbar spine. Severe destructive spondyloarthropathy must be differentiated from vertebral osteomyelitis. Deposits of β_2-microglobulin amyloid have been demonstrated in paravertebral ligaments and intervertebral disks of patients with this spondyloarthropathy. Cystic deposits of β_2-microglobulin amyloid within the odontoid process and the vertebral bodies of the upper cervical spine and periodontoid soft-tissue masses of β_2-microglobulin amyloid, termed "pseudotumors," have also been demonstrated.

The initial symptom of destructive spondyloarthropathy is pain, typically in the neck when the cervical spine is involved. However, most patients who have radiographic abnormalities in the cervical spine have no neck pain. Although neurologic compromise occurs infrequently, significant myelopathy has resulted from β_2-microglobulin amyloid deposits in the cervical and lumbar spinal canal.

5. Bone cysts. Cystic bone lesions may develop in the appendicular skeleton of patients undergoing long-term hemodialysis. Subchondral amyloid cysts, most commonly found in the carpal bones, may also occur in the acetabulum and in long bones, such as the femoral head or neck, the humeral head, the distal radius, and the tibial plateau. Unlike brown tumors of hyperparathyroidism, these bone cysts typically occur adjacent to joints. On plain radiographs, they appear as well-defined radiolucencies, with occasional disruption of the bony cortex but no periosteal reaction. Cysts vary in size, ranging from 2 to 3 mm diameter in the carpal bones to as large as 40 mm in the acetabulum. Even in the absence of radiographic features of hyperparathyroidism, these cysts increase in number and enlarge with time. Some reports suggest that bone cysts characteristic of dialysis-related amyloidosis occur less frequently among patients dialyzed against hydrophobic synthetic polymer membranes, such as polyacrylonitrile (AN69), than among those dialyzed against cellulose-based Cuprophane membranes. However, this topic remains controversial.

    6. Pathologic fractures, especially of the femoral neck, may occur through areas of bone weakened by amyloid deposits.

    7. Systemic manifestations of β_2-microglobulin amyloidosis. Although β_2-microglobulin amyloid deposits predominantly in osteoarticular tissue, visceral deposits of β_2-microglobulin amyloid have been identified in patients receiving long-term dialysis. Most such patients have undergone hemodialysis for 10 years or longer and also have carpal tunnel syndrome or arthropathy. The amount of visceral β_2-microglobulin amyloid deposition increases with longer duration of dialysis; however, the extent of systemic involvement remains controversial. In contrast to osteoarticular β_2-microglobulin amyloid, which is deposited predominantly in the interstitium, visceral β_2-microglobulin amyloid is deposited predominantly in blood vessels. Although gastrointestinal tract and cardiovascular complications have been reported, visceral β_2-microglobulin amyloid deposits usually do not cause symptoms.

C. Diagnosis. The diagnosis of dialysis-related amyloidosis is suggested primarily by its clinical appearance. Radiographic findings, such as bone cysts, narrowing of the intervertebral disk space, and vertebral end-plate erosion, serve to corroborate the diagnosis. Diagnostic ultrasonography detects changes in articular and periarticular soft-tissue structures that are characteristic of β_2-microglobulin amyloidosis in patients undergoing long-term hemodialysis: thickening of the rotator cuff to larger than 8 mm and interposition of echogenic pads between muscle groups of the rotator cuff. However, histologic identification of β_2-microglobulin amyloid by Congo red and immunohistochemical staining in biopsy specimens remains the "gold standard" for diagnosis.

D. Treatment. The treatment of pain caused by β_2-microglobulin amyloid deposits in patients undergoing dialysis is symptomatic. Heat and range-of-motion exercises for the shoulder increase mobility. The intra-articular injection of corticosteroids or the application of 10% hydrocortisone cream to the shoulder using phonophoresis may greatly decrease the pain associated with the shoulder periarthritis of dialysis-related amyloidosis and thereby permit increased shoulder function. Nonsteroidal anti-inflammatory drugs (NSAIDs) are useful in treating symptoms of pain involving multiple joints. Because of the increased risk of bleeding in patients undergoing dialysis, consideration should be given to the use of a specific cyclooxygenase-2 (COX-2) inhibitor or the concurrent use of a prostaglandin analog, such as misoprostol. Joint pain and restriction of motion may improve in patients with β_2-microglobulin amyloidosis who are treated with oral prednisone, up to 8 mg per day, although symptoms recur within 48 hours upon the discontinuation of prednisone. However, the potential risks of corticosteroid-induced bone loss and atherosclerosis limit the use of low-dose prednisone to the treatment of β_2-microglobulin amyloidosis that has not responded to other forms of medical therapy. Surgery may be necessary for symptomatic patients with large deposits of β_2-microglobulin amyloid. Patients with β_2-microglobulin amyloidosis who undergo successful renal transplantation experience a marked reduction in joint pain and stiffness.

E.   Prevention. Although hemodialysis with more biocompatible membranes does not necessarily reduce the incidence of β_2-microglobulin amyloidosis, it may postpone the onset of clinical manifestations. Carpal tunnel syndrome and bone cysts have developed later in patients undergoing hemodialysis with more biocompatible membranes than in those receiving hemodialysis with Cuprophane membranes. Early renal transplantation in appropriate candidates, before significant β_2-microglobulin amyloid deposition has occurred, may be the most effective preventive measure currently available for this condition without a definitive cure. β_2-Microglobulin amyloid deposits do not progress and may regress in patients who have undergone successful renal transplantation. Following renal transplantation, subchondral bone cysts do not increase in size or number. Because AGEs appear to play a pivotal role in the pathogenesis of this condition, future treatment strategies directed toward inhibition of AGE formation might interfere with the development of this condition.

II.   Other forms of arthritis in dialysis patients

A.   Crystal-induced arthritis in patients receiving dialysis treatment for chronic renal failure may be caused by one of several different intra-articular crystals: calcium pyrophosphate dihydrate, monosodium urate, hydroxyapatite, or calcium oxalate. The clinical presentations of these entities are often similar, requiring synovial fluid examination for crystals to distinguish among these conditions.

1.   Pseudogout. Attacks of pseudogout occur when calcium pyrophosphate dihydrate (CPPD) crystals are shed from cartilage into joints or periarticular tissues, inducing a sterile inflammatory response. CPPD crystals are more likely to cause painful joint inflammation in the dialysis patient than monosodium urate crystals, especially when hyperparathyroidism is poorly controlled.

Pseudogout usually affects large- or medium-sized joints, most commonly the knees, although small joints such as the first metatarsophalangeal joint may also be involved. Acute attacks of pseudogout present with the sudden onset of severe joint pain with swelling, erythema, and warmth of the overlying soft tissues. Joint aspiration reveals an exudative synovial fluid containing many neutrophils. The finding of weakly positively birefringent rod-shaped crystals in a joint fluid aspirate makes the diagnosis. Radiography of involved joints may demonstrate chondrocalcinosis.

Although episodes of arthritis associated with CPPD crystals may resolve spontaneously without treatment, joint aspiration (with or without injection of microcrystalline corticosteroid esters) or NSAID therapy may be helpful.

2.   Gout. Gouty arthritis occurs when monosodium urate crystals deposit in tissues in and around joints and induce a sterile inflammatory response. Although common in patients with renal insufficiency before the initiation of dialysis treatment, acute attacks of gouty arthritis are uncommon among hyperuricemic individuals with uremia. The inflammatory response to monosodium urate crystals is diminished in patients with uremia compared to individuals with normal renal function. In patients in whom preexisting acute gouty arthritis continues after the onset of uremia, symptoms are milder than before its onset.

The clinical presentation of gout is similar to that of pseudogout, although small joints, such as the first metatarsophalangeal joint, are most commonly affected by gouty arthritis. Finding needle- or rod-shaped crystals, which are strongly negatively birefringent when viewed under compensated polarized light, in a joint fluid aspirate makes the diagnosis of gout.

Patients respond rapidly to treatment with NSAIDs, oral or intra-articular corticosteroids, intramuscular adrenocorticotropic hormone gel (40–80 IU), intramuscular triamcinolone hexacetonide (60 mg), or colchicine. Oral colchicine (0.6 mg) given every hour until the patient experiences relief of symptoms often results in debilitating diarrhea with accompanying fluid and electrolyte losses. Intravenous colchicine (1.0–2.0 mg initially with an additional 1.0 mg 8–12 hours later, if needed) is less likely to induce gastrointestinal symptoms (Table 37-3). Allopurinol may be used in dialysis patients with persistent hyperuricemia and recurrent attacks of gouty arthritis. Because allopurinol elimination depends on renal excretion, the drug should be given in a reduced dosage of 100 mg daily.

3.   Arthropathy associated with hydroxyapatite crystals. Hydroxyapatite crystals may also cause joint pain and swelling in patients undergoing dialysis, especially when the serum calcium–phosphorus product exceeds 75 mg^2 per dL^2. The inciting event is presumed to be migration of microspherular crystals of calcium hydroxyapatite into the joint to induce inflammation. However, with better control of hyperphosphatemia and hyperparathyroidism in recent years, calcific periarthritis is no longer as prevalent as it was during the early era of hemodialysis.

The shoulder is the joint most commonly involved; deposits also may occur around the small joints of the hand, the hip, the wrist, the ankle, and the elbow. These deposits, which appear on radiographs of the shoulder as "multiloculated," nodular, periarticular calcifications, may enlarge to become palpable and visible masses (called "tumoral calcinosis"). Limited calcification in tendons, ligaments, and the joint capsule may be associated with acute attacks of painful peri-articular inflammation. Although crystals usually are not seen when synovial fluid is examined by compensated polarizing light microscopy, they may be visualized when the fluid is stained with alizarin red S.

Treatment involves immobilization of the involved area and short-term administration of NSAIDs or oral colchicine. Injection of microcrystalline corticosteroid esters and local anesthetic, with or without aspiration of hydroxyapatite, may provide symptomatic relief and hasten recovery. Reduction of serum phosphorus levels by limiting dietary intake of phosphate, discontinuing vitamin D supplementation, and administering phosphate binders has been associated with marked decreases in both shoulder pain and periarticular calcification on radiographs. When conservative therapy has failed, surgical removal of the soft-tissue calcification may lead to the resolution of pain and functional improvement. Parathyroidectomy may be necessary for patients in whom calcific periarthritis does not respond to other therapy and who are not candidates for renal transplantation.

4. Arthropathy associated with calcium oxalate crystals. Calcium oxalate crystals can cause acute and chronic synovitis in individuals receiving hemodialysis or peritoneal dialysis. Although the small joints of the distal extremities are more commonly affected, large joints also may become inflamed. Chondrocalcinosis may be evident on radiographs of involved joints. Characteristic strongly birefringent bipyramidal crystals are seen with compensated polarized light microscopy on examination of synovial fluid. Positive staining with alizarin red S confirms the presence of calcium in the crystals. Calcium oxalate crystals also may deposit in vascular smooth muscle, resulting in acrocyanosis and livedo reticularis.

Patients with calcium oxalate–associated arthritis have responded poorly or not at all to treatment with colchicine, NSAIDs, intra-articular microcrystalline corticosteroid ester injections, or increased frequency of hemodialysis. Because ascorbic acid (vitamin C) is metabolized to oxalate, the administration of vitamin supplements containing ascorbic acid increases the plasma oxalate concentration in patients with chronic renal failure and may exacerbate manifestations of oxalosis. Thus, caution should be observed in prescribing vitamin supplementation for these patients.

B. Septic arthritis. Bacterial infections of joint spaces and bursae occur more frequently among individuals undergoing hemodialysis, in whom percutaneous vascular access is established several times each week, than in the general population and are most commonly caused by *Staphylococcus aureus.*

1. Diagnosis. Typically, an individual with septic arthritis experiences pain, swelling, warmth, and decreased range of motion in the affected joint. Septic arthritis may be present in the absence of fever, leukocytosis, or radiographic abnormalities. Thus, the diagnosis of septic arthritis may be missed unless fluid from the affected joint is aspirated and cultured for bacteria, mycobacteria (typical and atypical), and fungi to confirm the presence of infection.

   2.   Treatment of an acutely infected joint includes parenteral administration of appropriate antimicrobial drugs for at least 2 weeks, followed by 2 weeks of oral antibiotic therapy. Septic joints should be drained regularly by repeated closed-needle aspiration. However, arthroscopic or open surgical drainage may be beneficial, especially in joints such as the hip, that are not easily accessible to closed-needle aspiration. The synovial fluid leukocyte count and culture should be assessed serially during the course of treatment for septic arthritis. Persistent elevation of the leukocyte count or positive cultures after several days of initial therapy should prompt consideration of surgical drainage of the infected joint.

C.   Osteonecrosis. The prevalence of osteonecrosis among patients receiving chronic hemodialysis has been estimated to range from 3% to 18%. Among patients with chronic renal failure, the femoral head is the site most commonly affected by osteonecrosis.

III.   Tendinitis/bursitis in dialysis patients

A.   Spontaneous tendon rupture. Tendons rupture spontaneously in up to 15% of patients undergoing chronic hemodialysis. The quadriceps femoris tendon is the one most commonly involved; ruptures of the Achilles, triceps brachii, and patellar tendons and the extensor tendons of the fingers also have been reported. Spontaneous tendon rupture is frequently associated with secondary hyperparathyroidism. The presence of bone erosion at the site of tendon insertion, weakening the tendon insertion, and higher levels of serum alkaline phosphatase than in patients without tendon rupture suggests that hyperparathyroid bone disease predisposes to spontaneous tendon rupture. Ruptured tendons should undergo prompt surgical repair. Medical therapy should be directed to control of secondary hyperparathyroidism, if present.

B.   Olecranon bursitis. The bursa overlying the extensor surface of the elbow may become inflamed in patients receiving chronic hemodialysis, usually on the same side as the vascular access. Sustained pressure on the elbow exerted by the arm rest during repeated dialysis treatments is the most likely cause of this "dialysis elbow." The swollen olecranon bursa may be aspirated to relieve symptoms, and the bursal fluid should be cultured to exclude septic bursitis. Recurrent bursitis should be treated by altering the position of the patient's arm during dialysis to avoid applying pressure to the elbow; intrabursal steroid injection may be performed. Surgical excision of the olecranon bursa should be reserved for patients whose condition is refractory to medical therapy.

IV.   Systemic rheumatic diseases

A.   Laboratory measures of the acute phase response

   1.   Erythrocyte sedimentation rate (ESR). The ESR is elevated (more than 25 mm per hour) slightly in many patients receiving dialysis (median 30 mm per hour; Brouillard et al, 1996). The predictive value of a markedly elevated ESR in patients whose anemia is adequately controlled (Hct 33%–36%) has not been well studied.

   2.   Hyaluronan (hyaluronic acid). Recently, hyaluronan, a marker of inflammatory reaction, has been found to be a risk predictor of poor survival in dialysis.

   3.   C-reactive protein (CRP). Levels of CRP are moderately elevated (10–50 mg per L) in up to 50% of patients undergoing dialysis who do not have active infection or inflammation. However, marked elevation of the CRP level (greater than 50 mg per L) is a more accurate indicator of active inflammation than the ESR in patients receiving dialysis. High serum CRP levels are an independent predictor of mortality in ESRD patients.

B.   Systemic lupus erythematosus (SLE). The overall activity of nonrenal manifestations of SLE decreases after the initiation of dialysis treatments, even as immunosuppressive drug therapy is withdrawn, but does not disappear completely. Persistent disease may be more common in African American women (Krane et al, 1999). Hydroxychloroquine (200–400 mg per day) should be given to patients with active SLE. Minor flares of disease activity, which typically manifest as arthritis, rash, or serositis, usually can be controlled with the addition of NSAIDs or low doses of prednisone (5–15 mg per day). Infrequently, higher doses of prednisone, alone or with azathioprine or cyclophosphamide, are required to control more severe manifestations of SLE, such as cerebritis or vasculitis.

C.   Rheumatoid arthritis (RA). Joint inflammation occurring in RA is treated initially with NSAIDs or small doses of prednisone (5–15 mg per day). Disease-modifying antirheumatic drugs (DMARDs), such as hydroxychloroquine (200–400 mg per day) or azathioprine (50–100 mg per day), are administered in combination with anti-inflammatory drugs to reduce disease activity. However, in patients with RA who are receiving dialysis therapy, gold compounds and methotrexate (which is not dialyzable) should be avoided (Table 37-3).

V.   Muscle weakness. Patients with chronic renal failure undergoing dialysis may develop diffuse muscle weakness, predominantly affecting the lower extremities and involving proximal muscles. Serum muscle enzyme levels are usually within the normal range. EMG reveals an abnormal increase in nonspecific polyphasic motor unit potentials. On muscle biopsy, type II fiber atrophy predominates. The cause of muscle weakness in this population is often multifactorial (Table 37-2).

Table 37-2.   Causes of muscle weakness in dialysis patients

Peripheral neuropathy
Vitamin D deficiency
Hyperparathyroidism
Carnitine deficiency
Aluminum intoxication
Hyperkalemia or hypokalemia
Acidosis
Iron overload
Severe hypophosphatemia
Drug toxicity (glucocorticoids, colchicine, clofibrate)
Muscle ischemia due to vascular calcification
Inactivity
Underlying systemic rheumatic disease

A. Vitamin D deficiency is the most common nonneuropathic cause of muscle weakness in dialysis patients. Vitamin D seems to be important for preservation of normal muscle fiber architecture and normal skeletal muscle function. Myopathy caused by vitamin D deficiency is suggested by the presence of diffuse weakness, asthenia, and coexisting osteopenia.

Muscle strength, EMG findings, and histologic changes usually improve after several weeks of therapy with 1,25-dihydroxyvitamin D_3 (0.5–1.5 µg per day). In most patients, the myopathy remits completely after a few months of vitamin D therapy; however, some patients may require 1–2 years of treatment. Hypercalcemia is a common complication of vitamin D therapy.

B. Hyperparathyroidism may be associated with proximal muscle weakness and impaired respiratory muscle strength. Some patients may regain muscle strength after subtotal parathyroidectomy.

C. Carnitine deficiency. L-Carnitine is involved in the transfer of long-chain fatty acids into mitochondria for oxidation, producing energy for muscle and other cells. In patients with chronic renal failure, carnitine production by the nonfunctioning kidney is reduced and dietary carnitine intake is decreased. Additionally, hemodialysis removes L-carnitine. Thus, muscle carnitine concentrations are low in dialysis patients. Intravenous L-carnitine supplementation may improve muscle strength, function, and mass in dialysis patients.

D. Aluminum intoxication. Muscle weakness in patients with aluminum intoxication has improved following chelation therapy with deferoxamine. The exact mechanism by which aluminum poisoning causes muscle weakness is unknown.

VI. Use of antirheumatic drugs in dialysis patients (Table 37-3).

A. NSAID. Traditional NSAIDs, including aspirin, ibuprofen, naproxen, indomethacin, sulindac, oxaprozin, and nabumetone, inhibit both COX-1 and COX-2. At therapeutic concentrations, the specific COX-2 inhibitors celecoxib and rofecoxib do not inhibit COX-1 and thus spare inhibition of thromboxane production by platelets and prostaglandin biosynthesis in the gastrointestinal tract. Accordingly, specific COX-2 inhibitors have no appreciable effect on bleeding and a lower risk of inducing gastric ulcers than traditional NSAIDs. Because dialysis patients are especially susceptible to gastrointestinal bleeding (for reasons discussed in Chapter 34), specific COX-2 inhibitors may be preferred over traditional NSAIDs in this patient population. However, all NSAIDs (including specific COX-2 inhibitors) inhibit prostaglandin production in the kidney and thus have the potential to cause reduced glomerular filtration, salt retention, and hyperkalemia (side effects that may be important in dialysis patients with residual renal function).

Little has been published about the chronic use of NSAIDs in dialysis patients. The liver primarily metabolizes all NSAIDs; very little (less than 10%) parent compound is excreted unchanged in the urine. An exception is indomethacin, 15%–25% of which is excreted unchanged in the urine. However, 40%–95% of NSAID metabolites are excreted in the urine, as glucuronide conjugates as well as in other forms. Few data are available regard-

Table 37-3.   Use of antirheumatic drugs in dialysis patients

Drug	Unique Toxicity	Renal Excretion (%)[a]	Dosage Adjustment for Dialysis Patients
Allopurinol	Exfoliative dermatitis Rare xanthine stones	50–75[a]	Decrease dose and lengthen dosing interval; administer dose after HD or administer 50% supplemental dose
Colchicine	Myopathy/neuropathy	10–20	50% of the usual dose; avoid prolonged use
Hydroxychloroquine	Retinopathy	15–20	No dose modification
Sulfasalazine	Dizziness/headache; reversible oligospermia	50–70	
Aurinofin	Diarrhea; stomatitis	60–90	Avoid use
Gold sodium thiomalate	Stomatitis; thrombocytopenia	60–90	Avoid use
Methotrexate	Hepatic cirrhosis and fibrosis; myelosuppression; pneumonitis	45–100	Avoid use (not dialyzable)
Penicillamine	Aplastic anemia; myasthenia gravis	30–60	Avoid use in CAPD

Azathioprine	Myelosuppression; increased risk of neoplasia	2–10	Slightly dialyzable (5%–20%) by HD; CAPD effects unknown; supplement 0.25 mg/kg after HD
Cyclophosphamide	Myelosuppression; hemorrhagic cystitis	50[b]–100[b]	Administer doses after HD or administer 50% supplemental dose
Cyclosporine	Hypertension; seizures and tremors	6	No dose modification
Corticosteroids	Cushingoid features		
Prednisone		20–35	No dose modification
Methylprednisolone		5	No dose modification (but administer supplemental dose after HD)
Hydrocortisone		5	No dose modification
Dexamethasone		3	No dose modification

[a] Of allopurinol and its principal active metabolite, oxypurinol. HD, hemodialysis; CAPD, continuous ambulatory peritoneal dialysis.
[b] Anecdotal evidence suggests that 50% dose reduction may be prudent initially.

ing the bioactivity and toxicity of these metabolites. Consequently, manufacturer product labeling suggests that NSAIDs be used with caution and at reduced doses in patients with renal failure. Because they are highly bound to proteins, NSAIDs are removed poorly by dialysis modalities; postdialysis supplemental doses are unnecessary.

B.   Drugs for gout. Colchicine and allopurinol doses must be reduced substantially when treating dialysis patients.

1.   Colchicine toxicity occurs more frequently in individuals with compromised renal function. Because its bioavailability is extremely variable in renal failure, prophylactic use of colchicine should be avoided. Prolonged administration of colchicine (0.6 mg twice daily) to patients with renal insufficiency or chronic renal failure has caused a severe lysosomal, vacuolar myopathy with marked elevation of serum creatine kinase (CK) levels. Fortunately, this myopathy resolves within 4 weeks of colchicine discontinuation. Severe heart failure has also been reported in patients with chronic renal failure who were taking colchicine.

2.   Allopurinol. Both allopurinol and its active metabolite oxypurinol are cleared by dialysis modalities. Because oxypurinol is excreted slowly by the kidneys, the dose of allopurinol should be reduced to 100 mg daily in patients undergoing dialysis.

C.   Corticosteroids. Purely pharmacokinetic considerations do not contraindicate the treatment of dialysis patients with corticosteroids. However, use of these drugs can result in sodium and fluid retention, hypertension, glucose intolerance, osteoporosis, osteonecrosis, increased susceptibility to infection, and worsened azotemia (due to catabolic effects). Thus, every effort should be made to avoid their use in dialysis patients or to administer the lowest dose for the shortest duration possible.

SELECTED READINGS

Bardin T. Low dose prednisone in dialysis-related amyloid arthropathy. *Rev Rheum (Engl. Ed)* 1994;61(9 Suppl):97S–100S.

Brouillard M, et al. Erythrocyte sedimentation rate, an underestimated tool in chronic renal failure. *Nephrol Dial Transplant* 1996 Nov; 11(11):2244–2247.

Chalmers A, et al. The arthropathy of maintenance intermittent peritoneal dialysis. *Can Med Assoc J* 1980;123:635–638.

Cruz C, Shah SV. Dialysis elbow: olecranon bursitis from long-term hemodialysis. *JAMA* 1977;238:243.

Gómez-Fernández P, et al. Effect of parathyroidectomy on respiratory muscle strength in uremic myopathy. *Am J Nephrol* 1987;7:466–469.

Hande KR, Noone RM, Stone WJ. Severe allopurinol toxicity: description and guidelines for prevention in patients with renal insufficiency. *Am J Med* 1984;76:47–56.

Jadoul M, et al. Histologic prevalence of β₂-microglobulin amyloidosis in hemodialysis: a prospective post-mortem study. *Kidney Int* 1997;51: 1928–1932.

Jadoul M, et al. Prevalence of histological β₂-microglobulin amyloidosis in CAPD patients compared with hemodialysis patients. *Kidney Int* 1998;54:956–959.

Jimenez RE, et al. Development of gastrointestinal β_2-microglobulin amyloidosis correlates with time on dialysis. *Am J Surg Pathol* 1998;22:729–735.

Jones M, Kjellstrand CM. Spontaneous tendon ruptures in patients on chronic dialysis. *Am J Kidney Dis* 1996;28:861–866.

Krane NK, et al. Persistent lupus activity in end-stage renal disease. *Am J Kidney Dis* 1999;33:872–876.

Kay J. β_2-Microglobulin amyloidosis. *Amyloid Int J Exp Clin Invest* 1997;4:187–211.

Kay J, et al. Utility of high resolution ultrasound for the diagnosis of dialysis-related amyloidosis. *Arthritis Rheum* 1992;35:926–932.

Koda Y, et al. Switch from conventional to high-flux membrane reduces the risk of carpal tunnel syndrome and mortality of hemodialysis patients. *Kidney Int* 1997;52:1096–1101.

Kuncl RW, et al. Colchicine myopathy and neuropathy. *N Engl J Med* 1987;316:1562–1568.

McCarthy JT, et al. Serum β_2-microglobulin concentration in dialysis patients: importance of intrinsic renal function. *J Lab Clin Med* 1994; 123:495–505.

McIntyre C, et al. Serum C-reactive protein as a marker for infection and inflammation in regular dialysis patients. *Clin Nephrol* 1997;48: 371–374.

Matsuo K, et al. Dialysis-related amyloidosis of the tongue in long-term hemodialysis patients. *Kidney Int* 1997;52:832–838.

Miyata T, et al. β_2-Microglobulin modified with advanced glycation end products is a major component of hemodialysis-associated amyloidosis. *J Clin Invest* 1993;92:1243–1252.

Mojcik CF, Klippel JH. End-stage renal disease and systemic lupus erythematosus. *Am J Med* 1996;101:100–107.

Montseny JJ, Meyrier A, Gherardi RK. Colchicine toxicity in patients with chronic renal failure. *Nephrol Dial Transplant* 1996;11: 2055–2058.

Owen WF, Lowrie EG. C-reactive protein as an outcome predictor for maintenance hemodialysis patients. *Kidney Int* 1998;54:627–636.

Prabhala, et al. Severe myopathy associated with vitamin D deficiency in western New York. *Arch Int Med* 2000;160:1199–1203.

Schreiner O, et al. Reduced secretion of proinflammatory cytokines of monosodium urate crystal-stimulated monocytes in chronic renal failure: an explanation for infrequent gout episodes in ESRD? *Nephrol Dial Transplant* 2000;15:644–649.

Siami G, et al. Evaluation of the effect of intravenous L-carnitine therapy on function, structure and fatty acid metabolism of skeletal muscle in patients receiving chronic hemodialysis. *Nephron* 1991;57: 306–313.

Stenvinkel P, et al. High serum hyaluronan indicates poor survival in renal replacement therapy. *Am J Kidney Dis* 1999;34:1083–1088.

Tan SY, et al. Long term effect of renal transplantation on dialysis-related amyloid deposits and symptomatology. *Kidney Int* 1996;50: 282–289.

van Ypersele de Strihou C, et al, and the Working Party on Dialysis Amyloidosis. Effect of dialysis membrane and patient's age on signs of dialysis-related amyloidosis. *Kidney Int* 1991;39:1012–1019.

Word-Sims WS, Hall CD. Carpal tunnel syndrome in the dialysis patient. *Semin Dial* 1990;3:47–51.

38

Sleep Disorders

Robert L. Benz and Mark R. Pressman

End-stage renal disease (ESRD) has long been associated with sleep complaints, especially by patients undergoing dialysis. Recent surveys of dialysis patients report that 41%–52% have one or more sleep complaints, and more than 50% studied in a sleep disorders laboratory have a sleep disorder objectively documented by polysomnography.

I. Patient complaints

A. Problems falling asleep or staying asleep, frequent awakenings. Dialysis patients complain frequently of "insomnia" independent of anxiety or depression. They may have difficulty falling asleep or staying asleep. Patients often complain of awakening frequently during the night without apparent cause.

B. Daytime fatigue and unplanned naps. Excessive daytime sleepiness (EDS) is a frequent complaint. It is common to enter a dialysis unit during the daytime and find many patients fast asleep while undergoing dialysis. Chronic daytime sleepiness may affect cognitive functioning, interfere with activities of daily living, and decrease quality of life. Daytime sleepiness may also interfere with the patient's ability to work and place him or her in danger while driving or operating heavy equipment.

C. Restless legs. One of the most common complaints among ESRD patients is restless legs syndrome (RLS) (Montplaisir and Godbout, 1989). RLS is a subjective complaint for which there is no objective test. Patients often describe an irritating sensation deep in the muscles of the lower leg, particularly in the calf muscle. Patients can relieve this sensation only by moving their legs and feet. The irritating sensation typically appears when patients are at rest, often in the hours prior to the patient's usual bedtime. RLS may significantly delay sleep onset.

II. Objective findings. Polysomnographic (sleep) studies of ESRD patients have demonstrated a very high incidence of both sleep apnea and periodic leg movements in sleep. These can occur in patients with or without sleep complaints.

A. Sleep apnea. Obstructive sleep apnea is a very common medical disorder resulting from a collapse of the upper airway during sleep in the presence of continuing respiratory effort. It is often associated with loud snoring, gasping, and snorting sounds during sleep. It is reported to occur in 4% of normal men and 2% of women 30–60 years of age. As many as 81% of elderly nursing home patients are reported to have sleep apnea. Obstructive sleep apnea has been reported to be associated with increased morbidity and mortality. This morbidity is most often related to cardiovascular and cerebrovascular pathophysiologic processes, as well as accidents due to sleepiness. Studies have found sleep apnea in 53%–75% of dialysis patients with sleep-related complaints. The sleep apnea found in the majority of dialysis patients may differ from that of the general population.

Some sleep laboratory studies of dialysis patients have reported that the sleep apnea is often of the central type. In central apnea, neither respiratory effort nor airflow is present, suggesting a malfunction in the respiratory centers of the brain. Mixed apneas, which refers to central sleep apnea with an obstructive component, are not uncommon in the dialysis population. Successful renal transplantation has been reported to improve ESRD-related sleep apnea.

B. Periodic leg movements in sleep (PLMS). PLMS is a common sleep disorder occurring with increased incidence with age and common in the elderly of the general population. It generally consists of a dorsiflexion of the foot or movement of the lower limb lasting 2–4 seconds and repeating every 20–40 seconds numerous times. It occurs primarily in the first third of the sleep period during non-REM sleep. Each movement may result in a brief arousal from sleep and can be the source of complaints about unrefreshing sleep and daytime fatigue. PLMS occurs in approximately 80% of patients who complain of RLS. PLMS is found in a very high percentage of ESRD patients. Dialysis patients with PLMS have a much higher number of movements per hour of sleep than patients in the general population with PLMS. In one case series of 45 dialysis patients, 71% had significant PLMS, with several patients having more than 1,500 leg movements in a single night. Many of the PLMS incidents were associated with repetitive arousals, resulting in very poor-quality sleep, daytime complaints of fatigue, and increased mortality.

III. Diagnosis

A. History. A sleep history can easily be obtained using a questionnaire or brief interview. Patients or bed partners should be questioned regarding quantity and quality of nocturnal sleep, number of awakenings from sleep, whether sleep is restorative, snoring, gasping, breathing pauses during sleep, lower-limb movements (kicking) while awake or asleep, daytime fatigue or inappropriate napping. A review of medications or social habits (e.g., excess caffeine) associated with excess irritability should be reviewed.

B. Polysomnography. Sleep disorders such as sleep apnea and periodic leg movements in sleep are easily identifiable via standard diagnostic polysomnography (sleep studies). These studies are usually performed in specially equipped laboratories found in many hospitals.

Polysomnography generally encompasses simultaneous electroencephalography, electrooculography, electromyography, electrocardiography, as well as monitoring of breathing sounds, respiratory effort and airflow, arterial oxygen saturation, and leg movements during the patient's usual sleep period.

IV. Treatment

A. Sleep apnea

1. Medication. Medication has not been shown to be effective in the treatment of obstructive sleep apnea. However, medications such as theophylline, acetazolamide, medroxyprogesterone, and clomipramine have been reported with variable results as a treatment for central sleep apnea but may not be appropriate for ESRD patients. Benzodiazepines are contraindicated for obstructive sleep apnea, as are other central nervous system depressants, because they may result in longer apneas, greater O_2 desaturation, and more severe sleep fragmentation with consequently greater daytime fatigue.

2. Nasal continuous positive airway pressure (NCPAP). Sleep apnea of ESRD is often more difficult to treat than in the usual patient with obstructive sleep apnea because many of the apneas found in ESRD patients are central or mixed apneas. However, administration of NCPAP has been shown to be an effective treatment for central apneas in this population. NCPAP consists of the administration of positive air pressure via the nares. The positive air pressure splints the upper airway open, effectively preventing obstruction. NCPAP has also been found to be an effective treatment for central apneas in the general population and in dialysis patients. Patients who use NCPAP treatment for obstructive sleep apnea are only 40%–60% compliant with this form of therapy.

3.   Surgery. Various surgical approaches have been used for the treatment of obstructive sleep apnea. These usually involve the surgical reduction or removal of the uvula and tissues of the soft palate. Surgeries for obstructive sleep apnea have been reported to have an overall success rate of 50%.

4. O_2. Administration of low-flow supplemental O_2 has been reported to be a successful treatment for central sleep apnea in some recent studies. However, if obstructive sleep apnea is also present, low-flow O_2 may result in a lengthening of apnea duration.

B.   RLS/PLMS
   1.   Medication
      a.   Dopamine precursors or agonists such L-dopa (e.g., Sinemet) have been shown to reduce the number and severity of both disorders and are considered the treatment of choice by many (Montplaisr and Godbout, 1989).
      b.   Benzodiazepines, such as clonazepam, have been used for many years. Controversy exists as to whether benzodiazepines actually reduce the number of movements or simply suppress arousal.
      c.   Opiate narcotics (e.g., propoxyphene) have also been reported to reduce the number of limb movements.

V.   Effects of dialysis. Maintenance hemodialysis has not been shown to have an effect on the frequency or severity of sleep apnea (Mendelson et al, 1990). However, a case report of initiation of dialysis in an elderly patient with renal failure documented improvement of sleep apnea. Effects on PLMS have not been reported. Sleep quality may be improved with long nocturnal dialysis (Pierratos et al, 1997).

VI.   Effects of transplantation. Complete resolution of both sleep apnea and RLS/PLMS have been reported following kidney transplantation.

VII.   Mortality. Dialysis patients have a high rate of mortality. On average, 24% of all dialysis patients die each year (Owen et al, 1993). Our research has shown that patients with a PLMS index of >35 per hour of sleep had a much higher mortality rate than other patients studied in the sleep laboratory. Albumin and urea reduction ratio levels for these patients did not predict the patient mortality and did not distinguish the surviving patients from the deceased. Only the presence of significant numbers of periodic leg movements during sleep predicted mortality in these patients.

ESRD patients have a high incidence of major organic sleep disorders resulting in fragmentation of sleep and decreased daytime alertness. The symptomatic treatment of sleep disorders in ESRD patients with hypnotic medication may be inappropriate without a complete differential diagnosis showing the absence of sleep apnea or PLMS. Sleep disorders appear to result from kidney failure per se, as well the inability of dialysis to normalize the uremic state. Sleep disorders of ESRD are easily diagnosable and often treatable. They are common and warrant appropriate investigation and therapy.

SELECTED READINGS

Benz RL, et al. Potential novel predictors of mortality in end-stage renal disease patients with sleep disorders. *Am J Kidney Dis* 2000; 35:1052–1060.

Benz RL, et al. A preliminary study of the effects of correction of anemia with recombinant human erythropoietin therapy on sleep, sleep disorders, and daytime sleepiness in hemodialysis patients (the SLEEPO study). *Am J Kidney Dis* 1999;34:1089–1095.

Hallet M, et al. Sleep apnea and end stage renal disease. *ASAIO J* 1995;41:S54.

Kimmel PL, Miller G, Mendelson WB. Sleep apnea syndrome in chronic renal disease. *Am J Med* 1989;86:308–314.

Langevin B, et al. Sleep apnea syndrome and end stage renal disease: cure after renal transplantation. *Chest* 1993;103:1330–1335.

Mendelson WB, et al. Effects of hemodialysis of sleep apnea syndrome in end-stage renal disease. *Clin Nephrol* 1990;33:247–251.

Millman RP, et al. Sleep apnea in hemodialysis patients: the lack of testosterone effect on its pathogenesis. *Nephron* 1985;40:407–410.

Montplaisir J, Godbout R. Restless legs syndrome and periodic leg movements in sleep. In: Kryger MH, Roth T, Dement WC, eds. *Principles and practice of sleep medicine*. Philadelphia: WB Saunders, 1989:402–409.

Owen WF Jr., et al. The urea reduction ratio and serum albumin concentration as predictors of mortality in patients undergoing hemodialysis. *N Engl J Med* 1993;329:1001–1006.

Pierratos A, et al. Nocturnal hemodialysis improves sleep quality in patients with chronic renal failure. *J Am Soc Nephrol* 1997;8:169a (abstr).

Pressman MR, Benz RL, Peterson DD. High incidence of sleep disorders in end stage renal disease patients. *Sleep Res* 1995;25:321.

Pressman MR, Benz RL. Sleep disordered breathing in ESRD: acute beneficial effects of treatment with nasal continuous positive airway pressure. *Kidney Int* 1993;43:1134–1139.

Yasuda T, et al. Restless legs syndrome treated successfully by kidney transplantation: a case report. *Clin Transplant* 1986;138.

Nervous System

Anthony J. Nicholls

Uremia is accompanied by disordered functioning of both the central and peripheral nervous systems. Neurologic problems also arise in dialyzed patients as a complication of treatment, from metabolic derangements, or from disordered homeostasis. This chapter is limited to cerebral disorders, neuropathy, and seizures; aluminum toxicity is considered in Chapter 31 and muscle weakness in Chapter 37.

I. Central nervous system abnormalities. Cerebral symptoms occur in four settings in the dialysis patient: (a) acute obtundation unassociated with dialysis itself, encountered either as a feature of advanced uremia or occurring in a previously stable dialysis patient; (b) disordered brain function during or immediately after dialysis; (c) chronic dementia in regular dialysis patients; and (d) subclinical disturbances of cognitive function in apparently adequately treated patients.

   A. Acute obtundation not associated with the dialysis procedure.

   1. Uremic encephalopathy. Encephalopathy is a cardinal feature of untreated uremia. Initial manifestations are subtle: flattened affect, irritability, and poor rapport with others. Formal evaluation at this stage may reveal patchy cognitive or psychomotor impairment, and event-related brain potentials [stimulus-evoked averaged electroencephalogram (EEG) waveforms] may be abnormal. As uremia advances, lassitude gives way to disorientation, confusion, delirium, stupor, and, preterminally, coma. There are accompanying motor disturbances: tremulousness, myoclonus, and asterixis (flapping tremor). These major signs of uremic encephalopathy will reliably regress within a week or so of initiation of regular dialysis; failure to do so should lead to an alternative or additional diagnosis.

   2. Acute aluminum intoxication. In patients taking aluminum along with citrate in any form (Shohl's solution, calcium citrate, or effervescent analgesics such as Alka-Seltzer), an acute neurotoxicity syndrome recently has been described characterized by agitation, confusion, seizures, myoclonic jerks, and coma. The acute syndrome also can be seen when dialysis solution is highly contaminated with aluminum or in the course of deferoxamine (DFO) therapy (see Chapter 31). The plasma aluminum level usually is more than 500 µg/L, and typical EEG changes (multifocal bursts of slow or delta wave activity, often accompanied by spikes) are present. Most of the reported patients have died, despite institution of DFO therapy.

   3. Other causes of acute obtundation. Table 39-1 lists the main conditions to be considered in such cases. Appropri-

Table 39-1.   Partial differential diagnosis of acute obtundation not associated with dialysis

Uremic encephalopathy
Acute aluminum toxicity (coingestion of citrate, highly contaminated dialysate)
CNS infection
  Meningitis
  Encephalitis
  Endocarditis
Hypertensive encephalopathy
Hemorrhage
  Subarachnoid
  Subdural
  Intracranial
Drug intoxication (by drugs renally excreted)
  Penicillin
  Cefazolin
Wernicke's encephalopathy (in patients with vomiting, poor food intake)

ate history, examination, and special investigations (including computed brain tomography) usually reveal the diagnosis.

B.   Acute cerebral dysfunction during or immediately after dialysis.

1.   Disequilibrium syndrome. Rapid correction of advanced uremia is sometimes complicated by a characteristic syndrome of neurological dysfunction appearing in the last part of dialysis or shortly afterward. Hemodialysis is usually involved, but disequilibrium can also occur with peritoneal dialysis. In its mildest form, the syndrome is limited to restlessness, headache, nausea, and vomiting; more severe manifestations include confusion and major seizures. The syndrome is believed to be caused by brain swelling due to a lag in osmolar shifts between blood and brain during dialysis, but changes in brain pH may also play a role. Disequilibrium occurs in a major form in previously undialyzed patients, but minor features may complicate chronic therapy. Infusion of 20% mannitol solution at a rate of 50 mL/h during initial hemodialysis, together with a single dose of an anticonvulsant (e.g., diazepam), will prevent the major manifestations of the syndrome. Disequilibrium is more likely to occur when patients with advanced states of uremia are dialyzed for excessive lengths of time during their first treatment sessions. The initial dialyses should be relatively short, so as to reduce elevated serum urea levels slowly over the course of several days.

2.   Intracranial bleeding. The most important differential diagnosis of dialysis disequilibrium syndrome is intracranial bleeding, precipitated or aggravated by anticoagulation during hemodialysis. Spontaneous subdural hemorrhage is typical, but intracranial or subarachnoid bleeds are not uncommon. This is a particular problem in patients with polycystic kidneys who may have intracranial aneurysms. Headache occurs in both disequilibrium and early cerebral hemorrhage, but the pattern of recovery is different. Thus, the patient whose clinical course is atypical for disequilibrium should be evaluated for possible intracranial hemorrhage by computed tomography (CT). Management is similar to that for nonuremic patients. Heparin-free dialysis should be used.

3.   Other causes. Metabolic disorders and hypotension also can mimic disequilibrium (Table 39-2). These may be excluded by measuring the blood pressure and requesting simple laboratory tests. Aluminum intoxication, in addition to the acute manifestations described above and the chronic syndrome discussed below, can give rise to subacute central nervous system symptoms similar to disequilibrium syndrome, which sometimes appear to be worse just after dialysis.

C.   Chronic dementia. Aluminum poisoning in dialysis patients causes a highly characteristic progressive myoclonic dementia. Typical early signs are stuttering and stammering (Table 31-1). Signs and symptoms may be exacerbated by dialysis and by DFO administration. The diagnosis of aluminum-related dementia should be pursued by performing an EEG, which may show the characteristic multifocal bursts of delta or theta activity, measuring serum aluminum levels, and performing a DFO infusion test to help assess the body aluminum burden. These are described in Chapter 31.

Dialysis patients with progressive dementia in whom aluminum poisoning has been excluded are likely to suffer from some form of progressive cerebrovascular disease. Table 39-3 lists a brief differential diagnosis of chronic dementia in this population. Widespread atheromatous plaques commonly found in dialysis patients predispose them to develop multi-infarct dementia. At autopsy, the brains of these patients are seen to

Table 39-2.   Conditions that may mimic dialysis disequilibrium syndrome

Intracranial bleeding
    Subdural
    Subarachnoid
    Intracranial
Metabolic disorders
    Hyperosmolar states
    Hypercalcemia
    Hypoglycemia
    Hyponatremia
Cerebral infarction
Hypotension
    Excessive ultrafiltration
    Cardiac arrhythmia
    Myocardial infarction
    Anaphylaxis
Aluminum intoxication (subacute)

Table 39-3.   Partial differential diagnoses of chronic dementia in dialysis patients

Aluminum encephalopathy (dialysis dementia)
Multiinfarct dementia
Chronic subdural hematoma
Hydrocephalus (possibly secondary to subarachnoid hemorrhage)
Metabolic disorders
   Hypercalcemia (autonomous hyperparathyroidism or iatrogenic)
   Hypoglycemic brain damage
   Demyelination syndrome secondary to hyponatremia
   Uremia (underdialysis)
   Thiamine deficiency (chronic Wernicke-Korsakoff syndrome)
Drug intoxication
Anemia
Presenile dementias
Depressive pseudodementia
Chronic infection

contain multiple lacunar infarcts in the basal ganglia, thalamus, internal capsule, pons, and cerebellum. Clinically, these patients present with a progressive stepwise decline in intellectual and neurologic functioning, and may have a variety of neurologic signs according to the site of the infarcts. The diagnosis of chronic subdural hematoma as a complication of anticoagulant treatment should always be borne in mind as the disease may present with pseudodementia, drowsiness, and confusion. The diagnosis is made by CT scanning. Metabolic disorders, including drug intoxication, are excluded by simple laboratory tests and a careful drug ingestion history.

D.   Subclinical cognitive dysfunction. Subclinical uremic encephalopathy may be present in chronic dialysis patients if inadequate dialysis is delivered. Possible reasons include noncompliance, vascular access recirculation, and impaired peritoneal transport. Alternatively, severe depression (and sometimes anxiety) can impair cognitive function, but these may be detected only if detailed and regular neuropsychological assessment is undertaken. With aluminum-induced dialysis dementia, subtle, unrecognized alterations in cerebral function due to aluminum accumulation can occur as a result of therapy with aluminum-containing phosphorus binders.

Recently, the widespread use of recombinant human erythropoietin (EPO) has led to the realization that some of the chronic cerebral disturbances of dialysis patients are attributable to anemia; both event-related potentials and neuropsychological test scores improve after treatment of anemia with EPO.

E.   Sleep disorders. Sleep disturbance is an integral feature of uremia, affecting 50% of hemodialysis and continuous ambulatory peritoneal dialysis (CAPD) patients. It is not related to total urea clearance (Kt/V) or other markers of dialysis delivery but may be worsened by caffeine intake, cigarette smoking, and anxiety. Chronic dependence on nocturnal hypnotics is common in the renal failure population. Sleep disorders in dialysis patients is discussed in Chapter 38.

F. Visual/auditory disturbances. A syndrome of acute visual or, more rarely, auditory loss has been described as a relatively frequent complication of DFO therapy, especially when higher dosages are used. Acute sight loss also has occurred due to retinal artery leukoembolization.

G. Atlanto-cervical spondylopathy. Progressive neck instability and cord compression has been described in long-term dialysis patients. The cause is destructive β_2-microglobulin-derived amyloidosis; the deposits may be seen by MRI. Early decompression is vital to avoid major disability. See Chapter 37 for a more complete discussion of amyloidosis and its complications.

II. Neuropathy

A. Uremic neuropathy. Uremic neuropathy is a distal, symmetric, mixed motor and sensory polyneuropathy. It typically involves the legs more than the arms. Clinical manifestations include paresthesia in the feet, painful dysesthesia, ataxia, and weakness. The sense of position and the vibratory threshold are often impaired. Physiologic studies show slowing of motor nerve conduction and sensory action potentials. The condition is thought to be due to one or more toxins retained in uremia and inadequately removed by hemodialysis.

With effective dialysis, clinical manifestations of uremic neuropathy are unusual, but subclinical manifestations can be detected in over 50% of dialysis patients. Serial electrophysiologic monitoring has been used to assess the adequacy of dialysis schedules but is not routinely employed. If clinical signs of peripheral neuropathy appear, then the adequacy of the dialysis treatment should be carefully evaluated using urea kinetic modeling. For hemodialysis patients being dialyzed three times per week, a Kt/V of at least 1.2–1.4 should be delivered and at least 1.4 if the dialysis session length is short. A 30-minute postdialysis serum urea value should be checked and the whole-body Kt/V using Fig. A-2 should be recomputed. This "equilibrated" Kt/V will better reflect the true amount of therapy being delivered and may identify the patient as one in whom a large degree of post-dialysis urea rebound normally occurs. A switch to a high-flux membrane to increase the removal of middle molecules may be of benefit. Whether short daily or long nocturnal dialysis benefit neuropathy has not been well studied. Symptoms may be improved by a switch to a continuous form of peritoneal dialysis. In the final analysis, clinical manifestations are most reliably reversed by successful renal transplantation.

B. Differential diagnosis. In many patients with polyneuropathy, uremic neuropathy has to be distinguished from disturbed peripheral nerve function due to an underlying systemic disease (e.g., amyloidosis or diabetes mellitus). Table 39-4 gives an abbreviated list of disorders to be considered in the differential diagnosis.

C. Mononeuropathies. Paresthesia in the extremities may also be due to a mononeuropathy. The most common mononeuropathy in dialysis patients affects the median nerve at the

Table 39-4. Principal differential diagnosis of uremic polyneuropathy

Diabetes mellitus
Ethanol abuse
Amyloidosis
Malnutrition
Polyarteritis
Lupus erythematosus
Multiple myeloma
Thiamine deficiency

wrist (carpal tunnel syndrome). This typically involves the fistula arm but may be bilateral. The pathogenesis and management of the carpal tunnel syndrome are discussed in Chapter 37. Occasionally, prolonged recumbency during the hemodialysis procedure may predispose to ulnar and peroneal nerve palsies.

D. Restless-legs syndrome. Patients typically complain of aching or discomfort in their legs, often during sleep or rest, which can be relieved only by moving the legs. It is unclear to what extent this common condition is related to uremic polyneuropathy. Restless-legs syndrome may respond to administration of benzodiazepines, particularly clonazepam.

E. Autonomic neuropathy. Autonomic neuropathy occasionally occurs in renal failure in the absence of diabetes and may contribute to the occurrence of hypotension during hemodialysis (controversial) and to impotence in the male. Tonically increased sympathetic nervous system activity, as measured by peroneal nerve microneurography, is present, and may contribute to hypertension.

III. Seizures

A. Etiology. Seizures are not uncommon in dialysis patients. Generalized seizures are an integral feature of advanced uremic encephalopathy. Seizures can also be a manifestation of severe disequilibrium syndrome, as discussed above. Table 39-5 lists the most common associated conditions. Intracranial hemorrhage commonly leads to focal seizures, while most of the other causes lead to generalized seizures.

B. Predisposing factors. Seizures characterize both aluminum-induced encephalopathy and severe hypertension. In children with renal failure, the incidence of seizures is higher than in adults. Predialysis hypocalcemia can result in seizures during or soon after dialysis due to the fall in serum ionized calcium level associated with rapid correction of acidosis. Hypoglycemia can occur if glucose-free dialysis solution is used.

The incidence of seizures in patients treated with EPO has come under close scrutiny; the risk appears to be 1 seizure per 13 patient-years of therapy, with the highest risk during the early months of treatment. There is little evidence of an excess of seizures in normotensive patients on EPO; however, when hematocrit rises, there is a tendency for a concomitant rise in

Table 39-5.   Seizures in dialysis patients

Etiology
Uremic encephalopathy (unlikely in dialysis patients)
Disequilibrium syndrome
Aluminum encephalopathy
Hypertensive encephalopathy
Intracranial hemorrhage
Alcohol withdrawal
Toxins (star fruit ingestion)
Other (metabolic)
  Hypocalcemia
  Hyperosmolality due to peritoneal dialysis
  Hypernatremia (accidental due to hemodialysis machine
    malfunction) or hyponatremia
  Anoxia
    Arrhythmia
    Anaphylaxis
    Severe hypotension
    Air embolism

Prevention
Identification of susceptible subgroups
  Predialysis serum urea nitrogen level > 130 mg/dl
  Severe hypertension
  Children
  Patients receiving erythropoietin (EPO)
  Previous seizure disorder
  Alcoholism
  Predialysis hypocalcemia (< 6 mg/dl) with acidosis
Limiting initial dialysis session length and blood flow rate
Maintenance of dialysis solution sodium concentration at or above
  plasma level
Use of 3.5 mEq/L or 4.0 mEq/L calcium bath in hypocalcemic
  patients; administration of IV calcium during dialysis if necessary
Scrupulous attention to blood pressure control during EPO therapy
Limiting exposure to ethanol and to "epileptogenic" drugs
  Penicillins
  Cyclosporine
  Meperidine (Demerol)
  Theophylline
  Metoclopramide
  Lithium

Therapy
Stopping dialysis
Maintenance of airway patency
Drawing blood for glucose, calcium, and other electrolytes
If hypoglycemia is suspected, administration of IV glucose
Administration of IV diazepam, and also phenytoin if required
Treatment of metabolic disturbance if present

blood pressure. This may provoke hypertensive encephalopathy and seizures if the rate of rise in blood pressure exceeds the capacity of the cerebral circulation to alter its autoregulatory thresholds.

Seizures tend to be more common in patients taking a variety of "epileptogenic" drugs. Penicillins and cephalosporins are common offenders, especially if high doses are given. A selection of other epileptogenic drugs is given in Table 39-5. A variety of poisonings in dialysis patients can present with seizures, including star fruit ingestion (numbness, weakness, obtundation, seizures; see Chang et al, 2000).

C. Diagnosis. Electroencephalography is of limited value in the evaluation of seizures in dialysis patients. Patients with renal failure rarely have a normal EEG, the most common abnormal findings being reduced voltage, loss of alpha activity, and the appearance of periodic, symmetric, and usually frontal delta wave slowing. In any case the EEG is unlikely to distinguish between the various causes of seizures listed in Table 39-5, and a search for aluminum poisoning, an underlying metabolic cause, a complication of the dialysis procedure, or a structural intracranial lesion is more appropriate.

D. Prevention. Susceptible patients can often be identified (see Table 39-5). The prevention of dialysis disequilibrium is discussed above. Patients with low serum ionized calcium levels can be given IV calcium at the start of dialysis, and a dialysate with a high calcium concentration can be used. Blood pressure needs to be monitored closely during initiation of EPO therapy, and the dosage of antihypertensive medication may need to be raised.

E. Management. The emergency treatment of convulsions should begin by stopping dialysis and ensuring patency of the airway. Blood should be sampled immediately and serum glucose, calcium, and other electrolyte values determined. IV glucose should be administered if hypoglycemia is suspected. If seizures persist, then 5 to 10 mg of diazepam can be infused slowly IV. Infusion can be repeated at 5-minute intervals to a maximum total dosage of 30 mg. Diazepam therapy can be followed by a loading dosage of phenytoin in a dose of 10 to 15 mg/kg given by slow IV infusion, at a rate no greater than 50 mg/min, during constant electrocardiographic monitoring to guard against phenytoin-induced bradycardia, atrioventricular conduction block, or other arrhythmias.

F. Drug prophylaxis. The prophylaxis of recurrent convulsions is usually effective with administration of phenytoin, carbamazepine, or sodium valproate. Fits of dialysis encephalopathy respond best to benzodiazepines, particularly clonazepam. Table 39-6 lists dosage schedules and other pharmacokinetic data for anticonvulsants in dialysis patients.

1. Phenytoin

a. Reduced plasma half-life. The half-life of phenytoin is reduced in dialysis patients, resulting in lower plasma levels at the usual therapeutic dosage.

b. Increased free fraction in uremia. Phenytoin is normally 90% protein bound, and drug effect is proportional to the free (unbound) drug level. Normal therapeutic blood

Table 39-6. Pharmacokinetics of anticonvulsants in dialysis patients

Drug	Renal excretion (%)	Nonuremic dosage range (mg/day)	Usual dosage for ESRD patients (%)	Plasma half-life (h) Nonuremic patients	Plasma half-life (h) ESRD patients	Removed by hemodialysis	Notes
Carbamazepine	3	600–1600	100	10–20	Same[a]	No	NU-TPL = 4–12 mg/L
Clonazepam	<1	0.5–20.0	100	17–28	Same[a]	No	
Diazepam	<1	5–10 (IV)[b]	?50	20–70	Same[a]	No	Active metabolites may accumulate in renal failure
Ethosuximide	>30	750–2000	100	50–60	Same[a]	Yes	NU-TPL = 40–100 mg/L
Phenobarbital	10–40	60–200	75	100	120–160	Yes	
Phenytoin	<5	300–600	100	10–30	Same[a]	±	NU-TPL = 10–20 mg/L; ESRD-TPL = 4–10 mg/L due to decreased protein binding
Primidone	40[c]	500–2000	Caution	5–15	Same[a]	Yes	Avoid in ESRD patients
Valproic acid	<4	750–2000	75–100	6–16	Same[a]	±	NU-TPL = 50–120 mg/L
Vigabatrin	50	2000–4000	25	7	14	Unknown	New drug; little experience in dialysis patients

ESRD, end-stage renal disease; NU-TPL, therapeutic plasma concentration in nonuremic subjects; ESRD-TPL, therapeutic plasma concentration in dialysis patients

[a] Inferred (estimated) from pharmacokinetic considerations.

[b] Initial dose.

[c] Extensive metabolism to PEMA and phenobarbital. Primidone and PEMA are excreted unchanged, and 10%–40% of phenobarbital is excreted by the kidneys.

levels of total (bound plus unbound) phenytoin are usually 10 to 20 mg per L, corresponding to about 1.0 to 2.0 mg per L of free phenytoin. In uremia, and also with low serum albumin, the unbound phenytoin fraction can increase from 10% to 15% to 30%, resulting in more marked drug effect for any given blood level of total phenytoin.

   c. **Falsely high levels with immunoassay methods in uremia.** In uremic patients, a number of inactive metabolites of phenytoin can accumulate that are picked up rather indiscriminately by the usual immunoassay methods (e.g., the enzyme multiplied immunoassay, or EMIT, procedure), resulting in inaccurately high readings. Chromatographic methods (e.g., gas-liquid chromatography) are not subject to this error. The amount of overestimation by the EMIT procedure, initially considerable, is now less due to improvements in the immunoassay procedure.

   d. **Therapeutic recommendations.** The usual loading and maintenance dosages of phenytoin should be given (see Table 39-6); one should give a divided daily maintenance dosage because of the reduced plasma half-life. Although the amount of drug given will depend on clinical response, a target blood level for total phenytoin measured by a chromatographic procedure should be in the range of about 4 to 10 mg per L.

G. **Other anticonvulsant drugs.** Carbamazepine, ethosuximide, and valproic acid can be given in 75% to 100% of the usual dosage to dialysis patients. Protein binding of valproic acid may be reduced in uremia. Carbamazepine is not well removed by dialysis. Valproic acid is slightly dialyzable (about 5% of a dose removed). Ethosuximide is substantially dialyzable, and a post-hemodialysis supplement may be required. Primidone is 40% renally excreted and is moderately dialyzable. Primidone should be used with extreme caution in dialysis patients; the need for a substantially reduced dosage should be anticipated, and a post-hemodialysis supplement may be required. Phenobarbital can be given in 75% to 100% of the usual dosage. Phenobarbital is dialyzable, and a dose should be scheduled after the dialysis treatment. Vigabatrin, a newly introduced GABA-transaminase inhibitor, is eliminated by the kidney; major dosage reduction is necessary in dialysis patients (see Table 39-6).

SELECTED READINGS

Altmann P, et al. Disturbance of cerebral function by aluminum in haemodialysis patients without overt aluminum toxicity. *Lancet* 1989;ii:7.

Apostolou T, Gokal R. Neuropathy and quality of life in diabetic continuous ambulatory peritoneal dialysis patients. *Perit Dial Int* 1999;19 Suppl 2:S242–S247.

Bazzi C, et al. Uremic polyneuropathy: a clinical and electrophysiological study in 135 short- and long-term hemodialyzed patients. *Clin Nephrol* 1991;35:176.

Biasoli S, et al. Uremic encephalopathy: an updating. *Clin Nephrol* 1986;25:57.

Bolton CF, Young GB, eds. *Neurological complications of renal disease.* Boston: Butterworth, 1990.

Chang JM, et al. Fatal outcome after ingestion of star fruit (Averrhoa carambola) in uremic patients. *Am J Kidney Dis* 2000;35:189–193.

Edmunds ME, Walls J. Pathogenesis of seizures during recombinant human erythropoietin therapy. *Semin Dial* 1991;4:163.

Glenn CM, et al. Dialysis-associated seizures in children and adolescents. *Pediatr Nephrol* 1992;6:182.

Hellden A, et al. Neurotoxic side effects of valacyclovir in hemodialysis (HD) patients with herpes zoster—high plasma levels of the metabolite CMMG differentiate from herpes encephalitis. *J Am Soc Nephrol* 1999;10:282 (abstr.).

Jungers P, et al. Incidence and risk factors of atherosclerotic cardiovascular accidents in predialysis chronic renal failure patients: a prospective study. *Nephrol Dial Transplant* 1997;12:2597–2602.

Jungers P, et al. Incidence of atherosclerotic arterial occlusive accidents in predialysis and dialysis patients: a multicentric study in the Ile de France district. *Nephrol Dial Transplant* 1999;14:898–902.

Kawamura M, et al. Incidence, outcome, and risk factors of cerebrovascular events in patients undergoing maintenance hemodialysis. *Am J Kidney Dis* 1998;31:991–996.

Kiley JE. Residual renal and dialyser clearance, EEG slowing, and nerve conduction velocity. *ASAIO J* 1981;4:1.

Lass P, et al. Cognitive impairment in patients with renal failure is associated with multiple-infarct dementia. *Clin Nucl Med* 1999; 24:561–565.

Lindholm B, et al. Progress of peripheral uremic neuropathy during continuous ambulatory peritoneal dialysis. *ASAIO Trans* 1982;28:263.

Marsh JT, et al. Electrophysiological indices of CNS function in hemodialysis and CAPD. *Kidney Int* 1986;30:957.

Marsh JT, et al. rHuEPO treatment improves brain and cognitive function of anemic dialysis patients. *Kidney Int* 1991;39:155.

Nissenson AR, et al. Central nervous system function in dialysis patients—a practical approach. *Semin Dial* 1991;4:115.

Savazzi GM, et al. Hypertension as an etiopathological factor in the development of cerebral atrophy in hemodialyzed patients. *Nephron* 1999;81:17–24.

Silver SM. Cerebral edema after hemodialysis: the "reverse urea effect" lives. *Int J Artif Organs* 1998;21:247–250.

Tattersall JE, et al. Rapid high-flux dialysis can cure uremic peripheral neuropathy. *Nephrol Dial Transplant* 1992;7:539.

Toepfer M, et al. Inflammatory demyelinating neuropathy in patients with end-stage renal disease receiving continuous ambulatory peritoneal dialysis. *Perit Dial Int* 1998;18:172–176.

Appendix A

Urea Kinetic Modeling: Tables and Figures

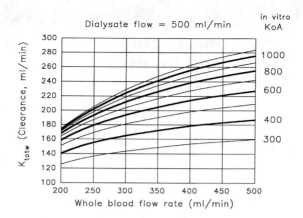

Fig. A-1.   Relationship between nominal blood flow rate (Q_B) and blood water urea clearance (k_{totw}) as a function of dialyzer efficiency (KoA). K_{totw} was computed as per the equations in Table A-1. These dialyzer clearance values still overestimate true in vivo values. To use, start with blood flow rate on the horizontal axis. Go up to intersect with the proper dialyzer KoA line, then go left for the dialyzer clearance, K_{totw}.

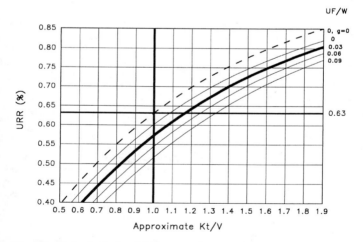

Fig. A-2.   Actual relationship between fractional urea clearance (Kt/V) and urea reduction ratio (URR), taking into account urea generation and the effects of volume contraction. To use, start with the URR on the vertical axis. Move right until you intersect with the proper UF/W line (e.g., for a 4.2 kg weight loss in a 70 kg patient, UF/W = 4.2/70 = 0.06). Then drop down to the horizontal axis for the Kt/V. (Reproduced with permission from Daugirdas JT. Urea kinetic modeling. *Hypertens Dial Clin Nephrol* (HDCN) http://www.hdcn.com)

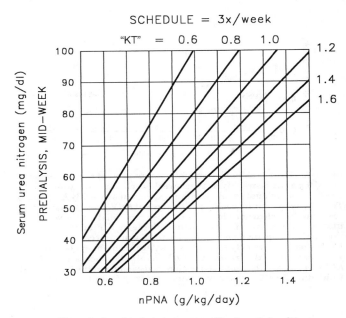

Fig. A-3. The relationship between normalized protein nitrogen appearance (nPNA), the midweek predialysis serum urea nitrogen (SUN), and Kt/V for patients undergoing thrice-weekly dialysis. A similar nomogram designed for first-of-the-week predialysis SUN sampling is given in Chapter 2. To use, find the predialysis SUN on the vertical axis, move right to the proper "KT" diagonal, then drop down to read nPNA on the horizontal axis. "KT" is the treatment Kt/V adjusted for Kru, using the equation "KT" = $Kt/V + 4.5 \times$ Kru/V, where Kru is the residual renal urea clearance in mL/min, and V is the urea distribution volume in L. If Kru = 0, then "KT" = Kt/V (Reproduced with permission from Daugirdas JT. Urea kinetic modeling. Hypertens Dial Clin Nephrol (HDCN) http://www.hdcn.com)

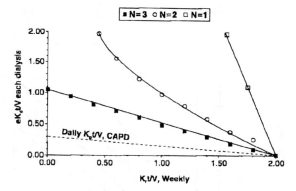

Fig. A-4.   The Gotch nomogram for computation of the treatment
e*Kt*/*V* for a thrice-weekly or twice-weekly schedule in patients with
substantial residual renal function (expressed as weekly *Kt*/*V*-urea).
To use, first compute weekly residual renal *Kt*/*V*-urea. Measure the
residual urea clearance in milliliters per minute, then convert to
liters per week (multiply by 10), then divide by *V*. Find this point on
the *x* axis and go up a perpendicular until you intercept the thrice-
weekly or twice-weekly treatment line. At this point, go left to the
y axis to read off the treatment e*Kt*/*V* required to increase weekly
Kt/*V*-urea to 2.0. (Reproduced with permission from the NKF–DOQI
Guidelines for PD Adequacy, National Kidney Foundation, 1997.)

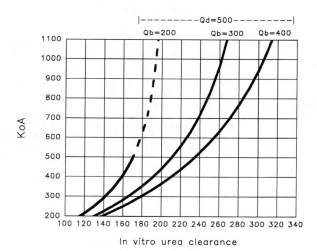

Fig. A-5.   Estimating the in vitro *KoA*-urea from a dialyzer specification sheet. In most cases, the in vitro urea clearance reported at
300 mL of "blood" flow, and preferably that reported at 400 mL per
minute, should be used. To find the *KoA*, first find the urea clearance
on the horizontal axis, rise vertically to the blood flow rate used, and
read the *KoA* off the vertical axis. The 200 mL per minute blood flow
line has been dotted deliberately in the range of high-*KoA* dialyzers;
use clearances at 300 or 400 mL per minute blood flow rate only.
(From Daugirdas JT, Depner TA. A nomogram approach to hemodialysis urea modeling. *Am J Kidney Dis* 1994;23:33–40.)

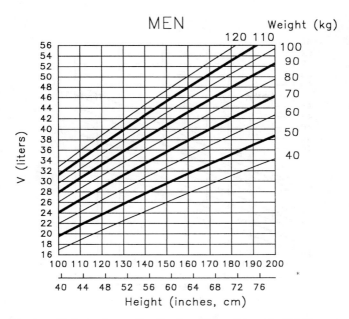

Fig. A-6.   Estimated urea distribution volume V in male dialysis patients. These data are based on the assumption that V = total-body water (TBW) as measured by tritium (actually V is somewhat lower than tritium TBW). The TBW was computed based on body surface area according to Hume and Weyers (*J Clin Pathol* 1971;24: 234–238), with body surface area derived according to Du Bois and Du Bois (*Arch Intern Med* 1916;17:863–871). To use, find the height on the horizontal axis, rise until the appropriate weight (postdialysis) line has been reached, and read V off the vertical axis. (From Daugirdas JT, Depner TA. A nomogram approach to hemodialysis urea modeling. *Am J Kidney Dis* 1994;23:33–40.)

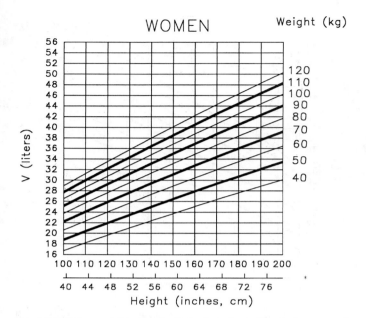

Fig. A-7.   Estimated *V* in female dialysis patients. The data are based on the same assumptions as noted for Fig. A-6. To use, follow the instructions in Fig. A-6. (From Daugirdas JT, Depner TA. A nomogram approach to hemodialysis urea modeling. *Am J Kidney Dis* 1994;23:33–40.)

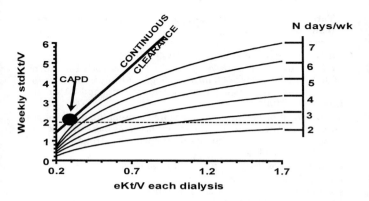

Fig. A-8. Relationship between equilibrated treatment *Kt*/*V* (e*Kt*/*V*) and weekly standard *Kt*/*V* [std (*Kt*/*V*)] (derived from Gotch adjusted eKru as described in Chapter 2) with different dialysis schedules. The weekly *Kt*/*V* line of 2.0 as recommended by DOQI for peritoneal dialysis is highlighted. Using the Gotch approach, one can see that, when using a 3x/week schedule, a weekly std (*Kt*/*V*) of 2.0 corresponds to an equilibrated treatment *Kt*/*V* (e*Kt*/*V*) of 1.0 (follow the 2.0 line until it intersects the 3x/week curve and drop down to the horizontal axis onto 1.0). With a 3x/week schedule, rebound averages about 0.20 *Kt*/*V* units (see discussin in Chapter 2), so this corresponds to the standard sp*Kt*/*V* of 1.2 for 3x/week dialysis. For a 6x/week schedule, the required treatment e*Kt*/*V* is about at 0.37 (follow the 2.0 line to the 6x/week curve and drop down onto the horizontal axis at 0.37). Because rebound with short daily dialysis is about 0.15 *Kt*/*V* units (Daugirdas, unpublished information), this e*Kt*/*V* value corresponds to an sp*Kt*/*V* of about 0.37 + 0.15 = 0.53. (Reproduced with permission from Gotch FA. Kinetic modeling of home dialysis. *Home Hemodial Int* 1998;237–240).

Table A-1.   Estimating dialyzer blood water clearance from *KoA*, Q_B, and Q_D

Step 1: Reduce industry-reported *KoA* by 10%.[a]

Step 2: Adjust resultant *KoA* upward by 3.3% for each 100 mL/min of dialysate flow rate >500 mL/min (e.g., multiply by 1.00 when $Q_D = 500$ mL/min, 1.033 when $Q_D = 600$ mL/min, and 1.1 when $Q_D = 800$ mL/min).

Step 3: Adjust blood flow to compensate for prepump negative pressure (the tubing in the pump segment becomes more oval as prepump negative pressure increases, reducing its stroke volume) and other factors.

Adjustment factor $F = 1.0 - (Q_B - 200)/2000$

Adjusted Q_B $(Q_{badj}) = Q_B F$
   (no adjustment when $Q_B < 200$ mL/min)
   Example: $Q_B = 400$ mL/min
   $F = 1 - (400 - 200)/2000 = 0.90$
   $Q_{badj} = 360$ mL/min

Step 4: Compute diffusive blood water clearance (K_{difw}) from adjusted *KoA* and adjusted Q_B. K_{difw} depends on KoA_{adj}, Q_B (Q_{badj}), and the dialysate flow rate Q_D, according to a fairly complicated equation.

To simplify writing it, we define an intermediate variable called Z. Then:

$Z = \exp [KoA_{adj}/Q_{badj} * (1 - Q_{badj}/Q_D)]$
$K_{difw} = 0.894 * Q_{badj} * (Z - 1)/(Z - Q_{badj}/Q_D)$

The 0.894 multiplier is to correct clearance for blood water, as discussed in text.

Step 5: Add convective clearance to diffusive clearance. First, we compute the ultrafiltration rate in milliliters per minute (Q_f), and then, compute the total blood water clearance (K_{totw}) from the diffusive clearance (K_{difw}), the blood flow rate (Q_{Badj}), and Q_f.

$Q_f = W_{tlosskg} * 1000/(t_{min})$
$K_{totw} = [1 - Q_f/(0.894 * Q_{badj})] * K_{difw} + Q_f$

---

*, asterisk, denotes multiplication; $\exp (x) = e^x$

[a] Actually, industry reported KoA should be reduced by 20%–30% for a true in vivo clearance, but this will vary by manufacturer, and then the urea distribution volume V will be 15–20% lower than anthropometrically estimated total body water.

Table A-2. Anthropometric estimates for total body water

Watson estimate of anthropometric volume:

    For men: V (L) = 2.447 + 0.3362 * W(kg) + 0.1074 * H(cm)

                − 0.09516 * Age(yr)

    For women: V = −2.097 + 0.2466 * W + 0.1069 * H

Hume-Weyers method:

    For men: V = −14.012934 + 0.296785 * W + 0.192786 * H

    For women: V = −35.270121 + 0.183809 * W + 0.344547 * H

For a nomogram of the Hume-Weyers methods, see Fig. A-6 and A-7.

Mellits–Cheek method for children:

    For boys:

        V (L) = −1.927 + 0.465 * W (kg) + 0.045 * H (cm),

           when H < 132.7 cm

        V = −21.993 + 0.406 * W + 0.209 * H, when H > 132.7 cm

    For girls:

        V = 0.076 + 0.507 * W + 0.013 * H, when H < 110.8 cm

        V = −10.313 + 0.252 * W + 0.154 * H, when H > 110.8 cm

---

*, asterisk, denotes multiplication.

References

Watson PE, Watson ID, Batt RD. Total body water volumes for adult males and females estimated from simple anthropometric measurements. *Am J Clin Nutr* 1980;33:27–39.

Hume R, Weyers E. Relationship between total body water and surface area in normal and obese subjects. *J Clin Pathol* 1971;24:234–238.

Mellits ED, Cheek DB. The assessment of body water and fatness from infancy to adulthood. *Monogr Soc Res Child Dev* (Serial 140) 1970;35:12–26.

Du Bois D, Du Bois EF. A formula to estimate the approximate surface area if height and weight are known. *Arch Intern Med* 1916;17:863–971.

Caveat:

1) Watson underestimates V in black people; Hume-Weyers overestimates V in older men (Daugirdas JT et al, *J Am Soc Nephrol* (Abstr.) 1996;7:1510).

Table A-3.   Equations for dialyzer *KoA* from in vitro clearances

Step 1: Compute the ultrafiltration rate (Q_{uf} in mL/min) at which the clearances were done.

Ignore this step if clearances were done at TMP = 0.

If not, find the ultrafiltration coefficient of the dialyzer in question. Compute Q_{uf} as follows:

Q_{uf} (mL/min) = (1/60) $*$ K_{Uf} (mL/hr/mm Hg) $\times$ TMP (mm Hg)

Example: Assume K_{Uf} = 20, and the clearance was done at TMP 40 mm Hg. Q_{uf} (mL/hr) = 20 $*$ 40 = 800 mL/hr = 800/60 = 13.3 mL/min.

Step 2: Read the clearance of the dialyzer spec sheet or clearance graph. Take at least two different blood flow rates, preferably >200 mL/min. This clearance is K_{totw}. Now subtract the ultrafiltration component of clearance from this as follows, to get the diffusive clearance:

$K_{dif} = (K_{totw} - Q_f) / (1 - Q_f/Q_B)$

Example: Assume clearance at Q_B = 300 mL/min is 240 mL/min from a spec sheet, but this was done using Q_{uf} of 13 mL/min. K_{tot} = 240 mL/min.

K_{dif} = (240 − 13)/(1 − 13/300) = 227/0.957 = 237 mL/min

Step 3: Compute in vitro *KoA* from K_{dif}, Q_B, and Q_D, using the uncorrected values for Q_B and Q_D on the dialyzer specification sheet based on the following equations:

$$N = \log ((K_{dif} / Q_D - 1) / (K_{dif} / Q_B - 1))$$
$$D = (1 - Q_B/Q_D)$$
$$KoA = 200 * N/D$$

$*$, asterisk, denotes multiplication in equations; log (x) denotes natural logarithm of x; N,D stand for intermediate variables (numerator, denominator) to make the overall equation simpler to write. Note that when reported clearances are obtained at a non-zero TMP, the values for KoA computed, by these equations will be somewhat lower than by using the nomogram in Fig. A-5, which does not make the ultrafiltration correction.

Appendix B

Molecular Weights and Conversion Tables

Table B-1.   Molecular weights and conversion tables

I.   Molecular weights of some nonionic substances

Substance	MW
Albumin	68,000
β_2-microglobulin	11,600
Serum urea nitrogen (SUN)	28
Creatinine	113
Dextrose (glucose monohydrate)	198
Ethanol	46
Ethylene glycol	62
Glucose	180
Hemoglobin	68,800
Light chains	23,000
Methanol	33
Myoglobin	17,800
Urea	60
Vancomycin	1,486
Vitamin B_{12}	1,355

II.   Converting between weight, valency, and molarity

A.   Number of milligrams in 1 milliequivalent or 1 millimole
     of substance

Substance	1 mEq	1 mmol
Na^+	23	23
K^+	39	39
Ca^{2+}	20	40
Mg^{2+}	12	24
Li^+ (lithium)	7	7
HCO_3^-	61	61
Cl^-	35.5	35.5
N (nitrogen)		14
P (phosphorus)		31
C (carbon)		12

B.   Changing milligrams to milliequivalents or millimoles
     1.   Sodium, potassium, chloride, bicarbonate

1 g NaCl	= 1,000 mg/(23 + 35.5) mg
	= 17 mEq or mmol of Na^+
1 g Na^+	= 1,000 mg/23 mg
	= 43 mEq or mmol of Na^+
1 g KCl	= 1,000 mg/74.5 mg
	= 14 mEq or mmol of K^+
1 g K^+	= 1,000 mg/39 mg
	= 26 mEq or mmol of K^+
1 g $NaHCO_8$	= 1,000 mg/84 mg
	= 12 mEq or mmol of Na^+
	= 12 mEq or mmol of HCO_3^-

continued

Table B-1.   *Continued*

2. Calcium
   Normal serum
   Ca level   = 10 mg/dL
                   = 100 mg/L
                   = 100/20 mEq/L, since 20 mg = 1 mEq
                   = 5 mEq/L
                   = 5/2 mM, since 2 mEq = 1 mmol
                   = 2.5 mM

3. Magnesium
   Normal serum
   Mg level   = 2.4 mg/L
                   = 24 mg/L
                   = 24/12 mEq/L, since 12 mg = 1 mEq
                   = 2 mEq/L
                   = 2/2 mM, since 2 mEq = 1 mmol
                   = 1 mM

4. Phosphorus (P)
   Normal serum
   inorganic P level   = 2.5 to 4 mg/dL
                   = 25 to 40 mg/L
                   = (25/31 to 40/31) mM,
                     since 1 mmol of P = 31 mg
                   = 0.8 to 1.3 mM

As P values when expressed in mEq/L change with alterations in pH, the mEq/L unit is not ordinarily used in clinical practice.

III. Estimating the serum ionized calcium level

Since 1 g/dL albumin binds with 0.8 mg/dL calcium, 4.5 g/dL albumin (normal serum albumin level) will bind with 3.6 mg/dL calcium.

Since 1 g/dL globulin binds with 0.16 mg/dL calcium, 2.5 g/dL globulin (normal serum globulin level) will bind with 0.4 mg/dL calcium.

Total serum protein-bound calcium level = 3.6 + 0.4
                                        = 4 mg/dL

In addition, about 6% of serum calcium is complexed with various anions, such as phosphorus. This complexed fraction can double when the serum phosphorus level is very high.

Ionized calcium = total calcium − protein-bound calcium
                                  − complexed calcium

Subject Index

A

Abdomen
  in peritoneal dialysis, 330,
    399–400, 400t
    distention of, 239
    hernias, 607
    pain in, 329–330
Abscesses
  myocardial and valvular, 593
  pancreatic, 608
  prostatic, 617
  renal, 618
  spinal epidural, 78
Access recirculation
  defined, 35
  impact of, 35–36
Access sites. *See* Vascular
    access
Acebutolol
  in hypertension, 471t
Acetaminophen
  poisoning treatment, 268
  removal by hemoperfusion,
    264t, 276t
Acetate
  in dialysis solution
    hypotension from, 153
    hypoventilation from, 165
    in peritoneal dialysis, 297
    reactions to, 160
  in predialysis acidosis cor-
    rection, 103
  in total parenteral nutrition,
    443t
Acetazolamide
  in glaucoma, 462
  in sleep apnea, 653–654
Acetylsalicylic acid. *See* Aspirin
Acid-base balance, 43–44
Acid-citrate dextrose for anti-
    coagulation in plasma-
    pheresis, 242–243
Acidosis
  in aspirin poisoning, 268
  hemodialysis in, 107
    in metabolic acidosis, 107
    in respiratory acidosis, 107
  metabolic
    dialysis-induced, 590
    as indication for dialysis,
      4t, 5, 107
    in infants and children, 578
  predialysis correction of, 107

respiratory, 107
  hemodialysis in, 107
Acquired renal cystic disease,
    611–612
Activated clotting time, 184, 186t
Acute dialysis
  choice of procedures in, 5–6
  indications for, 3
  in infants and children,
    562–565, 567
  peritoneal. *See* Acute peri-
    toneal dialysis
Acute hemodialysis, 102–119
  air detection in, 117
  anaphylactoid reactions in
    with AN69 membrane and
      ACE inhibitors, 104
  anticoagulation orders in, 102
  blood flow rate in, 102–103
  dialysis solution in, 105
  dialyzer choice in, 104–105
  excessive inflow suction in, 115
  fluid removal plan in, 102,
    109–110
  heparin administration in, 113
  high venous pressure in,
    116–117
  hypernatremia in, 108
  hyponatremia in, 107
  in infants and children,
    563–565, 567
  infections in, from cellulose
    membranes, 104
  initiation of, 113
  monitoring of, 114–117
    blood circuit, 117
    dialysis solution circuit,
      117–118
    in hyponatremia, 107
    patient in, 118
  postdialysis evaluation of,
    118–119
  prescription for, 102–119
  rinsing and priming of
    dialyzer in, 113
  session length in, 102–103
  sterilization of dialyzer in,
    104–105
  termination of, 118
  ultrafiltration coefficient in,
    105
  vascular access in, 113–114